ONCOLOGY INFORMATICS

ONCOLOGY INFORMATICS

Using Health Information Technology to Improve Processes and Outcomes in Cancer

Edited by

BRADFORD W. HESSE, PhD
*Health Communication and Informatics Research Branch,
Division of Cancer Control and Population Sciences,
National Cancer Institute, Rockville, MD, United States*

DAVID K. AHERN, PhD
*Health Communication and Informatics Research Branch, Healthcare Delivery Research Program,
National Cancer Institute, Rockville, MD, United States; Program in Behavioral Informatics and eHealth,
Department of Psychiatry, Brigham & Women's Hospital, Boston, MA, United States;
Harvard Medical School, Boston, MA, United States*

ELLEN BECKJORD, PhD MPH
*Population Health Program Design and Engagement Optimization, UPMC Health Plan,
Pittsburgh, PA, United States*

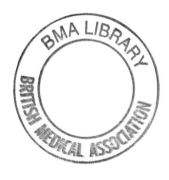

AMSTERDAM • BOSTON • HEIDELBERG • LONDON
NEW YORK • OXFORD • PARIS • SAN DIEGO
SAN FRANCISCO • SINGAPORE • SYDNEY • TOKYO
Academic Press is an imprint of Elsevier

Academic Press is an imprint of Elsevier
125 London Wall, London EC2Y 5AS, UK
525 B Street, Suite 1800, San Diego, CA 92101-4495, USA
50 Hampshire Street, 5th Floor, Cambridge, MA 02139, USA
The Boulevard, Langford Lane, Kidlington, Oxford OX5 1GB, UK

British Library Cataloguing-in-Publication Data
A catalogue record for this book is available from the British Library.

Library of Congress Cataloging-in-Publication Data
A catalog record for this book is available from the Library of Congress.

ISBN: 978-0-12-802115-6

For Information on all Academic Press publications
visit our website at http://www.elsevier.com/

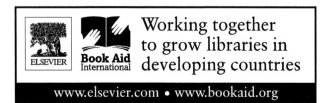

Publisher: Mica Haley
Acquisition Editor: Catherine Van Der Laan
Editorial Project Manager: Lisa Eppich
Production Project Manager: Melissa Read
Designer: Greg Harris

Typeset by MPS Limited, Chennai, India

Dedication

This book is dedicated to two courageous women—Dr Jessie Gruman and Dr Abagail Prestin—whose work, which they completed during their own cancer journeys, survives them and will inspire and empower all who take part in the fight against cancer.

Contents

List of Contributors   xi
Foreword   xiii
Preface   xvii
Introduction   xix

I

AN EXTRAORDINARY OPPORTUNITY

1. Creating a Learning Health Care System in Oncology
RICHARD L. SCHILSKY AND ROBERT S. MILLER

1.1 The Challenges of Delivering Quality Cancer Care   4
1.2 Overview of Traditional Learning in Cancer Medicine   7
1.3 The Interface of Quality, Value, and Learning   9
1.4 ASCO's Vision for a Rapid Learning System in Oncology: CancerLinQ   10
1.5 CancerLinQ Data Architecture   10
1.6 History and Current Status of CancerLinQ Implementation   12
1.7 CancerLinQ Solution Operating Characteristics   13
1.8 Regulatory Underpinnings of CancerLinQ   17
1.9 Summary and Conclusions   19
List of Acronyms and Abbreviations   19
Acknowledgments   19
References   19

2. Reducing Cancer Disparities Through Community Engagement: The Promise of Informatics
APRIL OH, WEN-YING SYLVIA CHOU, DEVLON JACKSON, SAMUEL CYKERT, NORA JONES, JENNIFER SCHAAL, EUGINIA ENG AND COMMUNITYRX

Section 1: Public Health Informatics: Implications on Cancer Health Disparities   24
2.1 Introduction   24
2.2 Cancer Health Disparities: An Overview   24
2.3 The Role of PHIs in Addressing Cancer Health Disparities   25
Section 2: CBPR to Inform the Practice of PHIs to Address Health Disparities   27
Section 3: Examples of Public Health and Health Informatics   29
2.4 Example 1: Community Engagement and the Accountability for Cancer Care Through Undoing Racism and Equity Trial (ACCURE Project)   29
2.5 Example 2: PHIs and the Chicago CommunityRx Innovation   32

Section 4: Discussion   34
2.6 Challenges for the Field   35
2.7 Strengths of PHI Applications in Health Disparities   36
List of Acronyms and Abbreviations   37
References   38

3. Cancer Clinical Research: Enhancing Data Liquidity and Data Altruism
WARREN KIBBE

3.1 Drivers   41
3.2 Data Liquidity   42
3.3 Data Science   42
3.4 Data Access   43
3.5 Translational Research   44
3.6 Capturing the Patient Experience Across the Continuum of Care   46
3.7 Empowering the Patient as a Full Participant in Research   46
3.8 Building a National Learning Health Care System for Cancer   46
3.9 Incentives for Data Sharing   46
3.10 Adaptive Instruments   47
3.11 Ontologies and Workflow Systems   47
3.12 Connected Health and Mobile Technologies   48
3.13 A Focus on Lowering Barriers to Data Access for Cancer Research   48
3.14 Precision Medicine Drivers   49
List of Acronyms and Abbreviations   51
References   51

4. Engaging Patients in Primary and Specialty Care
ALEX H. KRIST, DONALD E. NEASE, GARY L. KREPS, LINDA OVERHOLSER AND MARC MCKENZIE

4.1 Introduction   56
4.2 Overview of Hit Tools to Engage Patients   61
4.3 Key Patient Engagement Activities   66
4.4 HIT Implementation to Promote Patient Engagement   73
4.5 Conclusions   77
List of Acronyms and Abbreviations   77
References   77

5. Coordination at the Point of Need
KATHERINE K. KIM, JANICE F. BELL, SARAH C. REED AND ROBIN WHITNEY

5.1 Introduction   81
5.2 Frameworks for Care Coordination   83
5.3 HIT Functions for Care Coordination   88

5.4 Current Efforts in Informatics and Coordination
     at the Point of Need   90
5.5 Opportunities for Oncology Informatics at the
     Point of Need   96
List of Acronyms and Abbreviations   97
References   97

II

SUPPORT ACROSS THE CONTINUUM

6. Prevention, Information Technology, and Cancer

GLEN D. MORGAN AND MICHAEL C. FIORE

6.1 Overview   104
6.2 Key Behaviors of Interest for the Prevention of Cancer 104
6.3 Current Use of Information Technology for Cancer
     Prevention   107
6.4 Electronic Health Records   108
6.5 Mobile, Web, and Wearable Applications   115
6.6 Summary and Future Directions   118
List of Acronyms and Abbreviations   119
Acknowledgments   119
References   119

7. Early Detection in the Age of Information Technology

EKLAND ABDIWAHAB, STEPHEN H. TAPLIN, GLORIA CORONADO,
HEATHER DACUS, MELISSA LEYPOLDT AND CELETTE SKINNER

7.1 Introduction   124
7.2 Epidemiology   124
7.3 Early Detection   125
7.4 The Process of Care   128
7.5 The Challenge of Early Detection   129
7.6 Communication Challenges   132
7.7 Evidence-Based Solutions   134
7.8 Challenges With Using IT   139
7.9 Overcoming Disparities   139
7.10 Looking to the Future   139
List of Acronyms and Abbreviations   140
Acknowledgments   140
References   140

8. Informatics Support Across the Cancer Continuum: Treatment

BRADFORD HIRSCH AND AMY P. ABERNETHY

8.1 Overview   145
8.2 Data Aggregation   148
8.3 Data Optimization   149
8.4 Patient Insights to Optimize Care   151
8.5 Genomics in the Care Continuum   153
8.6 The Tooling Required   153
8.7 Novel Organizational Approaches   155
8.8 Summary   155
List of Acronyms and Abbreviations   155
References   156

9. Survivorship

ELLEN BECKJORD, G.J. VAN LONDEN AND RUTH RECHIS

9.1 Cancer Survivorship   159
9.2 Challenges in Survivorship   162
9.3 Opportunities for Informatics-Based Solutions 167
9.4 Envisioning a Future State   174
9.5 Conclusions   176
List of Acronyms and Abbreviations   176
References   176

10. Advanced Cancer: Palliative, End of Life, and Bereavement Care

LORI L. DUBENSKE, DEBORAH K. MAYER AND DAVID H. GUSTAFSON

10.1 Introduction   182
10.2 Opportunities for eHealth to Address Needs in
      Advanced Cancer Care   184
10.3 A Case Example: CHESS—The Comprehensive
      Health Enhancement Support System   190
10.4 Future Directions for Research   197
10.5 Future Directions for Development and
      Implementation   200
10.6 Conclusion   200
List of Acronyms and Abbreviations   201
Acknowledgments   201
References   201

III

SCIENCE OF ONCOLOGY INFORMATICS

11. Data Visualization Tools for Investigating Health Services Utilization Among Cancer Patients

EBERECHUKWU ONUKWUGHA, CATHERINE PLAISANT AND
BEN SHNEIDERMAN

11.1 Introduction   208
11.2 Methods and Data Visualization Tools   209
11.3 Applications of Data Visualization in the
      Cancer Setting   214
11.4 Case Studies   219
11.5 Conclusion   227
List of Acronyms and Abbreviations   228
References   228

12. Oncology Informatics: Behavioral and Psychological Sciences

DAVID K. AHERN, ILANA M. BRAUN, MARY E. COOLEY
AND TIMOTHY W. BICKMORE

12.1 Introduction   232
12.2 Role of Behavioral/Psychological Science in
      Advancing Informatics   232
12.3 Definition and Role of Behavioral Informatics 239
12.4 Applications of Behavioral Informatics Resources
      and Tools in Cancer Care   241
12.5 Conclusions   248

List of Acronyms and Abbreviations 249
References 249

13. Communication Science: Connecting Systems for Health

BRADFORD W. HESSE, NEERAJ K. ARORA AND WILLIAM KLEIN

13.1 The Communication Revolution 253
13.2 Using Communication Science to Improve Quality of Cancer Care 260
13.3 A Functional Approach to Patient-Centered Communication 263
13.4 Conclusion 271
List of Acronyms and Abbreviations 272
References 272

14. Cancer Surveillance Informatics

LYNNE T. PENBERTHY, DEBORAH M. WINN AND SUSAN M. SCOTT

14.1 Background on Cancer Surveillance 277
14.2 Current Status and Opportunities for Informatics in Cancer Surveillance: NLP, Automation, and Linkages 280
14.3 New Areas for Cancer Surveillance Supported Through Informatics 282
14.4 Conclusion 284
List of Acronyms and Abbreviations 284
Acknowledgments 284
References 284

15. Extended Vision for Oncology: A Perceptual Science Perspective on Data Visualization and Medical Imaging

TODD S. HOROWITZ AND RONALD A. RENSINK

15.1 Introduction 287
15.2 How Vision Works (and How It Can Fail) 288
15.3 Visualization and Data Exploration 292
15.4 Example 1: Human Number Perception and Quantitative Data 294
15.5 Example 2: Visual Attention and Medical Images 294
15.6 Frontiers of Perceptual Science and Oncology Informatics 299
15.7 Conclusions 300
List of Acronyms and Abbreviations 300
References 301

IV

ACCELERATING PROGRESS

16. Crowdsourcing Advancements in Health Care Research: Applications for Cancer Treatment Discoveries

EMIL CHIAUZZI, GABRIEL EICHLER AND PAUL WICKS

16.1 Introduction 307
16.2 The Crowdsourcing Concept 308
16.3 Crowdsourcing in Health Care 312
16.4 Methodological and Ethical Issues in Crowdsourcing 320
16.5 The Future of Crowdsourcing 323
16.6 Conclusion 326
List of Acronyms and Abbreviations 326
Acknowledgments 326
References 326

17. Patient-Centered Approaches to Improving Clinical Trials for Cancer

RONI ZEIGER AND GILLES FRYDMAN

17.1 While Trials Are Important, Trial Participation Rates Are Dismal 331
17.2 Barriers to Trial Participation 332
17.3 Patients Searching for Trials Online 333
17.4 Current Use of the Internet and Online Cancer Communities 334
17.5 How the Internet Shaped Online Cancer Communities, and Vice Versa 334
17.6 What Do Patients Talk About in Online Cancer Communities? 336
17.7 Impact of Online Patient Communities 336
17.8 Participatory Research 337
17.9 Borrowing From Silicon Valley and User-Centered Design 337
17.10 Participatory Clinical Trial Design 338
17.11 What If Trial Participants Discuss the Trial in Online Communities? 339
17.12 Challenges and Next Steps 339
List of Acronyms and Abbreviations 339
References 340

18. A New Era of Clinical Research Methods in a Data-Rich Environment

WILLIAM T. RILEY

18.1 Transition From a Data-Poor to Data-Rich Science 343
18.2 Traditional Trial Designs: What's Wrong With Continuing to Do What We Do? 344
18.3 Data-Rich Biomedical and Behavioral Research Environment 345
18.4 The Vision of a Data-Rich Biomedical and Behavioral Research Enterprise 348
18.5 Recent Advances That Poise Clinical Research to Become a Data-Rich Research Enterprise 348
18.6 New Approaches to Treatment Testing in Preparation for a Comprehensive Health Data Research Infrastructure 350
18.7 Conclusion 352
List of Acronyms and Abbreviations 353
References 353

19. Creating a Health Information Technology Infrastructure to Support Comparative Effectiveness Research in Cancer

SUSAN K. PETERSON AND KEVIN PATRICK

19.1 Introduction 358
19.2 Cancer CER: Gaps and Opportunities 358
19.3 Health Information Technology Infrastructure for Improving CER 359

19.4 Enhancing the Collection of Evidence to Inform Patient
      Care and CER Through Distance Medicine Technology   360
19.5 Distance Medicine Technology in Cancer Care and
      Research   361
19.6 CYCORE: CYberinfrastructure for Cancer
      COmparative Effectiveness REsearch   361
19.7 Application of CYCORE Across the Cancer
      Prevention and Control Continuum to
      Accelerate CER   364
19.8 Strengthening the Capacity of the CER Infrastructure
      Through EHRs   367
19.9 Conclusion   369
List of Acronyms and Abbreviations   369
Acknowledgments   369
References   370

20. Editors' Conclusion: Building for Change
BRADFORD W. HESSE, DAVID K. AHERN AND ELLEN BECKJORD

20.1 Introduction   373
20.2 The Bright Spots in Oncology Informatics   375
20.3 Living in a Post HITECH World   380
20.4 Building the Future Together   382
20.5 Conclusion   384
List of Acronyms and Abbreviations   385
References   385

Glossary   **387**
Index   **395**

List of Contributors

Ekland Abdiwahab MPH Healthcare Delivery Research Program, Division of Cancer Control and Population Science, National Cancer Institute, Rockville, MD, United States

Amy P. Abernethy MD, PhD Flatiron Health, New York, NY, United States

David K. Ahern PhD Health Communication and Informatics Research Branch, Healthcare Delivery Research Program, National Cancer Institute, Rockville, MD, United States; Program in Behavioral Informatics and eHealth, Department of Psychiatry, Brigham & Women's Hospital, Boston, MA, United States; Harvard Medical School, Boston, MA, United States

Neeraj K. Arora PhD Improving Healthcare Systems, Patient-Centered Outcomes Research Institute, Washington, DC, United States

Ellen Beckjord PhD MPH Population Health Program Design and Engagement Optimization, UPMC Health Plan, Pittsburgh, PA, United States

Janice F. Bell PhD, MPH, MN Betty Irene Moore School of Nursing, University of California Davis, Sacramento, CA, United States

Timothy W. Bickmore PhD College of Computer and Information Science, Northeastern University, Boston, MA, United States

Ilana M. Braun MD Dana-Farber Cancer Institute, Harvard Medical School, Boston, MA, United States

Emil Chiauzzi PhD PatientsLikeMe, Inc., Cambridge, MA, United States

Wen-ying Sylvia Chou PhD, MPH Health Communication and Informatics Research Branch, Division of Cancer Control and Population Science, National Cancer Institute, Rockville, MD, United States

CommunityRx University of Chicago Medicine, University of Chicago, Chicago, IL, United States

Mary E. Cooley PhD, RN, FAAN Phyllis F. Cantor Center, Research in Nursing and Patient Care, Dana-Farber Cancer Institute, Boston, MA, United States; College of Nursing and Exercise Health Science, University of Massachusetts-Boston, Boston, MA, United States

Gloria Coronado PhD Kaiser Permanente Center for Health Research, Portland, OR, United States

Samuel Cykert MD NC AHEC Program, UNC School of Medicine, Chapel Hill, NC, United States

Heather Dacus DO, MPH New York State Department of Health, Albany, NY, United States

Lori L. DuBenske PhD Department of Psychiatry, School of Medicine and Public Health, University of Wisconsin–Madison, Madison, WI, United States

Gabriel Eichler PhD PatientsLikeMe, Inc., Cambridge, MA, United States

Euginia Eng PhD, MPH Gillings School of Global Public Health, University of North Carolina Chapel Hill, Chapel Hill, NC, United States

Michael C. Fiore MD, MPH, MBA Center for Tobacco Research and Intervention, University of Wisconsin School of Medicine and Public Health, Madison, WI, United States

Gilles Frydman BSc Smart Patients, Mountain View, CA, United States; Association of Cancer Online Resources, Mountain View, CA, United States

David H. Gustafson PhD Center for Health Enhancement Systems Studies, University of Wisconsin–Madison, Madison, WI, United States

Bradford W. Hesse PhD Health Communication and Informatics Research Branch, Division of Cancer Control and Population Sciences, National Cancer Institute, Rockville, MD, United States

Bradford Hirsch MD, MBA Flatiron Health, New York, NY, United States

Todd S. Horowitz PhD Behavioral Research Program, Division of Cancer Control and Population Sciences, National Cancer Institute, Rockville, MD, United States

Devlon Jackson PhD, MPH Health Communication and Informatics Research Branch, Division of Cancer Control and Population Science, National Cancer Institute, Rockville, MD, United States

Nora Jones MS The Partnership Project, Greensboro, NC, United States

Warren Kibbe PhD Center for Biomedical Informatics and Information Technology, National Cancer Institute, Rockville, MD, United States

Katherine K. Kim PhD, MPH, MBA Betty Irene Moore School of Nursing, University of California Davis, Sacramento, CA, United States

William Klein PhD Behavioral Research Program, Division of Cancer Control and Population Sciences, National Cancer Institute, Rockville, MD, United States

Gary L. Kreps PhD Center for Health and Risk Communication, Department of Communication, George Mason University, Fairfax, VA, United States

Alex H. Krist MD, MPH   Department of Family Medicine and Population Health, Virginia Commonwealth University, Richmond, VA, United States

Melissa Leypoldt RN   Division of Public Health, Nebraska Department of Health and Human Services, Lincoln, NE, United States

Deborah K. Mayer PhD   School of Nursing, University of North Carolina Lineberger Comprehensive Cancer Center, Chapel Hill, NC, United States

Marc McKenzie BS, MBA   Retired Computer Industry Senior Executive, Survivor of Cancer and Stem-Cell Transplant, Windsor, CO, United States

Robert S. Miller MD, FACP, FASCO   CancerLinQ, American Society of Clinical Oncology, Alexandria, VA, United States

Glen D. Morgan PhD   Tobacco Control Research Branch, Behavioral Research Program, Division of Cancer Control and Population Sciences, National Cancer Institute, Rockville, MD, United States

Donald E. Nease MD, MPH   Department of Family Medicine, University of Colorado, Denver, CO, United States

April Oh PhD, MPH   Health Communication and Informatics Research Branch, Division of Cancer Control and Population Science, National Cancer Institute, Rockville, MD, United States

Eberechukwu Onukwugha MS, PhD   Department of Pharmaceutical Health Services Research, School of Pharmacy, University of Maryland, Baltimore, MD, United States

Linda Overholser MD, MPH   Department of General Internal Medicine, University of Colorado, Denver, CO, United States

Kevin Patrick MD, MS   Department of Family Medicine and Public Health, The Qualcomm Institute/Calit2, University of California-San Diego, San Diego, CA, United States

Lynne T. Penberthy MD, MPH   Surveillance Research Program, Division of Cancer Control and Population Sciences, National Cancer Institute, Rockville, MD, United States

Susan K. Peterson PhD, MPH   Department of Behavioral Science, University of Texas MD Anderson Cancer Center, Houston, TX, United States

Catherine Plaisant PhD   Human-Computer Interaction Lab, UMIACS, University of Maryland, College Park, MD, United States

Ruth Rechis PhD   Programs & Strategy, LIVESTRONG Foundation, Austin, TX, United States

Sarah C. Reed MSW, MPH   Betty Irene Moore School of Nursing, University of California Davis, Sacramento, CA, United States

Ronald A. Rensink PhD   Departments of Computer Science and Psychology, University of British Columbia, Vancouver, BC, Canada

William T. Riley PhD   Office of Behavioral and Social Sciences Research, National Institutes of Health, Bethesda, MD, United States

Jennifer Schaal MD   The Partnership Project, Greensboro, NC, United States

Richard L. Schilsky MD, FACP, FASCO   CancerLinQ, American Society of Clinical Oncology, Alexandria, VA, United States

Susan M. Scott MPH   Surveillance Research Program, Division of Cancer Control and Population Sciences, National Cancer Institute, Rockville, MD, United States

Ben Shneiderman PhD   Computer Science Department, Human-Computer Interaction Lab, UMIACS, University of Maryland, College Park, MD, United States

Celette Skinner PhD   Department of Clinical Sciences, UT Southwestern Medical Center, Dallas, TX, United States

Stephen H. Taplin MD, MPH   Healthcare Delivery Research Program, Division of Cancer Control and Population Science, National Cancer Institute, Rockville, MD, United States

G.J. van Londen MD, MS   Division of Hematology-Oncology, Department of Medicine, University of Pittsburgh, Pittsburgh, PA, United States

Robin Whitney RN   Betty Irene Moore School of Nursing, University of California Davis, Sacramento, CA, United States

Paul Wicks PhD   PatientsLikeMe, Inc., Cambridge, MA, United States

Deborah M. Winn PhD   Office of the Director, Division of Cancer Control and Population Sciences, National Cancer Institute, Rockville, MD, United States

Roni Zeiger MD, MS   Smart Patients, Mountain View, CA, United States; Santa Clara Valley Medical Center, Santa Clara, CA, United States

Foreword

The anatomy of a decision, decision making under stress and uncertainty by providers and patients, the visualization and interpretation of data to support clinical reasoning, gleaning insight from big data, correlating with gene variants and the various "omics"—these are the overarching subjects of oncology informatics to be addressed in this text—*Oncology Informatics*. Many envision a future state where health information technology (health IT) is supportive of much higher order clinical reasoning than possible in today's systems—where the interaction between the computer, providers, and their patients will be intuitive and integrated seamlessly in the clinical workflow, where increasing data enhances understanding and insight, rather than confounding clinicians and their patients. This future health IT will deemphasize the technology itself, and restore the focus appropriately on patients, evidence-based clinical goals, and outcomes.

This evolution toward a more informed future state of clinical decision making is perhaps most especially relevant in oncology. Studies of health IT have demonstrated its ability to reduce medication errors [1], improve patient safety [2], improve the quality of care [3], and lower costs [4–6]. Health IT may cause unintended adverse consequences, however, and negatively impact clinical processes and outcomes [7]. The overarching critical challenge for the successful design and effective use of health IT is to fundamentally reorient the current model of use [8]: from one where the user of health IT is obliged to support health IT—to laboriously enter, search, retrieve, and manually interpret patient data, to execute and manage transactions in the system—to one where health IT supports the user. In the current model, the user must interact with a system that has a fundamentally different (machine) model of the patient's data, organized for transactions and billing, with little or no intrinsic model of the care process, and desired clinical goals. Rather, health IT should truly support its users, informing the clinician's and patient's mental models of disease, wellness, and care delivery, as well as their shared care goals and objectives and the processes they engage in together to pursue these goals and objectives [9]. Unless health IT systems are adapted to provide such advanced patient-centered cognitive support capabilities, the effective and transformative use of health IT will remain a vision rather than a reality.

A concurrent revolution is underway with the advent of a truly patient-centered care model in the era of genomic medicine—based broadly on the subject matter of this book: applied oncology informatics. Clinical practice is on the cusp of an evolution from George Engel's biopsychosocial model [10] to one informed by personalized medicine [11–14]—characterized by decision making informed by patient personal history, family history, social/environmental factors, and clinical data along with genomic data and patient preferences. To achieve this vision, clinical decision making will need to be patient-centered in new ways, bringing the best evidence at the genetic level to bear on many clinical scenarios [15–18], and an understanding of patient preferences for genetic information [19–22]. The relevance to oncology practice and care is clear. Personalized genetic medicine [23] is expected to generate data that will outstrip the information and knowledge processing capabilities of most practitioners, and many clinicians feel overwhelmed by this impending tsunami of additional knowledge they must master [21,24,25]. One-on-one genetic counseling will not be available to all: primary care and specialist practitioners alike will need to manage their patients with basic genomic test interpretation and guidance at the point of care [26–28].

The practicing clinician may be supported with health information technologies, however, which enable a personalized approach especially to clinical genetic medicine [29–33]. Key to personalized medicine will be tools to support "prospective" medicine [34,35]—health risk assessments, acquisition of a detailed family history, genomic information, and clinical decision support (CDS) in an electronic medical record (EMR) [36,37]. CDS has been shown to impact physician behavior [38,39], diagnostic test ordering and other care processes [40,41], the costs of care [6,42–45], and clinical outcomes [46–49]. While there is great promise with health IT and CDS, it is not without potential peril: health IT poorly designed or implemented, or misused, may generate unintended consequences [50–52], and new types of medical error [53].

Why is this important now? The goal of oncology informatics may be fundamentally to bring genomic-, and patient preference-based, personalized medicine CDS to any provider receiving genetic sequencing test results at the point of care in EMRs, and eventually to the patient via a personal health record. Whole genome sequencing will soon be available to almost any patient and their physician, and with it will come enormous potential for return of incidental genetic findings [54]. The molecular laboratory will make choices of which incidental findings to analyze and report to the physician, and the physician in turn, will make choices as to which of these to return to the patient. The choices of which reported variants to return to each individual patient will require contextualization by the physician and preference setting by the patient [55]. However, scalable solutions for dealing with incidental information by both clinicians and patients have not yet been addressed. As described in this text, the field of oncology informatics will leverage large-scale whole genome sequencing and is developing scalable CDS tools that can support the era of genomic medicine.

Oncology informatics will address four related questions (originally conceived by PCORI) of particular relevance to the cancer patient:

"Given my personal characteristics, conditions, and preferences, what should I expect will happen to me?"

Oncology informatics will provide the caregiver and patient insight on the current knowledge base with respect to gene sequencing and personalized medicine, tailored to the patient's own expressed preferences. If patients choose to know, oncology informatics can help inform them of their own unique expected outcomes given the best evidence to date.

"What are my options and what are the benefits and harms of those options?"

Oncology informatics will help the patient and provider understand unique diagnostic and therapeutic options given the patient's incidental genomic findings and preferences for return of genomic information. Patient's will be able to make more informed choices about knowing, or not knowing specific genetic test results, and make more informed decisions when sequence data are known about specific treatment options.

"What can I do to improve the outcomes that are most important to me?"

Oncology informatics will help patients and providers understand better the patient's unique profile, and tailor both care plans, and identify patient behaviors that may mitigate risk, or improve health outcomes. Better understanding of the options is the first step to patient activation and engagement.

"How can the health care system improve my chances of achieving the outcomes I prefer?"

Oncology informatics helps the patient and provider, and care team, act in concert with respect to a shared understanding of patient preferences for personalized genomic information in designing and pursuing an individually tailored care plan.

Assessment of patient preferences for genetic testing has found that patients are more likely to wish to obtain incidental genetic results than expected [56–58], but that concerns exist about quality of the information provided, misunderstanding the significance of information disclosed, maintaining the confidentiality of genetic information [59,60], and restricting access to results by insurers [61]. Prior research suggests that four key themes exist among patients, with several important subthemes [61], including understanding source of information, experiences with conventional prescribing, pharmacogenomic-based testing issues (access, discomfort, test reliability and validity, costs, etc.), and several issues surrounding targeted therapeutics (effectiveness, adverse effects, increase treatment options, prevention, preferences for tailored therapy, costs, quality of life, access, and compliance or adherence). The multidimensionality of the preference problem for genetic test information [62] necessitates consideration of another important dimension to the traditional doctor–patient relationship [63] around clinical significance, and patient-preferences: that of communicability [62]. The communicability dimension addresses issues around health literacy, comprehensible message, appropriateness of message for participant, and clarity of message. Even traditional notions of "clinical utility" may be challenged in communicating about genetic test results [64–66]. Traditional notions of clinical utility may need to be broadened to consider ethical, legal, and social implications [67,68].

While the scientific and applied foundations of oncology and informatics are advancing in the United States, we are in the midst of a profound sea change in how clinical care is delivered, measured, and rewarded. Health IT will both enable a better understanding and assessment of clinical processes and outcomes, and should serve as the foundation with which clinicians and health systems can accept more financial risk or stake in the value of the care being provided [69,70]. This may in fact be the most important goal of oncology informatics, and all of clinical medicine—to advance the state-of-the-art such that we fundamentally transform care to achieve the Triple Aim of better patient experience, improved population health, and reduced cost [71].

Blackford Middleton MD, MPH, MSc,
FACP, FACMI, FHIMSS
Chairman, American Medical Informatics
Association, Past-Chair, Healthcare Information
Management and Systems Society, Past-Chair,
Computer-based Patient Record Institute, Harvard
T.H. Chan School of Public Health, Stanford Clinical
Excellence Research Center (adjunct)

References

[1] Bates DW. Preventing medication errors: a summary. Am J Health Syst Pharm 2007;64(14 Suppl 9):S3–S9.

[2] Einbinder JS, Bates DW. Leveraging information technology to improve quality and safety. IMIA Yearb 2007:22–9.

[3] Bates DW. The quality case for information technology in healthcare. BMC Med Inform Decis Mak 2002;2:7.

[4] Amarasingham R, Plantinga L, Diener-West M, Gaskin DJ, Powe NR. Clinical information technologies and inpatient outcomes: a multiple hospital study. Arch Intern Med 2009;169:108–14.

[5] Fischer MA, Vogeli C, Stedman M, Ferris T, Brookhart MA, Weissman JS. Effect of electronic prescribing with formulary decision support on medication use and cost. Arch Intern Med 2008;168:2433–9.

[6] Walker J, Pan E, Johnston D, Adler-Milstein J, Bates DW, Middleton B. The value of health care information exchange and interoperability. Health Aff 2005(Suppl Web Exclusives) W5–10–W5–18.

[7] Campbell EM, Sittig DF, Ash JS, Guappone KP, Dykstra RH. Types of unintended consequences related to computerized provider order entry. J Am Med Inform Assoc: JAMIA 2006;13:547–56.

[8] Lin HS, Stead WW. Computational technology for effective health care: immediate steps and strategic directions. Washington, DC: National Academies Press; 2009.

[9] Schnipper JL, Linder JA, Palchuk MB, Einbinder JS, Li Q, Postilnik A, et al. "Smart Forms" in an electronic medical record: documentation-based clinical decision support to improve disease management. J Am Med Inform Assoc: JAMIA 2008;15:513–23.

[10] Engel G. The need for a new medical model: a challenge for biomedicine. Science 1977;196:129–36.

[11] Sriram KB, Larsen JE, Yang IA, Bowman RV, Fong KM. Genomic medicine in non-small cell lung cancer: paving the path to personalized care. Respirology 2011;16:257–63.

[12] Ginsburg GS, Willard HF. Genomic and personalized medicine: foundations and applications. Transl Res 2009;154:277–87.

[13] Sander C. Genomic medicine and the future of health care. Science 2000;287:1977–8.

[14] Hamburg MA, Collins FS. The path to personalized medicine. N Engl J Med 2010;363:301–4.

[15] Shim E-J, Lee K-S, Park J-H, Park J-H. Comprehensive needs assessment tool in cancer (CNAT): the development and validation. Support Care Cancer 2011;19(12):1957–68.

[16] Davis K, Schoenbaum SC, Audet A-M. A 2020 vision of patient-centered primary care. J Gen Intern Med 2005;20:953–7.

[17] Coulter A, Entwistle V, Gilbert D. Sharing decisions with patients: is the information good enough? BMJ 1999;318:318–22.

[18] Robinson A, Thomson R. Variability in patient preferences for participating in medical decision making: implication for the use of decision support tools. Qual Health Care 2001;10(Suppl 1):i34.

[19] Shiloh S, Gerad L, Goldman B. Patients' information needs and decision-making processes: what can be learned from genetic counselees? Health Psychol 2006;25:211–9.

[20] Liu Y, Yu X, Wang L, Li C, Archacki S, Huang C, et al. Mutation p. Leu354Pro in EDA causes severe hypohidrotic ectodermal dysplasia in a Chinese family. Gene 2012;491:246–50.

[21] Fargher EA, Eddy C, Newman W, Qasim F, Tricker K, Elliott RA, et al. Patients "and healthcare professionals" views on pharmacogenetic testing and its future delivery in the NHS. Pharmacogenomics 2007;8:1511–9.

[22] Haga SB, Kawamoto K, Agans R, Ginsburg GS. Consideration of patient preferences and challenges in storage and access of pharmacogenetic test results. Genet Med 2011;13:887–90.

[23] Chan IS, Ginsburg GS. Personalized medicine: progress and promise. Annu Rev Genomics Hum Genet 2011;12:217–44.

[24] Baars MJH, Henneman L, Kate ten LP. Deficiency of knowledge of genetics and genetic tests among general practitioners, gynecologists, and pediatricians: a global problem. Genet Med 2005;7:605–10.

[25] Scheuner MT, Sieverding P, Shekelle PG. Delivery of genomic medicine for common chronic adult diseases: a systematic review. JAMA 2008;299:1320–34.

[26] Ali-Khan SE, Daar AS, Shuman C, Ray PN, Scherer SW. Whole genome scanning: resolving clinical diagnosis and management amidst complex data. Pediatr Res 2009;66:357–63.

[27] Elwyn G, Edwards A, Kinnersley P, Grol R. Shared decision making and the concept of equipoise: the competences of involving patients in healthcare choices. Br J Gen Pract 2000;50:892–9.

[28] Elwyn G, Edwards A, Kinnersley P. Shared decision making and the concept of equipoise: the competences of involving patients in healthcare choices. Br J Gen Pract 1999;49:477.

[29] Lesko LJ. Personalized medicine: elusive dream or imminent reality? Clin Pharmacol Ther 2007;81:807–16.

[30] Shabo A. The implications of electronic health record for personalized medicine. Biomed Pap Med Fac Univ Palacky Olomouc Czech Repub 2005;149(suppl):251–8.

[31] Glaser J, Henley DE, Downing G, Brinner KM. Advancing personalized health care through health information technology: an update from the American health information community's personalized health care workgroup. J Am Med Inform Assoc: JAMIA 2008;15:391.

[32] Downing GJ, Boyle SN, Brinner KM, Osheroff JA. Information management to enable personalized medicine: stakeholder roles in building clinical decision support. BMC Med Inform Decis Mak 2009;9:44.

[33] Ullman-Cullere MH, Mathew JP. Emerging landscape of genomics in the electronic health record for personalized medicine. Hum Mutat 2011;32:512–6.

[34] Snyderman R, Sanders Williams R. Prospective medicine: the next health care transformation. Acad Med 2003;78:1079.

[35] Langheier JM, Snyderman R. Prospective medicine: the role for genomics in personalized health planning. Pharmacogenomics 2004;5:1–8.

[36] Hoffman MA, Williams MS. Electronic medical records and personalized medicine. Hum Genet 2011;130:33–9.

[37] Overby CL, Tarczy-Hornoch P, Hoath JI, Kalet IJ, Veenstra DL. Feasibility of incorporating genomic knowledge into electronic medical records for pharmacogenomic clinical decision support. BMC Bioinformatics 2010;11:S10.

[38] Lindgren H. Decision support system supporting clinical reasoning process—an evaluation study in dementia care. Stud Health Technol Inform 2008;136:315–20.

[39] Schedlbauer A, Prasad V, Mulvaney C. What evidence supports the use of computerized alerts and prompts to improve clinicians' prescribing behavior? J Am Med Inform Assoc: JAMIA 2009;16(4):531–8.

[40] Blumenthal D, Glaser JP. Information technology comes to medicine. N Engl J Med 2007;356:2527.

[41] Bates DW, Gawande AA. Improving safety with information technology. N Engl J Med 2003;348(25):2526–34.

[42] Wang SJ, Middleton B, Prosser LA, Bardon CG, Spurr CD, Carchidi PJ, et al. A cost-benefit analysis of electronic medical records in primary care. Am J Med 2003;114(5):397–403.

[43] Parente S, McCullough J. Health information technology and patient safety: evidence from panel data. Health Aff 2009;28:357–60.

[44] Raths D. A mandate in Mass. Massachusetts wants CPOE in place by 2012. Will CIOs be willing and able to comply? Healthc Inform 2008;25:46–7.

[45] Haynes RB, Wilczynski NL. Computerized Clinical Decision Support System (CCDSS) Systematic Review Team. Effects of computerized clinical decision support systems on practitioner performance and patient outcomes: methods of a decision-maker-researcher partnership systematic review. Implement Sci 2010;5:12.

[46] Baron RJ. Quality improvement with an electronic health record: achievable, but not automatic. Ann Intern Med 2007;147:549–52.

[47] Cebul RD, Love TE, Jain AK, Herbert CJ. Electronic health records and quality of diabetes care. N Engl J Med 2011;365:825–33.

[48] Ahrq AFHRAQ Costs and benefits of health information technology. Evid Rep Technol Assess 2006;132:1–154.

[49] Stead WW, Lorenzi NM. Health informatics: linking investment to value. J Am Med Inform Assoc: JAMIA 1999;6:341–8.

[50] Harrison MI, Koppel R, Bar-Lev S. Unintended consequences of information technologies in health care—an interactive sociotechnical analysis. J Am Med Inform Assoc: JAMIA 2007; 14:542–9.

[51] Ash JS, Berg M, Coiera E. Some unintended consequences of information technology in health care: the nature of patient care information system-related errors. J Am Med Inform Assoc: JAMIA 2004;11:104–12.

[52] Ash JS, Sittig DF, Poon EG, Guappone K, Campbell E, Dykstra RH. The extent and importance of unintended consequences related to computerized provider order entry. J Am Med Inform Assoc: JAMIA 2007;14:415–23.

[53] Institute of Medicine Health IT and patient safety: building safer systems for better care. Washington, DC: The National Academies Press; 2012.

[54] Kohane IS, Masys DR, Altman RB. The incidentalome: a threat to genomic medicine. JAMA 2006;296:212–5.

[55] Berg JS, Khoury MJ, Evans JP. Deploying whole genome sequencing in clinical practice and public health: meeting the challenge one bin at a time. Genet Med 2011;13.

[56] Schwartz LM, Woloshin S, Fowler FJ, Welch HG. Enthusiasm for cancer screening in the United States. JAMA 2004;291:71–8.

[57] Hauskeller C. Direct to consumer genetic testing. BMJ 2011;342:d2317.

[58] Salz T, Brewer NT. Direct-to-consumer genomewide profiling. N Engl J Med 2011;364:2074.

[59] Vaszar LT, Cho MK, Raffin TA. Privacy issues in personalized medicine. Pharmacogenomics 2003;4:107–12.

[60] Kollek R, Petersen I. Disclosure of individual research results in clinico-genomic trials: challenges, classification and criteria for decision-making. J Med Ethics 2011;37:271–5.

[61] Issa AM, Tufail W, Hutchinson J, Tenorio J, Baliga MP. Assessing patient readiness for the clinical adoption of personalized medicine. Public Health Genomics 2009;12:163–9.

[62] Kohane IS, Taylor PL. Multidimensional results reporting to participants in genomic studies: getting it right. Sci Transl Med 2010;2:37–9.

[63] Levinson W, Kao A, Kuby A, Thisted RA. Not all patients want to participate in decision making. A national study of public preferences. J Gen Intern Med 2005;20:531–5.

[64] Foster MW, Mulvihill JJ, Sharp RR. Evaluating the utility of personal genomic information. Genet Med 2009;11:570–4.

[65] Grosse SD, Kalman L, Khoury MJ. Evaluation of the validity and utility of genetic testing for rare diseases. Adv Exp Med Biol 2010;686:115.

[66] Grosse SD, McBride CM, Evans JP, Khoury MJ. Personal utility and genomic information: look before you leap. Genet Med 2009;11:575–6.

[67] McGuire AL, Caulfield T, Cho MK. Research ethics and the challenge of whole-genome sequencing. Nat Rev Genet 2008;2008:152–6.

[68] Clayton EW, Smith M, Fullerton SM, Burke W, McCarty CA, Koenig BA, et al. Confronting real time ethical, legal, and social issues in the Electronic Medical Records and Genomics (eMERGE) Consortium. Genet Med 2010;12:616–20.

[69] Burwell SM. Setting value-based payment goals—HHS efforts to improve U.S. health care. N Engl J Med 2015;372:897–9.

[70] McClellan M. Accountable care organizations and evidence-based payment reform. JAMA 2015;313:2128–30.

[71] Berwick DM, Nolan TW, Whittington J. The triple aim: care, health, and cost. Health Aff (Millwood) 2008;27:759–69.

Preface

When we were approached by the acquisition editor at Elsevier to submit a proposal for an edited volume on *Oncology Informatics*, we jumped at the opportunity. Our enthusiasm for the topic stemmed from our observation of several trends that were manifesting themselves in the winter of 2014. First, attestations for Stage I of the Centers for Medicare and Medicaid Services (CMS) Meaningful Use incentive program were rolling in and we knew that adoption of at least a basic Electronic Health Record (EHR) was soaring. Yet at the same time as EHR adoption climbed, we saw early indications that the markets had not yet been able to rectify problems related to full interoperability (precipitated by reports of "data-blocking" by some proprietary health systems), and we'd heard reports of how user-unfriendly some of these early implementations were. Still, for us, that was all the more reason for compiling an edited volume with contributions by the thought-leaders, scientists, and practitioners in oncology who were struggling with exactly these issues and leading efforts to resolve them. Finding these "bright spots" on the oncology landscape, we anticipated, would give others insight on how to move forward and take advantage of benefits that a fully connected medical system would offer to clinical teams, hospital administrators, patients, and their families.

Little did we know at the time, though, how other events might make the timing of this volume seem even more propitious. On January 20, 2015, the President of the United States announced a concerted effort toward making the advantages of Precision Medicine a reality. Against all odds, many of our authors became deeply involved in the mechanics of that effort while staying engaged in the writing, internal conversations, and strategic thinking that would be represented in their chapters. At around the same time, the President's Cancer Panel—the independent body tasked with evaluating the breadth of the National Cancer Program and then delivering recommendations to the President on gaps needing attention—became engaged in a review of connected-health technologies and how they could contribute to improvements in the quality of cancer care. Again, many of the authors contributing to this volume were tapped by the panel to contribute their expertise in public town hall meetings. They did so unselfishly, while at the same time staying vigilant to the steps necessary for completing their contributions to this cornerstone volume. On January 12, 2016, the President of the United States upped the ante even

further by announcing a "moon shot" for doubling the nation's progress against cancer over the next decade. As details of the Administration's efforts emerge, it has become clear that a robust electronic infrastructure and improved policies for data sharing will be central to the moon shot efforts. Also important in the equation would be a reinvigoration of the clinical trials enterprise in cancer, building on the good will and data altruism of fully engaged patients. We were happy to recognize that these topics were front-and-center in our authors' minds as we reviewed their contributions to the volume.

For all of their work at this extraordinary time, then, we offer our deepest gratitude to the authors and contributors whose work comprise this book. Each worked tirelessly to ensure that their chapters would represent a window into the state-of-the-science for at least one crucial aspect of oncology informatics from their field's perspective. By doing so, the authors ensured that the chapters in this book would form an integrative whole that is distinct from other informatics texts. Rather than focus on the technologies of the moment, which often become obsolete just a short time after publication, the authors emphasized lessons from the accumulating knowledge base on how the affordances these technologies offer can be optimized to reduce the burden of cancer in the population. They were also forthright in recognizing the limits of current knowledge, and were visionary in laying a course for further research into the self-improving implementation of informatics structures to improve processes of care and to optimize patient outcomes. In this sense, their contributions are timeless, informing the ongoing collaborative efforts of many dedicated professionals in the field of oncology informatics for years to come.

Of course, an effort such as this could not be possible without the dedicated service of a team of professionals who worked behind the scenes to make this volume a reality. In particular, we are especially grateful to Lisa Eppich, who was our "go to" person at Elsevier for production of the book; and to Catherine Van Der Laan, who was our original contact in reaching out to us with the opportunity. They, along with many others, made working with Elsevier an absolute pleasure. We would also like to acknowledge the contributions of Jocelyn Marrow, Scott Finley, Nadia Zaghal, Patricia Kelley, Julie Ehrhart, and Alexandra Cardy, who worked with us as internal and external consultants in preparing the integrative content of each of the chapters.

On a personal note, we would each like to acknowledge the invaluable contributions that enriched our own personal investigations into the interdisciplinary area of oncology informatics. Nicola Hesse, who as an obstetrician/gynecologist worked in the trenches to convert a hospital-based practice from paper to an informatics-supported system, offered invaluable insight into the realities and challenges associated with workflow conversion in a high-volume clinical practice. She also offered personal support that in any effort such as this was just as valuable as any experiential contribution. Louise Hope Burke offered steady injections of enthusiasm, energy, and reminders of the joy that children bring to life. Carolyn Ahern continued to offer her unwavering support during the many weekend days and evenings this effort required knowing the important contribution it would make to those individuals and families touched by cancer, including our own. Each helped to fuel our efforts during the preparation of this book, and reminded us that our commitment to the fight against cancer is rooted in wanting to end the devastation that this disease causes families around the world.

Perhaps the most important contribution for all of us, though, came from the personal stories of cancer patients and survivors who freely shared their care experiences with us over the course of compiling this book. Through their stories, we gained better insight into the personal courage and unyielding hope that these patients, their families, and their care teams maintain in spite of the complexities of a care system under strain. These were patients, we learned, who became emboldened by the opportunities to use modern information technologies to improve care, both for themselves but also for others. For these patients and for their care teams, we were inspired to work with our authors in offering a vision of *deep support* that would bring the best that science can offer to every decision and every exchange these teams can make to improve outcomes and relieve burden. Improving care systems through leadership and thoughtful design, we came to understand, would mean more than improving systemic efficiencies. For each of those waging their own personal battle against cancer, it may mean the difference between exhaustion and relief, or literally between life and death. It is to these patients and their relentless care teams that we offer our greatest acknowledgment, and to whom we pledge our steadfast support and respect.

Bradford W. Hesse PhD
David K. Ahern PhD
Ellen Beckjord PhD, MPH

Introduction

*Bradford W. Hesse PhD[1], David K. Ahern PhD[2,3,4]
and Ellen Beckjord PhD MPH[5]*

[1]Health Communication and Informatics Research Branch, Division of Cancer Control and
Population Sciences, National Cancer Institute, Rockville, MD, United States
[2]Health Communication and Informatics Research Branch, Healthcare Delivery Research Program,
National Cancer Institute, Rockville, MD, United States [3]Program in Behavioral Informatics and
eHealth, Department of Psychiatry, Brigham & Women's Hospital, Boston, MA, United States
[4]Harvard Medical School, Boston, MA, United States [5]Population Health Program Design and
Engagement Optimization, UPMC Health Plan, Pittsburgh, PA, United States

In the United States, approximately 14 million people have had cancer and more than 1.6 million new cases are diagnosed each year. By 2022, it is projected that there will be 18 million cancer survivors and, by 2030, cancer incidence is expected to rise to 2.3 million. However, more than a decade after the Institute of Medicine (IOM) first addressed the quality of cancer care in the United States; the barriers to achieving excellent care for all cancer patients remain daunting. The growing demand for cancer care, combined with the complexity of the disease and its treatment, a shrinking workforce, and rising costs, constitute a crisis in cancer care delivery. **Institute of Medicine, 2013 [1]**

I.1 WHY THIS BOOK NOW?

In 2013, the Board on Health Care Services within the Institute of Medicine (IOM) published a report titled *"Delivering High-Quality Cancer Care: Charting a New Course for a System in Crisis."* The implications of the report were sobering and warrant action. Cancer, as a disease associated with aging, was rarely diagnosed in the first part of the last century, but now competes with cardiovascular disease as a leading cause of mortality in North America. As people live longer, the report emphasized, the more likely they are to experience the cumulative effect of genetically influenced mutations or to be exposed to the epigenetic stress of sedentary lifestyles, environmental stressors (such as tobacco smoke), or encroaching adiposity from unhealthy body habitus.

More crucially, as people live longer lives the more likely it will be that they will need to encounter the complex web of services that comprise the modern cancer care system. Inefficiencies in that convoluted web of services will drive up costs, while gaping discontinuities may mean missed opportunities to intervene preemptively to save lives and reduce suffering. To the degree that the current system cannot adapt to the stresses of an increasing number of cancer patients, or that health systems buckle under the changing realities of 21st century cancer care, the cancer care system will be headed for a crisis [1].

I.1.1 The Cancer Care Crisis

Estimates cited by the IOM placed incidence rates for new cancer cases up to 2.3 million by 2030, a marked increase over the 1.6 million new cases anticipated in 2014 [2]. The American Cancer Society (ACS) reports that about 77% of all cancer cases are diagnosed among people aged 55 years or older, which is why an aging cohort causes concerns regarding the projected number of new cancers expected to interact with the health care system in the future [2]. In addition, cancer is a complex disease requiring interactions with multiple health care service providers and utilizing services that can be costly to administer [3,4]. The complexity of the disease can create inefficiencies in the handoffs between the many professionals and laboratories needed to diagnose the disease, to prescribe and administer treatment, to support posttreatment survivorship, and in terminal cases to negotiate hospice and end-of-life care [5].

Discontinuities in these transitions in care can lead to further expense and can increase risk for medical errors [5]. In the United States the cost of cancer care is rising faster than any other sector in medicine, with economic analyses showing an increase from $72 billion spent on cancer care in 2004 to $125 billion spent in 2010; and a projected increase of another 39% to $173 billion by 2020 [1,4]. The presence of comorbidities, a distinct likelihood within an aging cohort, expands the number of health care providers seeing cancer patients, thus further escalating risks for inefficiencies and discontinuity [6–8]. Finally, the IOM projects a marked shortfall in the number of trained professionals to deal with the impending surge in cancer cases in the years to come [1], meaning fewer health care providers will have to do more to meet the demands of the growing population of people diagnosed with and who survive cancer.

The United States is not alone when confronting the realities of projected deficits in health care service delivery. In his book "Shock of Gray," author Ted Fishman explained how the paradox of modern medicine—which has been "cheating death, one molecule at a time"—may actually be creating an unsustainable path for the future in which aging populations throughout the world may find a dearth of health care professionals who are ready and trained to take care of the diseases that are naturally associated with aging [9]. The World Health Organization (WHO) noted that the global population aged 60 years or older in 2012 had doubled since 1980; while projections show a quadrupling in the number of people 80 years and older expected to be alive in 2050 up to 395 million worldwide [10].

With this rise in an aging population globally, the WHO projects a concomitant rise in the number of health complications attributable to noncommunicable diseases (NCDs), especially if care is not taken to improve prevention and support for these aging demographic cohorts within the countries' public health systems [11]. "More than 87% of the burden of disease for older adults comes from NCDs—conditions such as diabetes, heart disease, chronic respiratory disease and cancer, among others that typically manifest later in life," warned the authors of the international agency's 2013 report on Aging (p. 11). These diseases can be devastating to families and economies, but can be reduced through effective interventions aimed at reducing multiple, shared risk factors such as tobacco use, unhealthy diet, obesity, physical inactivity, and harmful use of alcohol. The WHO estimates that approximately 40% of cancer cases worldwide could be eliminated through preventive interventions alone. The exhortation is that good health, along with personal engagement in preventive care, will not just add years of life to individuals' outlook but will "add life to years." According to the international organization, there is an urgent need to "innovate in the areas of health technology and health services delivery" to minimize the gap between "life expectancy"—the average number of years an individual may be expected to live in a developing or developed economy—and "healthy life expectancy"—the average number of years an individual will be expected to live without serious disease or disability [10].

One way to extend lives while at the same time extending expectancies for healthy living, suggested National Institutes of Health (NIH) director Elias Zerhouni to a US Congressional appropriations committee, is to move away from a 20th century *industrial age* approach to medicine into a 21st century *information age* approach [12]. Industrial age medicine, he explained, was often focused on the mass production of a "one-size-fits-all" set of remedies applied too late in the disease process to prevent irreparable tissue damage or to avoid irreversible loss of function. In contrast, information age technologies will allow care teams to adopt an approach to care that will be *predictive, preemptive, precise,* and *participative* in nature.

In the information age, a deep understanding of molecular processes will give care teams the ability to make predictive assessments of disease risk and then intervene preemptively in the disease process early before permanent damage results. In cancer, the ability to identify variations in disease processes at the subcellular level is catalyzing an era of precision medicine in which treatment can be oriented to the genetic disruptions of an individuals' specific cancer cell and then optimized to target the molecular drivers of an individual patient's unique expression of the disease. Information age technologies are also allowing cancer treatment to become more participative in nature as engineers find ways to engage patients more proactively in their own care through patient-facing tools, while contributing their data back to the research enterprise in an expression of citizen science.

Paradoxically, this shift to predictive, preemptive, precision, and participative medicine may be contributing further to the perceived sense of crisis in cancer care unless something is done to accommodate the complexities of these approaches in practice. Fig. I.1, presented by William Stead to an IOM working committee on October 8, 2007, illustrates the magnitude of the problem. Fig. I.1 presents the average number of "facts" needed to reach a diagnostic or treatment decision for individual patients during an era of industrial age, "one-size-fits-all" medicine. Over time, the average number of individual data points needed to personalize treatment is expected to climb almost exponentially as practitioners avail themselves of information made available first through advances in structural genetics (Single Nucleotide Polymorphisms, haplotypes), then to a more sophisticated use of gene expression profiles, and

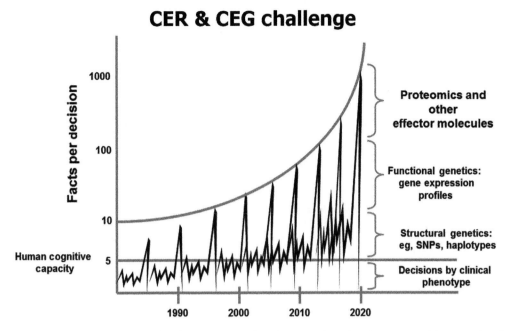

FIGURE I.1 Growth in facts affecting provider decisions over time juxtaposed against human cognitive capacity. *Source: Courtesy of William Stead.*

finally to the inclusion of molecular information made available through proteomics. Research on human cognitive capacity has suggested that it is only possible to retain up to seven (plus or minus two) individual facets of new information in working memory at a time—a threshold indicated by a horizontal line on the graph. Needless to say, informatics technologies and solutions must be designed to reduce the complexity of precision medicine into actionable displays for human decision making.

The complexity of cancer care delivery under rapidly evolving assumptions in precision medicine is directly relevant to one of the main reasons for compiling this book. As NIH Director Francis Collins declared in a January 13, 2015, commentary in the *Journal of the American Medical Association*, cancer is "at the leading edge of this new era of precision medicine" [13]. Investments in the Cancer Genome Atlas and other related projects are revealing that even for the same types of cancers, individual tumors can be differentially receptive to treatment based on the distinct profile of genes influencing the mechanisms of malignant growth within individuals. "Cancer death rates have decreased about 1% annually for … 15 years," Collins explained. Opening up a new frontier in cancer prevention and treatment based on the knowledge made possible through increases in capacity and falling prices for gene sequencing technologies represents an era of "exceptional opportunities for medical science" in the years to come [13]. On January 20, 2015, President Obama added further heft to the NIH

Director's words in his annual State of the Union speech. This is how he put it to the US Congress and people of the United States: "*Tonight, I'm launching a new Precision Medicine Initiative to bring us closer to curing diseases like cancer and diabetes—and to give all of us access to the personalized information we need to keep ourselves and our families healthier*" [14].

Another prevailing reason for compiling this edited volume now is the recognition that without the connective support of care teams and families, cancer can be a "long and lonely road" [15] for patients. As oncologist Patricia Ganz cautioned in her forward to the IOM's *Delivering High Quality Cancer Care* report, cancer patients "often endure protracted periods of primary and adjuvant therapies, multimodal treatments with substantial toxicities and comorbidities, years to recover physically and psychologically, with great financial hardship and social disruption" [1]. Moreover, cancer treatments have soared in expense, with the "punishing cost of cancer care" [16] crippling personal savings accounts and bankrupting social insurance funds. The complexity of the disease outstrips the capacity of many of our current support systems, with the average cancer survivor interacting with scores of independent service providers, the majority of which do not communicate with each other or have the availability of reliable, secure informatics infrastructures to efficiently share and exchange information about patient care [7]. Informatics engineering will be needed to provide a new support system that will coordinate work flows across care teams, and will serve as a repository of the data and information needed to support situational awareness among every member of the care team [17]. Opening up those structures to patients, families, and their caregivers, under the right circumstances, should help reduce costs further by putting patients at the leading edge of preemptive medicine [18,19].

Even for those patients who make it through the cancer care process and who can subsequently declare themselves to be survivors, their journeys can continue to be fraught with confusion and fragmentation [20]. Survivors struggle with the transition as they move back into the primary care environment, but yet must carry with them the fears of recurrence, secondary cancer, or even the risk of late-term side effects from their cancer treatments. Subsequent downstream health care providers, who may not have the full record of treatment given during cancer care, may be at risk of missing signs or symptoms, or of prescribing treatments that may be contraindicated from an oncologic perspective. In a very positive vein, the number of cancer survivors estimated to be alive in the United States in 2012 was up to 12 million with that number rising to 18 million by 2020 [21]. On the more cautious side of that projection, the capabilities of a fragmented and overburdened primary and specialty care system to provide vigilance and deep support for the health needs of this growing cohort will become strained unless efforts are made to improve quality across—as well as within—systems [1].

I.1.2 The Indispensable Role of Informatics

As the IOM has repeatedly affirmed, the promise of "omics-informed" medicine in cancer care cannot be enabled without significant participation from the informatics community [22–24]. Participation is needed to create the necessary technologies for collecting and processing the vast amounts of information required to inform clinical decision making in close to real-time, to create a distributed platform for sharing information with multiple members of a patient's care team, to improve quality of care delivery, to inform research, and to empower patients and families. As NIH Director and genomics pioneer Francis Collins puts it, we are only going to succeed (in medicine) if we work closely together—between those with biological sophistication and those with computational sophistication [25]. Phillip Sharp, past president of the American Association for the Advancement of Science and faculty member at the Koch Institute for Integrative Cancer Research at the Massachusetts Institute of Technology, put it this way: "Increasing the quality of health care in a cost-effective fashion is dependent upon using information technology (IT) and advances in life sciences and medicine to assess, inform, and modify lifestyles and better treat

individuals … Innovation along these lines will require a broad convergence of social, mathematical, physical, and engineering sciences with the medical, regulatory, and financial communities" [26].

This convergence of disciplinary perspectives to achieve better care, at lower costs, with better patient satisfaction (ie, the triple aim in health care) has been a theme in the series of reports compiled by the IOM on the topic of improving safety and quality in medicine. In the first report, *To Err is Human*, authors provided the alarming statistic that an estimated 44,000–98,000 die annually from avoidable medical errors [8]. Subsequent analyses placed the price tag for avoidable medical errors at roughly $17.1 billion per year [27]. Blame for these errors should not be placed on individuals in the system, argued the authors of the reports; doing so would be anathema to lessons learned from safety improvement success in other industries. Rather, the etiology of avoidable error is best viewed through an interdisciplinary lens at the systems level, where converging sets of expertise can be integrated to engineer error-prevention protocols upstream in the process before the serious errors create irreparable consequences. This is the approach the aviation industry took when assuming the imperative task of turning a very complex, potentially dangerous, and technology-dependent industry into a safe and reliable mode of public transportation following a spate of crew-induced errors during World War II. To do this, industry leaders and policy makers used converging perspectives from human factors—engineers, physicists, psychologists, mathematicians, industrial designers, and organizational specialists—to engineer a sociotechnical environment with safety as a first priority. Today, the aviation industry has a remarkable safety record with the number of fatalities from air travel approaching zero in many of the postwar years.

In IOM's follow-up report, *Crossing the Quality Chasm: A New Health System for the 21st Century*, lead scientist Don Berwick and his colleagues highlighted the changes that must occur within the fabric of the modern health care system to improve the quality of care delivery across its many facets [28]. Similar to the perspective taken in the aviation and other high-risk industries, Berwick and his colleagues assumed that quality must be considered to be a system property. Improving the quality of health care would mean reengineering the health care environment to support better outcomes for the many dedicated health care workers who operate within the system. The objective must be to create a new care environment that is by design safe; effective (ie, adherent to evidence); patient-centered; timely; efficient; and equitable across all patient populations. Because medicine is inherently an information-based science, health information technology (HIT) was seen as a necessary platform upon which to achieve this goal [1,28,29]. The prediction was that HIT could be used to reengineer care processes, support a more timely and effective workflow, serve as a platform for evidence implementation, collect data on care effectiveness as input to quality improvement efforts, and could be used to help connect and coordinate the expanding palette of specialized services needed to treat patients over their lives [1,30]. Indeed, in many other sectors IT has led to marked improvements in quality and efficiencies, but for a number of sector-specific reasons its utilization had lagged in hospitals and physicians' offices [31].

On April 27, 2004, President George W. Bush issued Executive Order # 13335 establishing the Office of the National Coordinator for Health Information Technology (ONC) within the US Department of Health and Human Services (DDS). The executive order directed the newly created office to coordinate efforts throughout the nation toward utilizing a mutually accessible health information infrastructure to ensure that the best medical information would be made available to the right people, at the right time, at the right place in order to guide evidence-based decision making. In conjunction with other agencies, the ONC would provide leadership in identifying best practices in utilizing HIT and it would facilitate interoperability of content while protecting patients from unwanted intrusions into their own individually identifiable personal health information. President George W. Bush set a national goal that year for the widespread use of electronic health records (EHRs) before a decade was out.

Adoption of EHRs proceeded fitfully during the first years after establishment of the ONC. Estimates placed adoption of "at least a basic EHR"—defined as implementing at least 10 essential computerized functions in at least one clinical unit in a hospital setting—at around 9% within hospitals in 2008 according to the American Hospital Association's Annual Survey on Information Technology Support. The 10 functions considered to be essential within a basic EHR included: patient demographics, physician notes, nursing assessments, patient problem lists, patient medication lists, discharge summaries, laboratory and radiologic reports, diagnostic test results, and order entry for medications. Estimates for a fully comprehensive EHR—defined as including the basic 10 functions plus 14 additional capabilities in conjunction with being implemented in all major clinical units of the hospital—were much lower at about 3% of US hospitals in 2008 [32].

Acknowledging this lag in adoption, the US Congress passed the Health Information Technology for Economic and Clinical Health (HITECH) Act as Title XIII of the American Recovery and Reinvestment Act (ie, the "stimulus package") in 2009. The HITECH Act gave the Centers for Medicare & Medicaid Services (CMS) the power to work with the ONC in awarding monetary incentives to those providers attesting to the "meaningful use" of HIT within the context of care. The meaningful use provision intended to go beyond the development of new technologies to stimulate a market-based ecosystem of technology products and services designed: (1) to improve safety and efficiency; (2) to engage patients and their families; (3) to encourage greater continuity of care; (4) to promote management of population health outcomes across the patient base; and (5) to ensure privacy and security [33,34].

I.1.3 Health IT Adoption and Uptake From the Provider's Perspective

A report funded by the Robert Wood Johnson Foundation (RWJ) and published in 2014 suggested that, in broad strokes, the meaningful use incentive payments have been effective in stimulating adoption of HIT [32]. Adoption of at least a basic EHR increased to an estimated 58.9% of US hospitals by 2013, essentially quadrupling adoption rates from 2010 at the beginning of the program. Adoption of a comprehensive EHR climbed to an estimated 25.5% of US hospitals by the same year, representing a seven fold increase over 3 years. As might be expected, adoption rates varied by hospital context. Hospitals were more likely to have at least a basic EHR if they were large (72.9%), urban (62.7%), not-for-profit (63%), or if they were classified as a major teaching hospital (76.6%). On the physician side of the equation, the report summarized 2013 data from the National Ambulatory Medicare Care Survey to show that nearly half the physicians included in the survey met the criteria for utilizing at least a basic EHR. That represented a doubling of adoption rates from 2009, and a 22% relative increase for physician adoption from 2009. Physicians who reported accessing at least a basic EHR were more likely to come from large practices, while physicians who practiced as part of a Health Maintenance Organization (HMO) had significantly higher rates of adoption as compared to physicians in solo practice [32].

Although these adoption rates were promising, there were significant challenges still persisting in the health care landscape that would prevent systems from taking full advantage of these new HIT capacities. Hospital administrators complained about the lack of true interoperability (ie, the ability to exchange data seamlessly between systems) that seemed to be creating added expense and complexity as different units in the hospital adopted incompatible technologies. Physicians complained that many of the technologies made available to them during the first phase of meaningful use attestation were not user-friendly, and were disruptive of work flows. In fact, the American Medical Association has written several letters on behalf of its members to the ONC urging government to reconsider its meaningful use program until issues of interoperability, usability, and work-flow compatibility were addressed. Given these observations, the President's Council of Advisors on Science and Technology (PCAST) published the second [35] of two reports [35,36] on HIT in May of 2014. The report's focus was on the importance of applying a systems engineering perspective to the challenge of converting HIT investments into better health care and lower costs. Noting some of the same issues, authors of the 2014 RWJ report concluded that "adopting EHRs is simply the first step in a long and complex journey to an IT-enabled health care system in which technology is effectively leveraged to address ongoing cost and quality challenges."

Of course, the first target in medical informatics is to create an environment that focuses on patient needs and optimizes resources for achieving medical or health objectives; that is, it is about a commitment to deliver high-quality, evidence-based care [37]. A 2011 review of published findings on the benefits and costs of HIT in terms of medical outcomes showed "primarily positive results" when taken as a whole [34]. Of the 154 studies included in a systematic review, 96 (62%) revealed positive findings, defined by the authors to mean that one or more aspects of the HIT intervention yielded positive results with no aspect of care worsening; while 142 (92%) of the studies yielded results that were either positive or mixed-positive. Dimensions for which findings were reported included: efficiency of care ($\approx 60/78$ positive; $\approx 10/78$ mixed positive/negative); effectiveness of care ($\approx 28/49$ positive, $\approx 10/49$ mixed); provider satisfaction ($\approx 14/48$ positive, $\approx 28/48$ mixed); patient safety ($\approx 21/30$ positive, $\approx 3/30$ mixed); patient satisfaction ($\approx 18/26$ positive, $\approx 6/26$ mixed); care process ($\approx 21/28$ positive, $\approx 4/28$ mixed); preventive care ($\approx 6/10$ positive, $\approx 3/10$ mixed); and access to care ($\approx 4/7$ positive, $\approx 2/7$ mixed).

Although the 2011 review concluded that effects were mostly positive, the authors were cautious in noting that there were not enough statistically quantified negative findings to go beyond making just a suggestive conclusion for the early efficacy of HIT. What they did note, however, was a very strong relationship between provider dissatisfaction and the presence of negative findings. "The stronger finding," they suggested, "may be that the 'human element' is critical to H.I.T. implementation." Some of the descriptions of failed implementations described situations in which clinical leadership was lacking, staff resentment was high, schedules were unrealistic, interfaces were poorly designed, and vendors were behind schedule. These negative conditions would often lead to increases in patient care errors, increases in cost, and confusion over professional responsibilities in the new environment. The authors of a RAND study published in 2013 worried that overall modern HIT systems had not yet been used effectively under the early

incentives of *meaningful use* and noted that the necessary changes in health care delivery needed to bend the cost curve had not yet taken effect. The authors concluded that more work would be needed to improve interoperability, patient-centeredness, and ease of use—all necessary preconditions for an efficient and effective health care system [38].

I.1.4 Health IT Adoption and Uptake From the Consumer's Perspective

In 2001, near the inflection point of the first "dot com" speculative bubble, NCI launched a general population survey called the Health Information National Trends Survey (HINTS). Its purpose was to give behavioral researchers and communication planners access to population data on how Americans 18 years or older accessed and utilized information relevant to cancer control and prevention in a rapidly changing information environment [39]. Anecdotally, program planners had heard stories of patients walking into their primary care and oncology care offices with "reams of printouts" from the World Wide Web related to their conditions. NCI wanted to know, first, if people were indeed flocking to new electronic media outlets for cancer information and, second, how well were people able to utilize the information and channels they encountered in this new environment to prevent disease, adhere to treatment, or maintain personal vigilances as a cancer survivor. The first administration of the national probability sample was fielded as a random digit dialing (RDD) telephone survey in 2003, with the second administration occurring in 2005. For the third administration, in 2007, the program split the sampling frame into a newly announced postal frame for paper-and-pencil administration in one arm to be compared with the traditional RDD sampling approach. A fourth administration began in 2012, with four cycles of the survey conducted in succession over the course of 3 years [40].

Fig. I.2 depicts some of the major trends in the public's use and perceptions of e-Health functionality from 2003 to 2013, where e-health can be defined simply as a set of activities "at the intersection of medical informatics, public health and business, referring to health services and information delivered or enhanced through the Internet and related technologies" [41]. In this case, HINTS began by tracking public access to the Internet in 2003 with a question asking if respondents had "gone online to access the Internet or World Wide Web, or to send and receive e-mail" [42]. In 2003 HINTS documented a 63% penetration rate for adults 18 years and older, which languished in 2005 down to 61% following the dot com implosion, but then increased steadily to 68% in 2008, 78% in 2012, and 80% in 2013. Also, in 2003 HINTS began tracking where people reported

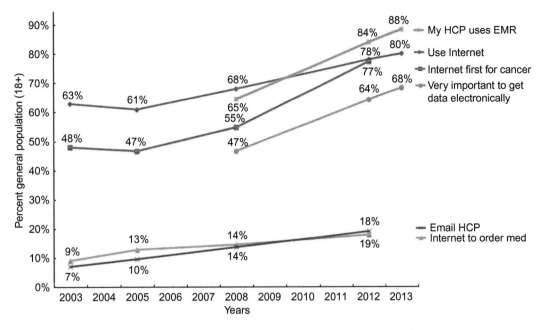

FIGURE I.2 Data from the Health Information National Trends Survey (HINTS) showing public use, or perceptions, of selected e-Health functionalities.

going first when looking for information about cancer (from the subset of people who said that they had looked for cancer information from any source). The estimated percentage of individuals who reported going to the Internet first (of those who looked for cancer information) in 2003 was 48%. That number has climbed steadily up to an estimated 78% who went online first to look for cancer information by 2012.

Beyond using the Internet for general information gathering, HINTS began tracking the use of eHealth functionality to order medications and to exchange email with health care providers. Estimates for both functions were low in 2003, with 7% reporting online ordering of medications and 9% using email. Reports of usage in both areas rose steadily across all 10 years of the survey with just a little under one-fifth of the population engaged in online utilization of both functions: that is, 18% of the population reported using the Internet to order medications while 19% reported interacting with their health care providers through email. Plans for engaging the American public in a goal to adopt EHRs or other forms of HIT had not yet been formulated when HINTS first started collecting data. Questions related to perceptions of EHR usage were added for the 2008 data collection. From those data, a little less than half or 47% of the general population reported that getting data electronically from their health care providers was important to them. About 65% reported that, to their knowledge, they believed their health care providers were already utilizing a system to exchange patients' health information electronically. By 2013, those numbers rose to 68% and

88%, respectively. It is interesting to note in this case that the general public's perceptions of their provider's utilization of EHRs may have exceeded percentages of actual implementation as described earlier.

Taken together, these data suggest an increase in demand from the general public for health services that can be provided through electronic means. Not surprisingly, consumers are accustomed to making travel reservations online or checking their bank accounts online, but when it comes to checking their personal health information that capacity and uptake has been limited. Phase 2 of the meaningful use incentive program sought to address this discrepancy by requiring attesting hospitals to show that 5% of their patient base had gone online to engage in their health information during the qualifying period. Patient engagement has been identified as a core component of high quality health care for patients with chronic disease, especially given the often-cited observation that the success of treatment depends heavily on patient adherence and vigilance. Data confirm that patients who are disengaged in their own health care are "the toughest group to manage and account for a disproportionate share of healthcare costs" [43].

But patient engagement is only half of the equation. According to health services researchers, health care systems need to be ready and responsive to patient engagement efforts in order to produce positive health outcomes. Just as HIT systems can be engineered to reduce errors and improve efficiency and effectiveness on the clinical side, the same can—and must—be done to include support for patients and their caregivers.

Authors of a report published by the National Research Council (NRC) embodied this perspective in a recommendation that investments in medical informatics be rebalanced "to place a greater emphasis on providing cognitive support for health care providers, patients, and family caregivers" [37]. Doing so, the authors of the report suggested, would require interdisciplinary work in at least three areas: (1) organizational systems-level research in the design of health care systems, processes, and workflow; (2) computable knowledge structures and models for medicine needed to make sense of available patient-data including preferences, health behaviors, and literacy level; and (3) human-computer interaction in the clinical context [37].

More recently, there has been a proliferation in the market place of consumer-facing applications and mobile devices designed to promote health. According to reports, almost one-third of US smartphone owners used apps downloaded from the health and fitness categories of online app stores [44]. Many of these are fitness apps built to connect with personally quantified data from a wearable sensing device. In June 2014, Apple Computer—arguably one of the most influential consumer electronics companies—announced a joint agreement with Epic Systems and the Mayo Clinic to design applications that would exploit features of the company's newly announced "HealthKit" platform released as part of their iOS 8 upgrade for mobile devices. The joint venture offers a potential bridge between physician care, as informed through EHRs, and patient self-care, as supported through personal access through mobile devices. In summing up the potential of this new shift in the marketplace, the Wall Street Journal declared on June 8, 2014, that the health care industry is engaged in a massive effort to "push patients to help themselves"; that is, to engage in the "last mile in the race to fix health-care—getting patients more involved."

Other innovations include extensions of support through the "Internet of Things," to create environmental supports for at-home care while nudging healthy behaviors. One commonly cited example is the development of smart scales that can transmit weight data into smartphone apps, and eventually even into EHRs, as a way of helping patients engage in active weight management. Another example is the implanted cardiac defibrillator received by cancer survivors with cardiotoxic secondary effects from chemotherapy. Wireless versions of these devices can be engineered to send signals to the cardiologists for remote monitoring, but are still not often engineered to deliver self-management back to patients. New devices are also under development to help with improved adherence and monitoring for cancer patients taking home-based oral chemotherapies by utilizing wireless signals from transponders placed in pharmaceutical bottles to track drug intake and body temperature sensors to achieve early identification of fever that can warn of serious complications like neutropenia. The US Food and Drug Administration (FDA), CMS, and other regulatory agencies are investigating the use of these sensors to save costs through reimbursements for telemedicine and at-home care.

I.2 THE PURPOSE OF THIS BOOK

The purpose of this book is to contribute a guiding vision to the broader cancer care community oriented toward leveraging progress in informatics toward achieving optimal results in cancer prevention, care, and survivorship. We have embarked upon this effort to create a knowledge product that is of value and service to the people who care for, study, and aim to help individuals affected by cancer. The content of the book should provide actionable guidance on the how to use informatics across the broad spectrum of "cancer"; what informatics applications are of use; and when informatics can improve research and practice. The book is also intended to serve as a platform for directing continued and future work, supporting convergence of important, foundational themes; and spurring innovation in this evolving field of study.

More importantly, the book is intended to build on the recommendations of the IOM in its prescription for *Delivering High Quality Cancer Care*. We review each of those recommendations as a backdrop to the book, starting with its most central recommendation: "Creating a system that supports all patients in making informed medical decisions consistent with their needs, values, and preferences in consultation with their clinicians who have expertise in patient-centered communication and shared decision making" [1]. We turn our attention at this time to a careful consideration of each of those recommendations in the context of oncology informatics.

I.2.1 Creating Deep Support for Engaged Patients

By emphasizing the goal of making a system that is patient-centered, the IOM has reiterated a common theme; that the focus of systems reengineering efforts should be on creating an underlying foundation of deep support for patients, their families, and the professionals who care for them [1,28,29,45]. In the early days of Internet-based technologies, explained Harvard business experts Zuboff and Maxmin, companies commonly made the egregious error of exploiting value solely from individual transactions—much in the same way that fee-for-service health care focused on exploiting value from individual consultations or treatments. These companies soon went out of business (part of the dot com implosion), but were replaced with companies who used their IT systems to create an enduring fabric of trust in their customers. Companies such as FedEx assure their clients that all services have been engineered to ensure prompt delivery of a valued parcel, even to point of providing real-time monitoring capabilities to customers to track progress of the parcel as it moves around the globe. Companies such as Amazon and Netflix made a name for themselves by recognizing their customers' tastes and purchasing habits, and in focusing all facets of their supply chain toward meeting the needs of their customers over time. Zuboff and Maxmin referred to this strategy as an effort to provide "deep support" through a relational, rather than transactional, engagement with customers over time [46].

Providing deep support for patients in oncology care will be crucial as well, especially as patients and their families are encouraged to cope with their chronic conditions by taking a more active role in their own care [18]. To get a sense for how the contributions of this book might speak to patients' needs, we spoke directly to cancer survivors about their thoughts regarding the role of HIT in their care. We heard their hopes for the ways informatics can improve the lives of people affected by cancer, but we also heard their frustrations over seeing how many well-meaning supports do not seem to help but may actually hinder their ability to take care of themselves or a loved one. Here is one patient's experience with information overload while trying to cope with a complex care regimen:

> Patient 1: "Because when you're a patient, and you're sick, and you don't feel well, and you're tired, and you're taking 10 medicines or whatever it is, you don't have time to read 40 pages of discharge [notes]."

That sentiment struck us as we thought through the importance of user-centered design, and the promise of HIT to deliver the right information, to the right person (in a language they can understand) at the right time [47,48]. This may seem far-off for IT in health care settings, but it is not far off from what patients have come to expect when interacting with the ubiquitous tools that enrich lives—from searches on the web for information on any facet of their lives, including health and cancer; to making their own travel reservations online; or even interacting effortlessly with a Geographic Positioning System that puts all of the mathematic calculations behind the scenes as it presents terabytes of localized data easily through an intuitive interface. In a similar vein, here is how two patients described their view for

how HIT can help them and help their providers get a more coordinated, personalized view of their own health conditions.

> Patient 2: "You know, when you have [an electronic medical record] EMR and can go out and look things up in a way that makes sense to an individual care provider ... whether it's blood work or former radiologists' reports, and even the actual images themselves, you give them a quicker, better way to really understand you as a patient without either having to try and remember it on your own or for them to try and piece it together."
>
> Patient 3: "Nobody ... and I can say this truthfully ... in the last 2 years-nobody is looking—except one physician who happens to be in the room—none of them are looking at the others' [clinical notes]. And I do resent that...when it is something that is right there in front of them. Even if it's their physician extender be it PA, be it a nurse—doesn't matter ... It is maddening, it is frustrating, and to the point that now I'm saying, 'Enough.'"

Notice how these patients' views paralleled observations from the report commissioned by the NRC on computational technology for effective health care as described earlier in this text. Based on observations of systems in action, authors of the NRC report called for interdisciplinary research to solve challenges in three critical areas: "(a) organizational systems-level research into the design of health care systems, processes, and workflow; (b) computable knowledge structures and models for medicine that help care teams make sense of all available patient data including preferences, health behaviors, and so on; and (c) human-computer interaction in a clinical context" [37]. Bringing these perspectives together within this book for the benefit of all users—patient care teams, laboratory/pathology teams, researchers, along with patients and their families—was a high priority of ours.

Moreover, a fourth patient emphasized for us the fact that we are no longer engaged in a solely academic exercise in informatics—with time to spare for slow, glacial translation of proven principles into the care system. With success in the consumer market around so many other facets of their daily lives, consumers are getting impatient with the slow progress in bringing them into their own care more effectively through technology. These were some of the lessons we learned in poring over the HINTS data. Patients and the general public were flocking to the Internet first, before being able to visit their providers, while hoping to interact with their providers in convenient ways online [49]. We were emboldened to see in 2012 and again in 2013 that the majority of American adults already thought that their providers were making use of EHRs to share information, and that a majority (91.4% in 2013) indicated that it would be very or somewhat important for doctors to share medical information with each other electronically. The fourth patient captured the upcoming surge of patient demand this way:

> Patient 4: "And yet the influx of new patients, I mean, they're more [tech] savvy than I'll ever be, and they're gonna demand it [i.e., access to their care through health I.T.]."

I.2.2 Augmenting and Coordinating an Adequately Trained Workforce

The second recommendation from the *Delivering High-Quality Cancer Care* report was to make a concerted effort to support an adequately staffed, trained, and coordinated workforce. We recognize that equipping such a traditional workforce of clinicians will be a challenge, if not an impossibility, given status quo expectations for service delivery. With the anticipated glut of demand from an aging population, more complicated treatment strategies, and a proliferation of cancer survivors, the cancer care delivery system will fall deeper into crisis unless something is done to improve the efficiency with which complex care is delivered. IT, the IOM report suggested, would be an important platform for extending the influence of highly effective care teams, drawing from a broader workforce including para-professionals such as community health workers and patient and family navigators.

Economist David Cutler sets the stage for this proposition in his book *The Quality Cure: How Focusing on Health Care Quality Can Save Your Life and Lower Spending Too* [31]. The book presented data on comparative gains in productivity growth across multiple sectors of the economy during the national rise in gross domestic product from 1995 to 2008. From these graphs, the Durable Goods and Information sectors appeared to lead productivity growth in economy with percentage growth measured in terms of output per hour up to +7% and +6%, respectively. The Health, Education, and Social Services sector fell on the negative side of the graph, with a loss in productivity at about −3% followed by Other Services at −1%, Construction at −1.2%, and Mining at −2%. That negative productivity estimate is actually an underestimate of loss in health care, Cutler argued, because the index did not adequately take quality into account—it was simply a matter of doing less with more over time with respect to the price of services. Factoring medical error and quality into the equation would have lowered the index even further.

What distinguished the leading producers from the laggards during the 1995–2008 period? One of the differentiating characteristics noted by Cutler was a strategic use of IT. All of the leading sectors achieved rapid productivity growth through an extensive use of IT to strengthen supply chains, shore up inefficiencies, automatic tedious processes, and expand reach of communications; while those in the trailing industries lacked a sustained use of IT. These observations fueled many of the legislative efforts to encourage a broad adoption of HIT from the 2004 inclusion of priorities in the State of the Union address by President George W. Bush, to the 2009 formulation of the HITECH Act passed by the 111th US Congress. Clauser and his colleagues illustrated how IT could be deployed throughout the systems of health care to augment workforce processes and achieve similar efficiencies. Their blueprint placed IT at the center of any organizational strategy designed to: (1) improve connections between providers; (2) support and empower patients; (3) strengthen connections between providers and patients; and (4) fortify information flow between providers and the health care system [50].

Throughout the book, chapter authors will repeatedly visit an overarching design notion that, for oncology informatics to be effective, it must serve to connect the expanded workforce in timely, safe, and efficient ways. The workforce should include members of the cancer care team, as well as members of the primary care and specialty care teams, and other medical care teams interlinked in support of the patients and their families. The archetypal cancer care team, according to the IOM depiction, will include the physicians providing oncology care, clinicians providing psychosocial care and spiritual support, palliative care clinicians (including hospice at end-of-life), rehabilitation centers, physician assistants, pharmacists, and nurses. To the degree that activated patients can help save resources by performing some care tasks for themselves, then they too should be considered as part of the "workforce" with attention given to supporting patient tasks and communication through informatics automation. For lower literacy and diverse populations, community health workers and patient navigators are likely to become part of the expanded cancer care team.

I.2.3 Serving as a Platform for Evidence Implementation

Most information scientists recognize that the days in which physicians would be expected to digest the original source materials for scientific articles touching on their area of general care or specialization are long gone. A quick search of Medline using the simple term "cancer" yielded an explosion of published articles over the years from 5767 papers published in 1950, to 134,591 new articles published in 2014 with an overall list of publications ranging up to 3,069,392 articles archived overall. Some speculations in 2001 were that in order to just stay up on current, basic knowledge in medicine by reading the latest randomized controlled trials, an internist would have to read roughly 20 articles a day for

365 days a year [51]. That would be an impossible task, and would be anathema to the proposition of engineering a fail-safe delivery system [29].

Rather, we take it as a goal of this book to describe frameworks that can serve to instantiate best evidence universally within the supported processes of care [52]. This can be engineered into the system in several ways: reminders based on evidence-based guidelines, just-in-time information support with links to the medical literature, checklists, error-checks for known complications or contraindications, filtered references, as well as data-driven decision algorithms, to name a few. It can also be reinforced through the tracking mechanisms made available through electronic infrastructure. We were heartened when reading the 2014 RWJ-led report on the status of HIT implementation to see that some 69.5% of large hospitals had implemented tracking mechanisms for guideline adherence by 2013, followed by reports that 64.8% of medium-sized hospitals and 61.0% of small hospitals had done the same. We were also encouraged to note that 84.9% of large hospitals had implemented organizational level dashboards for tracking patient status, followed by 81.7% of medium-sized and 73.0% of small-sized hospitals. The systems are starting to be put in place for ensuring a reliable adherence to evidence-based guidelines [32].

The importance of creating systems to ensure reliable diffusion of evidence-based treatment in cancer cannot be overstated. In 2006, the directors of NCI's Comprehensive Cancer Centers jointly produced a report declaring that nationally the burden of cancer could be diminished dramatically if only known recommendations for prevention, early detection, and treatment were implemented with equal fidelity across hospitals. Citing an economic report from the University of Chicago, even a 1% reduction in mortality achieved by improvement to systems could translate into savings worth over $400 billion to the national economy [53].

Not only will informatics technology allow for a more reliable instantiation of evidence, but if deployed in ways that integrate well with hospital clinical practices, the technologies can be restructured to reinforce workflows that are more consistent with evidence-based principles for care delivery [54]. This is the observation made by Friedberg and colleagues who evaluated several organizational approaches for reducing barriers to cancer screening among patients. From all of the organizational changes they observed, it was the inclusion of a fully functional EMR that accounted for the most progress in reducing barriers to screening [55]. The problem is at this stage that many organizations find themselves in the throes of enforced organizational restructuring, catalyzed by incented adoption of EHRs, without knowledge of best practice. To the extent possible, we have asked our authors to report on evidence-based practices

from health services research to inform the deployment, maintenance, and ongoing calibration of informatics tools within the context of their chapters.

I.2.4 Enabling a Learning Health Care System in Cancer

On February 27 and 28, 2012, the National Cancer Policy Forum of the IOM conducted a public workshop on informatics needs and challenges in cancer research. A principal theme of the workshop was that as oncology moves toward genomically informed, precision care, opportunities will emerge to accelerate research and inform discovery by exploiting the data streams made available through clinical informatics applications. Not only will informatics solutions reinforce a standard of evidence-based care, but they will also open up an opportunity for care-based evidence. The vision is to create a learning health care system in cancer, one that exploits interoperable data streams for accelerating discovery through data mining; one that informs observation on what works and what does not in the increasingly nuanced forms of precision oncology care; one that can be used to shore up efficiencies and improve quality through principles of statistical process control; and one that can be used to explore cost savings through comparative effectiveness evaluations. A major recommendation from the workshop was for the oncology community to "embrace cancer informatics" in order to improve the efficiency of the "discovery engine" in cancer research, while bridging the gap between discovery and health [22].

The theme of a learning health care system in oncology was similarly reinforced by the American Society of Clinical Oncology (ASCO) in its 2011 Blueprint [56]. The report acknowledged that cancer research is in a period of revolutionary change as more is learned about the molecular triggers that cause abnormal growth and proliferation from normal cells. Clinicians' abilities to choose therapies that have been carefully engineered to target these molecular triggers will only be enabled if researchers follow a new model of accelerated therapeutic development, enabled by an electronic health information infrastructure, and catalyzed by new "big data" analytics. The "network effect," of channeling parallel discovery in a coordinated way through distributed computer networks, has begun to accelerate discovery in astrophysics, oceanography, and proteomics [57]. Its potential for accelerating discovery in cancer research is equally promising, and will drive a new era of precision medicine [22,58].

The collective objective from all of these emerging efforts is to create a self-calibrating evidence base, based on data and not conjecture, for improving the quality of cancer care in all of its facets. Of course, the full promise of a learning health care system will not be realized until standards are set in place to guide interoperability and to harmonize data inputs [58]. The ONC has been investing heavily in efforts to achieve interoperability of data across health care systems since its inception. Even before instantiating its meaningful use incentive program, the ONC announced its multimillion dollar Strategic Health IT Advanced Research Projects (SHARP) program to conduct some of the essential research needed during a period of anticipated scale-up. Foci of the program included grants aimed at securing privacy and confidentiality of personal health information, creating patient centered decision support technologies, advancing designs to achieve information exchange, and developing strategies for utilizing data stored in EHRs for improving the overall quality of health care. Confronted with the persistent challenges of full interoperability well within meaningful use implementation, the US Department of Health and Human Services Secretary announced a $28 million investment in grants to boost interoperability efforts further during the ONC's annual meeting on February 3, 2015. At around the same time, the ONC released its draft interoperability roadmap for public comment.

Though the pragmatic reality of a fully interoperable data system may not have been realized at the time in which we are compiling this book, we have oriented our view toward the goal of achieving the benefits of a learning health care system in cancer through the concerted efforts of all who read these chapters.

I.2.5 Speeding Up Processes in Translational Medicine

The "network effect," enabled by an interconnected lattice of HIT, should not only be instrumental in accelerating basic discoveries; it should also play a role in speeding up the translational process by which discoveries are turned into effective treatments. The oft-cited statistic of taking 17 years, on average, to move the discovery of a new therapeutic into practice following industrial age traditions [59,60] will be untenable in an era of precision medicine in which new, molecularly oriented therapies are being introduced in rapid succession across a wide array of newly discovered, and increasingly localized, targets. New strategies are needed, which has become the raison d'être for private sector companies such as PatientsLikeMe and the Smart Patients networks. Both companies are striving to use the accelerative effects of a massively connected "patient powered research network" to create a platform for citizen engagement in biomedical science.

Examples of these nontraditional, innovative applications in oncology informatics are included in the last section of this book. The purpose is to suggest new ways of thinking and to stimulate further innovation in technologies that may represent creative disruptions on standard practices. In our estimation, the companies represent some of the cutting edge of disruptive technologies in medicine and oncology; they may represent to biomedical research what the ride-sharing company "Uber" represented to the transportation industry. The PatientsLikeMe network operates by allowing patients with similar diagnoses to compare experiences, and share data on the course of their treatments. Pharmaceutical companies are explicitly invited—with the acquiescence and support of patients—to mine these data to gain invaluable surveillance on potential side effects and to generate knowledge on the effectiveness of therapeutic agents across different patient types and populations. The Smart Patients network grew out of early observations that cancer patients were adept at finding each other online, and through participative venues such as the Association of Cancer Online Resources, contributed greatly to each other's knowledge on treatment options and expected course. The Smart Patients network is striving to facilitate more efficient connections between patients and clinical trials. It is capitalizing on patients' desires to give back to the scientific enterprise; in essence, to give more than charitable contributions at the grocery store but to become directly engaged in supporting the scientific enterprise. Patients, in turn, benefit from the "wisdom of the crowds" to find the best fit for themselves.

This approach, of using distributed networks to engage lay citizens who are nevertheless dedicated to the principles of the scientific enterprise and want to help scientists solve problems of personal relevance, has been referred to as "citizen science" by the National Science Foundation. The FDA adopted a version of this type of platform through its mini-sentinel program. The mini-sentinel program uses a platform of distributed networks to monitor the safety of FDA-regulated medical products. The Patient-Centered Outcomes Research Institute (PCORI) recognized that patient participation would be integral to their mission in comparatively evaluating the effectiveness of similarly situated treatments in terms of compatibility with patient values. The National Patient-Centered Clinical Research Network (PCORnet), established by the institute, was built to serve as the platform through which multiple cohorts of *patient powered research networks* could volunteer to reduce costs and improve quality in health care delivery [61,62].

Also on the quality improvement front, the ASCO-funded Institute for Quality has introduced the Cancer Learning Intelligence Network for Quality (CancerLinQ) as a cutting-edge HIT platform aimed at revolutionizing how oncologists care for people with cancer [63]. The system takes advantage of nationally recognized quality metrics in cancer care delivery, and then compiles those data for feedback to providers, hospitals, and health care systems. The objective is to introduce a self-regulating culture of quality in cancer care using (close to) real-time dashboards for immediate feedback on the effectiveness of treatment protocols, policy, and systems. At a much broader level, the NCI's Surveillance Epidemiology and End Results (SEER) program has been tasked with the responsibility of monitoring the overall effectiveness of cancer control efforts in the general population. The program has been exploiting the use of clinical informatics systems to expedite the compilation of electronic pathology reports through cancer registries. Representatives from both the ASCO CancerLinQ and SEER programs offer their respective visions as part of this volume.

I.2.6 Promoting Accessible, Affordable Cancer Care

The market forces driving up the costs associated with the delivery of aggressive cancer care, especially near end-of-life, are substantial; while the unequal burdens of cancer are socially alarming. Much of this unequal and expanding financial burden of cancer can be traced back to a fragmented system of care that is unequal in its application of evidence-based medicine, explained the ACS Chief Medical Officer, Otis Brawley, and his coauthor Paul Goldberg, editor of the Cancer Letter, in their book *How We Do Harm* [64]. At the beginning of the book, Brawley draws a comparison between two patients. One patient, low in socioeconomic status and abandoned by the prevention system, walked into a clinic with a late stage breast cancer so severe that it had resulted in a naturally occurring, automastectomy—the breast had detached. Metastases had been so extensive that it was not long before she passed away.

In comparison, Brawley related his experience with another patient who had been professionally successful and had the money to pursue the best care possible. This patient detected a lump in her breast early enough in the process that she could be proactive in doing something about it. She went to a well-respected oncologist and showing full trust in the medical system accepted an aggressive course of chemotherapy followed by a bone-marrow transplant and adjuvant postsurgical therapy. The side effects from this aggressive course were much more serious than she anticipated or that her care team had predicted. She was in and out of care routinely over the course of several years for severe nausea, vomiting, diarrhea, dehydration, continued low platelet counts, and anemia. Nine years after her bone marrow transplant, the patient was newly diagnosed with an adenocarcinoma. At that time, though, she received a letter from her insurance company explaining that she had exceeded her lifetime maximum for health insurance

and was now uninsurable. Left without many financial options, she too succumbed to her cancer and eventually passed away.

Both of these contrasting cases speak to the variability of inconsistent quality in care. In the first case, a more reliable investment in preventive services aided by the failsafe tracking systems of a patient-centered medical system would likely have prevented the fatal, late-stage breast cancer through early detection. In the second case, an independent physician and treating hospital adopted a course of treatment that has since been discredited by evidence as undesirable for standard of care. This is why it is imperative, reiterated health economist David Cutler cited earlier in this chapter, to address the issue of rising health care costs by reengineering the health care system to deliver higher quality care. In cancer, high quality care means beginning with evidence-based prevention and screening strategies, adhering equitably across all populations to accepted recommendations from the US Preventive Services Task Force. It continues by creating a coordinated, patient-centered, delivery platform for evidence-based treatment throughout care, and follows with an accessible and clear plan for survivorship. At end of life, it also means creating an environment that will protect patient values, ameliorate pain, and allow for providers and patients to "choose wisely" in order to improve care while eliminating unnecessary tests and procedures. All of these phases along the cancer care continuum are treated in-depth in the second section of the book.

Innovation in HIT may also play a role in reducing costs and driving accessibility of care. In 2014, the President's Cancer Panel—a presidentially appointed body of advisors who are asked to provide routine assessments related to the state of the "national cancer program"—announced its intention to produce a report on the topic of "Connected Health." The concept of connected health as used by the Panel is an umbrella term for using technologies to enable remote delivery of medical services under the traditional rubric of "telemedicine"; remote access to tools for healthy living as embodied under the rubric of "telehealth"; along with a rapidly developing use of wireless sensors and smartphones to provide ubiquitous access to the public for distributed care under the more recently introduced rubric of "mHealth." Several policy makers and health care administrators have argued that as we age connected health technologies will be needed to deal with the expected strains on the medical system as well as changes brought about through insurance reform.

Used effectively, connected health technologies can help keep health care costs down for both patients and physicians by allowing virtual consultations to replace more expensive face-to-face visits [43,65]. Just as EMRs can prompt physicians, these technologies can also be used to prompt patients; set up appointments for screening; or serve as a motivational aid for diet, exercise, smoking cessation, and medication adherence. The "Aging in Place" movement, in which communication and information technologies can be used to extend the time that seniors spend in their own homes to reduce assisted nursing home costs while preserving autonomy, is another manifestation of how these connected health technologies can be utilized to extend services beyond the clinical environment. Internationally, the National Health Service in the United Kingdom has made a concerted effort to reduce health care costs by equipping citizens and patients with the tools they need to be more proactive in their own health and subsequent care. Doing so, authorities within the service have argued, will be the only way the United Kingdom will be able to protect the health of its own aging citizenry while protecting its financial reserves [43].

Taken together, EHRs and connected health extenders will only work if they reinforce the goals of improving quality consistently and equitably throughout the US population. This means paying close attention to the ways in which the science of oncology informatics can be brought to bear on the right questions in oncology to make a sustained difference. Throughout the book, we have carefully selected authors who can successfully place the extraordinary promise of these technologies within the rigorous boundaries of science and evidence.

I.3 ORGANIZATION OF THE BOOK

Undoubtedly, there is much at stake in addressing the pending crises in cancer care preemptively as identified repeatedly by IOM and ASCO. Fortunately, investments in information infrastructure incented by Congress through the HITECH Act have begun to accelerate the adoption of EHRs and other aspects of HIT throughout the oncology sector. Navigating the disruptive forces that are inevitable within any sector encountering a massive paradigm shift in the way it conducts its core business; however, will require some insightful planning. The history of informatics projects has been littered with interventions that fail to scale-up, or that work under controlled conditions but create unexpected damage once they are incorporated into the larger organizational environment. Sometimes this happens from asking the wrong questions for technology to solve; for example, seeking to replace human capabilities rather than augmenting them [66–68]. Other times it happens from not taking into account the interdisciplinary expertise needed to ensure that interventions adhere to evidence-based practice in medicine, computer science, communication science, behavioral science, and cognitive research. Failure to take into account the interdisciplinary nature of these interventions has resulted in systems that have been perceived as being unusable, costly, inefficient, and disruptive.

Nevertheless, moving forward thoughtfully and with evidence at this crucial time is essential. Failure to act is not an option. Now is the time when standards of care and best practices will begin to settle out into a template for hospitals and private practices. If the designs are inferior, they will, at the very least, fail to deliver on their promise to address the predicted demands on an already strained health care system; at the very most, they may do incalculable damage to fragile systems by driving up costs and disrupting safe workflows, essentially violating the first edict of the Hippocratic Oath to "do no harm." Reports have already been coming in during the initial phases of meaningful use implementation decrying unanticipated expenses and in some cases being responsible for systemic harm. We as editors and authors feel the pressure to "get it right" in oncology, so that our collective efforts can serve to benefit, and not harm, the individuals whose cancers we can prevent as well as the patients and their families whose lives we can touch with the best care possible.

The good news is that the knowledge base is beginning to emerge across all facets of cancer care and research that can begin to guide our implementations in more thoughtful, innovative, and evidence-based ways. In this book, we have assembled a cadre of interdisciplinary experts whose knowledge and experience make them the best minds to consult as we collectively seek to leverage HIT to build a better delivery system in cancer. We have worked closely with these experts to ensure that their contributions are interconnected and complementary. We have also asked them to focus on a broad conceptual and process level, rather than tout the features of a particular, ephemeral, technology. In the technology space, individual products and features come and go rapidly. In compiling this book, we are looking to highlight the generalizable principles supported by a mounting knowledge base; we are looking for the best science and the best medicine. To provide coverage of the appropriate waterfront in oncological care, we have selected authors' contributions to fit within one of four major sections: (1) An Extraordinary Opportunity, (2) Support across the Continuum, (3) Science of Oncology Informatics, and (4) Accelerating Progress.

I.3.1 An Extraordinary Opportunity

Everyone here has the sense that right now is one of those moments when we are influencing the future. This is one of the many inspirational quotes uttered by Steve Jobs when speaking about the team that created the Macintosh computer. He was not only a visionary and insanely successful entrepreneur but also a philosopher for the digital age. As reflected in his words, we too believe we have assembled an extraordinary group of authors for this book who are not only experts in their respective disciplines but who collectively believe that this time is one of *those moments we are influencing the future*. This first section of the book, *An Extraordinary Opportunity*, highlights the unique moment in time for informatics to dramatically address the crisis in cancer care we face today and to alter the course ahead for the better. The authors of the chapters for this opening section represent a cross-section of disciplines including oncology informatics, primary care, computer and data science, nursing informatics, and communication science. These first five chapters lay the ground work and a solid foundation for subsequent chapters of the book.

In Chapter 1, "Creating a Learning Health Care System in Oncology," Richard Schilsky and Robert Miller describe how the field of oncology presents a prime opportunity to develop and deploy rapid learning health care systems that effectively use real-world, clinical data. They begin with a discussion of the complexity of contemporary cancer care and the limitations of the traditional approach to learning in cancer medicine. Societal pressures to control the cost of cancer care, the variety of treatment options, and the diversity of the cancer population all combine to drive the pursuit of a more cost-effective, equitable, and sustainable learning health system. To achieve the IOM's vision for delivering high quality cancer care will require that a learning HIT system be developed that enables real-time analysis of data from cancer patients in a variety of care settings. As leaders in the field of medical oncology, they describe the goals and potential community benefits of CancerLinQ, an example of an oncology rapid-learning system being developed and implemented by ASCO.

Chapter 2, "Reducing Cancer Disparities Through Community Engagement: The Promise of Informatics" is written by April Oh and coauthors Sylvia Chou, Devlon Jackson, Samuel Cykert, Nora Jones, Jennifer Schaal, and Euginia Eng and focuses on the potential for informatics approaches to reduce disparities and promote equity and engagement through community involvement. Here the authors describe how public health informatics can enable participatory health communication and knowledge acquisition and meet the needs of diverse communities. Applying general principles of community engagement to the design and implementation of public health informatics approaches can enhance usability, acceptability, and uptake. Community-based participatory research is highlighted as a means to not only engage individuals as "citizen scientists," but to also increase community trust and sustained engagement with the outcome of reducing disparities. Importantly, the authors focus on the issues of trust, privacy, ownership, and barriers to data sharing, especially for diverse populations. They note that sensitivity and awareness of historical experiences with discrimination and disempowerment by researchers and government agencies, among others, must be considered. *Syndemics*, the interactions between multiple diseases and outcomes and their relationships, is introduced as a potential mediator of disparities in cancer control. The authors conclude with the notion that a new day is dawning for engagement in public health, with informatics serving as a catalyst.

Warren Kibbe in Chapter 3, "Cancer Clinical Research: Enhancing Data Liquidity and Data Altruism" discusses how informatics technology may address current challenges and gaps in engaging and using data from research participants and patients participating in clinical trials. He describes how informatics may improve areas such as the streamlining of consent practices, increasing meaningful engagement with participants/patients, and measuring the broader context of participants'/patients' experiences across the care continuum. The benefits to science are enormous if patients can be empowered through unfettered data access and patients become true partners in the research enterprise.

In Chapter 4, "Engaging Patients in Primary and Specialty Care," Alex Krist, Donald Nease, Gary Kreps, Linda Overholser, and Marc McKenzie discuss the important role of informatics in enabling the process of engaging patients in the evolving landscape of primary and specialty care. According to the authors, patient-centered IT has multiple benefits and can: (1) enable collection of patient reported information; (2) organize and aggregate existing clinical information; (3) translate medical content into comprehensible language for patients; (4) provide individualized, evidence-based recommendations; and (5) stimulate patient activation. With respect to cancer care, this process can: (1) empower patients and clinicians with information; (2) engage patients in the medical decision-making process; (3) promote the adoption of healthy behaviors to prevent cancer; (4) encourage screening to identify cancer at an earlier stage when it is more amenable to treatment; (5) facilitate transitions in care; and (6) support treatment of cancer patients, and enhance survivorship planning. The authors discuss in some detail how HIT can enable optimal decisions in the context of cancer via evidence-based decision aids. They go on to highlight that the next generation of patient educational material and decision aids will focus on personalizing information to fully support precision medicine. Using existing evidence, modeling, and predictive analytics, generic information can be transformed to present personalized risks and benefits. This will require careful integration of decision aids with clinical information, as well as ensuring that models and analytics accurately portray an individual's risks.

In Chapter 5, "Coordination at the Point of Need," Katherine Kim, Janice Bell, Sarah Reed, and Robin Whitney focus on the promise of informatics in supporting coordination of care at the point of need. They begin with a definition of "point of need" by explaining that health decisions are made and health actions are taken throughout a person's day, and across time. The point of care is an important weigh station in this process as it represents only one snapshot in time. Relevant and accurate information is needed during the critical times when health decisions are being made throughout the process, and coordination of actions among all stakeholders is needed during those times. The points of transition are particularly important, for example, between sites and providers, during changes in treatment regimen, and across phases such as from active treatment to survivorship. The authors expand the focus to include family and caregiver perspectives along with the patient. As an example, in hospice for cancer care the "patient" is considered to be the whole "family" surrounding the individual with illness. They introduce the "Community-Wide Care Coordination" model and compare and contrast it with other approaches such as care and disease management. The necessity for creating a broader workforce of caregivers is articulated and they site examples including the association of Oncology Nurse Navigators. The role and need for informatics in the integrated Community-Wide Care Coordination framework is delineated for each aspect including within and across care teams, across the community, longitudinally, and person-centered. Case examples are provided to illustrate diverse perspectives of those involved in care and for diverse populations. The authors conclude with a discussion of the role of oncology informatics in providing support and solutions for Community-Wide Care Coordination efforts.

I.3.2 Support Across the Continuum

The cancer care continuum begins with primary prevention (preventing cancer from occurring in the first place), then moves to secondary prevention (identifying cancer at its earliest stages so that treatment may be delivered with curative intent), then to tertiary prevention (treatment to prevent mortality), and concludes with end-of-life care [69]. Traditionally, the continuum has been represented in a linear fashion, suggesting that individuals enter their experience of the continuum at primary prevention, proceed through secondary prevention if they are adherent to recommended guidelines for cancer screening for their age and gender, and, if they become one of the 50% of individuals diagnosed with cancer in his or her lifetime [2], go on to experience treatment and possibly end-of-life care depending on the success of curative intervention.

More recently this continuum has been revisited in a way that is reflected in the chapters that comprise Part II of this book. Two enhancements to the continuum have been suggested within the past decade [70]. First, "survivorship"—a phase that encompasses life after the completion of primary treatment but during which most individuals diagnosed with cancer continue to experience significant cancer-related physical, emotional, and practical concerns [71–73]—is given a dedicated place within the cancer continuum. Second, the continuum has been reconceived to have a cyclical, rather than a linear, organization [70]. In this way, the cancer continuum now reflects the fact that a large and growing percentage of people diagnosed with cancer will go on to live the balance of their lives for a duration that makes their reentry into the primary and secondary prevention components of the continuum not only relevant, but critical, due to their increased risks of cancer (either recurrence or new primary diagnosis) given their history of the disease [21].

Chapter 6, "Prevention, Information Technology, and Cancer" addresses primary prevention. Glen Morgan and Michael Fiore tackle the important questions around how many cancer diagnoses and deaths could be avoided if robust informatics-enhanced primary prevention efforts were to become a widely adopted reality. Morgan and Fiore cover the full spectrum of cancer risk factors and primary preventions strategies, including relatively recent strategies such as vaccinations for infectious agents known to cause certain types of cancer. They use tobacco as an exemplar to detail conceptual frameworks for and empirical evidence from both system- and individual-level informatics-based interventions to improve primary prevention of cancer and reduce cancer incidence and mortality at a population level.

Chapter 7, "Early Detection in the Age of Information Technology" covers the area of early detection in an age of IT, and is contributed by Ekland Abdiwahab, Stephen Taplin, Gloria Coronado, Heather Dacus, Melissa Leypoldt, and Celette Skinner. These authors segment early detection into two critical functions: screening tests to identify the presence of cancer; and health care intervention to address symptoms caused early in the onset of cancer to minimize morbidity and reduce mortality from the disease. Both of these functions, the authors argue, involve complex processes of care. Ultimately, the simplification of these processes will be instrumental to their success, and in this chapter, the authors outline how informatics applications are being and can be used to simplify processes in secondary prevention to optimize the impact of early detection. Covering all approved screening modalities, including the most recently approved screening test by the US Preventive Services Task Force—lung cancer screening—this chapter will give illustrative examples of and future visioning for how informatics can positively impact all stakeholders involved in secondary prevention of cancer.

Chapter 8, "Informatics Support Across the Cancer Continuum: Treatment" covers the area of treatment and is authored by Bradford Hirsch and Amy Abernethy. Hirsch and Abernethy detail the essential role of informatics in providing an actionable foundation for the delivery of data-driven cancer care. Using the treatment of kidney cancer as a case study, the Treatment chapter discusses how a robust informatics infrastructure can support a learning cancer care system to allow for data from clinical trials, precision medicine initiatives, and studies of best practices to be seamlessly integrated into clinical decision tools used by oncologists on the front lines providing care to patients. Additionally, the authors demonstrate how that same informatics infrastructure can be leveraged to elevate the voice of the patient toward aligning care delivery with patient behavior, preferences, needs, and values.

Chapter 9, "Survivorship," written by Ellen Beckjord, Gisberta van Londen, and Ruth Rechis, covers the area of informatics for cancer survivors. The authors begin by describing the needs and characteristics of the 14 million cancer survivors alive in the United States today, and highlight predictions of how that will continue to rise as treatments improve. They discuss how informatics at the system, provider, and individual levels is and will continue to be instrumental to bringing about the enhancements in survivorship care planning that are desperately needed to provide optimal care to this "booming population" [21,74,75]. The Survivorship chapter will consider what is known about how cancer survivors currently use informatics in the context of managing their health, but will also suggest a roadmap for pushing the field further ahead to a state where technology is used in multiple ways to positively affect people at this critical point in the cancer continuum.

In Chapter 10, "Advanced Cancer: Palliative, End of Life, and Bereavement Care," Lori DuBenske, Deborah Mayer, and David Gustafson address the role of informatics in palliative and end-of-life care and bereavement. With the recognition that cancer is truly a disease that affects the entire family, this chapter will describe how informatics can be used to keep multiple lines of communication open and functional over what is often an enormously difficult time—when curative treatment transitions to symptom management and difficult, though critical, conversations must be held to address how to balance quantity and quality of life.

I.3.3 The Science of Oncology Informatics

The American Medical Informatics Association (AMIA) described the "science of informatics" [76] as being made up of an interdisciplinary mix of contributions from medicine, the information sciences, cognitive research, computer science, organizational theory, and behavioral medicine, as well as contributions from allied health fields. Numerous volumes have been written on the many manifestations of IT in medicine, from overarching texts on the theory and applications of biomedical informatics [77], to the clinical trials emphasis of cancer informatics [78], to the patient-centered focus of consumer informatics [79], and to the population focus of public health informatics [80]. Each has brought together the optimal mix of scientific perspectives to cover the topic area in a way that is compatible with this book's objective and historical context. In addition, we have invited authors to describe the science needed to augment capacity in cancer care at a time of increasing precision, swelling demand, rising complexity, growing sense of patient engagement, and soaring costs. These are the challenges set forth by the IOM's Cancer Policy Forum [1,4,58] as well as evaluation reports by federal [35,36] and nongovernmental organizations [32,56].

In Chapter 11, "Data Visualization Tools for Investigating Health Services Utilization Among Cancer Patients," authors Eberechukwu Onukwugha, Catherine Plaisant, and Ben Shneiderman combine a scientific focus taken from medical decision-making with a computer science focus on human system integration to explore how cutting edge techniques in data visualization can improve the timely application of evidence within a learning oncology system. We anticipate that the science of data visualization will become more valuable as medical decision making becomes more reliant on data and, following the tenets of meaningful use, anticipate that those data streams will become useful across levels of decision-making from individual patient diagnosis and treatment, to office-wide management of patient medical needs, to hospital-based interventions to improve population health, and even to regionally-based depictions of data for policy refinement. The authors begin by presenting a review of what data visualization tools are currently available, and how they have already been applied in oncology. They then turn their attention to the implications for research and practice that are implied by the necessary utilization of data-intensive decision tools, but then complete their chapter with a valuable set of case studies to illustrate the potential these tools hold for improving the effectiveness and usability of data visualization.

In Chapter 12, "Oncology Informatics: Behavioral and Psychological Sciences," David Ahern, Ilana Braun, Mary Cooley, and Timothy Bickmore describe how a robust knowledge base from the behavioral sciences can be leveraged to advance oncology informatics and to improve cancer control efforts. Their writings come at a time when the economic incentives of value-based medicine have begun to favor the science of behavior and behavior change as a way of reducing the costs of late stage disease through effective prevention, and at a time when the professional associations have emphasized the importance of identifying and reducing patients' distress across the course of treatment and survivorship. The authors relate case examples taken directly from clinical care to illustrate how fundamental behavioral and psychological constructs can be utilized to inform the design and evaluation of patient-centered support systems. Consistent with exhortations from the Office of the National Coordinator and from Congressional subcommittee hearings, the authors describe how the future of effective and usable informatics systems will rely heavily on the findings from behavioral science to improve scalability and effectiveness.

Chapter 13, "Communication Science: Connecting Systems for Health," authored by Bradford Hesse, Neeraj Arora, and William Klein, turns its focus on the role of communications within the evolving ecosystem of oncology informatics systems. The authors cite data from the Joint Commission on Accreditation, Health Care, and Certification suggesting to acknowledge that communication breakdowns account for up to 63% of all reported mishaps as recorded in their Sentinel database. Fortunately, an evolution in advanced communication technologies along with a systems level view of communication flow and error has enabled other industries to make great strides in error-proofing their systems. Innovations relevant to oncology include: (1) management systems to ensure that no one is left out of the loop on essential communications; (2) secure messaging systems to promote timely responses to patients' questions; (3) patient-portals to serve as a trusted, one-stop-shop for care needs; (4) multiuser notes to keep all parties on the "same page" for collaborative care; (5) wireless sensors and medication adherence tools to support remote care; (6) self-management and personal coaching tools; and (7) interactive video and telephone conferencing. Each of these innovations is explored within the context of building an oncology system that is safe, effective, patient-centered, timely, efficient, and equitable.

In Chapter 14, "Cancer Surveillance Informatics," Lynn Penberthy, Deborah Winn, and Susan Scott turn their attention to the role of oncology informatics in supporting a more responsive surveillance system for cancer. Many researchers, decision makers, and policy makers depend on the yearly announcement that surveillance data will be made publically available to the cancer community from the SEER data program. Information demands on those data will be increasing as we learn more about the relevance of molecular subtypes for tracking and treating under an evolution of precision medicine principles. Penberthy, Winn, and Scott describe how advances in automated processing techniques can improve the breadth and timeliness of cancer registry data as extracted from the EHR. They also describe how advanced techniques in natural language processing and the use of newly formed, interoperable linkages between data sources can be used to expand the breadth as well as the depth of cancer surveillance.

Chapter 15, "Extended Vision for Oncology: A Perceptual Science Perspective on Data Visualization and Medical Imaging" completes this section with a chapter by Horowitz and Rensink on the role of perceptual science for improving data visualization and medical imaging. In many respects this final chapter serves as a book-end to the Onukwugha, Plaisant, and Shneiderman chapter at the beginning of the section. The difference is that this chapter builds from the perspective of cognitive and perceptual science to give an evidentiary underpinning to the ways in which individual users perceive and apprehend the types of information portrayed to them across a variety of the user interfaces comprising a typical oncology system. The chapter should be especially instructive for developers, as they seek to optimize the visual look-and-feel of devices and interfaces; for clinical staff who are reliant on biomedical imaging for any aspect of patient care; for administrators who seek to prevent visually conveyed errors throughout their health system; and for researchers wishing to understand basic perceptual science as it intersects with medical decision-making.

I.3.4 Accelerating Progress

In January 2013, the PCAST released a follow-up report in its ongoing summary of opportunities under the rubric of *Designing a Digital Future*. The report began with an energizing summary declaring that: "the impact of networking and information technology (NIT) is stunning. Virtually every human endeavor is affected as advances in NIT enable or improve domains such as scientific discovery, human health, education, the environment, national security, transportation, manufacturing, energy, governance, and entertainment" [81]. We recognize that the pace of disruptive innovation in medicine is rapidly altering our conceptualizations of what can be done in the biomedical sciences to accelerate discovery and conquer disease [82]. In this last section, we have invited some of the thought leaders who are at the cutting edge of the digital revolution to describe their vision for how innovations in oncology informatics can accelerate progress against cancer.

Chapter 16, "Crowdsourcing Advancements in Health Care Research: Applications for Cancer Treatment Discoveries," written by Emil Chiazzu, Gabrial Eichler, and Paul Wicks, is written from the perspective of biomedical scientists working within the context of one of the more cutting-edge and revolutionary platforms for crowdsourcing medical discovery with the help of patients: PatientsLikeMe. Like Wikipedia, PatientsLikeMe represents an experiment in what the National Science Foundation has referred to as technology-mediated social participation [83]. Patients who join the platform are encouraged to share data related to the progression of their conditions, the prevalence of side-effects from treatments, and even their feelings and thoughts for the benefit of other patients struggling with the same disease and, unreservedly, for the benefit of science and the faster pursuit of cures. In essence, the authors describe a change in ethos from patients as subjects of research, to patients as motivated collaborators in the research enterprise. The new ethos is firmly instantiated within the patient-driven research networks supported by the Patient-Centered Outcomes Research Network (PCORNET) and is embedded within the DNA of the National Institute of Health's precision medicine initiatives.

Roni Zeiger and Gilles Frydman continue the theme of accelerating research through active patient participation in clinical research in Chapter 17, "Patient-Centered Approaches to Improving Clinical Trials for Cancer." Citing findings from extant research, the two authors point out that barriers to clinical trial recruitment stem from unfounded fears related to the randomization process in clinical trials, a sense of distrust of the research process, the perceived complexity of the protocol, a simple lack of awareness, or a fear of jeopardizing the trusting relationship patients have with their oncologists. Internet communities, though, have been very good at addressing these types of concerns by offering a mechanism for correcting misperceptions and by offering social support for overcoming initial fears and misgivings. The two authors then go on to describe how community-based sites such as their SmartPatients platform can be utilized to remove barriers and to drive greater participation in clinical trials.

In Chapter 18, "A New Era of Clinical Research Methods in a Data-Rich Environment," William Riley picks up the thread of accelerated research by describing the new research methods and analytic techniques available in an informatics-rich environment to move from Big Data to Knowledge at a faster pace. He begins his chapter by explaining how many of the traditional research designs we use today were actually forged in data-poor environments. As a result, historical methods placed a big emphasis on a linear process of moving from theory, to prospective research designs based on sampling and painstaking protocol for measurement, and finally to statistical analysis designed to compensate for the sampling limitations imposed by the research design. Informatics technologies are creating a new era in which data are plentiful, are collected routinely as part of care, are collected passively though automated collection systems, and can be retained and shared for further analysis. Riley then chronicles for the reader a documented list of emerging new research designs and analytic methods that are being developed within data-rich environments to accelerate discovery. Methods include new approaches in epidemiology that will do a better job in creating longitudinal views of population trends; new ways of conducting clinical trials to cull data from single cases and from rapid learning systems; and new computational processes for turning data back into rapid revisions of theory.

The section concludes in Chapter 19, "Creating a Health Information Technology Infrastructure to Support Comparative Effectiveness Research in Cancer" with illustrations brought forward through a unique partnership between MD Anderson Cancer Center and the University of California at San Diego's Supercomputer Center to envision what the oncology data environment of tomorrow might look like. In this final chapter, Susan Peterson and Kevin Patrick offer a vision for big data in oncology that is inclusive of signals from wireless sensors, mobile devices, EHR data, and even data from geophysical mapping arrays. Their project is using a cloud-based structure to integrate data from these multiple structures, and then to provide those data back to researchers for an entirely new view on disease processes. Enriched by investments in Genome-Wide Association Studies, their Cyberinfrastructure for Comparative Effectiveness Research [84] extends Big Data techniques beyond the genome to evaluate influences from the "exposome" [85].

I.4 CONCLUSION

When a field of study is moving quickly, wonderful things can happen; but much like cancer itself—which arises from the unbridled proliferation of cells—there are risks that appear when there is a lack of an organizing framework or vision to guide something that is growing quickly. Without a guiding vision, a fast-paced field can result in confusion and in a proliferation of products so disparate and disconnected that the opportunity for making real progress is lost. Informatics in oncology is moving at an unparalleled pace, and the opportunities to capitalize upon this pace to make exponential progress in reducing pain and suffering from cancer are real. Without a guiding framework, the benefits of seizing these opportunities at a time when evidence-based designs are most needed will be lost.

We are creating this book to help oncology informatics reach its full potential in achieving a preemptive remedy to the "cancer care crisis" as identified by the IOM. But more importantly, we are creating this book with the primary purpose of preventing the disease when at all possible, and to improve the lives of all those people who would otherwise be affected by cancer when not.

Again, this book is not intended to showcase the "latest and greatest" informatics applications from the marketplace or the laboratories, practices, or businesses of the authors contributing chapters to this book. We know that a book that focuses on specific products will be outdated before it is read by anyone. But these authors, having been on the frontlines of the field making some of the most important contributions to date, are in the best position to describe the foundational elements of what "oncology informatics" means to them in a way that will guide continued development toward a robust, high-impact, and innovative area of inquiry.

LIST OF ACRONYMS AND ABBREVIATIONS

ACS American Cancer Society
ACA Affordable Care Act
AMIA The American Medical Informatics Association
CMS Centers for Medicare & Medicaid Services
EHR Electronic Health Record
EMR Electronic Medical Record
FDA US Food and Drug Administration
HINTS Health Information National Trends Survey
HIT Health information technology
HITECH Health Information Technology for Economic and Clinical Health Act of 2009
IOM Institute of Medicine
NCDs Noncommunicable diseases
NCI National Cancer Institute
NIH National Institutes of Health
NRC National Research Council
ONC The Office of the National Coordinator for Health Information Technology
PCAST President's Council of Advisors on Science and Technology
SHARP Strategic Health IT Advanced Research Projects
SEER Surveillance Epidemiology and End Results System
WHO World Health Organization

References

[1] Levit LA, Levit E, Nass SJ, Ganz P, Institute of Medicine (U.S.). Committee on improving the quality of cancer care: addressing the challenges of an aging population. Delivering high-quality cancer care: charting a new course for a system in crisis. Washington, DC: National Academies Press; 2013. xxviii, 384 pp.

[2] American Cancer Society Cancer facts & figures 2014. Atlanta, GA: American Cancer Society; 2014.

[3] Patlak M, Balogh E, Nass SJ, National Cancer Policy Forum (U.S.) National Coalition for Cancer Survivorship (U.S.) Institute of Medicine (U.S.). Patient-centered cancer treatment planning: improving the quality of oncology care: workshop summary. Washington, DC: National Academies Press; 2011. xii, 66 pp.

[4] Balogh E, Patlak M, Nass SJ, National Cancer Policy Forum (U.S.), Institute of Medicine (U.S.). Board on health care services. delivering affordable cancer care in the 21st century: workshop summary. Washington, DC: National Academies Press; 2013. xiv, 80 pp.

[5] Taplin SH, Rodgers AB. Toward improving the quality of cancer care: addressing the interfaces of primary and oncology-related subspecialty care. J Natl Cancer Inst Monogr 2010;2010(40):3–10.

[6] Tinetti ME, Fried TR, Boyd CM. Designing health care for the most common chronic condition—multimorbidity. JAMA 2012;307(23):2493–4.

[7] Hesse BW, Hanna C, Massett HA, Hesse NK. Outside the box: will information technology be a viable intervention to improve the quality of cancer care? J Natl Cancer Inst Monogr 2010;2010(40):81–9.

[8] Kohn LT, Corrigan J, Donaldson MS. To err is human: building a safer health system. Washington, DC: National Academy Press; 2000. xxi, 287 pp.

[9] Fishman TC. Shock of gray: the aging of the world's population and how it pits young against old, child against parent, worker against boss, company against rival, and nation against nation, 1st Scribner hardcover ed. New York, NY: Scribner; 2010. 401 pp.

[10] World Health Organization Global health and aging. Washington, DC: National Institute on Aging; 2011. Contract No.: NIH Publication no. 11-7737.

[11] World Health Organization Global status report on noncommunicable diseases 2010. Geneva: World Health Organization; 2010.

[12] Zerhouni E. Extracting knowledge from science: a conversation with Elias Zerhouni. Interview by Barbara J. Culliton. Health Aff (Millwood) 2006;25(3):w94–103.

[13] Collins FS. Exceptional opportunities in medical science: a view from the National Institutes of Health. JAMA 2015; 313(2):131–2.

[14] Collins FS, Varmus H. A new initiative on precision medicine. N Engl J Med 2015;372(9):793–5.

[15] Hoffman J. Awash in information, patients face a lonely, Uncertain Road. New York Times. 2005 August 14, 2005;Sect. Health.

[16] Sekeres MA. The punishing cost of cancer care. New York Times. 2014 December 11, 2014;Sect. Well.

[17] Karsh B-T. Clinical practice improvement and redesign: how change in workflow can be supported by clinical decision support. Rockville, MD: Agency for Healthcare Research and Quality; June 2009. Report No.

[18] Cayton H. The flat-pack patient? Creating health together. Patient Educ Couns 2006;62(3):288–90.

[19] Finkelstein J, Knight A, Marinopoulos S, Gibbons MC, Berger Z, Aboumatar H, et al. Enabling patient-centered care through health information technology. Rockville, MD: Johns Hopkins University Evidence-based Practice Center; 2007. Evidence Report/Technology Assessment No. 206.

[20] Hewitt ME, Ganz PA, Institute of Medicine (U.S.) American Society of Clinical Oncology (U.S.). From cancer patient to cancer survivor: lost in transition: an American Society of Clinical Oncology and Institute of Medicine Symposium. Washington, DC: National Academies Press; 2006. vi, 189 pp.

[21] Parry C, Kent EE, Mariotto AB, Alfano CM, Rowland JH. Cancer survivors: a booming population. Cancer Epidemiol Biomarkers Prev 2011;20(10):1996–2005.

[22] Nass SJ, Wizemann TM, National Cancer Policy Forum (U.S.). Informatics needs and challenges in cancer research: workshop summary. Washington, DC: National Academies Press; 2012. xvi, 129 pp.

[23] Olson S, Institute of Medicine (U.S.) Roundtable on Translating Genomic-Based Research for Health Institute of Medicine (U.S.) Board on Health Sciences Policy Integrating large-scale genomic information into clinical practice: workshop summary. Washington, DC: National Academies Press; 2012. xx, 92 pp.

[24] National Research Council (U.S.) Committee on a Framework for Developing a New Taxonomy of Disease Toward precision medicine: building a knowledge network for biomedical research and a new taxonomy of disease. Washington, DC: National Academies Press; 2011. xiii, 128 pp.

[25] Collins FS. Research agenda. Opportunities for research and NIH. Science 2010;327(5961):36–7.

[26] Sharp PA, Leshner AI. Meeting global challenges. Science 2014;343(6171):579.

[27] Van Den Bos J, Rustagi K, Gray T, Halford M, Ziemkiewicz E, Shreve J. The $17.1 billion problem: the annual cost of measurable medical errors. Health Aff (Millwood) 2011;30(4):596–603.

[28] Institute of Medicine (U.S.) Committee on Quality of Health Care in America Crossing the quality chasm: a new health system for the 21st century. Washington, DC: National Academy Press; 2001. xx, 337 pp.

[29] Reid PP, Compton WD, Grossman JH, Fanjiang G, National Academy of Engineering Institute of Medicine (U.S.). Building a better delivery system: a new engineering/health care partnership. Washington, DC: National Academies Press; 2005. xiv, 262 pp.

[30] Institute of Medicine. Health IT and patient safety: building safer systems for better care. Washington, DC: The National Academies Press; 2012.

[31] Cutler DM. The quality cure: how focusing on health care quality can save your life and lower spending too. Berkeley, CA: University of California Press; 2014. xviii, 214 pp.

[32] DesRoches CM, Painter MW, Jha AK. Health information technology in the United States: progress and challenges ahead. Princeton, NJ: Robert Wood Johnson Foundation; 2014.

[33] Blumenthal D, Tavenner M. The "meaningful use" regulation for electronic health records. N Engl J Med 2010;363(6):501–4.

[34] Buntin MB, Jain SH, Blumenthal D. Health information technology: laying the infrastructure for national health reform. Health Aff (Millwood) 2010;29(6):1214–9.

[35] President's Council of Advisors on Science and Technology. Better health care and lower costs: accelerating improvement through systems engineering. Washington, DC: The White House; 2014.

[36] President's Council of Advisors on Science and Technology. Realizing the full potential of health information technology to improve healthcare for Americans: the path forward. Washington, DC: Executive Office of the President of the United States; 2010.

[37] Stead WW, Lin HS, editors. Computational technology for effective health care: immediate steps and strategic directions. Washington, DC: National Academies Press; 2009.

[38] Kellermann AL, Jones SS. What it will take to achieve the as-yet-unfulfilled promises of health information technology. Health Aff (Millwood) 2013;32(1):63–8.

[39] Nelson DE, Kreps GL, Hesse BW, Croyle RT, Willis GB, Arora NK, et al. The Health Information National Trends Survey (HINTS): development, design, and dissemination. J Health Commun 2004;9(5):443–60.

[40] Finney Rutten LJ, Davis T, Beckjord EB, Blake K, Moser RP, Hesse BW. Picking up the pace: changes in method and frame for the health information national trends survey (2011–2014). J Health Commun 2012;17(7):979–89.

[41] Eysenbach G. What is e-health? J Med Internet Res 2001;3(2):E20.

[42] Hesse BW, Nelson DE, Kreps GL, Croyle RT, Arora NK, Rimer BK, et al. Trust and sources of health information: the impact of the Internet and its implications for health care providers: findings from the first Health Information National Trends Survey. Arch Intern Med 2005;165(22):2618–24.

[43] Kvedar J, Coye MJ, Everett W. Connected health: a review of technologies and strategies to improve patient care with telemedicine and telehealth. Health Aff (Millwood) 2014;33(2):194–9.

[44] Fox S, Rainie L. The web at 25 in the U.S. Washington, DC: Pew Research Center; 2014.

[45] Institute of Medicine. Patients charting the course: citizen engagement and the learning health system: workshop summary. Washington, DC: National Academies Press; 2011. xxv, 310 pp.

[46] Zuboff S, Maxmin J. The support economy: why corporations are failing individuals and the next episode of capitalism. New York, NY: Viking; 2002. xvii, 458 pp.

[47] Shneiderman B, Plaisant C. Designing the user interface: strategies for effective human-computer interaction, 5th ed. Boston, MA: Addison-Wesley; 2010. xviii, 606 pp.

[48] Finn NB, Bria WF. Digital communication in medical practice. London: Springer; 2009. xviii, 171 pp.

[49] Hesse BW, Moser RP, Rutten LJ. Surveys of physicians and electronic health information. N Engl J Med 2010;362(9):859–60.

[50] Clauser SB, Wagner EH, Aiello Bowles EJ, Tuzzio L, Greene SM. Improving modern cancer care through information technology. Am J Prev Med 2011;40(5 Suppl. 2):S198–207.

[51] Shaneyfelt TM. Building bridges to quality. JAMA 2001;286(20): 2600–1.

[52] Abernethy AP, Hesse BW. Information technology and evidence implementation. Transl Behav Med 2011;1(1):11–14.

[53] Cancer Center Directors Working Group. Accelerating successes against cancer. Washington, DC: U.S. Department of Health and Human Services; 2006.

[54] Hesse BW, Ahern DK, Woods SS. Nudging best practice: the HITECH act and behavioral medicine. Transl Behav Med 2011;1(1):175–81.

[55] Friedberg MW, Coltin KL, Safran DG, Dresser M, Zaslavsky AM, Schneider EC. Associations between structural capabilities of primary care practices and performance on selected quality measures. Ann Intern Med 2009;151(7):456–63.

[56] American Society of Clinical Oncology. Accelerating progress against cancer: ASCO's blueprint for transforming clinical and translational cancer research. Alexandria, VA: American Society of Clinical Oncology; 2011.

[57] Nielsen MA. Reinventing discovery: the new era of networked science. Princeton, NJ: Princeton University Press; 2012. 264 pp.

[58] Institute of Medicine. A foundation for evidence-driven practice: a rapid learning system for cancer care. Workshop summary. Washington, DC: The National Academies Press; 2010.

[59] Westfall JM, Mold J, Fagnan L. Practice-based research—"Blue Highways" on the NIH roadmap. JAMA 2007;297(4):403–6.

[60] Morris ZS, Wooding S, Grant J. The answer is 17 years, what is the question: understanding time lags in translational research. J R Soc Med 2011;104(12):510–20.

[61] Fleurence RL, Beal AC, Sheridan SE, Johnson LB, Selby JV. Patient-powered research networks aim to improve patient care and health research. Health Aff (Millwood) 2014;33(7): 1212–9.

[62] Fleurence RL, Curtis LH, Califf RM, Platt R, Selby JV, Brown JS. Launching PCORnet, a national patient-centered clinical research network. J Am Med Inform Assoc: JAMIA 2014;21(4):578–82.

[63] Schilsky RL, Michels DL, Kearbey AH, Yu PP, Hudis CA. Building a rapid learning health care system for oncology: the regulatory framework of CancerLinQ. J Clin Oncol 2014;32(22):2373–9.

[64] Brawley OW, Goldberg P. How we do harm: a doctor breaks ranks about being sick in America, 1st ed. New York, NY: St. Martin's Press; 2012. vi, 304 pp.

[65] Kvedar JC, Herzlinger R, Holt M, Sanders JH. Connected health as a lever for healthcare reform: dialogue with featured speakers from the 5th annual connected health symposium. Telemed J E Health 2009;15(4):312–9.

[66] Shneiderman B. Leonardo's laptop: human needs and the new computing technologies. Cambridge, MA: MIT Press; 2002. xi, 269 pp.

[67] Hesse BW, Shneiderman B. eHealth research from the user's perspective. Am J Prev Med 2007;32(5 Suppl):S97–S103.

[68] Zuboff S. In the age of the smart machine: the future of work and power. New York, NY: Basic Books; 1988. xix, 468 pp.

[69] Adami H, Hunter D, Trichopoulos D, editors. Textbook of cancer epidemiology. New York, NY: Oxford; 2002.

[70] Rowland JH, Bellizzi KM. Cancer survivors and survivorship research: a reflection on today's successes and tomorrow's challenges. Hematol Oncol Clin North Am 2008;22(2):181–200.

[71] Beckjord EB, Reynolds KA, van Londen GJ, Burns R, Singh R, Arvey SR, et al. Population-level trends in post-treatment cancer survivors' concerns and associated receipt of care: results from the 2006 and 2010 LIVESTRONG surveys. J Psychosoc Oncol 2014;32(2):125–51.

[72] Ganz PA. Survivorship: adult cancer survivors. Prim Care 2009;36(4):721–41.

[73] Rechis R, Reynolds KA, Beckjord EB, Nutt S, Burns RM, Schaefer JS. "I Learned to Live With It" is not good enough: challenges reported by post-treatment cancer survivors in the LIVESTRONG surveys. Austin, TX: LIVESTRONG; 2011.

[74] Forsythe LP, Parry C, Alfano CM, Kent EE, Leach CR, Haggstrom DA, et al. Use of survivorship care plans in the United States: associations with survivorship care. J Natl Cancer Inst 2013;105(20):1579–87.

[75] Parry C, Kent EE, Forsythe LP, Alfano CM, Rowland JH. Can't see the forest for the care plan: a call to revisit the context of care planning. J Clin Oncol 2013;31(21):2651–3.

[76] American Medical Informatics Association. The science of informatics 2015 [cited 2015 February 9, 2015]. Available from: <http://www.amia.org/about-amia/science-informatics>.

[77] Shortliffe EH, Cimino JJ. Biomedical informatics: computer applications in health care and biomedicine, 3rd ed. New York, NY: Springer; 2006. xxvi, 1037 pp.

[78] Silva JS. Cancer informatics: essential technologies for clinical trials. New York, NY: Springer; 2002. xxvi, 377 pp.

[79] Nelson R, Ball MJ. Consumer informatics: applications and strategies in cyber health care. New York, NY: Springer; 2004. xix, 166 pp.

[80] O'Carroll PW. Public health informatics and information systems. New York, NY: Springer; 2003. xxvii, 790 pp.

[81] President's Council of Advisors on Science and Technology. Designing a digital future: federally funded research and development in networking and information technology. Washington, DC: Executive Office of the President of the United States; 2013.

[82] Topol EJ. The creative destruction of medicine: how the digital revolution will create better health care, 1st pbk. ed. New York, NY: Basic Books; 2013. xi, 319 pp.

[83] Shneiderman B, Preece J, Pirolli P, Smith MA, Marchionini G, Lazar J. An open letter to Obama, in support of social participation. GCN: Technology, Tools and Tactics for Public Sector IT [Internet]. 2009. Available from: <http://gcn.com/Articles/2009/08/03/Commentary-Shneiderman-letter-to-Obama.aspx>.

[84] Patrick K, Wolszon L, Basen-Engquist KM, Demark-Wahnefried W, Prokhorov AV, Barrera S, et al. CYberinfrastructure for COmparative effectiveness REsearch (CYCORE): improving data from cancer clinical trials. Transl Behav Med 2011;1(1):83–8.

[85] Coughlin SS. Toward a road map for global -omics: a primer on -omic technologies. Am J Epidemiol 2014;180(12):1188–95.

PART I

AN EXTRAORDINARY OPPORTUNITY

CHAPTER

1

Creating a Learning Health Care System in Oncology

Richard L. Schilsky MD, FACP, FASCO and
Robert S. Miller MD, FACP, FASCO

CancerLinQ, American Society of Clinical Oncology, Alexandria, VA, United States

OUTLINE

1.1 The Challenges of Delivering Quality Cancer Care	4
1.1.1 Diversity of Cancer and the Cancer Patient Population	5
1.1.2 The Need for Multidisciplinary Cancer Care	5
1.1.3 The Complexity and Cost of Cancer Care Delivery	6
1.2 Overview of Traditional Learning in Cancer Medicine	7
1.2.1 Clinical Trials as the Foundation of Evidence-Based Medicine in Cancer	7
1.2.2 Limitations of Conventional Clinical Trials	8
1.3 The Interface of Quality, Value, and Learning	9
1.4 ASCO's Vision for a Rapid Learning System in Oncology: CancerLinQ	10
1.5 CancerLinQ Data Architecture	10
1.6 History and Current Status of CancerLinQ Implementation	12
1.6.1 Background and Prototype Development 2011–12	12
1.6.2 CancerLinQ Development 2013–15	12
1.6.3 CancerLinQ and SAP	13
1.7 CancerLinQ Solution Operating Characteristics	13
1.7.1 Data Ingestion	13
1.7.2 CancerLinQ Portal	14
1.7.3 User Types	14
1.7.4 Quality Benchmarking	14
1.7.5 Clinical Decision Support	14
1.7.6 Other Secondary Uses of Deidentified and/or Limited Data Sets	16
1.8 Regulatory Underpinnings of CancerLinQ	17
1.8.1 Data Governance Guiding Principles and Policies	18
1.9 Summary and Conclusions	19
List of Acronyms and Abbreviations	19
Acknowledgments	19
References	19

B. Hesse, D. Ahern & E. Beckjord: Oncology Informatics.
DOI: http://dx.doi.org/10.1016/B978-0-12-802115-6.00001-X

1.1 THE CHALLENGES OF DELIVERING QUALITY CANCER CARE

More than 1.6 million Americans are diagnosed with cancer each year [1]. By 2030, the incidence of cancer in the United States will rise to 2.3 million per year [2]. Some 14 million people in the United States are cancer survivors, and that number will rise to 18 million by 2030 [1]. These cancer patients and survivors have complex medical and psychosocial needs. They rely on multiple health care specialists, often practicing in different care settings, to apply an ever changing body of scientific evidence about the best way to manage their disease. Not surprisingly then, cancer care providers are increasingly challenged to deliver high-quality care at a time when the burden of cancer is growing, the treatments options are expanding but costly, and health care systems are demanding high value treatments.

The Institute of Medicine (IOM) of the US National Academies and other organizations has addressed these issues in a series of workshops and committee reports extending over many years. In 1999, the National Cancer Policy Board (NCPB) described quality care as "providing patients with appropriate services in a technically competent manner, with good communication, shared decision making, and cultural sensitivity" [3]. The NCPB provided a series of recommendations to achieve quality cancer care including that:

- patients undergoing technically complex procedures receive care in highly experienced centers;
- care be guided by systematically developed guidelines based on the best available evidence;
- efforts be made to measure and monitor the quality of care delivered using a core set of quality measures;
- health care systems, health plans, and physicians be held accountable for delivering high-quality care; and
- each individual with cancer receives treatment recommendations from experienced professionals; a care plan that clearly outlines the goals of care; and access to all necessary resources to implement the care plan, including access to clinical trials, a mechanism to coordinate care among necessary medical specialists, and psychosocial and other supportive care services—particularly management of cancer-related pain and timely referral to palliative care specialists and hospice services.

The NCPB also stressed the need for those patients without insurance to have equitable access to the cancer care system and called for the development of a "cancer data system" to provide quality benchmarks to providers.

In 2006, the American Society of Clinical Oncology (ASCO) and the European Society of Medical Oncology (ESMO) jointly issued a consensus statement on quality cancer care [4]. This statement incorporated many of the key recommendations of the NCPB report, including that:

- patients have access to information about their illness, possible interventions, and the known benefits and risks of treatment options;
- patients have access to their medical records;
- access to care be provided without discrimination;
- patients be empowered to participate in decision making about their treatment and have access to a multidisciplinary care team that comprises all appropriate oncology specialists as well as palliative care experts; and
- patients be offered the opportunity to participate in clinical trials.

The consensus statement called for survivorship care planning as an element of quality cancer care and stressed the importance of pain management, palliative care, and end-of-life discussions in the management of all cancer patients.

In September 2013, the IOM released a seminal report entitled "Delivering High-Quality Cancer Care: Charting a New Course for a System in Crisis" [5]. The report identifies six components of a cancer care delivery system that are integral to achieving high-quality care for all cancer patients:

- engaged patients and patient-centered communication;
- interprofessional cancer care teams integrated with noncancer care teams and caregivers;
- evidence-based care, including clinical trials and comparative effectiveness research (CER);
- a learning health information technology (HIT) system for cancer;
- translation of evidence into clinical practice, quality measurement, and performance improvement; and
- affordable care accessible to all patients.

The report highlights the interconnectivity of these six components. To bring about the new system, the report recommends that a "learning health care information technology system" be developed that enables real-time analysis of data from cancer patients in a variety of care settings. The IOM committee expressed the view that a learning health care system supports patient–clinician interactions by providing patients and clinicians with the information and tools necessary to make well-informed medical decisions. It plays an integral role in developing the evidence base that supports clinical decisions by capturing data from real-world care settings that researchers can then analyze to generate new hypotheses and insights. Further, it can be used to deliver point of care education and to collect and report quality metrics, implement performance improvement initiatives, and allow payers to identify and reward high-quality care. A key recommendation of the committee was that "Professional organizations should design and implement the digital infrastructure and analytics necessary to enable continuous learning in cancer care."

1.1.1 Diversity of Cancer and the Cancer Patient Population

Successful implementation of these many facets of quality cancer care is often challenging in view of the enormous diversity of the cancer patient population, the complexity and risks of contemporary cancer treatment, the need to coordinate care among the many specialists who comprise the multidisciplinary cancer care team, and the fragmented health care delivery system in the United States. Recent recognition of the biological, spatial, and temporal diversity of cancer further complicates clinical evaluation and management of the cancer patient and challenges physicians to assimilate more information than ever before.

Oncologists have recognized for many years that cancer is not a single disease but it has only been recently that the enormous biological diversity of cancer has been revealed through sophisticated molecular profiling studies of human tumors [6]. It is probable that no two cancers are alike in their genomic and proteomic profiles or microenvironment. This biological heterogeneity gives rise to cancers that, while histologically similar, vary in clinical presentation, natural history, prognosis, and response to treatment. Indeed, recent studies suggest that histologically disparate cancers such as transitional cell carcinoma of the bladder and squamous cell carcinoma of the lung may have molecular subtypes that are highly concordant, perhaps requiring similar treatment approaches [7]. Such observations suggest that the traditional histological classification of cancer may soon give way to a molecular classification that will require new approaches to cancer diagnosis, treatment selection and monitoring disease response and progression. The clinical assessment of a patient's cancer is further complicated because cancers are spatially heterogeneous [8] and evolve over time in response to treatment and attack by the host immune system [9]. That is, different regions of any tumor nodule in a patient likely harbor different malignant clones that can be identified by unique genomic profiles. The tumor itself is not static but changes under the selection pressures of treatment such that clones of sensitive cells regress while those of resistant cells emerge giving rise to the familiar clinical scenario of initial response to treatment followed by disease progression and drug resistance. Increasingly then, successful management of a patient with cancer requires comprehensive and repeated molecular profiling of the tumor each time a clinical decision is to be made. This new paradigm of cancer care requires that oncologists acquire or have ready access to information about the genomics of cancer and the molecular pharmacology of targeted cancer drugs to supplement their clinical insights that stem from knowledge of the natural history of each cancer type and the clinical assessment of the patient. Increasingly, oncology professionals are challenged to recognize the molecular subsets of common cancers, interpret results of complex molecular diagnostic tests, develop appropriate treatment plans, and deliver state of the art care when clinical guidelines and clinical decision support (CDS) services are either lacking or outdated [10].

1.1.2 The Need for Multidisciplinary Cancer Care

Contemporary cancer care is, of necessity, highly multidisciplinary, involving medical specialists from medical, surgical and radiation oncology, pathology, radiology, palliative care, rehabilitation medicine, and many other disciplines. As cancer treatment decisions are increasingly influenced by the results of sophisticated molecular testing, new specialists, such as molecular pathologists, genomics experts, and bioinformaticians, are being added to the cancer care team. Due to the severity of the underlying illness, the necessary treatments for cancer are often associated with significant morbidity and reduced patient quality of life. The recent introduction of a large number of oral therapies for cancer heightens the risk of multiple drug interactions and raises concerns about patient adherence with treatment, both factors that can negatively impact patient outcomes. Thus, the management of cancer, its complications, and the side effects of treatment requires the frequent interaction and communication among multiple medical specialists, often practicing in different care settings, challenging the provider community to coordinate care in an efficient and cost-effective fashion. Furthermore, as the number of cancer survivors continues to grow and transition their care from oncologists to primary care physicians, sharing of data, treatment summaries, and survivorship care plans between care teams will be essential to ensure that cancer survivors are not "lost in transition" as described in a recent IOM report [11]. Indeed, several reports point to the fragmentation of care for cancer patients, gaps in transition from treatment to survivorship, and failures in communication between multiple providers and specialists involved in the patient's care [5,12,13].

For all of these reasons, delivery of quality cancer care is challenging to achieve. While cancer can occur in individuals of any age, it is most prevalent among older individuals, many of whom have multiple comorbid illnesses that complicate coordination of their cancer care, increase their risks of treatment, and may limit their access to specialized treatment and to participation in clinical trials [14,15]. As a consequence, we often have scant evidence to guide treatment recommendations for the older individuals who comprise the largest segment of the population affected by cancer. Creation of a learning HIT system will potentially remedy many of these problems by permitting physicians to share data and learn from the experience of treating each individual.

1.1.3 The Complexity and Cost of Cancer Care Delivery

Efficient health care delivery in the United States is plagued by fragmented delivery systems, siloed medical information, variable insurance coverage, and disparities in access to care across the population. Even with the advent and broad adoption of electronic health records (EHRs), complete clinical information about a patient is not always integrated into a single clinical record as some information may reside in separate pathology, radiology, or pharmacy record systems that do not interface easily with the primary EHR. For providers who see patients at multiple locations, sometimes owned by different health systems and using different EHRs, delivery of well-coordinated care remains a challenge even with the best of intentions. The result is often poor information exchange among providers that leads to repetitive and unnecessary testing, polypharmacy, and treatment plans that are not developed, communicated, or applied in a coordinated way resulting in excessive expenditures and administrative burdens. These challenges are magnified in patients with cancer by many factors, including the multidisciplinary nature of cancer care, the high cost of many cancer drugs and other treatments, cultural diversity in patients' goals, expectations following a cancer diagnosis, and the suboptimal use of palliative care throughout treatment and of hospice services near the end of life. Apart from unnecessary or wasteful spending, poorly managed disease can lead to complications for patients, such as unnecessary side effects, disease progression, unplanned hospitalizations, avoidable visits to the emergency room, and chronic disability from disease or treatment [16–18].

Health care costs in the United States have been rapidly escalating for decades and, while cancer care comprises only a small proportion of overall spending for health care, the costs of cancer care are rising at a more rapid rate than in other areas of medicine. Drugs costs have been a major focus in the discussion about cost and value in

cancer care particularly since recently introduced cancer drugs are among the most costly to Medicare. Indeed, 8 out of the 10 of the most expensive drugs reimbursed by Medicare are cancer drugs. As the prospects for using combinations of targeted agents grows—concerns about affordability, both for patients and the US health care system overall, are growing.

Alarming statistics about drug costs have emerged in recent years:

- The average monthly cost of a branded cancer treatment has more than doubled to $10,000 over the past decade [19].
- Cancer drug costs are steadily increasing over time, with some approaching nearly $40,000 per patient per month in 2014 dollars [20].
- Targeted drugs are especially expensive, reaching up to $270,000 annually per patient [21].
- The United States spends $37.2 billion annually on cancer drugs and supportive therapies, more than 40% of worldwide expenditures [22].
- Spending on oral oncology drugs is growing with a 37% increase in average quarterly spending from $940 million in 2006 to $1.4 billion in 2011 (in 2012 dollars) [23].

Despite these booming expenditures, little information exists about how best to use many oncology drugs in large segments of the cancer patient population as patients with significant comorbidities are often excluded from clinical trials and many older patients are unaware of or choose to not participate in trials [24]. Important information on issues such as tolerance of treatment, adherence to therapy, and effectiveness in real-world cancer patient populations is desperately needed to optimize the use of these expensive agents. Furthermore, as multiple therapies become available within a particular indication, information on their comparative effectiveness, toxicity, and cost becomes essential to guide treatment recommendations. While information pertaining to these issues can sometimes be gleaned from insurance claims data, such information is often fraught with inaccurate or incomplete information and often lacks clinical nuance to enable complete understanding of how and why treatment decisions are made.

Although drugs are one of the fastest growing costs in the health care delivery system, they are not the largest contributors to overall spending on cancer care in the United States. A large national insurance company recently reported that hospitals and outpatient facilities account for more than half of spending on cancer care [25]. The nearly 5 million cancer-related hospitalizations each year in the United States represent a cost of more than $20 billion [26] and as many as one-fifth of those hospitalizations are potentially avoidable with better planning, communication, and patient education [27].

Cancer care providers also contribute to the overall costs of care when they recommend diagnostic tests, treatment strategies, or supportive care measures that are not well supported by evidence. ASCO identified 10 common clinical practices that should be discouraged due to lack of sufficient evidence to support their use and contributed these to the Choosing Wisely Campaign sponsored by the American Board of Internal Medicine Foundation [28,29]. Preliminary evidence suggests that oncology providers are reluctant to curtail some long-standing practices despite recommendations to do so [30] and it will only be through careful analysis of clinical practice patterns, revision of quality measures, and feedback to physicians at the point of care that such practices are likely to change. Deployment of a rapid learning HIT system for cancer has the potential to spur such practice change through rapid feedback to clinicians regarding their adherence to recommended practices and quality measures.

1.2 OVERVIEW OF TRADITIONAL LEARNING IN CANCER MEDICINE

Information to guide the delivery of optimal cancer care has traditionally been developed through the conduct of prospective clinical trials sponsored by public agencies such as the National Cancer Institute (NCI) or by commercial entities, that is, the pharmaceutical industry. The results of these trials form the evidence base for clinical practice guidelines, treatment pathways, drug compendia listings, and other care standards that support reimbursement policies and, hence, access to care. Where evidence from clinical trials is lacking, reimbursement policies and clinical decision making are typically supported by data from observational studies, tumor registries, or analysis of outcomes derived from insurance claims data. As treatment options for cancer patients continue to expand, all of these mechanisms will likely be necessary to understand how treatments compare and which treatment works best in which patients. The potential to learn from the experiences and outcomes of each cancer patient through development of a rapid learning HIT system could greatly expand and enhance these traditional learning mechanisms and shorten the time required to develop clinically useful information about rare cancer subtypes or outcomes of patients who are excluded from participation in clinical trials.

1.2.1 Clinical Trials as the Foundation of Evidence-Based Medicine in Cancer

Randomized clinical trials (RCTs) provide the highest level of evidence to establish the efficacy of the intervention being studied. Oncology RCTs conducted by both the academic research community and commercial sponsors have provided data to support the regulatory approval of new drugs or new indications for existing drugs that can potentially cure or improve survival of cancer patients; refine the methods of delivery, scheduling, and dosing of oncology drugs; identify subpopulations of patients that are most likely to benefit (or be harmed) from a specific therapy; and establish the utility of combining different therapeutic modalities to treat patients [31,32]. Many of these studies, often conducted by the NCI-sponsored National Clinical Trials Network, fulfill the goals and spirit of CER laid out by the IOM [33]. CER is defined as "the generation and synthesis of evidence that compares the benefits and harms of alternative methods to prevent, diagnose, treat, and monitor a clinical condition or to improve the delivery of care. The purpose of CER is to assist consumers, clinicians, purchasers, and policy makers to make informed decisions that will improve health care at both the individual and population levels." Research that is compatible with the aims of CER has six defining characteristics:

- It aims to inform a specific clinical question.
- It compares at least two alternative interventions, each with the potential to be a "best practice."
- It addresses and describes patient outcomes at both a population and subgroup level.
- It measures outcomes that are important to patients, including harms and benefits.
- It uses research methods and data sources that are appropriate for the question of interest.
- It is conducted in settings as close as possible to the settings in which the intervention will be used.

CER can be conducted using multiple research methodologies, including clinical trials as well as observational research and systematic reviews. The appropriate methodology depends on the question the research aims to answer. An advantage of RCTs is that they provide a context and infrastructure that enables investigators to also prospectively collect biospecimens or images that can be used to answer important questions about the benefits (and harms) of therapies in subgroups of patients as well as to develop new prognostic and predictive tests. The results of correlative studies have the potential to define patient subgroups that benefit more or less from the study treatment and to provide insights into mechanisms of drug resistance. Randomized trials also provide investigators with a platform to prospectively study patient-reported outcomes (PROs) and quality of life, as well as to collect economic data for cost-effectiveness analyses and economic modeling. Thus RCTs can be considered not only the gold standard of efficacy research but also the cornerstone of CER [34].

Publically sponsored trials in particular often seek to directly compare the effectiveness of various treatment options. They may combine and/or compare drugs developed by different commercial sponsors, develop multimodality therapies, such as the combination of chemotherapy and radiation, or develop novel treatment schedules or routes of drug administration, such as intraperitoneal chemotherapy for ovarian cancer [31]. Publicly sponsored trials are more likely to focus on therapies for rare diseases and to study survivorship and quality of life, as these areas may not be a priority for commercial entities. Given the public nature of the funding, investigators are expected to publish their results, even if the outcome is unfavorable for the investigational therapy. Finally, screening and prevention strategies have been developed almost exclusively by the public sector given the large sample size and long follow-up needed to complete the trial.

1.2.2 Limitations of Conventional Clinical Trials

While RCTs have clearly advanced the care of cancer patients, they have significant limitations (see Chapter 18, "A New Era of Clinical Research Methods in a Data-rich Environment" in Part IV by Riley et al.). An RCT is costly to develop and conduct. The process of developing and activating an RCT is slow and plagued by a burdensome infrastructure and substantial regulatory oversight [35]. These trials often require large numbers of patients to identify modest differences between treatments and can take years to accrue and reach the primary endpoint being studied. RCTs often require complex protocols and the collection of large amounts of patient data and documentation, which increases the workload and costs for participating sites. Recent studies suggest that a substantial proportion of phase III oncology trials are never completed, wasting both financial and patient resources [36]. As the treatment of cancer advances and new findings are discovered, the delays in start-up and completion of RCTs may lead to results that are no longer relevant by the time they are reported due to changing standards of care. Furthermore, all RCTs have eligibility criteria to define the patient population necessary to address the trial's objectives. Eligibility criteria, by their nature, limit the applicability of the trial results. Thus, critics of RCTs argue that the patient population studied often does not reflect the "real-world" practice of medicine as the inclusion criteria may lead to the selection of only the healthiest patients and may exclude patients with medical comorbidities or borderline organ function. Thus, while an RCT may adequately assess the efficacy of an intervention (ie, what can work); the "real-world" effectiveness that is seen once the intervention is deployed in community practice (ie, what does work) may be substantially different. The disparity between efficacy and effectiveness is often most apparent in trials designed to

obtain regulatory approval for a drug or device, where the selection criteria may be particularly strict and the comparison arm may not reflect current standard practice [37]. RCTs developed in the public sector and/or conducted in a community-based practice are more likely to represent real-world effectiveness as their inclusion criteria may be less stringent compared with RCTs developed by commercial entities; however, the patient selection criteria will always limit the generalizability of results obtained from RCTs.

In addition, RCTs often evaluate therapies under idealized clinical conditions including protocol-specified dose modifications and toxicity management; thus the results generated from an RCT may not be replicated when the therapy is translated to general practice settings and to real-world patients. Furthermore, the efficacy endpoints traditionally employed in cancer clinical trials may not reflect outcomes that are most important to patients, such as relief of symptoms, improvement in quality of life, or achievement of personal goals. Better measures of these PROs are urgently needed and must be incorporated in clinical trials to better assess the impact and value of a new treatment.

Tumor heterogeneity also challenges our ability to develop new cancer treatments through traditional prospective clinical trials. As common tumors are divided into rare molecular subtypes, it is increasingly challenging to identify eligible patients and complete recruitment to clinical trials in a timely fashion. Rates of enrollment of adult cancer patients in clinical trials remain stagnant at no more than 3–5%. Drug development remains risky and inefficient with the vast majority of agents that enter human testing failing to achieve approval for marketing [38]. With more tumor types, more drugs, fewer eligible patients, and strained research budgets, it is no longer possible to learn everything that still needs to be learned in cancer treatment through the conduct of conventional, prospective clinical trials. The introduction of targeted treatments that are highly effective in biomarker-defined populations now often provides evidence of treatment efficacy sufficient to support regulatory approval to be developed with small patient cohorts [39]. Indeed, some new cancer drugs have been approved under the Food and Drug Administration's (FDA) Breakthrough Designation based on results of phase I clinical trials [40]. While this rapid approval process is able to deliver new drugs to the market with remarkable speed, it does so based on the experience of small patient populations and limited safety data sets. Thus, some drugs now enter clinical practice with limited clinical experience that is restricted to patients who meet the eligibility criteria for the registration trials leaving much to be learned from exposure of a more heterogeneous real-world population to the drug [41]. Postmarketing studies and registries are mechanisms to fill gaps in knowledge about drug performance in the general population but a rapid learning HIT system has the potential to not only collect information but to use the insights gained from its analysis to rapidly modify clinical practice guidelines and inform physician treatment recommendations.

Sharing research results typically occurs through a number of well-established mechanisms, such as presenting study results at professional meetings, publishing study results in medical journals, or revising clinical practice guidelines. Each of these methods of dissemination has inherent limitations in that not all members of a professional society attend its meetings, journal publications are typically delayed 6–12 months from when research results are first presented, a significant fraction of cancer clinical trials are never published [42], and clinical practice guidelines may not be updated in a timely fashion. These limitations in traditional mechanisms of knowledge transfer are particularly troubling when information has the potential to immediately impact clinical practice, such as new data about toxicity of a marketed drug in a high-risk population or potential new uses of marketed products. In such cases, rapid delivery of reliable information to physicians at the point of care has great potential to improve the quality of care delivery. To be sure, commercially available decision support tools such as Up-To-Date or Adjuvant! Online are frequently updated by content experts and are readily available at the point of care but even such valuable products may suffer from lacking information that is directly pertinent to the patient sitting in the examination room. The potential for a rapid learning health care system to query a large patient database and return clinically useful information about patients similar to the patient before the physician adds an important new dimension to point of care information that can impact clinical practice.

1.3 THE INTERFACE OF QUALITY, VALUE, AND LEARNING

The variety of treatment options and the diversity of the cancer population viewed in the context of mounting societal pressures to control the cost of care demand continuous assessment of quality to assure that all patients receive the best possible care and are neither overtreated nor undertreated.

Recent legislative action has focused the attention of both health care providers and payers on strategies to improve the quality of medical care in the United States by emphasizing outcomes achieved rather than services provided as a basis for payment and by providing incentives to adopt quality measurement and improvement activities as an integral component of care delivery. For example, the Physician Quality Reporting System (PQRS), originally included in the Tax Relief and Healthcare Act of 2006, uses a combination of incentive payments and negative payment adjustments to promote reporting of quality information by eligible professionals. Providers participating in PQRS have multiple routes to submit quality data to the Centers for Medicare & Medicaid Services (CMS), including through Medicare Part B claims, EHRs, and CMS-approved registries [43]. CMS is also driving increased visibility of quality assessment by making PQRS participation information publicly available through its Physician Compare website [44].

In addition, Medicare's Hospital Value-Based Purchasing Program employs a pay-for-performance approach that provides payment incentives for meeting certain performance measures. Hospitals are scored based on their performance on each measure relative to other hospitals and on how their performance on each measure improves over time. By rewarding the higher of achievement or improvement on measures, the Hospital Value-Based Purchasing Program gives hospitals the financial incentive to continually improve how they deliver care. The Prospective Payment System (PPS) Exempt Cancer Hospital Quality Reporting Program, initiated by the Affordable Care Act, requires participating hospitals to submit data on their performance on quality measures to CMS as well as to publically report such information. The first round of reporting for this program began in 2014 with five measures, three of which are cancer specific.

In January 2015, the Secretary of the US Department of Health and Human Services (HHS) announced a new initiative to improve the quality of care and control health care costs through [45] the following:

- Using incentives to motivate higher value care;
- Tying payment to value through alternative payment models;
- Changing the way care is delivered through greater teamwork and integration;
- Coordinating providers more effectively across settings;
- Greater attention by providers to population health; and
- Harnessing the power of information to improve care for patients

Furthermore, efforts will be made to advance EHR interoperability through the alignment of HIT standards with payment reform. Notably, the HHS announcement highlighted that Medicare will develop and test new payment models for specialty care beginning with oncology care [46]. Certainly the near ubiquitous adoption of EHRs by oncologists will greatly facilitate data aggregation and sharing to advance these initiatives through near real-time quality assessment, detection of trends in medical practice and outcomes in unique populations, and generation of hypotheses for research studies.

The many complexities of cancer and the challenges of multidisciplinary cancer care call for new approaches to learning about cancer, disseminating new information, assessing the effectiveness of treatment, and monitoring the quality of care. With the rapid uptake of EHRs in the medical community and the extraordinary computational power and data storage capacity now available, it will soon be feasible to learn from every encounter with every patient. Information technology vastly expands the information that can inform medical decision making, drive innovation, and improve quality. Lynn Etheredge, who is widely credited with developing the concept of the rapid learning health care system, defines it as "one that generates as rapidly as possible the evidence needed to deliver the best care for each cancer patient" [47]. As information technology has evolved, the oncology community has begun to focus on the possibilities and benefits of harnessing electronic health care data to power a rapid learning information technology system for cancer. ASCO is building a system known as CancerLinQ to make Dr Etheredge's vision a reality.

1.4 ASCO'S VISION FOR A RAPID LEARNING SYSTEM IN ONCOLOGY: CANCERLINQ

CancerLinQ (Cancer *Learning Intelligence Network for Quality*) (CLQ) is a physician-led initiative representing a fundamental evolution of ASCO's core mission of supporting the delivery of quality cancer care. Designed as an oncology rapid learning health care system as envisioned by the IOM [48], CancerLinQ is a groundbreaking HIT platform with the potential to revolutionize how oncology care is delivered. CancerLinQ harnesses the power of Big Data to "learn" from every patient. Building on the success of ASCO's Quality Oncology Practice Initiative (QOPI), a grassroots, oncologist-led, practice-level quality assessment program available to US oncology practices since 2006 [49], CancerLinQ meets the need for more effective, adaptable, and comprehensive quality improvement tools at the point of care. It compares the process and outcomes of care against the best standards available to rapidly feed information back to practices on the quality of care achieved.

CancerLinQ gathers data through direct electronic feeds from the EHRs and practice management systems (PMSs) of participating oncology practices. This obviates the need for manual chart abstraction, making the system more flexible and attractive to providers than existing systems. CancerLinQ attempts to ingest all data contained within the source systems, not just selected fields, and stores the data in a series of progressive databases within the architecture.

CancerLinQ's primary objectives include the following:

- *Provide real-time quality feedback*: CancerLinQ enables oncology practices to measure how their care compares against guidelines and to their peers based on aggregated reports of quality, so they may use the information in their own quality improvement process, thereby furthering a culture of self-examination and improvement.
- *Provide personalized insights*: CancerLinQ provides CDS to prompt physicians to choose the right therapy at the right time for each patient, based on published treatment guidelines and other knowledge bases.
- *Uncover patterns that can improve care*: Powerful analytic tools reveal new, previously unseen patterns in patient characteristics, treatments, and outcomes that can lead to improvements in care and suggest new research hypotheses. Insights gained in this process, once verified, have the potential to contribute to a virtuous cycle of learning that ultimately will improve practice guidelines.

The long-term vision for CancerLinQ has a number of additional objectives:

- Help providers assess patient eligibility for clinical trials and match patients to available trials.
- Help providers create longitudinal treatment plan documents at the start of an episode of care and treatment summary documents at the conclusion to facilitate communication among members of the health care team and between patients and providers.
- Improve the signal-to-noise ratio of CDS tools for oncologists by providing CDS that is more specific to the characteristics of individual patients.
- Improve risk stratification for patients when considering treatment, either standard of care or care delivered in the context of a clinical trial.
- Monitor the performance and safety of drugs after introduction into routine clinical practice to discover new signals and potentially inform the regulatory process and drug labeling.
- Assess patient outcomes following off-label prescribing of approved drugs.
- Generate a longitudinal database of PROs through the deployment of a patient portal.

1.5 CANCERLINQ DATA ARCHITECTURE

CancerLinQ ingests and stores data from a set of core and associated/federated data sources and possesses the ability to query within and across these data sources in a rapid and effective manner. The core data sources are EHRs for the capture of clinical data, and PMSs for business and financial transactions in a practice. Most commonly, these are commercially available vendor systems, and in some cases, a single system may perform both functions in an integrated suite. Additional associated and/or federated data sources may include: (1) ASCO internal databases and document repositories, such as those containing membership information as well as publications from ASCO journals; (2) medical payor/claims databases or data warehouses; (3) national, state, or private tumor registries; and (4) molecular diagnostics/genomics data source(s). Other local, regional, or national data sources will likely become candidates for integration by CancerLinQ depending on their availability and relevance as the platform matures.

The EHRs and PMSs from participating practices are connected electronically to CancerLinQ, thereby minimizing the burden and workflow impact of manual data collection and submission. The data are uploaded via either a continuous feed or an intermittent, regular connection strategy. These collected data contain protected health information (PHI) and personally identifiable information (PII). The information extracted from these practice systems by CancerLinQ are stored both as structured and unstructured data (see Section 1.7.1).

CancerLinQ will also be able to collect and process unstructured information from clinician notes using natural language processing (NLP) techniques.

The CancerLinQ data model is illustrated in Fig. 1.1. CancerLinQ comprises a series of cloud-based logical database classes through which data flows and undergoes a series of transformations, including progressive deidentification. Clinical data (made up of PHI and PII from practices), practice management data, and potentially data from other sources flow through an ingestion gateway into a storage database also known as a "data lake" [50]. The data lake receives and saves all incoming data from all sources, and sufficient controls ensure transmissions are complete and accurate and no data are lost. Use, disclosure, and protection of the data are governed and protected by the regulatory requirements of the Privacy Rule [51] and Security Rule [52] promulgated under the Health Insurance Portability and Accountability Act (HIPAA) of 1996 [53] and the Health Information Technology for Economic and Clinical Health (HITECH) Act [54]. Further, a number of more stringent state laws may apply to the use and disclosure of the data.

The raw collected data in the data lake is then cleansed and standardized and flows into the next database of processed data. To facilitate analytics on health care data from disparate sources, it is necessary

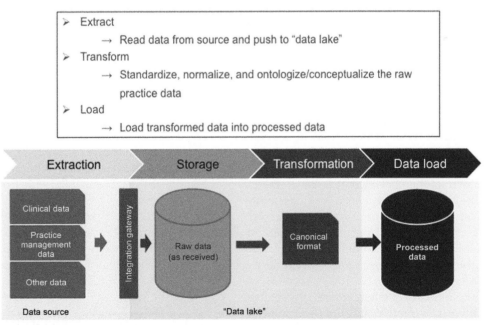

FIGURE 1.1 CancerLinQ data ingestion. Data from electronic health records, practice management systems, and other sources enter a data lake as protected health information and personally identifiable information. All data received from practices are stored and maintained in the data lake. CancerLinQ moves codified data from the first database (data lake) to the second (the "processed data"). In this process the data are standardized and normalized. The knowledge source (content) for the standardization is the NCI Metathesaurus.

to provide a tool that enables the system to interoperate with different vocabularies, since several are used, sometimes simultaneously, in the health care domain. The NCI Metathesaurus was chosen as the unified medical language system (UMLS) for CancerLinQ [55]. It is based on the UMLS of the National Library of Medicine [56], which is a large multipurpose vocabulary database that contains information about biomedical and health-related concepts, such as the Systematized Nomenclature of Medicine-Clinical Terms [57]. The NCI Metathesaurus is a cancer-centric extension of UMLS that additionally includes a growing number of cancer-related biomedical vocabularies. The database receiving processed data from the data lake also stores PII/PHI and is governed by and protected in accordance with HIPAA, HITECH, and various state laws.

Patient/provider record matching must be performed on the processed data prior to any downstream data redaction. The current lack of a national patient identifier number within the US health care system is a barrier for many aspects of care, research, and quality improvement. Since maintaining a complete longitudinal record for patients is essential to the success of CancerLinQ by enabling patient-level quality reporting, collected data within CancerLinQ are associated with a particular patient via an enterprise master patient index (EMPI), which enables patient verification using a specified minimum number of data fields. Treating providers will also be identified in an enterprise master provider index.

CancerLinQ will employ a third party tool to remove or mask individual identifiers from the collected data to create redacted data sets, which are then stored in a downstream database. There are multiple instances of this database, which feeds downstream secondary uses, such as analytical reports. Redacted data are longitudinal in nature and comprise *limited data sets* and *deidentified data sets*. A limited data set is defined under HIPAA in 45 CFR 164.514(e) as containing PHI minus 16 specific identifiers, such as names and phone numbers [58]. A deidentified data set is defined in Section 164.514(a) of the HIPAA Privacy Rule and is achieved by one of two methods: the "expert determination" method (also known as the statistical opinion method) or the "safe harbor" method [59]. CancerLinQ uses the "expert determination" method, under which a person with appropriate knowledge and experience applies accepted principles and methods to deidentify the data and determines the risk of identifying an individual in such a data set is very small [60].

CancerLinQ employs robust safeguards to protect the anonymity of patient information and the deidentification process. No individuals with access to the redacted data sets have any access to the fully identifiable collected data. The only exception is the treating provider who has access to the data for his or her own patients,

although not simultaneous access to redacted data and identifiable data. A variety of administrative, technical, and physical measures will be used to enhance data security.

1.6 HISTORY AND CURRENT STATUS OF CANCERLINQ IMPLEMENTATION

1.6.1 Background and Prototype Development 2011–12

Inspired by the work of IOM, the ASCO Board of Directors developed guiding principles for an oncology-specific rapid learning health care system at a 2011 strategy meeting. A separate Quality Department within ASCO was formed to house the CancerLinQ project management office, and a CancerLinQ business plan was developed. A working group staffed by ASCO volunteers and supported by ASCO staff and expert consultants was created, and development of a prototype to demonstrate the feasibility of CancerLinQ and obtain insights for the full system was begun in 2012. The prototype had five goals:

1. Demonstrate the ability to capture and aggregate complete longitudinal patient records from any source, in any format, and make use of the data.
2. Demonstrate ASCO's capability to develop rapid, real-time, CDS based on clinical guidelines and integrate them into a demonstration EHR system.
3. Demonstrate value-added tools, such as the ability to measure a clinician's performance on a subset of QOPI measures in real-time.
4. Create new ways of exploring clinical data and generating hypotheses.
5. Provide "lessons learned" about the technological and logistical challenges involved in a full-scale CancerLinQ implementation.

The prototype was constructed in 5 months from open source software and one commercially available analytics package. It included more than 170,000 deidentified medical records of breast cancer patients from several oncology practice groups of various sizes around the United States. The prototype demonstrated that the five goals identified prospectively were indeed feasible. Moreover, it showed that oncology practices were willing to sign data use agreements and share actual patient data to be able to participate in a rapid learning system [61].

1.6.2 CancerLinQ Development 2013–15

Following the demonstration of the prototype, ASCO systematically put the infrastructure in place to support the further development of the full CancerLinQ platform.

In 2013, Data Governance and Advisory Committees were established, composed of leading thinkers from an array of relevant fields engaged to advise on design and implementation. Advisors included leading oncologists, patient advocates, privacy advocates, health outcomes researchers, ethicists, HIT experts, and others. In 2014, the key functional requirements of CancerLinQ were established and a search for suitable technology and expertise began. Also in 2014, a CancerLinQ Request for Proposals was released, and both vendor build and organizational teaming responses were received. The ASCO Board of Directors decided to pursue a collaborative teaming path with the global technology organization SAP to create CancerLinQ. The ASCO Board of Directors approved the creation of a separate limited liability company within ASCO to provide governance and strategic direction to CancerLinQ, and thus CancerLinQ, LLC was born. The organization has its own Board of Governors, officers, executive leadership, and committee structure and was charged to bring CancerLinQ to fruition and oversee its deployment and growth.

1.6.3 CancerLinQ and SAP

In January 2015, ASCO announced a strategic technical partnership with the global software company SAP to create the big data software platform on which CancerLinQ was built [62]. CancerLinQ was developed using SAP's HANA, a flexible, multipurpose in-memory data management and application platform, which provides predictive text analytics, spatial processing, and data virtualization on the same architecture. SAP's HANA had already been employed in other global health care settings, including the National Center for Tumor Diseases in Heidelberg, Germany, where its real-time data analytics helped accelerate cancer research and improve clinical trial matching for patients treated at that institution [63].

The first fully functional version of CancerLinQ is scheduled for release in late 2015 to early 2016. Fifteen US oncology practices, representing more than 500,000 patient records, are expected to be in the vanguard group to deploy the first version of CancerLinQ. The CancerLinQ, LLC will continue to provide governance and drive the overall development of the platform, with input from physicians, patients, and experts in relevant disciplines including quality improvement, health outcomes, epidemiology, and HIT. ASCO will maintain control over the data, services, and products that stem from the platform including CDS tools and analyses. SAP will provide access to customized technologies based on HANA, along with engineering and other technical support from both their standard development ranks and their team specialized in custom application

development, to help enrich CancerLinQ's versatility for providers.

CancerLinQ is supported by the ASCO's Conquer Cancer Foundation [64].

1.7 CANCERLINQ SOLUTION OPERATING CHARACTERISTICS

1.7.1 Data Ingestion

An essential initial step in order to realize the vision of CancerLinQ is the extraction of data from the electronic systems of a participating practice, a process known as data ingestion. The extract, transform, and load functions in CancerLinQ consist of the following steps:

1. Data Extraction. The practice produces a package of clinical data from the EHR and business/financial/operations data from the PMS containing all information as both structured and unstructured elements. The clinical extract contains common data concepts incorporated into oncology EHRs. This is a dynamic set of elements, ranging from patient demographics to medication lists to treatment-specific elements such as date of last chemotherapy. There have been a number of attempts to create a common data model to represent the richness and multidisciplinary nature of cancer care, one of which was a collaboration between ASCO, the National Cancer Institute Center for Biomedical Informatics and Information Technology, and the National Community Cancer Centers Program in 2009, which produced the Clinical Oncology Requirements for the EHR document [65]. However, penetration of this model was minimal, and a universally agreed upon standard does not currently exist. CancerLinQ ideally ingests the universe of data elements found in the EHR, especially those of fundamental interest to oncologists. The data will be extracted from the source systems using a multipronged approach most applicable to the practice site. Each practice is asked to provide any standards-based documents that are currently in use or produced per compliance with Federal meaningful use requirements. Examples include the Continuity of Care Document (CCD), an Extensible Markup Language (XML)-based mark-up standard used for the exchange of patient summaries [66], and the Health Level Seven (HL7) Consolidated-Clinical Document Architecture (C-CDA) [67]. Another candidate document is the Clinical Oncology Treatment Plan and Summary (eCOTPS), recently described by Warner et al., the first oncology-specific CDA standard to achieve HL7 Draft Standard for Trial Use (DSTU) status [68]. Customized solutions developed in cooperation

with EHR vendors may also be used. Most sites will require a combination of these techniques.

2. **Data Transfer.** The practice securely transmits the files to CancerLinQ for consumption.
3. **Data Load and Storage #1:** All data received from practices are initially stored and maintained in the data lake.
4. **Data Processing.** CancerLinQ moves codified data from the first database (data lake) to the second (the "processed data"). In this process the data are standardized and normalized. As noted above, the knowledge source (content) for the standardization is the NCI Metathesaurus.
5. **Ontology Services.** Custom-built ontology services are implemented deeply at the database level to make them available to several layers, including analytics, data ingestion, and NLP. NLP of unstructured data (eg, free text fields in a file or text/PDF/Microsoft Word binary documents) will find a "Fact", eg, a Diagnosis Fact or a Biomarker Fact. Here too ontologies can be applied to the results of the NLP to infer facts and conduct reasoning.
6. **Data Transfer and Storage #2.** The data are written to the processed database.

1.7.2 CancerLinQ Portal

The portal is a central "gateway" providing access for all practice users and CancerLinQ staff to administrative services, reporting functionality, dashboards, and quality measures, while conforming to the highest levels of security and compliance. It is accessed via the Internet using a web browser. Most modern browsers are supported. Mac OS, Microsoft Windows, and various mobile platforms are supported. The portal possesses functionality for standard analytic reports, graphical displays for quality reporting, and a data exploration tool.

1.7.3 User Types

Target users represent the primary users and consumers of CancerLinQ. At the practice level these include clinical users, clinical supervisors, practice managers, and primary account users. CancerLinQ staff users include informaticists, statisticians, data staff, and privacy and security staff. Each role has a defined set of access rights to the system meeting minimum necessary standards under HIPAA. For example, the clinical supervisor role—typically a practice's lead physician—has privileges to explore the practice management data and individually identified health information for patients at the subscriber practice down to the individual record level, whereas the individual clinical user is only able to view PHI on his/her own patients. For the CancerLinQ staff, the data staff role will have access to deidentified patient records but no access to PHI.

1.7.4 Quality Benchmarking

Providing real-time quality feedback to practices is one of the fundamental objectives of CancerLinQ. CancerLinQ enables oncologists to measure and document their adherence to clinical care guidelines without manual extraction of data from paper files or the EHR, thereby reaching a greater number of physician practices and offering analysis based on far more patients than was previously available. CancerLinQ's data architecture permits faster, more current, and more robust feedback to providers on the quality of their care.

CancerLinQ will support clinical quality measures (CQMs), which are tools consisting of numerator and denominator patient counts, giving a ratio of patients satisfying the definition of the measure. Denominator exclusions, factors supported by the clinical evidence that should remove a patient from inclusion in the measure population, are represented in CancerLinQ. CancerLinQ provides the ability to define a categorized set of electronic CQMs, or eCQMs (eg, based on disease type or domain); and users are able to select from a categorized list of core guidelines in order to visualize and evaluate CQMs using real-time data from their own set of patients. Users have the ability to drill down to see individual patient data. Measures can be compared against other practice data, but users cannot see the detailed patient data if they are not authorized. Users can see aggregated data from all participating practices and are able to compare their performance on each measure to the whole population. However, they are not able to identify any characteristics (eg, individual patient counts or practice identity) outside of their own practice.

In CancerLinQ, eCQMs are displayed in graphical format using the Clinical Measure Analysis (CMA) application, which resides in the SAP HANA Enterprise Cloud as part of the user-facing portal. Within HANA, CancerLinQ informaticists use a Clinical Measurement Library (CML) to create formal measure definitions, which are standards-based and machine readable representations of a CQM. The eCQM definitions in CancerLinQ are supplied in Health Quality Measures Format (HQMF), Release 2, an HL7 Version 3 DSTU [69].

1.7.5 Clinical Decision Support

CDS systems can be defined as "HIT applications that relate individual patient health data to established knowledge bases and thereby assist in clinical decision making and health management" [70]. Providing personalized insights to oncologists with CDS is one of the primary objectives of CancerLinQ. There are countless areas in oncology where data are needed to make clinical decisions but are largely absent. As the number of new molecular diagnostic tests proliferates, propelled in part by the explosion of cancer panomics, and the number of therapeutic agents expands proportionally, it will become increasingly challenging to practice high-quality cancer medicine without computerized CDS.

At the time of publication of this text, a specific CDS solution has not been determined. It is anticipated that the ASCO clinical practice guidelines [71], derived from high-quality evidence by expert ASCO panels and addressing disease-specific clinical situations or modalities, such as tests or procedures, may serve as a robust source of content knowledge for the development of CDS in CancerLinQ. CancerLinQ will include a feature that will identify relevant guidelines to present CDS that is relevant to the characteristics of an individual patient to assist physicians in treating specific patients. Furthermore, the clinical insights gained by oncologists from the redacted data sets in the system may be used as feedback to inform the refinement of existing guidelines and suggest new clinical areas where guidelines may be necessary.

CancerLinQ will also include observational CDS, which will enable a physician to query the system about a specific case to learn about the treatments and outcomes for similar patients. CancerLinQ will match a particular patient's data against the experience of similar cancer patients whose data reside within the system and provide the oncologist with aggregate information pertinent to the possible treatments available to the patient and the range of outcomes experienced by other similar patients. Boxes 1.1 and 1.2 provide representative use cases of the CDS capabilities envisioned for CancerLinQ.

BOX 1.1

PERSONALIZED MEDICINE CDS USE CASE

Phillip Alk is a 72-year-old white male who presents to his primary care physician with nonproductive cough and pleuritic chest pain. He is otherwise healthy except for high cholesterol, for which he takes atorvastatin, mild hypertension, and gastroesophageal reflux treated with omeprazole. He has no fever or weight loss and a Karnofsky performance status (PS) of 90. Mr Alk smoked cigarettes for a few years during college but has not smoked in the last 50 years. A routine chest X-ray reveals a 3 cm nodule in the right middle lobe (RML) confirmed by follow-up chest computerized tomography scan that also demonstrates scattered 1 cm nodules in the left lung and ground glass opacities in the right lower lobe. Routine blood chemistries are normal except for a serum creatinine of 1.8 mg/dL. A core needle biopsy of the RML nodule is performed and reveals malignancy consistent with adenocarcinoma. Upon receiving the diagnosis, the patient is referred to a local oncologist for discussion of treatment options.

Dr Gene Profile is a practicing general oncologist in a group of six oncologists. He has been in practice for 20 years. His practice was a participant in ASCO's QOPI program for the last 8 years and transitioned to participation in CancerLinQ when offered the opportunity to do so. The practice's QOPI reports revealed high adherence with measures of adjuvant chemotherapy use and appropriate antiemetic use but also demonstrated need for improvement in chemotherapy use in the last 2 weeks of life and counseling patients about smoking cessation. During his initial visit with Mr Alk, Dr Profile reviews the pathology reports and wonders if the diagnosis of adenocarcinoma reflects a primary lung cancer or metastases from another organ. The patient's medical history and review of systems do not suggest other problems. A positron emission tomography (PET) scan is performed for staging purposes and demonstrates the RML lung nodule as well as several smaller nodules scattered throughout the left lung. No other areas of increased fluorodeoxyglucose (FDG) uptake are noted. Dr Profile recalls seeing some literature in the office from a lab that offers gene expression profiling to assess carcinomas of unknown primary. He considers ordering the test but first consults the CancerLinQ clinical decision support system. He immediately receives a link to an ASCO guideline on carcinoma of unknown primary that recommends against use of commercially available RNA expression profiling panels due to lack of evidence of clinical utility in helping to establish a more definitive diagnosis. Dr Profile ultimately concludes that primary adenocarcinoma of the lung is the most likely diagnosis and records that diagnosis in the patient's EMR. He immediately receives a guidance notification from CancerLinQ recommending a standard molecular work-up of the tumor to include testing for sensitizing and resistance mutations to epidermal growth factor receptor (EGFR) inhibitors, *EML4-ALK* translocation, *ROS1* and *KRAS* mutation. The notification includes a link to ASCO's provisional clinical opinion (PCO) on integration of palliative care into standard oncology care as well as a link to ASCO's PCO on *EGFR* mutation testing for

---

BOX 1.1 (Cont'd)

patients with nonsmall cell lung cancer. Dr Profile orders the recommended tests to be performed on the patient's tumor biopsy. Mr Alk is anxious to begin treatment but is advised to wait for the molecular test results to see if they impact Dr Profile's treatment recommendation. Two weeks later, Dr Profile receives a report from a commercial laboratory of a 400 gene mutation panel that was performed on the biopsy. His hospital's pathology department had determined that it is more cost-effective to obtain the multigene panel rather than the individual tests for the mutational analysis recommended by CancerLinQ. The report describes an L858R mutation in exon 21 of the *EGFR* gene, wild type *KRAS*, mutation in the *p53* gene, mutation at the V600E locus of the *BRAF* gene, as well as alterations in other genes. Uncertain of how to proceed, Dr Profile uses the CancerLinQ physician portal to submit the molecular profiling test results and a brief case summary to the ASCO University Molecular Oncology Tumor Board. Two days later, he receives an explanation of the molecular profiling results that confirm his plan to prescribe an *EGFR* inhibitor drug for Mr Alk. Upon entering the order for erlotinib in the patient's EHR, Dr Profile receives a notification from CancerLinQ of a possible drug interaction with omeprazole and is advised to discontinue that medication. He is also advised to carefully monitor the patient's renal function in view of the toxicity profile of erlotinib and the patient's preexisting renal insufficiency.

After 3 months on treatment, Mr Alk's cough and chest pain have fully resolved and his CT scan reveals complete resolution of all pulmonary nodules. He continues on treatment but 3 months later notices a return of his cough. When these new symptoms are recorded in his EHR, Dr Profile receives a message from CancerLinQ advising him to consider erlotinib-induced interstitial lung disease as a possible complication of treatment. A repeat CT scan reveals new pulmonary nodules consistent with recurrent and progressive lung cancer. Dr Profile recalls that the molecular testing of Mr Alk's tumor had revealed a *BRAF* V600E mutation. He wonders if a new *BRAF* inhibitor, recently approved to treat melanoma, could possibly benefit his patient. He uses CancerLinQ's observational clinical decision support function to query the CancerLinQ database and receives a report of 30 patients in the system with adenocarcinoma of the lung and a *BRAF* V600E mutation. Of these, 20 had been treated with vemurafenib and 10 had experienced significant tumor shrinkage. Dr Profile prescribes off-label vemurafenib for his patient. Within 2 months, Mr Alk's symptoms have worsened, his performance status has declined, and his cancer has progressed on CT scan. He consults Dr Profile about other treatment options, particularly whether he should give chemotherapy a try. He is advised to transition to hospice care at this point in his illness.

1.7.6 Other Secondary Uses of Deidentified and/or Limited Data Sets

Other potential uses of redacted data sets in CancerLinQ include:

1. Trend Discovery: CancerLinQ will employ machine learning algorithms and artificial intelligence to uncover trends in the redacted data sets, such as unanticipated adverse events, that may require further analysis, development, and exploration.
2. Off-Label Use: A significant minority of oncology drug use is for an indication that is not reflected on the FDA-approved label. Although such off-label use is often sound medical practice, it can be based on small studies and even case reports. There is no organized system to aggregate these experiences and understand what actually works and in what setting. CancerLinQ will be able to supply this information to enable more comprehensive and in-depth analysis of off-label uses and associated patient outcomes. This may also inform decisions by drug manufacturers to seek regulatory approval for expansion of a drug's label and contribute data to the regulatory review process.
3. Risk Stratification: There is tremendous heterogeneity within each cancer patient population. Variables such as age, gender, comorbid conditions, current medications, specific organ function, performance status, and a host of other factors influence cancer outcome. Increasingly, molecular characteristics will be incorporated into risk stratification schemes. CancerLinQ will be able to analyze tens or hundreds of thousands of cases and produce findings that enable treating oncologists to begin to risk stratify patients with far more precision, hopefully leading to better selection of therapy and improved patient outcomes.

BOX 1.2

OBSERVATIONAL CDS USE CASE

Mr Jones is a 72-year-old African American man with advanced prostate cancer whose disease has been well controlled with conventional antiandrogen treatment. However, during the past month he has developed increased skeletal pain, rising prostate-specific antigen (PSA), and new visceral metastases detected on CT scan. Mr Jones consults his oncologist about treatment options and receives a recommendation to change treatment to abiraterone acetate, a recently approved *CYP17* inhibitor that inhibits the extragonadal conversion of pregnenolone to testosterone, a pathway frequently exploited by castrate-resistant prostate cancer. Abiraterone was approved by the FDA in 2011 based on a randomized clinical trial that compared abiraterone plus prednisone to prednisone alone and demonstrated an improvement in median overall survival from 10.7 to 14.8 months. Mr Jones is inclined to proceed with this new treatment until his oncologist tells him that the cost of treatment is about $6000/month. Mr Jones is concerned that he cannot afford the expected copayment of $1200/month and will have to forego further treatment. His oncologist recalls that the antifungal drug ketoconazole inhibits the same enzyme as abiraterone and has been reported in several small clinical trials to have activity in advanced prostate cancer. He explains to Mr Jones that ketoconazole was commonly used off-label to treat patients with castrate-resistant prostate cancer until the FDA approval of abiraterone. A generic drug, ketoconazole is considerably less expensive than abiraterone, costing approximately $500/month. No clinical trials have ever been performed that directly compare the effectiveness of ketoconazole and abiraterone. Mr Jones wonders if ketoconazole might be an acceptable alternative to abiraterone in his case and one that he could much more easily afford.

Mr Jones' oncologist is a participant in ASCO's CancerLinQ learning health care system. Using the observational clinical decision support function of CancerLinQ, he enters Mr Jones' characteristics into the system and requests a report on treatment administered to similar patients and the outcomes achieved. Minutes later, CancerLinQ provides a report on several thousand similar patients in the system. Of these, 15% had received treatment with ketoconazole and 25% treatment with abiraterone over the past 4 years. The patients in each group experienced similar survivals of about 12 months, although patients receiving ketoconazole experienced higher rates of fatigue and nausea. Upon learning of these data, Mr Jones opts for treatment with ketoconazole and receives a prescription from his oncologist to begin immediately.

---

4. Drug Safety Monitoring: CancerLinQ will enable the monitoring of safety and efficacy signals in real-world populations, overcoming the current limitations of drug registration trials, which often treat patient populations not representative of patients in practice, who are often older with a higher number of comorbidities. CancerLinQ's data model will support the capture of adverse events in near real time, meaning that the time to insight should be dramatically shortened compared to conventional adverse event reporting systems.

5. Research: CancerLinQ will make redacted data sets available for research activities pursuant to established policies and procedures. Where appropriate, individual investigators will be able to propose specific research questions for review and approval, and the system will use the redacted data sets to generate either a report or a data set necessary to address the question.

1.8 REGULATORY UNDERPINNINGS OF CANCERLINQ

For CancerLinQ to be successful as a rapid learning system, both the patients who contribute data and the physicians who make use of it must be confident that the PHI in the system is being stored securely and used only for the intended purposes, in a manner compliant with all applicable state and federal statutes and regulations. To this end, ASCO developed a transparent regulatory framework to validate CancerLinQ's compliance with the requirements of HIPAA, HITECH, and those of the "Common Rule," a policy addressing the protection of human subjects participating in federally funded research (45 CFR part 46) [72]. Schilsky et al., on behalf of ASCO, presented this regulatory framework for CancerLinQ, along with a description of the CancerLinQ data model and the principles of data governance [73]. In discussing HIPAA, the authors noted that PHI can be used or disclosed by a provider to a business associate—a relationship governed by a formal business associate agreement—if the use falls under the broad category of "health care operations." Health care operations encompass a number of acceptable activities, among them being quality assessment and improvement, evaluation of outcomes, and development and maintenance of clinical practice guidelines. Since CancerLinQ was designed for the primary purpose of collecting the data necessary to support and improve physician efforts at quality assessment, care coordination, rapid identification of treatment alternatives, real-time feedback and benchmarking, and other quality improvement activities, it falls squarely into the HIPAA definition of health care operations. Furthermore, the creation of limited data sets and deidentified data sets also falls under the category of health care operations as opposed to research. Therefore, it was the authors' conclusion that patients participating in CancerLinQ would not need to give individual consent for their data to be added to the CancerLinQ data lake and subsequently undergo processing, deidentification, and secondary use. This is in contradistinction to the collection of data for the purposes of research, which would require the patient to give individual consent.

Regarding the applicability of the Common Rule, the authors again drew the distinction between *research*, where data collection is performed as part of a systematic investigation used to test a hypothesis or otherwise contribute to generalizable knowledge, versus *health care operations*, inclusive of quality improvement activities and care coordination. The generation of the redacted data sets in CancerLinQ was felt not to invoke the definition of research under HIPAA or the Common Rule since the initial data collection was done exclusively for quality reasons and not investigation and because deidentified data may be used for research without patient consent. To further validate this argument, ASCO requested a review of CancerLinQ by an independent institutional review board (IRB) in 2013. The IRB opined that collecting PHI for these purposes did not constitute research and that the creation and use of redacted data sets downstream for research-related activities did not render the initial data collection itself a research activity governed by the Common Rule.

1.8.1 Data Governance Guiding Principles and Policies

CancerLinQ is deeply committed to the appropriate, secure, and ethical usage of health information entrusted to it and has adopted three basic guiding principles:

1. Stewardship: The data that are collected must be accurate, valid, and usable for performance evaluation and quality improvement. This requires adherence to rigorous standards to evaluate and govern the use of all data and to constantly monitor and protect the security of health information. The principle of stewardship means that requests for redacted data sets must adhere to a set of ethical principles respectful of the patients who have contributed data to the system. It also implies a level of nimbleness and willingness to adapt to environmental changes in the scientific and technological landscape that might impact the ethical principles upon which operational decisions are made.

2. Protection: CancerLinQ must strive to prevent harm and risk to others by maintaining, using, and sharing data in compliance with applicable law and regulations and with appropriate oversight. Data must be protected against unauthorized access and misuse throughout its life cycle, wherever it resides in the system. Strict standards for data collection and storage must be followed, and there must be a brisk and complete response to any threat to data security.

3. Transparency and accountability: CancerLinQ must be accountable to patients, providers, and the public for high standards for the ethical management of data and making information about the data governance policies available to all stakeholders.

CancerLinQ operationalized these principles in the following ways:

- Creation of a Data Governance Oversight Committee consisting of CancerLinQ volunteers and staff, including ethicists and patient advocates to provide input on the design, review, and implementation of data governance policies and procedures.
- Implementation of administrative, physical, and technical safeguards to protect against unauthorized access to patient information throughout all stages of the CancerLinQ lifecycle.
- Appointing a CancerLinQ Privacy and Security Officer to oversee implementation of and compliance with the HIPAA policies and procedures.

Requests for the use of redacted data sets for research purposes will be assessed in the light of the above guiding principles, carefully considering whether the value derived from their use is consistent with the expectation that their analysis will ultimately improve the health of individual patients and populations and contribute to the generalization of knowledge to improve cancer care more globally.

1.9 SUMMARY AND CONCLUSIONS

In this chapter we have addressed the urgent need, as recommended by the IOM, for enabling a learning health care system to improve the quality of cancer care. Many of the other chapters in this text also describe efforts underway to improve the state of cancer care through learning health care systems. We described the rationale, objectives, and early development of CancerLinQ, one example of an HIT-enabled rapid learning system for oncology created by the ASCO. The overarching goal of CancerLinQ is to enable oncologists to learn from every encounter with every cancer patient and to rapidly gain insights that can benefit all cancer patients. Rather than relying exclusively on traditional mechanisms of generating medical evidence, such as clinical trials, CancerLinQ, by capturing the longitudinal record of each patient's experience, will enable insights that are more broadly applicable and more clinically nuanced than can be determined from clinical trials, registries, or claims data sets and that can be generated in far less time by posing queries to an enormous database containing millions of patient records. Over time, the value of the CancerLinQ data will be further enhanced by incorporating genomic data, imaging data, and PROs that will be collected via a patient portal to be included in future versions of the system. Linkage of the CancerLinQ data to insurance claims data and cancer registry data in the future will provide a rich portrait of the characteristics, experiences, preferences, goals, outcomes, and resource utilization of every cancer patient and provide the ability "to generate as rapidly as possible the evidence needed to deliver the best care for each cancer patient" [47].

LIST OF ACRONYMS AND ABBREVIATIONS

ASCO American Society of Clinical Oncology
CCD Continuity of Care Document
C-CDA Consolidated-Clinical Document Architecture
CDS Clinical decision support
CER Comparative effectiveness research
CLQ CancerLinQ
CMA Clinical Measure Analysis
CML Clinical Measurement Library
CMS Centers for Medicare & Medicaid Services
CQMs Clinical quality measures
eCOTPS Electronic Clinical Oncology Treatment Plan and Summary
EHR Electronic health records
EMPI Enterprise master patient index
ESMO European Society of Medical Oncology
HHS US Department of Health and Human Services
HIPAA Health Insurance Portability and Accountability Act
HIT Health information technology
HITECH Health Information Technology for Economic and Clinical Health
HL7 Health Level Seven
HQMF Health Quality Measures Format
IOM Institute of Medicine
NCI National Cancer Institute
NCPB National Cancer Policy Board
NLP Natural language processing
PHI Protected health information
PII Personally identifiable information
PMSs Practice management systems
PPS Prospective Payment System
PQRS Physician Quality Reporting System
RCTs Randomized clinical trials
XML Extensible Markup Language

Acknowledgments

The authors thank Andrej Kolacevski and Alaap Shah for their invaluable assistance in reviewing this manuscript and Sara da Silva for expert editorial support.

References

[1] American Cancer Society (US). Cancer facts and figures 2015 [Internet]; 2015. Available from: <http://www.cancer.org/acs/groups/content/@editorial/documents/document/acspc-044552.pdf> [accessed 15.02.16].

[2] Smith B, Smith G, Hurria A, Hortobagyi GN, Buchholz TA. Future of cancer incidence in the United States: burdens upon an aging, changing nation. J Clin Oncol 2009;17:2758–65.

[3] Institute of Medicine (US). Ensuring quality cancer care [Internet]; 1999. Available from: <http://www.iom.edu/Reports/1999/Ensuring-Quality-Cancer-Care.aspx>.

[4] American Society of Clinical Oncology ASCO-ESMO consensus statement on quality cancer care. J Clin Oncol 2006;24:3498–9.

[5] National Academies Press (US). Delivering high-quality cancer care: charting a new course for a system in crisis [Internet]; 2013. Available from: <http://www.nap.edu/catalog.php?record_id=18359>.

[6] MacConnail LE, Garraway LA. Clinical implications of the cancer genome. J Clin Oncol 2010;28:5219–28.

[7] Hoadley KA, Yau C, Wolf DM, Cherniack AD, Tamborero D, Ng S, et al. Multiplatform analysis of 12 cancer types reveals molecular classification within and across tissues of origin. Cell 2014;158:929–44.

[8] Gerlinger M, Rowan AJ, Horswell S, Larkin J, Endesfelder D, Gronroos E, et al. Intratumor heterogeneity and branched evolution revealed by multiregion sequencing. N Engl J Med 2012;366:883–92.

[9] Sequist LV, Waltman BA, Dias-Santagata D, Digumarthy S, Turke AB, Fidias P, et al. Genotypic and histological evolution of lung cancers acquiring resistance to EGFR inhibitors. Sci Trans Med 2011;3(75) 75ra26.

[10] Gray SW, Hicks-Courant K, Cronin A, Rollins BJ, Weeks JC. Physicians' attitudes about multiplex tumor genomic testing. J Clin Oncol 2014;32:1317–23.

[11] Committee on Cancer Survivorship: Improving Care and Quality of Life National Cancer Policy Board Hewitt M, Greenfield S, Stovall E, editors. From cancer patient to cancer survivor: lost in transition. Washington, DC: National Academies Press; 2006.

[12] Ayanian JZ, Zaslavsky AM, Guadagnoli E, Fuchs CS, Yost KJ, Creech CM, et al. Patients' perceptions of quality of care for colorectal cancer by race, ethnicity, and language. J Clin Oncol 2005;23:6576–86.

[13] Aubin M, Giguere A, Martin M, Verreault R, Fitch MI, Kazanjian A, et al. Interventions to improve continuity of care in the follow-up of patients with cancer. Cochrane Database Syst Rev 2012. <http://dx.doi.org/10.1002/14651858.CD007672.pub2>.

[14] Hurria A, Dale W, Mooney M, Rowland JH, Ballman KV, Cohen HJ, et al. Designing therapeutic clinical trials for older and frail adults with cancer: U13 conference recommendations. J Clin Oncol 2014;32:2587–94.

[15] Wildiers H, Heeren P, Puts M, Topinkova E, Janssen-Heijnen MJ, Extermann M, et al. International Society of Geriatric Oncology consensus on geriatric assessment in older patients with cancer. J Clin Oncol 2014;32:2595–603.

[16] Neuss M, Malin J, Chan S, Kadlubek PJ, Adams JL, Jacobson JO, et al. Measuring the improving quality of outpatient care in medical oncology practices in the United States. J Clin Oncol 2013;31:1471–7.

[17] Blayney D, Severson J, Martin C, Kadlubek P, Ruane T, Harrison K. Michigan oncology practices showed varying adherence rates to practice guidelines, but quality interventions improved care. Health Aff 2012;31:718–28.

[18] Campion F, Larson L, Kadlubek P, Earle CC, Neuss MN. Advancing performance measurement in oncology: quality oncology practice initiative participation and quality outcomes. J Clin Oncol 2011;7:31–5.

[19] IMS Institute for Healthcare Informatics (US). Innovation in cancer care and implications for health systems [Internet]; 2014. Available from: <http://www.imshealth.com/deployed-files/imshealth/Global/Content/Corporate/IMS%20Health%20Institute/Reports/Secure/IMSH_Oncology_Trend_Report.pdf>.

[20] Memorial Sloan Kettering Cancer Center (US). Cost of cancer drugs [Internet]; 2014. Available from: <http://www.mskcc.org/research/health-policy-outcomes/cost-drugs>.

[21] Kantarjian HM, Fojo T, Mathisen M, Zwelling LA. Cancer drugs in the United States: justum pretium—the just price. J Clin Oncol 2013;31:3600–4.

[22] Mulcahy AW, Armstrong C, Lewis J, Mattke S. The 340B Prescription drug discount program [Internet]; 2014. Available from: <http://www.rand.org/pubs/perspectives/PE121.html>.

[23] Conti RM, Fein AJ, Bhatta SS. National trends in spending on and use of oral oncologics, first quarter 2006 through third quarter 2011. Health Aff 2014;33:1721–7.

[24] Conti R, Bernstein A, Villaflor V, Schilsky RL, Rosenthal MB, Bach PB. Prevalence of off-label use and spending in 2010 among patent-protected chemotherapies in a population-based cohort of medical oncologists. J Clin Oncol 2013;31:1134–9.

[25] Newcomer LN. Innovative payment models and measurement for cancer therapy. J. Oncol Pract 2014;10:187–9.

[26] Anhang Price R, Stranges E, Elixhauser A. Cancer hospitalizations for adults [Internet]; 2009. Available from: <http://www.hcup-us.ahrq.gov/reports/statbriefs/sb125.jsp>.

[27] Brooks GA, Abrams TA, Meyerhardt JA, Enzinger PC, Sommer K, Dalby CK, et al. Identification of potentially avoidable hospitalizations in patients with GI cancer. J Clin Oncol 2014;32:496–503.

[28] Schnipper LE, Smith TJ, Raghavan D, Blayney DW, Ganz PA, Mulvey TM, et al. American Society of Clinical Oncology identifies five key opportunities to improve care and reduce costs: the top five list for oncology. J Clin Oncol 2012;30:1715–24.

[29] Schnipper LE, Lyman GH, Blayney DB, Hoverman JR, Raghavan D, Wollins DS, et al. American Society of Clinical Oncology 2013 top five list in oncology. J Clin Oncol 2013;34:4362–70.

[30] Simos D, Hutton B, Clemons M. Are physicians choosing wisely when imaging for distant metastases in women with operable breast cancer? J Oncol Pract 2015;11:62–8.

[31] Hahn O, Schilsky RL. Randomized controlled trials and comparative effectiveness research. J Clin Oncol 2012;30:4194–201.

[32] Schilsky RL. Publically funded clinical trials and the future of cancer care: the 2012 Pinedo Lecture. Oncologist 2013;18:232–8.

[33] Institute of Medicine (US) Initial national priorities for comparative effectiveness research. Washington, DC: National Academies Press; 2009. [Internet]. Available from: <http://www.iom.edu/~/media/Files/Report%20Files/2009/ComparativeEffectivenessResearchPriorities/CER%20report%20brief%2008-13-09.ashx>.

[34] Lamont E, Schilsky RL, He Y, Muss H, Cohen HJ, Hurria A, et al. Generalizability of trial results to elderly Medicare patients with advanced solid tumors (Alliance 70802). J Natl Cancer Inst 2015;107:1–7.

[35] Institute of Medicine A national cancer clinical trials system for the 21st century: reinvigorating the NCI cooperative group program. Washington, DC: National Academies Press; 2010.

[36] Dilts DM, Cheng SK, Crites JS, Sandler AB, Doroshow JH. Phase III clinical trial development: a process of chutes and ladders. Clin Cancer Res 2010;16:5381–9.

[37] Meyerhardt JA, Li L, Sanoff HK, Carpenter IV W, Schrag D, et al. Effectiveness of bevacizumab with first-line combination chemotherapy for Medicare patients with stage IV colorectal cancer. J Clin Oncol 2012;30:608–15.

[38] DiMasi JA, Reichert JM, Feldman L, Malins A. Clinical approval success rates for investigational cancer drugs. Clin Pharmacol Therap 2013;94(3):329–35.

[39] Sharma MR, Schilsky RL. Re-examining the role of randomized phase III trials in an era of effective targeted therapies. Nature Rev Clin Oncol 2012;9:208–14.

[40] Merck & Co., Inc (IE) Highlights of prescribing KEYTRUDA® (pembrolizumab) [Internet]; 2015. Available from: <http://www.merck.com/product/usa/pi_circulars/k/keytruda/keytruda_pi.pdf>.

[41] Kesselheim AS, Darrow JJ. FDA designations for therapeutics and their impact on drug development and regulatory review outcomes. Clin Pharm Ther 2015;97:29–36.

[42] Tam VC, Tannock IF, Massey C, Rauw J, Krzyzanowska MK. Compendium of unpublished phase III trials in oncology: characteristics and impact on clinical practice. J Clin Oncol 2011;29:3133–9.

[43] Centers for Medicare & Medicaid Services (US). Group practice reporting option [Internet]; 2014. Available from: <http://www.cms.gov/Medicare/Quality-Initiatives-Patient-Assessment-Instruments/PQRS/Group_Practice_Reporting_Option.html>.

[44] Centers for Medicare & Medicaid Services (US). Official physician compare data [Internet]; 2015. Available from: <https://data.medicare.gov/data/physician-compare>.

[45] Burwell SM. Setting value-based payment goals—HHS efforts to improve U.S. health care. N Engl J Med 2015 [Internet]. Available from: <http://www.nejm.org/doi/full/10.1056/NEJMp1500445>.

[46] Kline RM, Bazell C, Smith E, Schumacher H, Rajkumar R, Conway PH. Centers for Medicare and Medicaid Services: using an episode-based payment model to improve oncology care. J Oncol Pract 2015. <http://dx.doi.org/10.1200/JOP.2014.002337>. epub ahead of print published February 17, 2015.

[47] Institute of Medicine A foundation for evidence-driven practice: a rapid learning system for cancer care: workshop summary. Washington, DC: The National Academies Press; 2010.

[48] Abernethy AP, Etheredge LM, Ganz PA, Wallace P, German RR, Neti C, et al. Rapid-learning system for cancer care. J Clin Oncol 2010;28:4268–74.

[49] Blayney DW, McNiff K, Eisenberg PD, Gilmore T, Jacobsen PB, Jacobson JO, et al. Development and future of the American Society of Clinical Oncology's quality oncology practice initiative. J Clin Oncol 2014;32:3907–13.

[50] Woods D. Big data requires a big, new architecture [Internet]; 2011. Available from: <http://www.forbes.com/sites/ciocentral/2011/07/21/big-data-requires-a-big-new-architecture/>.

[51] US Code of Federal Regulations. Applicability. 45 C.F.R. § 164.500 et seq.

[52] US Code of Federal Regulations. Applicability. 45 C.F.R. § 164.302 et seq.

[53] Health Insurance Portability and Accountability Act of 1996, Subtitle F, Public Law 104-191. The implementing regulations can be found at 45 C.F.R. §§ 160, 162 and 164.

[54] Title XIII of the American Recovery and Reinvestment Act of 2009, Subtitle I, Part D, Public Law 111-5.

[55] National Cancer Institute (US). NCI Metathesaurus [Internet]; 2015. Available from: <http://ncimeta.nci.nih.gov/ncimbrowser/>.

[56] U.S. National Library of Medicine. Unified medical language system [Internet]; 2015. Available from: <http://www.nlm.nih.gov/research/umls/>.

[57] U.S. National Library of Medicine. SNOMED clinical terms [Internet]; 2015. Available from: <http://www.nlm.nih.gov/research/umls/Snomed/snomed_main.html>.

[58] US Code of Federal Regulations. Other requirements relating to uses and disclosures of protected health information. 45 C.F.R. § 164.514(e)(1).

[59] US Code of Federal Regulations. Other requirements relating to uses and disclosures of protected health information. 45 C.F.R. § 164.514(b)(2).

[60] US Code of Federal Regulations. Other requirements relating to uses and disclosures of protected health information. 45 C.F.R. § 164.514(b)(1).

[61] Sledge G, Hudis C, Swain S, Yu PM, Mann JT, Hauser RS, et al. ASCO's approach to a learning health care system in oncology. J Oncol Pract 2013;9:145–8.

[62] American Society of Clinical Oncology (US). ASCO teams with multinational software corporation, SAP, to develop CancerLinQ™ [Internet]; 2015. Available from: <https://connection.asco.org/magazine/features/cancerlinq%E2%84%A2-takes-big-leap-forward>.

[63] SAP (US). Medical research insights. [Internet]; 2015. Available from: <http://www.sap-innovationcenter.com/2013/09/19/medical-research-insights/>.

[64] Conquer Cancer Foundation (US) [Internet]; 2015. Available from: <http://www.conquercancerfoundation.org/>.

[65] Miller RS. Electronic health record certification in oncology: role of the certification commission for health information technology. J Oncol Pract 2011;7:209–13.

[66] Health Level Seven International (US). HL7/ASTM implementation guide for CDA® R2 -Continuity of Care Document (CCD®) release 1 [Internet]; 2015. Available from: <http://www.hl7.org/implement/standards/product_brief.cfm?product_id=6>.

[67] Consolidated CDA Overview. Available from: <http://www.healthit.gov/policy-researchers-implementers/consolidated-cda-overview>. [accessed 05.03.15].

[68] Warner JL, Maddux SE, Hughes KS, Krauss JC, Yu PP, Shulman LN, et al. Development, implementation, and initial evaluation of a foundational open interoperability standard for oncology treatment planning and summarization. J Am Med Inform Assoc 2015;22:577–86.

[69] Health Level Seven International (US). HL7 version 3 standard: representation of the health quality measure format (eMeasure) DSTU, release 2 [Internet]; 2015. Available from: <http://www.hl7.org/implement/standards/product_brief.cfm?product_id=97>.

[70] Yu PP. Knowledge bases, clinical decision support systems, and rapid learning in oncology. J Oncol Pract 2015;11:e206–11.

[71] American Society of Clinical Oncology, Institute for Quality (US). Practice guidelines [Internet]; 2015. Available from: <http://www.instituteforquality.org/practice-guidelines>.

[72] U.S. Department of Health & Human Services. Federal policy for the protection of human subjects ("common rule"). [Internet]; 2015. Available from: <http://www.hhs.gov/ohrp/humansubjects/commonrule/>.

[73] Schilsky RL, Michels DL, Kearbey AH, Yu PP, Hudis CA. Building a rapid learning health care system for oncology: the regulatory framework for CancerLinQ™. J Clin Oncol 2014;32:2373–9.

2

Reducing Cancer Disparities Through Community Engagement: The Promise of Informatics

April Oh PhD, MPH[1], Wen-ying Sylvia Chou PhD, MPH[1], Devlon Jackson PhD, MPH[1], Samuel Cykert MD[2], Nora Jones MS[3], Jennifer Schaal MD[3], Euginia Eng PhD, MPH[4] and CommunityRx[5]

[1]Health Communication and Informatics Research Branch, Division of Cancer Control and Population Science, National Cancer Institute, Rockville, MD, United States [2]NC AHEC Program, UNC School of Medicine, Chapel Hill, NC, United States [3]The Partnership Project, Greensboro, NC, United States [4]Gillings School of Global Public Health, University of North Carolina Chapel Hill, Chapel Hill, NC, United States [5]University of Chicago Medicine, University of Chicago, Chicago, IL, United States

OUTLINE

Section 1: Public Health Informatics: Implications on Cancer Health Disparities — 24

2.1 Introduction — 24

2.2 Cancer Health Disparities: An Overview — 24

2.3 The Role of PHIs in Addressing Cancer Health Disparities — 25

Section 2: CBPR to Inform the Practice of PHIs to Address Health Disparities — 27

Section 3: Examples of Public Health and Health Informatics — 29

2.4 Example 1: Community Engagement and the Accountability for Cancer Care Through

Undoing Racism and Equity Trial (ACCURE Project) — 29

2.5 Example 2: PHIs and the Chicago CommunityRx Innovation — 32

Section 4: Discussion — 34

2.6 Challenges for the Field — 35

2.7 Strengths of PHI Applications in Health Disparities — 36

List of Acronyms and Abbreviations — 37

References — 38

B. Hesse, D. Ahern & E. Beckjord: Oncology Informatics.
DOI: http://dx.doi.org/10.1016/B978-0-12-802115-6.00002-1

SECTION 1: PUBLIC HEALTH INFORMATICS: IMPLICATIONS ON CANCER HEALTH DISPARITIES

2.1 INTRODUCTION

Cancer is a major cause of death in the United States, causing nearly one in four deaths [1]. Although overall cancer mortality rates have decreased, significant disparities in outcomes across the care continuum continue to persist. From delayed diagnosis to poorer survival rates, cancer health disparities across racial/ethnic and socioeconomic groups exist for numerous cancer sites. These differences in incidence, prevalence, mortality, and overall burden of cancer can be addressed through public health and cancer control efforts, such as screening or lifestyle behavior (smoking, diet, exercise) modifications for lung, colorectal, breast, and cervical cancers [1,2]. With the growth in technology, widespread use of the Internet, mobile technology, and changing technology policies in the United States, public health informatics (PHIs) offers a unique lever to identify, address, and reduce cancer health disparities. Defined as "the systematic application of information and computer science and technology to public health practice, research, and learning," [3] PHIs can support real-time data collection to immediately target health disparities when they occur; foster new approaches to health communication; and accelerate implementation and delivery of cancer control interventions. With the goal of addressing cancer health disparities using PHIs, principles, and lessons learned in community-based participatory research (CBPR)—an approach that employs community engagement for social justice and equality—we are poised to inform the use and adoption of these applications.

In this chapter, we will (1) provide an overview of cancer health disparities and describe the role of PHIs in addressing disparities; (2) discuss the application of the CBPR approach and its underlying principles to improve the use and adoption of informatics tools and platforms; and (3) present two case examples demonstrating the use of CBPR approaches in the development and deployment of PHIs to address cancer health disparities. The discussion highlights a new paradigm of PHIs that promotes community–clinical linkages to address health disparities and social determinants of health. This paradigm hinges on community engagement to enable informatics to act as a bridge between traditional public health and health care sectors with community partners. Engagement can create opportunities to identify, address, and promote participation with disparate communities. This type of engagement can be achieved by providing greater access to health information, identifying system efficiencies to address health needs, reducing information inequalities, surveillance of root causes of health disparities, and enhancing acceptability and effectiveness of public health and health care interventions.

2.2 CANCER HEALTH DISPARITIES: AN OVERVIEW

Data on national, state, and local levels continue to document cancer disparities across a variety of outcomes. On the national level, the Centers for Disease Control and Prevention (CDC) and the American Cancer Society (ACS) both monitor the trends and patterns of cancer incidence and mortality and identify populations disproportionately affected by the disease. According to the widely cited ACS 2015 Cancer Facts and Figures report, education attainment—a proxy measure for socioeconomic level—continues to be a predictor of cancer outcomes. For instance, among both Black and non-Hispanic White men, those with 12 or fewer years of education have nearly three times higher cancer mortality rates than those of college graduates for all cancers combined and four to five times higher for lung cancer. Moreover, racial and ethnic minorities are disproportionately affected by cancer burden: for example, non-Hispanic Black (henceforth Black) men and women are more likely to die from cancer than any racial or ethnic group. Hispanics and Asian and Pacific Islanders (APIs) have the highest rates for cancers of the liver and stomach due to a higher prevalence of infection with hepatitis B virus and *Helicobacter pylori*, respectively. Geographic location is another factor contributing to disparities. For example, lung cancer shows the most striking variation by state: death rates are more than threefold higher in Kentucky than in Utah (27 and 16 per 100,000 in men and women, respectively) [4].

Cancer health disparities are found across the cancer control continuum from prevention and early detection (eg, colorectal cancer (CRC) screening uptake); to treatment (eg, collecting patient-reported outcomes and physicians treatment recommendations to clinical trial participation); and to cancer survivorship and end-of-life care. Below we highlight a few examples to illustrate the wide range of disparities and possible ways informatics can help address the identified problems.

Differences in the utilization of cancer screening tests contribute to disparities in cancer outcomes. In the United States, African Americans have the highest incidence and mortality from CRC among all racial/ethnic groups, and studies have shown that this alarming rate is largely attributable to lower CRC screening uptake. A recent systematic review identified barriers to CRC screening in African Americans across patient-, provider-, and system-levels [5]. Technology-mediated opportunities (such as provider reminders based on electronic medical records (EMRs)) can potentially address these barriers.

Another domain of cancer health disparities lies in inequitable care and poor communication during treatment. Patients with limited health literacy tend to have lower self-efficacy in health care settings, and at the same time, providers are less effective in communicating with limited health literacy individuals. For example, disparities in breast cancer treatment have been documented, and much of the disparities are attributable to suboptimal patient–provider communication about treatment options [6].

Providers' recommendation/discussion of available clinical trial options is another domain of communication with documented disparities, particularly across race/ethnicity groups and geographic locations [7,8]. Moreover, failure to accurately and timely assess symptoms and measure patient's health-related quality-of-life (HRQOL) during treatment also result in disparities in outcomes. In the case of prostate cancer treatment, for example, many men feel uneasy or embarrassed to report bothersome urinary, sexual, and bowel symptoms. As a solution to address these barriers in communication, a user-centered, web-based design was used to develop graphic dashboards for symptoms reporting [9]. However, while such informatics-based solutions are beginning to be tested in clinical settings, they have not been tested on or tailored for patients who could potentially benefit most from technology-mediated, low-barrier reporting format and platform, namely those with limited health literacy. The next logical step is to extend such dashboards for symptoms reporting to limited health literacy patients and caregivers.

Equally important to note are the cancer health disparities that persist after the posttreatment phase. Evidence-based recommendations, such as survivorship care planning [10]. and efforts at integrating palliative care into routine cancer care tend to be adopted and implemented first in clinical settings and communities dominated with higher socioeconomic status and better support systems. Alternatively, underserved populations, often of limited digital and health literacy, may be less likely to benefit from technology-mediated cancer survivorship support.

While the above-mentioned examples illustrate the extent and persistence of cancer health disparities, much of the evidence is superficial at best in that they focus on downstream effects rather than root causes. Over the last decade, the field of social epidemiology has shed light on many of the fundamental causes of health disparities, and they tend to be multilevel and multifactorial [11,12]. Essentially, social determinants of health are the "root" or fundamental causes of many racial/ethnic and socioeconomic health disparities. These social determinants pertain to the circumstances in which people are born, grow up, live, work, and age, and include the systems put in place to deal with health and illnesses. These circumstances are in turn shaped by a wider set of forces, including economics, social policies, and politics. For example, social epidemiologists have found that poverty, low levels of education, lower social status, and income inequality are linked with higher mortality and poor health, with stronger evidence regarding some conditions [13–15]. Neighborhood conditions (including deprivation, poor housing, violence, and other stressors) are also associated with worse health status [16,17].

Documented social inequalities, availability, affordability, and quality of health care, plus increasing income gaps in the United States have all contributed to cancer health disparities. Indeed, taking a social epidemiologic view, access to mammography facilities [18]; cancer information inequalities [19]; differential cancer knowledge and awareness [20] (eg, clinical trials [21]); and cancer preventative behaviors [22] have all been observed to vary systematically by socioeconomic characteristics (eg, income, education and employment); social structure (eg, discrimination [23]); and social policies and institutions. Not surprisingly, the quality of the social and built environment is significantly associated with disparities in cancer outcomes including survival (eg, access to health facilities, social capital) [24].

While there is ample documentation of cancer health disparities including federal reports, what remains understudied are ways to reduce disparities through innovative, technology-mediated approaches in public health [25,26]. Reducing disparities through public health practice and applied prevention research, enabled by PHIs, requires multilevel intersecting factors. In a review of cancer control interventions, Simmons argues that the length of time it takes for public health research findings to be translated into practice has created a national urgency to design and deliver effective interventions and apply prevention research that engages disparities communities. This emphasis for research translation, implementation, and application has also been emphasized by the US Department of Health and Human Services (DSS) on public health importance and impact [27] and at the National Cancer Institute (NCI) [28–30]. In the following section, we will illustrate the crucial role PHI is poised to play in facilitating programs and services toward the goal of reducing cancer health disparities.

2.3 THE ROLE OF PHIs IN ADDRESSING CANCER HEALTH DISPARITIES

PHI has the potential to create a positive effect on the determinants across the cancer care continuum—etiology, prevention, early detection, treatment, and posttreatment survivorship. Broadly conceptualized, these effects can be the result of a wide range of activities from helping individuals avoid exposure to risky substances, affecting positive behavioral change, and enabling and optimizing cancer treatment to offering social and psychological support that are essential to both decision making and quality of life for cancer survivors. The section begins by outlining the context of current applications of PHI, moving to define and characterize PHI, and ending with an illustration of the four domains in which PHI plays a key role. Challenges to implement PHI will be discussed at the conclusion of the section.

Several current trends in communication and policy environment support a timely application of PHI endeavors. Specifically, the communication environment has exploded with growing penetration of the Internet and mobile technologies. As of 2014, the US Internet penetration rate was reported at 87%; more than 90% of adults have a cell phone and 58% of adults have a smartphone; and 84% of households own a computer, with 73% of US households having broadband connection [31,32]. A recent review of Internet communication pointed to a growing number of areas where technology has enabled communication via e-mail, instant messaging, voice-over Internet protocol, multimedia web-based information, chat rooms, bulletin boards, and e-commerce [33]. In addition to general technology-mediated opportunities, there is evidence that the "digital divide" by race and ethnicity is decreasing in the advent of Internet and mobile technologies and there are narrower gaps in cell phone and computer ownership across populations. For example, US Latino and Black adults are equally likely as Whites to own a smartphone—49%, 50%, versus 46%, respectively [34]. Latino and Black internet users are more likely than White internet users to go online through a mobile device—76% and 73% versus 60%, respectively. Among internet users, similar shares of Latinos (68%), Whites (66%), and Blacks (69%) say they use social networking sites such as Twitter and Facebook. These trends suggest great promises in using PHI to reach and engage with minorities and underserved populations.

In addition to the changing communication environment, the health policy environment is also supportive of PHI, particularly through greater support of clinical–community linkages. Current federal policies and programs related to health information technology (HIT) emphasize the role of disease prevention and control and access to health care and health information for all communities. The passage of the Patient Protection and Affordable Care Act (ACA) in 2010, regulatory pressures, federal incentives for electronic health record (EHR) adoption, and meaningful use in combination with market demand have helped push toward development,

integration, and application of IT tools; improve the flow of health information; and reduce systems-related inefficiencies. The reorganization of delivery and payment systems for value-based accountability in health care service delivery is helping drive the demand for increased HIT to support care coordination and care management. Providers will be increasingly accountable for managing and coordinating the care provided to patients across multiple settings.

Moreover, the ACA emphasizes a shift toward population health perspectives and greater integration of clinical and community environments. As part of the ACA, all nonprofit hospitals are required to conduct a Community Health Needs Assessment (CHNA) once every 3 years to maintain their tax-exempt status and avoid a financial penalty.[1] Hospitals conducting a CHNA are required to take into account input from persons who represent the broad interests of the community served by the hospital, including those with public health expertise. The rules also require that each hospital make its CHNA widely available to the public.[2] Additionally, the CHNA must be accompanied by a Community Health Implementation Plan (CHIP) based on the needs that emerge from the assessment. This plan must address the identified needs or explain why those needs are not addressed in the CHIP. Ultimately, this legislation forges a new role for health care to move toward population health and greater linkage between clinical and community settings for which PHI can help to facilitate.

In light of this favorable communication and policy environment, there are several ways that PHI can be leveraged to alleviate disparities. These include: (1) identifying health disparities in real time by offering surveillance tools for collecting community and population health needs; (2) disseminating health information to reduce disparities and associated information inequalities; and (3) redistributing deidentified personal information and health data previously collected for other purposes. Public health seeks to intervene on the social conditions and systems that affect everyone within a community. It also identifies and serves communities suffering disproportionately from disparities [3,35–37]. The collection and processing of population health data creates the information basis for knowledge in public health. Knowledge about disease trends, inequalities, and disparities in health behaviors, outcomes, and other threats to community health can improve program

[1]http://www.irs.gov/Charities-&-Non-Profits/Charitable-Organizations/New-Requirements-for-501(c)(3)-Hospitals-Under-the-Affordable-Care-Act.

[2]78 Fed, Reg, 20523 (proposed April 5, 2013) (to be codified at 26 CFR pts 1,53).

planning, decision making, and care delivery. With the advance in technology and the greater connectivity of racial and ethnic populations, the reach and potential for broader engagement of populations that were traditionally thought of as "unreachable" or "hidden" populations, can now be engaged to exchange information and reduce inequalities in information access. In PHI, it is also possible that in real time, targets can be identified across the cancer control continuum. This information is critical for identifying where, when, and with whom disparities occur across the cancer control continuum and possibly causes that are modifiable. It can also serve to monitor progress and improvements of public health interventions to reduce disparities. Health information systems, facilitated by PHI, offer the capacity to collect, store, analyze, monitor, interpret, and communicate population health data and information. Furthermore, because the causes of health disparities span multiple sectors, the ability of informatics to process and integrate multiple data sources offers an advantage to elucidate causes of disparities, beyond what one source of data could do alone.

PHI focuses on the promotion of health and disease prevention in populations and communities. Information technology (web, mobile, HIT) is a key part of PHI efforts as it provides resources and enabling tools for data integration and analysis of multiple sources (eg, geospatial, temporal, health) over time and in "real time" to inform intervention development that is context-specific and timely [38]. Informatics allows data from multiple sources to more efficiently and quickly identify major health threats, needs, and gaps so that communities can then benefit from opportunities for early intervention.

Benefits of PHI can span across community, hospital, and population levels. For hospitals, informatics can process individual clinical and other health information on patients that can be evaluated at the community level by public health departments. For population surveillance, PHI can improve population health data collection, rapidly and routinely deliver timely and emergent information to community clinicians on urgent public health issues, and assist and facilitate cross-organizational, institutional, and jurisdictional data collection and sharing. For providers, PHI can be a source of population-based analysis of individual disease data to provide improved trends to providers. For communities, PHI can return information from previously collected data sets into accessible forms of information for personal or community benefit [39].

There are several issues in PHI that can challenge its implementation. These challenges include issues of data privacy and security with individual-level data. Systems need to have enough security parameters in place to ensure privacy protection. Hospitals and physicians may also be reluctant to share data because of concerns of competition with other hospitals or provider networks. Some hospitals may perceive their clinical data as proprietary and essential to internal strategic planning. There are also data processing challenges, including identifying algorithms, decision tools, or types of data and queries that particular stakeholders and communities need. CBPR offers an approach that could potentially address these challenges throughout the identification, development, and implementation of PHIs. Section 2 illustrates how principles of CBPR can inform PHI practice.

SECTION 2: CBPR TO INFORM THE PRACTICE OF PHIs TO ADDRESS HEALTH DISPARITIES

Leveraging PHIs in addressing cancer health disparities requires "putting the public first" [40]. Public health approaches can help enhance the reach and utility of informatics platforms. In particular, a well-known and widely adopted public health framework, CBPR, emphasizes "equitable" engagement of partners throughout the research process from problem definition, data collection and analysis, dissemination, and use of findings to affect change [41,42]. This extensive collaboration between researchers and community members (individuals, organizations, agencies, etc.) is the hallmark of CBPR. Grounded in values of social justice and human rights, this approach has been applied in the promotion of health equity. CBPR combines culturally relevant knowledge and action for social change and social justice [43–46]. Applying these approaches within the design, delivery, and implementation of informatics-based interventions blends social determinants, communications, and engaged research methodologies to address cancer health disparities.

CBPR orientation to research has been well described and documented in numerous publications [41,47,48]. For addressing cancer health disparities, CBPR offers a strategy for addressing both "distributive justice" (equal protection and equitable and fair distribution of burdens and resources) and procedural justice (fairness in decision-making processes, especially with traditionally marginalized communities) [47]. It involves researcher-community collaboration from the onset and conceptualization of the goals and purposes of the collaboration and project, continuing throughout the project, and extending through the dissemination of the findings. The underlying rationale for community-engaged research includes ecological perspectives that recognize that lifestyles, behaviors, and disease incidence and epidemiology are shaped by social, physical, and policy environments. Important principles to consider in applying CBPR in cancer informatics include: (1) defining the community;

(2) developing a shared trust and goals in community partners; and (3) shared values for continuous engagement and collaboration by all partners. CBPR's focus on community engagement offers several advantages to improve application of PHIs, as illustrated below.

Agenda Setting and Role of Informatics—CBPR at its core seeks to contextualize interventions to enhance external and internal validity. It does so by incorporating local cultural knowledge to the social ecological models that recognize the intersection and bidirectional relationship with multiple levels of intersecting factors to influence health. Community engagement through outreach, consultation, and involvement can direct the focus of the project from the initiation process to identifying funding sources. Because informatics is an approach that extends beyond one-to-one to one-to-many, there is also the advantage that broader input on agenda and faster consensus can be reached.

Design and Delivery—PHI systems can have greater uptake and be more effective if there is enhanced usability and design. Challenges in informatics systems include developing a system that can handle a large volume of data inputs and outputs while also considering the usability of the design at the start of development. Usability facilitates use and systems adoption into existing workflows and delivery platforms. To develop and test platform usability, community partners and end users need to be engaged early in the process to inform design, tools, types of data collected, quality, analysis and dissemination, and implementation. The platforms are likely to be more rapidly adopted and implemented if "buy-in" by stakeholders and community members has already occurred. This is where principles of "user-centered design" are key: the design and evaluation process that focuses centrally on the intended user—what they will do with the product, where and how they will use it, and what features will be the most essential [49]. Incorporation of cultural beliefs and practices [50], mental models of illness, power differentials, and language barriers will all influence the design of any user-focused HIT system and its success [51]. Recognition of local culture, expertise, capacity, and history will enhance the usability of technology within the contexts and sociocultural norms and behaviors to promote a more community-focused design, versus a "one size fits all" approach that may not acknowledge local assets or barriers to implementation and ultimate effectiveness of the technology. If these factors are not included or considered in the design of patient- and community-focused platforms, then it is possible that the platform, at worse, could exacerbate disparities and at minimum, result in failure for minority and/or racial ethnic groups to use the platform and understand its purpose.

Implementation and Continuous Improvement—CBPR can improve the way PHI is implemented to achieve joint goals for change, organizational and community capacity for change, and maintenance or sustainability. One of the advantages of informatics systems, particularly those that collect and process data, is that there is the possibility to collect information in real time. For example, with EHRs, informatics can process medical record data to determine how many patients have received the human papillomavirus (HPV) vaccination and those that have not. Taking this data back to community members, providers, and patients is a way to understand barriers to vaccination. Sharing and discussing platforms may also identify new needs and can inform continuous quality and performance improvement. Sharing data collected and allowing for shared ownership of information may identify new strategies for improvement and can provide qualitative data context to quantitative data outcomes and reduce disparities in information access.

Ethical Considerations—Exchange of health and personal information data raises privacy, legal, and security concerns. In fact, this remains a key barrier in implementation [52]. In a survey of patients who were repeat users of personally controlled health records, reluctance for public health data sharing was associated with concerns that information would not remain anonymous (47.2%), lack of trust in government agencies to treat information with sensitivity (41.5%), and possible discrimination (24%) [53]. For disparate communities, to acknowledge the historical experience with racism, discrimination (racial/ethnic, religious, immigration, gender, sexual orientation), and inequalities in information and power can help to build relationships and trust. Recognition of these factors can be a part of a conversation to ensure that there is equality in the process and that data used and processed in informatics will be used for community and patient benefit.

For African Americans, the past injustices that include slavery, segregation, distrust of the health care system as a consequence of a 40-year-long Tuskegee Syphilis research study [54], distrust between minority communities and research institutions [55], and documented experiences of racism, bias, and discrimination in science and ethics of using personal data [56] and health care treatment [25] all influence the power dynamic between organizations and agencies and community members. These dynamics can influence the nature or relationships between research and health institutions and the community members, ultimately impacting the acceptability of any PHI intervention. Involving the community can ensure that PHI efforts appropriately and sensitively acknowledge the legacy of these negative lived experiences. Other racial, ethnic, sexual orientation, and religious discrimination in this country can impact trust in data and information systems for other racial/ethnic minority groups. Fear of deportation among undocumented Hispanics can also create distrust between Hispanic patients and providers, and in a study comparing communications-related factors between patients and providers, Asian Americans were the least likely to feel doctors understood their beliefs and that their doctors looked down on them [57]. These two examples in Hispanic and Asian American communities illustrate some challenges in trust and acceptability of sharing and exchanging health information.

Public Involvement in Health, Research, and Science— Community engagement in PHIs offers the ability to broadly engage the public in their health, research, and science. Relationships developed can build capacity to improve health. This includes developing skills, sharing, and exchanging resources. Capacity building can also include sharing knowledge, and leadership. Capacity building is especially important in informatics, as there may be inequalities in availability of technological expertise, financial resources, and staffing. Power imbalances will have to be acknowledged in the history, culture, social, political, and economic environments in which partners are embedded. Incorporating this knowledge and using this to build local capacity to inform, use, and deliver informatics-based cancer interventions will be instrumental to local acceptance, implementation, and buy-in.

Community Organizations and Movement Toward Population Health—PHIs core function lies in its reliance to be able to share and communicate information across organizations, individuals, hospitals at the local and state levels, and partnerships with multiple organizations. Collaboration with multiple organizations will require some new organizational capacity and there is the opportunity to build shared leadership, pool resources and expertise, and share reporting requirements and organizational burden. Today, with greater advances in technology, adoption of EHRs, and growing familiarity and acceptance of technology, more hospitals, community groups, and public health departments are exchanging information internally and externally. This trend has been increasing since 2008 [58].

SECTION 3: EXAMPLES OF PUBLIC HEALTH AND HEALTH INFORMATICS

The following section illustrates two PHI initiatives using a CBPR approach to address two major social determinants of health disparities: institutional racism and information inequalities. *Community Engagement and the Accountability for Cancer Care through Undoing Racism and Equity Trial* (ACCURE) uses a CBPR approach to develop an informatics platform to identify cases of unequal treatment or medical bias based on race. In *Public Health Informatics and the Chicago CommunityRx Innovation*, community engagement is employed for

data collection, and implementation and delivery of this information back to the community members to reduce information inequalities.

2.4 EXAMPLE 1: COMMUNITY ENGAGEMENT AND THE ACCOUNTABILITY FOR CANCER CARE THROUGH UNDOING RACISM AND EQUITY TRIAL (ACCURE PROJECT)

The "Accountability for Cancer Care through Undoing Racism and Equity" (ACCURE) study is an ongoing intervention trial designed to maximize care for all and attenuate treatment disparities between White and African American patients with Stage 1 or 2 breast or lung cancer. The project was created through an ongoing collaborative effort of a CBPR partnership, called the Greensboro Health Disparities Collaborative (GHDC). The partners are Hillman Comprehensive Cancer Center in Pittsburgh, Pennsylvania; Cone Health Cancer Center in Greensboro, North Carolina; The Partnership Project (TPP), an antiracism training organization in Greensboro; and investigators affiliated with the University of Pittsburgh Medical Center and the University of North Carolina's (UNC) Gillings School of Global Public Health and School of Medicine. ACCURE represents the latest step along a journey of community and academic engagement that was initiated by citizens of Greensboro concerned about "Unequal Treatment" as reflected in the 1999 Institute of Medicine (IOM) Report and their own lived experiences with race-specific inequities in care access, treatment, and outcomes among loved ones, friends, and neighbors.

As a result of adverse experiences with the health care system, and the support of the IOM report, TPP, a community organization dedicated to the work of antiracism led by the executive director Nettie Coad, decided to focus its energies on using the principles of Undoing Racism to address health disparities and began exploring how to do this. Although armed with strong observations and expertise in an historical perspective, provided by Undoing Racism Training, TPP was not equipped with the research training needed to focus the question, measure rigorously, and perform the analytics to thoroughly develop the case or methods for change.

As a first step in starting the health disparities research, TPP explored how to find a research partner. The Executive Director of the Moses Cone Community Foundation, who had completed the Undoing Racism Training, introduced Nettie Coad and her TPP staff to several investigators at UNC as potential academic collaborators. Dr. Eugenia Eng, a leader in the field of CBPR with a record of federally funded studies to understand and address health disparities, agreed to collaborate with TPP.

Together, they applied to the Moses Cone Community Foundation and received a planning grant to form a new collaborative that would integrate the principles of CBPR and Undoing Racism to design a study and apply for National Institutes of Health (NIH) funding that would engage community and academic partners in addressing racial disparities in health outcomes. With this planning grant, they convened local academic and community leaders, church leaders, and health care professionals to: (1) complete Undoing Racism training together; (2) apply the resulting common vocabulary to identify relevant concepts; (3) brainstorm research questions regarding poor health outcomes suffered by people of color in Greensboro, NC and the surrounding area; and (4) establish the GHDC.

The fledgling GHDC's first task was to promote relationship building among its diverse members (via age, race, religion, and profession) that included structured personal sharing, a memorandum of understanding (Full Value Contract) that emphasized safe and respectful communication, and a common language regarding race and ethnicity. This common language was built around the requirement that all GHDC members participate in formal Undoing Racism Training developed by The People's Institute for Survival and Beyond [59]. This highly rated workshop consists of 2 days of intensive, interactive dialogue and learning in five phases: (1) an exercise in shifting paradigms; (2) examination of the historical and present relationship of institutions with communities, power analysis, and creating a visual description of power relationships; (3) gatekeeping, accountability, and internalized racial oppression; (4) examination and definition of race and racism, and manifestations in our institutions linguistically, culturally, and individually; and (5) identification of institutional imposition of its values and culture on the communities they serve, and examination of internalized racial superiority. After 6 months of training in Undoing Racism and CBPR and an additional 6 months of exploring specific health concerns, GHDC forged a unanimous consensus that generating new knowledge on *why* disparities persist in cancer treatment and outcomes represented an important area of community and public health concern. Given the disproportionate breast cancer death rate among African American women despite a lower disease incidence, breast cancer was identified as the first GHDC research target. When approached about involvement in the research, the leadership of Cone Health Cancer Center enthusiastically supported the study and committed the Executive Director of its Cancer Center to GHDC membership.

Cone Health's commitment to GHDC allowed access to their cancer registry as a source of pilot data for more comprehensive work. These data were used to support an application to NCI for funding through the R21 mechanism to study the issue with more granularities by using the cancer registry more extensively and interviewing breast cancer patients about their breast cancer care interactions, experiences, and their ultimate completion of recommended care.

As a result, NCI funded the Cancer Care and Racial Equity Study (CCARES). Findings from the cancer registry portion of CCARES included:

- No significant difference between the 59% of African American women who received a lumpectomy compared to the 54% of Whitewomen.
- Likewise, the percentage of women who received a mastectomy was not significantly different by race (African American: 36%; White: 39%).
- However, uninsured women and women receiving Medicaid, regardless of race, were less likely to receive a lumpectomy (breast conserving surgery).

CCARES could not determine if the treatments received would be categorized as "reasonable care" as described in the National Comprehensive Cancer Network (NCCN) because the cancer registry for 2001 and 2002 did not record:

- Dates when chemotherapy and/or radiation started and ended, delayed, or discontinued care; and
- Each woman's comorbid illnesses.

At the same time, findings from qualitative Critical Incident Technique interviews with 52 White and African American patients revealed large gaps in information they received that contributed to delay or early termination of treatment completion and follow-up. CCARES findings were useful for two purposes: (1) Cone closed many of the information gaps in their cancer registry; and (2) the preliminary findings pointed to the need to increase transparency in cancer care.

In parallel to CCARES, Dr. Sam Cykert, a general internist and GHDC member, conducted an ACS-funded prospective cohort study exploring reasons for differences in lung cancer surgery between White and African American patients with early stage lung cancer. Cykert, a participant in Undoing Racism training, used principles of the training and GHDC advice in the design of the study. Findings, in this multicentered study with both community and academic health systems revealed an 11% difference in surgical rates between White and African American patients for this life-threatening and rapidly fatal disease. Published in the *Journal of the American Medical Association* in 2010, the results showed that there was no difference in treatment refusal according to race. Instead, African American patients with comorbid conditions almost never received surgery while similar White patients did, and African American patients without a regular source of care were only one-fifth as likely to pursue surgery. African American patients were also less likely to go to surgery if they perceived more difficult communication with their providers [60]. These findings revealed the need for increasing accountability for equity in cancer treatment outcomes.

The findings of CCARES and the Lung Cancer Surgery study were shared in detail with GHDC. Given the lack of documentation of breast cancer therapy completion in cancer registries, GHDC felt lack of transparency contributed substantially to cancer care disparities. With the discovery that African American patients with early stage lung cancer systematically received less aggressive therapy than their White counterparts, a lack of accountability and implicit bias were felt to also be component causes of more limited care for African Americans.

So how did informatics become a part of community engagement and the solution calculus for cancer disparities? When GHDC was applying the findings from these two studies to inform the design of a system change interventional approach to cancer disparities, several GHDC members were aware of the Health Information Technology for Economic and Clinical Health (HITECH) Act, the anticipated spread of EHRs, and the development of measures for EHR "meaningful use." GHDC's impression was that (1) transparency regarding the completion of cancer care needed to be measured, (2) a system of accountability needed to be established around achievement of care milestones, and (3) open communication of these measures to the providers and staff members of cancer centers needed to be established. By incorporating these change strategies and considering the new availability of digital data to aid systems of care and create measures, the intervention components for the ACCURE Trial were designed.

First, EHR and cancer registry data were combined to establish a 5-year baseline of treatment completion for African American and White patients that included completion of radiation and chemotherapy. Second, for prospectively enrolled patients, a real-time registry and warning system was established to track patients and identify both missed appointments and missed milestones of care. Third, a nurse navigator trained in the principles of antiracism and the literature on barriers to care for people of color was employed to reengage patients when any appointment was missed and submit inquiries to physician champions and specific providers regarding patients who had not met expected milestones of care. Fourth, all data, controlled for comorbidity, insurance status, and other important factors using quality improvement techniques are reported back to providers and cancer center staff to create an environment of total accountability and transparency. This feedback system is interwoven into a series of Healthcare Equity and Education Trainings for cancer center staff that include

not only the data described above but elements of antiracism training, vignettes on implicit bias, aggregate reports of prospective whole cancer center data, and results of qualitative surveys about patients' perceptions of their cancer care experience at crucial points of their care according to race. By including data on enrolled patients, qualitative data, and whole population data, it not only shows whether interventions improve the system of care for enrolled patients, but, more importantly, it measures whether the system is changing for everyone with the dose of exposure to feedback and Healthcare Equity and Education Training over time.

Another difficulty is that providers and staff are poorly informed about health disparities. They often attribute differences in care solely to insurance status or other socioeconomic factors. They cannot believe that disparities exist in their care environment and are generally altruistic and believe that race does not matter. With data feedback and Healthcare Equity and Education Training, this barrier tends to dissipate. Therefore, having EHRs and informatics systems that produce accurate, transparent, and reproducible measurement is paramount to establishing a culture of buy-in and change.

Part of the transparency of this process is that all data from GHDC community-engaged studies are presented periodically to the GHDC and less frequently aggregated data are presented to community stakeholders. Note that CCARES and ACCURE have led to the presentation of many abstracts at national meetings and several publications to date. As part of the initial memorandum of understanding, a publication committee as a subgroup of the GHDC was formed and every presentation and publication, including this chapter of this book, must be reviewed by the committee. This requirement to include partners in all aspects of research formulation, proposal writing, and dissemination ensures that GDHC produce work that is likely to move and affect the community, creates a learning environment for academic partners and community members, and maintains a relationship of equity and trust that nurtures continued research and needed solutions for system change [61]. The soundness of these methods has been borne out by the duration of this partnership as it move into its second decade of work. The image in Fig. 2.1 illustrates the joint involvement of partners in discussions of ACCURE data and information.

In conclusion, ACCURE is a product of a community–academic–medical CBPR partnership that began with the simplicity of open communication, personal sharing, and the unity of Undoing Racism Training. It has evolved into a research team that has incorporated EHRs and designed a sophisticated electronic, real-time registry system and Healthcare Equity and Education Training curriculum to combat multiple factors that perpetuate health disparities. Early results suggest that we

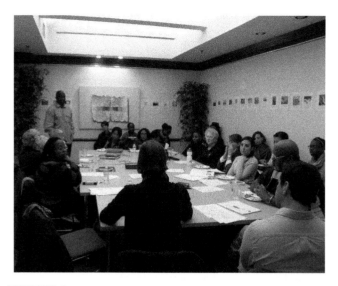

FIGURE 2.1 GHDC reviewing the latest ACCURE information. *Source: ACCURE.*

are on the right track but the full answer awaits further accrual and the full deployment of the ACCURE interventions.

2.5 EXAMPLE 2: PHIs AND THE CHICAGO COMMUNITYRX INNOVATION

CommunityRx Partners Alliance of Chicago Community Health Services, Chicago Health Information Technology Regional Extension Center at Northwestern University, Centers for New Horizons, Chicago Family Health Center, Friend Family Health Center, Greater Auburn Gresham Development Corporation, Near North Heath Services Corporation, and the University of Chicago. Gillian Feldmeth, Karen Lee, Stacy Lindau (Director, CommunityRx), and Doriane Miller contributed to authoring this chapter on behalf of the CommunityRx team. http://healtherx.org/about/project-staff for more information.

CommunityRx is an innovative multilevel program that provides patients, during the clinical encounter, with local and tailored community health resource information. At the core of this project is the application of informatics platforms that facilitate tailored access to data on community resources to meet health needs. This initiative also makes strides in the use of informatics to reduce health information inequalities, engage youth, and fuel economic development. This case example illustrates how an asset-based community-engaged research approach [62] facilitated the creation and delivery of an informatics platform to infuse personalized community resource information into the patient–provider clinical

encounter to address community health and vitality on the South Side of Chicago, IL.

The South Side of Chicago is approximately 95 square miles with 34 communities and more than 860,000 residents, with the predominant population identifying as African American (71%) [62]. The South Side has a rich history in African American culture, music, and community organizing. Despite its rich history, the community suffers from inequalities in access to basic resources and health compared to other areas in the City of Chicago [62].

In 2008, a multidisciplinary team of researchers with the South Side Health and Vitality Studies, supported by the University of Chicago Medicine Urban Health Initiative, partnered with community members and leaders toward the vision that Chicago's South Side would be a model of urban health by 2025. This model was envisioned to include a coordinated system of health care while actively engaging the community as a partner [62]. This partnership has been cultivated over time through a variety of engagement strategies, including outreach by the University of Chicago Center for Community Health and Vitality, and ongoing, collaborative meetings that were open to university researchers and community members, practitioners, and leaders. Community engagement was promoted via social networks, e-mail, social media, websites, earned and sponsored media, and data sharing. Following a series of community meetings in 2008–09, the group generated three major principles for partnership: (1) adopt a broad definition of health that incorporates economic vitality; (2) engage and employ local youth in scientific research; and (3) produce and quickly deliver meaningful data back to the community. These principles undergird all of the work of the South Side Health and Vitality Studies and led to the creation of CommunityRx (see Fig. 2.2).

The asset-based community-engaged research approach [62] was adopted as a blend of principles from CBPR and the Asset-Based Community Development (ABCD) approach widely used by community practitioners for urban development [63]. The relationships between partners and the continuous relationship and trust building are the kinetic energy that drive the actions of the collaboration. Once priorities are articulated, assets must be identified that can be leveraged to benefit the community's health and vitality. In contrast to the asset-based approach, the typical approach focuses on deficits and deprivation. The asset-based approach requires periodic reassessment of both community priorities and the quality of community engagement. Resolution of a priority happens when a sustainable solution is implemented.

Early on, when community and university collaborators with the South Side Health and Vitality Studies identified a desire to reach the 2025 goal, the team

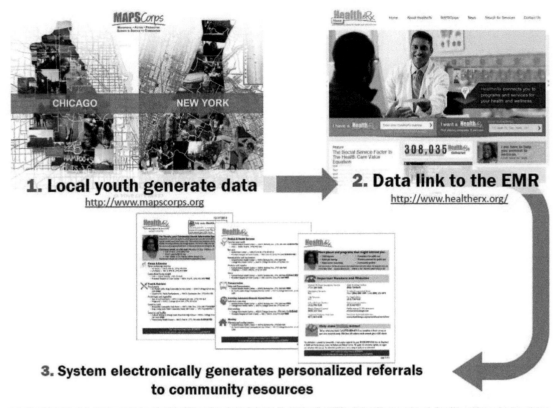

CommunityRx (ST Lindau, PI) is funded in part by a Health Care Innovation Award to the University of Chicago from the Department of Health and Human Services, Centers for Medicare and Medicaid Services (1C1CMS330997-02-00) and by Grant Number 1R01 AG 047869-01 from the National Institutes of Health/National Institute of Aging.

FIGURE 2.2   The Process to Generate a HealtheRx.

determined that it needed high-quality data on available assets, specifically on the community's built environment. The group decided that every business and organization, open and operating to serve the public, would be the target of a census to identify assets that could have a role in promoting health and/or vitality in the region. Everything was mapped—clinics, churches, grocery stores, schools, dry cleaners, liquor stores, and industrial parks. In the first year, 2009, students were employed to conduct the asset census. From these activities and the asset-based model, the Meaningful, Active, Productive Science in Service to Community (MAPSCorps) program emerged. MAPSCorps is one of two main components of CommunityRx (see Fig. 2.2, step 1).

MAPSCorps is a youth employment and science, technology, engineering, and mathematics (STEM) training program that pairs local high school youth with science-oriented college students to conduct an annual census of all open and operating businesses in the CommunityRx demonstration area on the South Side of Chicago [64]. The vision of MAPSCorps is to cultivate scientific minds, healthy bodies, and invested citizens from the assets of the community. The mission of MAPSCorps is to actively engage youth to produce meaningful asset data everyone can use [65]. MAPSCorps embodies the unifying principles of the community–university collaboration created by the South Side Health and Vitality Studies: hire and train youth, apply a broad definition of health, and gather and share meaningful data that everyone can use with the goals of advancing both health and economic vitality in the region.

To conduct the asset census, researchers and college student mentors train high school students to collect and classify community asset data. Students are equipped with web-enabled cell phones and use a custom MapApp™ tool for data entry. The MapApp™ tool includes an interface for data entry of each community asset identified, is searchable, and allows for real-time summaries of data collected. Within a 6-year period, this initiative has produced more than 100 square miles of data identifying active local businesses on the South and West sides of Chicago and has provided work experience and science training to 259 youth and 116 college students since 2009. MAPSCorps has also been replicated in Harlem and the Bronx, New York City in partnership with the Mount Sinai Adolescent Health Center and the New York State Health Foundation. In addition to employment and training in the data collection methods over a 6-week summer period, MAPSCorps stimulates youth interest in STEM fields through direct experience and mentorship.

By 2011, when the US Centers for Medicare & Medicaid Services (CMS) released the Health Care Innovation Challenge [66], the South Side Health and Vitality Studies team had accumulated 4 years of experience and data in large-scale urban asset mapping. The Innovation Challenge called for ideas that would improve health, improve health care, reduce health care costs, and contribute to developing the health care workforce of the future. The University of Chicago South Side Health and Vitality Studies team partnered with the Alliance of Chicago Community Health Services and the Chicago Health Information Technology Regional Extension Center at Northwestern University to develop CommunityRx. CommunityRx had two main components: technology and workforce. MAPSCorps was envisioned as the "workforce of the future" part of the innovation. The technology component was envisioned as "HealtheRx," an electronic prescribing technology that would integrate data about community assets with EMR platforms. In 2012, The University of Chicago received a Centers for Medicare & Medicaid Services Health Care Innovation Award (1C1CMS330997-01-00), leveraging MAPSCorps as the data engine for the health informatics solution, HealtheRx (see Fig. 2.2, step 2).

HealtheRx produces an electronically generated prescription for community services through an interface between the patient's EMR and the database of community health resources driven by MAPSCorps. Through an automated system, the patient's diagnoses, individual characteristics, and home address are matched with health and self-care programs and services in the CommunityRx database to generate a personalized list of local resources (Fig. 2.2, step 3). The HealtheRx prescription prints from the EMR during the regular medical workflow and is handed to the patient by a member of the health care team. Patients who live in 1 of 16 zip codes in the CommunityRx demonstration area can receive a HealtheRx from a physician or other health care provider at 33 clinical sites including outpatient clinics, community health centers, and emergency departments. Anyone can directly search for services on the public-facing HealtheRx website, www.healtherx.org.

In addition, anyone requiring assistance to understand their HealtheRx or in need of additional resources can contact a "community health information specialist" in their community. In the current CommunityRx model, information specialists are available by phone, e-mail, text, and for in-person consultation at one of two partnering community-based organizations, the Centers for New Horizons and the Greater Auburn Gresham Development Corporation. Besides providing support to people using a HealtheRx prescription or the HealtheRx website, the information specialists are responsible for keeping current the program and service information for every asset identified by MAPSCorps. Providing this additional support helps mitigate potential barriers in HIT, such as health literacy and access to Internet service. The Information Specialist Support Service, HealtheRx and MAPSCorps (www.mapscorps.org) websites and HealtheRx prescriptions are also provided in Spanish, according to the preference of the consumer.

During the Health Care Innovation Award demonstration period (2012–15), the CommunityRx innovation required several key steps that used the principles of rapid cycle iteration (RCI) and continuous quality improvement (CQI) to achieve a sustainable model: (1) iteration and expansion of MAPSCorps, including educating youth about HealtheRx and the impact of the data they collect on helping patients stay healthy; (2) continuous relationship and trust building with community-based partners, including execution of subcontracting arrangements, engagement in RCI and CQI processes, collaboration on building the sustainability model [67]; and (3) joint study and optimization of clinical workflows, including efficient training methods, to facilitate workflow redesign that aligned with other organizational priorities and adoption of the new HealtheRx prescribing function. In the current instance of CommunityRx, the HealtheRx prescription is printed and delivered with the after-visit/clinical visit summary. By providing these documents in tandem, patients' medical information is complemented by a practical list of resources near their homes that they can use to affect their wellness, self-care, caregiving, and disease self-management goals.

SECTION 4: DISCUSSION

The principles and approaches of CBPR can be challenging to implement or translate into practice, but the two case examples above offer concrete and practical approaches to facilitate the adoption of a CBPR approach in development and application of PHI to address health disparities, specifically focusing on two social determinants of cancer health disparities: institutional discrimination and information inequalities. In the following, we outline common themes that facilitated successful project implementation.

First, *transparency* was a major goal of both teams. Investing time to develop relationships, identify expectations and definitions, and establish values and systems for transparency and responsibility, while time intensive and at times, uncomfortable, are crucial to success. Both projects actively leveraged community partners in all activities (eg, using a community board for all decision making and actions, securing funding support) and activated partners in aspects of the design and implementation of projects. Transparency requires having defined expectations for members' respective roles and contributions, and continuous reevaluation of the roles and progress to build trust and capacity within communities. In both cases studies, the teams emphasized the relationship between partners at the crux of project initiation, development, and implementation. The ACCURE project used a memorandum of understanding between partners to establish goals, common language, and an emphasis on "safe and respectful communication." In the writing of this book chapter, both case studies emphasized that community partners would have the opportunity to review and comment on this chapter as authors.

Another major objective in both cases was *making data relevant* to community users. Both projects enabled the users access to informatics-informed data and the ability to interpret the data in the context of their own lives and experiences. In the case of CommunityRx, the team met with the community partners to determine that economic development was a key value, and the team incorporated this as one of the goals of the community partnership. This value resulted in the conceptualization of the MAPSCorps to promote job opportunities for students and residents of the community in data collection. Dissemination of available neighborhood services, in turn, stimulated the local economy by connecting residents with services and resources available within their community. In the ACCURE project, the EHR data were leveraged to produce accurate and transparent measurement of treatment disparities. Data produced from informatics systems that provided accurate, transparent, and reproducible information facilitated buy-in and changed provider attitudes about race and racism. Making "data talk" in this way was essential, as this was a community of providers who are generally altruistic and having data was the best way to communicate and dissipate any biases. In both cases, development of the informatics platforms both had an end-use target, but through the CBPR approach, dialogue with the community partners informed what data was important and how it was delivered.

A *capacity-building* component in both case studies was a common theme with training and learning opportunities embedded within the projects. Capacity building seeks to include the development of skills, resources, and organizational structure with an eye toward sustainability. It includes building leadership across all partners to represent the interests and local culture of where the work is taking place. In the ACCURE project, training and open dialogue to learn from content experts (from health care provider to community partners) to discuss and learn about health care bias and discrimination were essential to problem identification, acceptance, and participation in health care bias training. Within the CommunityRx case study, the emphasis on building the local economy and engagement of students and

youth within a research enterprise built local capacity and knowledge in conducting research. These capacity-building efforts fostered greater academic and local community partnerships. Too often, well-meaning community-based interventions cease as soon as the research period or financial resources diminish. Emphasis in both case studies on capacity-building offer opportunities for a new "pipeline" of interventions as well as potential momentum to continue projects post intervention.

The above themes all illustrate the importance of a *bottom-up approach* to data communication. Grassroots-oriented communication that share features of a CBPR approach have parallels with the emergence and rapid growth of social media, characterized by user-generated content. Many have argued that on social media platforms, information is increasingly "democratized" as individuals' voices are expressed and shared, and opinions crowdsourced without traditional information gatekeepers. Social marketing approaches have leveraged this new environment in delivering interventions (eg, health promotion messages) through existing networks and online influencers. Future PHI efforts may consider capitalizing on the changing communication environment to broaden and sustain community engagement. In this way, lessons from a CBPR approach have distinct and valuable parallels to the emerging social media landscape.

2.6 CHALLENGES FOR THE FIELD

Using PHIs to address cancer health disparities can be challenging for a number of reasons. First, some communities and geographic locations may not have adequate technology access, such as broadband and smartphones (eg, broadband access for rural hospitals, public health departments, and communities in those areas). Pew Research Center data show that in 2013, 15% of US adults did not use the Internet [68]. Older age, less education, lower income, and rural location are some of the significant factors associated with non-Internet access/use [68]. In addition to these factors, broadband availability can considerably affect an individual's Internet access. As of 2013, 20% of the US adult population does not have home broadband [69] and 19 million Americans reside in areas where broadband is not present [70]. Mobile technology is poised to serve as a link to connect individuals without Internet access—with more than 90% of cell phone penetration among US adults and high prevalence of using mobile phones to access the Internet, racial/ethnic populations often disproportionately affected by health disparities are more likely to have mobile access to the Internet [71]. One caveat is that those living in a rural location are less likely to have mobile phones, hence hindering the opportunity to access the Internet via these technologies [71]. Efforts are currently underway within the Federal Communications Commission (FCC) to modernize and expand its existing Lifeline Program to expand broadband access for low-income consumers [72].

Secondly, the community's overall health literacy and digital literacy may be limited. Individuals who lack digital health literacy may face additional obstacles in navigating health informatics platforms. Digital health literacy is defined as "meaning-making with health texts mediated by new technologies" [73]. Research has identified that factors such as low literacy and poor health status are associated with limited health literacy [74]. Considering the "Double Divide" due to gaps both in health literacy and Internet access/use, health disparities may potentially be exacerbated. Prior research has found that some populations' willingness to use PHI platforms is lower in comparison to other groups (racial/ethnic, gender-specific, etc.) [75]. Some reasons that may be attributed to low willingness to use the platforms are lack of time, feeling the platform is unnecessary, not user-friendly, etc. [76,77]. The CommunityRx project offers one example for addressing challenges with digital health literacy, where multiple avenues for disseminating community data are made available: during the clinical encounter, on the HealtheRx website, and information specialists who use and disseminate information during one-to-one encounters. The CommunityRx also offers a Spanish version so that the data could be accessed by Spanish language speakers. Informatics platform developers can identify potential digital health literacy barriers through community engagement as part of discussions in user-centered designs. These conversations can include aspects of readability, visual simplicity, language, and the logistics of Internet access [78]. Ideally, multiple options, as budget constraints allow, to share data across levels of literacy can be identified and modes of communication that facilitate access to informatics related data can be developed.

Moreover, there are challenges in sustained community investment, especially as the rapid advancement of technologies can be costly for communities to maintain. Logistical challenges exist for community health centers (many within a urban health care safety net system) in the development and implementation of informatics platforms. These include: availability of resources for informatics; organizational culture; disposition and capacity for HIT and implementation; HIT systems design and adaptability within extant workflows; provider and staff perceptions of utility; and unintended consequences of HIT implementation which slow the rate of deployment. The ACCURE project shared its early experiences with integration of multiple EHR systems from different vendors and some of the challenges of working with multiple provider groups. As the project evolved, solutions were developed to automate a system that included appropriate data downloads and processing, but the team learned to integrate intermittent manual checks. Interoperability challenges can be a barrier to automation of systems, however, with changing policies around meaningful use of EHR, new software and models for natural language processing, and emerging interoperability platforms, this barrier will likely diminish in the future [79]. Yet, for projects that may have budget constraints, this can be a timely process, and systems integration delays can create barriers and delays.

As PHI platforms become more widely adopted in multiple stakeholder settings, it is important to continuously evaluate the utility of systems in achieving intended goals and offering partners the voice and ability to give feedback on the systems as they use interfaces to ensure that the technology does not disrupt extant and evolving workflows. Successful community engagement would set the groundwork for buy-in from these stakeholders and ease the input of the organizational integration of the informatics system and on the output, the acceptability, and usability of data generated and disseminated from the system. The CommunityRx Project also offers a Spanish version.

2.7 STRENGTHS OF PHI APPLICATIONS IN HEALTH DISPARITIES

This chapter illustrates two major strengths of CBPR approaches to PHI applications to address health disparities in cancer control. The first is facilitation of community and clinical linkages (a well-established goal of CBPR but one that deserves renewed emphasis in PHI) to improve population health and the second is facilitation of a learning community health system.

PHI can expand the reach of traditional person-to-person interventions and data collection and dissemination efforts to a wider audience of individuals, communities, and organizations using information technology. There are many data sources that could be integrated and combined to generate and inform public health, from administrative, financial, and facility sources (eg, clinic, health system, community-based organizations) to clinical encounter, screening, registry, laboratory, and surveillance data. CBPR can be leveraged to identify what the right data, intervention, and target for PHI would be most appropriate to enhance buy-in. Efforts in developing PHI approaches can introduce new innovations and approaches that would previously not have been conceptualized without the partnership between PHI, hospitals, researchers and communities. CommunityRx provides one such example, but there are other examples and initiatives particularly in the area of integrating EMR data with community-level data to enhance community and clinical linkages. At the Ohio State University Wexner Medical Center, EHR data were enriched with community-level data on socioeconomic and obesogenic environmental factors to examine overweight and obesity in the patient population. Rather than collecting health data separately, which can be expensive, the data from two systems were integrated. The combination of these two systems created an opportunity for integrated data analysis to consider the patient's local environment in identifying clinical and nonclinical factors contributing to overweight and obesity. This type of information also offered the potential to enhance comparative effectiveness research by providing insights into why certain treatments were more or less effective based on patient context [80]. Contextual data like this at the individual level can enhance patient and provider communication and delivery of health information as socioeconomic and other factors within a patient's environment will likely influence, at minimum, adherence to any treatment recommendation. They also provide more information at a population level of the clinical and nonclinical factors that contribute to positive cancer outcomes.

A learning community health system is a system that incorporates multiple data sources to generate ongoing cycles of analysis for new knowledge to allow communities to have updated and tailored community health system feedback. The system is dynamic and will grow and change as it gains and responds to new knowledge. Similar to a learning *health* system, it is grounded in the recognition that community stakeholders have the power and expertise to get the right services and programs to communities when they need it and recognizes they are the owners of the data used to identify areas of improvement as well as areas of strengths. The secondary use of EHR data for identifying cases of racism in the ACCURE project and use of HER data to match patients with community resources to be healthy in their communities facilitate a learning health care system where the collective data from EHR and other outside data and resources were used to develop new insights and knowledge to directly address health disparities. In the CommunityRx case example, merging two systems—community data with patient EMR information—provided tailored information for each patient. In this learning community health system, the users were able to receive up-to-date and tailored information which received feedback and updates from community members working as part of MAPSCorps. A learning community health system also offers the potential for systems to be dynamic and spur innovation as new information and data are processed and knowledge is fed back to the system. One example of this potential is to identify syndemics or interactions between multiple diseases (eg, diabetes and cancer) and outcomes for disparities populations, in real time, with the contextual information of the community to identify the needs, and the assets that can be leveraged within communities to address these needs. This has been discussed as a new direction and key advantage of informatics platforms within public health.

As illustrated in this chapter, use of a CBPR model enhanced two PHI approaches that addressed social determinants and inequalities in cancer prevention and control. Success of partnerships cannot be assumed, most especially in dynamic health and community systems where varying budgets, diversity in regulations and accountability, and competing priorities will push and pull partners based on their demands. The sum total of these cases is that the choice to enter into PHI for addressing health disparities and inequalities, in itself should be community driven. Partnership and engagement enhances the success and acceptability for PHI interventions and allows for shared learning within community systems to address social determinants of health in cancer prevention and control.

LIST OF ACRONYMS AND ABBREVIATIONS

ABCD Asset-Based Community Development
ACA Affordable Care Act
ACCURE Accountability for Cancer Care through Undoing Racism and Equity
ACS American Cancer Society
API Asian and Pacific Islander
CBPR Community-based participatory research
CCARES Cancer Care and Racial Equity Study
CDC Centers for Disease Control and Prevention
CHIP Community Health Implementation Plan
CHNA Community Health Needs Assessment
CMS Centers for Medicare & Medicaid Services
CQI Continuous quality improvement
CRC Colorectal cancer
DHHS Department of Health and Human Services
EHR Electronic health record
EMR Electronic medical record
FCC Federal Communications Commission
GHDC Greensboro Health Disparities Collaborative
HIT Health information technology
HITECH Health Information Technology for Economic and Clinical Health
HPV Human papillomavirus
HRQOL Health-related quality-of-life
IOM Institute of Medicine
IT Information Technology
NCCN National Comprehensive Cancer Network
NCI National Cancer Institute
NIH National Institutes of Health
PHI Public health informatics
RCI Rapid cycle iteration
STEM Science, technology, engineering, and mathematics
TPP The Partnership Project
UNC University of North Carolina

References

[1] Siegel R, Ma J, Zou Z, Jemal A. Cancer statistics, 2014. CA Cancer J Clin 2014;64(1):9–29.

[2] Ward E, Jemal A, Cokkinides V, Singh GK, Cardinez C, Ghafoor A, et al. Cancer disparities by race/ethnicity and socioeconomic status. CA Cancer J Clin 2004;54(2):78–93.

[3] Yasnoff WA, O'Carroll PW, Koo D, Linkins RW, Kilbourne EM. Public health informatics: improving and transforming public health in the information age. J Public Health Manag Pract 2000;6(6):67–75.

[4] American Cancer Society. Cancer facts & figures 2015. Atlanta: American Cancer Society; 2015.

[5] Bromley EG, May FP, Federer L, Spiegel BM, van Oijen MG. Explaining persistent under-use of colonoscopic cancer screening in African Americans: a systematic review. Prev Med 2015;71C:40–8.

[6] Penner LA, Eggly S, Griggs JJ, Underwood III W, Orom H, Albrecht TL. Life-Threatening Disparities: The Treatment of Black and White Cancer Patients. J Soc Issues 2012;68(2).

[7] Battaglia TA, Ash A, Prout MN, Freund KM. Cancer prevention trials and primary care physicians: factors associated with recommending trial enrollment. Cancer Detect Prev 2006;30(1):34–7.

[8] Ramirez A, Wildes K, Talavera G, Napoles-Springer A, Gallion K, Perez-Stable E. Clinical trials attitudes and practices of Latino physicians. Contemp Clin Trials 2008;29(4):482–92.

[9] Izard J, Hartzler A, Avery DI, Shih C, Dalkin BL, Gore JL. User-centered design of quality of life reports for clinical care of patients with prostate cancer. Surgery 2014;155(5):789–96.

[10] Hewitt ME, Ganz PA, Institute of Medicine (U.S.) American Society of Clinical Oncology (U.S.) From cancer patient to cancer survivor: lost in transition: an American Society of Clinical Oncology and Institute of Medicine Symposium. Washington, DC: National Academies Press; 2006. vi, 189 pp.

[11] Warnecke RB, Oh A, Breen N, Gehlert S, Paskett E, Tucker KL, et al. Approaching health disparities from a population perspective: the National Institutes of Health Centers for Population Health and Health Disparities. Am J Public Health 2008;98(9):1608–15.

[12] Taplin SH, Anhang Price R, Edwards HM, Foster MK, Breslau ES, Chollette V, et al. Introduction: understanding and influencing multilevel factors across the cancer care continuum. J Natl Cancer Inst Monogr 2012;2012(44):2–10.

[13] Berkman LF, Kawachi I. Social epidemiology. New York, NY: Oxford University Press; 2000. xxii, 391 pp.

[14] Daniels N, Kennedy B, Kawachi I. Is inequality bad for your health?. Boston, MA: Beacon Press; 2001.

[15] Marmot MG, Wilkinson RG. Social determinants of health, 2nd ed. Oxford; New York, NY: Oxford University Press; 2006. x, 366 pp.

[16] Yen IH, Kaplan GA. Poverty area residence and changes in depression and perceived health status: evidence from the Alameda County Study. Int J Epidemiol 1999;28(1):90–4.

[17] Macintyre S, Ellaway A. Neighborhoods and health: an overview Kawachi I, Berkman L, editors. Neighborhoods and health. New York, NY: Oxford University Press; 2003.

[18] Zenk SN, Tarlov E, Sun JM. Spatial equity in facilities providing low- or no-fee screening mammography in Chicago neighborhoods. J Urban Health 2006;83(2):195–210.

[19] Ackerson LK, Viswanath K. The social context of interpersonal communication and health. J Health Commun 2009;14(Suppl. 1):5–17.

[20] Viswanath K, Breen N, Meissner H, Moser RP, Hesse B, Steele WR, et al. Cancer knowledge and disparities in the information age. J Health Commun 2006;11(Suppl. 1):1–17.

[21] Langford A, Resnicow K, An L. Clinical trial awareness among racial/ethnic minorities in HINTS 2007: sociodemographic, attitudinal, and knowledge correlates. J Health Commun 2010;15:92–101.

[22] Oh A, Shaikh A, Waters E, Atienza A, Moser RP, Perna F. Health disparities in awareness of physical activity and cancer prevention: findings from the National Cancer Institute's 2007 Health Information National Trends Survey (HINTS). J Health Commun 2010;15(Suppl. 3):60–77.

[23] Williams DR, Mohammed SA. Discrimination and racial disparities in health: evidence and needed research.. J Behav Med 2009;32(1):20–47.

[24] Shariff-Marco S, Yang J, John EM, Sangaramoorthy M, Hertz A, Koo J, et al. Impact of neighborhood and individual socioeconomic status on survival after breast cancer varies by race/ethnicity: the Neighborhood and Breast Cancer Study. Cancer Epidemiol Biomarkers Prev 2014;23(5):793–811.

[25] Smedley BD, Stith AY, Nelson AR. Unequal treatment: confronting racial and ethnic disparities in health care. Washington, DC: The National Academies Press; 2003.

[26] Quality AfHRa 2014 National healthcare quality and disparities report. Rockville, MD: Agency for Healthcare Research and Quality; 2015.

[27] 2020 HP. HealthyPeople.gov. Available from: <http://www.healthypeople.gov/>.

[28] Steinwachs D, Allen JD, Barlow WE, Duncan RP, Egede LE, Friedman LS, et al. NIH state-of-the-science conference statement: enhancing use and quality of colorectal cancer screening. NIH Consens State Sci Statements 2010;27(1):1–31.

[29] Neta G, Sanchez MA, Chambers DA, Phillips SM, Leyva B, Cynkin L, et al. Implementation science in cancer prevention and control: a decade of grant funding by the National Cancer Institute and future directions. Implement Sci 2015;10(1):4.

[30] Glasgow RE, Chambers DA, Cynkin L. News from the NIH: highlights in implementation science from the National Cancer Institute and the National Institute of Mental Health. Transl Behav Med 2013;3(4):335–7.

[31] Rainie LC, D'Vera. Census: Computer ownership, internet connection varies widely across U.S.; 2014 [cited 2014]. Available from: <http://www.pewresearch.org/fact-tank/2014/09/19/census-computer-ownership-internet-connection-varies-widely-across-u-s/>.

[32] Center PR. Mobile technology fact sheet; 2014. Available from: <http://www.pewinternet.org/fact-sheets/mobile-technology-fact-sheet/>.

[33] Eysenbach G. The impact of the Internet on cancer outcomes. Cancer J Clin 2003;53(6):356–71. Epub June 1, 2004.

[34] Lopez M, Gonzalez-Barrera A, Patten E. Closing the digital divide: Latinos and technology adoption; 2013 [cited 2013]. Available from: <http://www.pewhispanic.org/2013/03/07/closing-the-digital-divide-latinos-and-technology-adoption/>.

[35] Kraft M, Androwich I. Using informatics to promotes community/population health Mastrian DMK, editor. Nursing informatics and the foundation of knowledge. Sudbury, MA: Jones and Bartlett Publishers; 2009.

[36] Yasnoff WA. Introduction to PH informatics O'Carroll P, editor. Public health informatics and information systems. New York, NY: Springer-Verlag; 2003.

[37] Yasnoff WA, Overhage JM, Humphreys BL, LaVenture M, Goodman KW, Gatewood L, et al. A national agenda for public health informatics. J Public Health Manag Pract 2001;7(6):1–21.

[38] Kopp S, Schuchman R, Strecher V, Gueye M, Ledlow J, Philip T, et al. Public health applications Bashshur R, Mandil S, Shannon G, editors. Telemedicine/telehealth: an international perspective. Larchmont, NY: Mary Ann Liebert, Inc.; 2002.

[39] Institute PHI. Resources; 2015. Available from: <http://phii.org/resources/browse/topics>.

[40] Barclay G, Sabina A, Graham G. Population health and technology: placing people first. Am J Public Health 2014;104(12):2246–7.

[41] Minkler M, Wallerstein N. Community-based participatory research for health: from process to outcomes, 2nd ed. San Francisco, CA: Jossey-Bass; 2008. xxxv, 508 pp.

[42] Wilson N, Minkler M, Dasho S, Wallerstein N, Martin AC. Getting to social action: the Youth Empowerment Strategies (YES!) project. Health Promot Pract 2008;9(4):395–403.

[43] McCracken JL, Friedman DB, Brandt HM, Adams SA, Xirasagar S, Ureda JR, et al. Findings from the community health intervention program in South Carolina: implications for reducing cancer-related health disparities. J Cancer Educ 2013;28(3):412–9.

[44] Seifer SD, Michaels M, Collins S. Applying community-based participatory research principles and approaches in clinical trials: forging a new model for cancer clinical research. Prog Community Health Partnersh 2010;4(1):37–46.

[45] Simonds VW, Wallerstein N, Duran B, Villegas M. Community-based participatory research: its role in future cancer research and public health practice. Prev Chronic Dis 2013;10:E78.

[46] Wallerstein NB, Duran B. Using community-based participatory research to address health disparities. Health Promotion Practice 2006;7(3):312–23. Epub June 7, 2006.

[47] Israel B, Coomble C, Cheezum R, Schulz A, McGranaghan R, Lichtenstein R, et al. Community-based participatory research: a capacity-building approach for policy advocacy aimed at eliminating health disparities. Am J Public Health 2010;100(11):2094–102.

[48] Green LW, George MA, Daniel M, Frankish CJ, Herbert CP, Bowie WR, et al. Study of participatory research in health promotion. Ottawa, Ontario: Royal Society of Canada; 1995. p. 43–50.

[49] Morales R, Casper G, Brennan PF. Patient-centered design. The potential of user-centered design in personal health records. J Am Health Inf Manage Assoc 2007;78(4):44–6.

[50] Maliski SL, Connor S, Fink A, Litwin MS. Information desired and acquired by men with prostate cancer: data from ethnic focus groups. Health Educ Behav 2006;33(3):393–409.

[51] Valdez R, Brennan P. Medical informatics Gibbons M, editor. eHealth solutions for healthcare disparities. New York, NY: Springer-Verlag; 2008.

[52] Hung M, Conrad J, Hon S, Cheng C, Franklin J, Tang P. Uncovering patterns of technology use in consumer health informatics. Computat Stat 2013;5(6):432–47.

[53] Weitzman ER, Kelemen S, Kaci L, Mandl KD. Willingness to share personal health record data for care improvement and public health: a survey of experienced personal health record users. BMC Med Inform Decis Mak 2012;12:39.

[54] Gamble VN. Under the shadow of Tuskegee: African Americans and health care. Am J Public Health 1997;87(11):1773–8.

[55] Dancy BL, Wilbur J, Talashek M, Bonner G, Barnes-Boyd C. Community-based research: barriers to recruitment of African Americans. Nurs Outlook 2004;52(5):234–40.

[56] Skloot R. The immortal life of Henrietta Lacks, 1st ed. New York, NY: Broadway Paperbacks; 2011. xiv, 381 pp.

[57] Collins KS, Hughes D, Doty M, Ives B, Edwards J, Tenney K. Diverse communities, common concerns: assessing health care quality for minority Americans: The Commonwealth Fund; 2002.

[58] Foundation RWJ. Health information technology in the United States: Progress and challenges ahead, 2014; 2014.

[59] Yonas M, Jones N, Eng E, Vines A, Aronson R, Griffith D, et al. The art and science of integrating undoing racism with CBPR: challenges of pursuing NIH funding to investigate cancer care and racial equity. J Urban Health 2006;83(6):1004–12.

[60] Cykert S, Dilworth-Anderson P, Monroe M, Walker PS, McGuire F, Corbie-Smith G, et al. Modifiable factors associated with decisions to undergo surgery among newly diagnosed patients with early stage lung cancer. JAMA 2010;303(23):2368–76.

[61] Yonas M, Aronson R, Coad N, Eng E, Petteway R, Schaal J, et al. Infrastructure for equitable decision making in research Israel B, Eng E, Schulz A, Parker E, editors. Methods for community-based participatory research for health. San Francisco, CA: Josey-Bass; 2013.

[62] Lindau ST, Makelarski JA, Chin MH, Desautels S, Johnson D, Johnson Jr. WE, et al. Building community-engaged health research and discovery infrastructure on the South Side of Chicago: science in service to community priorities. Prev Med 2011;52(3-4):200–7.

[63] Kretzmann JP, McKnight JL. Building communities from the inside out: a path toward finding and mobilizing a community's assets. Chicago, IL: ACTA Publications; 1997.

[64] HealtheRx. About MAPSCorps. HealtheRx2013.

[65] MAPSCorps. Video file; 2014. Available from: <https://www.youtube.com/watch?v=Wi0MFaSl6L8>.

[66] Press Release: We Can't Wait: Health Care Innovation Challenge Will Improve Care, Save Money, Focus on Health Care; 2011.

[67] Health care innovation challenge cooperative agreement initial announcement; 2010.

[68] Zickuhr K. Who's not online and why. Washington, DC: Pew Research Center; 2013.

[69] Zickuhr K, Smith A. Home broadband 2013. Washington, DC: Pew Research Center; 2013.

[70] Commission FC. Eighth broadband progress report. Washington, DC; 2012.

[71] Duggan M, Smith A. Cell Internet use 2013. Washington, DC: Pew Research Center; 2013.

[72] Commission FC. FCC Takes Steps to Modernize and Reform Lifeline for Broadband; 2015 [cited 2015 September 22, 2015].

[73] Mein E, Fuentes B, Soto Mas F, Muro A. Incorporating digital health literacy into adult ESL education on the US-Mexico border. Rhetor Prof Commun Glob 2012;3(1):162–74.

[74] Weiss BD. Health literacy: an important issue for communicating health information to patients. Zhonghua Yi Xue Za Zhi (Taipei) 2001;64(11):603–8.

[75] Smith SG, O'Conor R, Aitken W, Curtis LM, Wolf MS, Goel MS. Disparities in registration and use of an online patient portal among adults: findings from the LitCog cohort. J Am Med Inf Assoc 2015;22(4):888–95.

[76] Kruse CS, Argueta DA, Lopez L, Nair A. Patient and provider attitudes toward the use of patient portals for the management of chronic disease: a systematic review. J Med Internet Res 2015;17(2):e40.

[77] Clark SJ, Costello LE, Gebremariam A, Dombkowski KJ. A national survey of parent perspectives on use of patient portals for their children's health care. Appl Clin Inform 2015;6(1):110–9.

[78] Davis O, Bean K, McBride D. Decreasing health disparities through technology: building a community health website. J Community Inform 2013;9(2).

[79] Foldy S, Grannis S, Ross D, Smith T. A ride in the time machine: information management capabilities health departments will need. Am J Public Health 2014;104(9):1592–600.

[80] Roth C, Foraker RE, Payne PR, Embi PJ. Community-level determinants of obesity: harnessing the power of electronic health records for retrospective data analysis. BMC Med Inform Decis Mak 2014;14:36.

I. AN EXTRAORDINARY OPPORTUNITY

3

Cancer Clinical Research: Enhancing Data Liquidity and Data Altruism

Warren Kibbe PhD

Center for Biomedical Informatics and Information Technology, National Cancer Institute, Rockville, MD, United States

O U T L I N E

3.1	Drivers	41	3.10	Adaptive Instruments	47
3.2	Data Liquidity	42	3.11	Ontologies and Workflow Systems	47
3.3	Data Science	42	3.12	Connected Health and Mobile Technologies	48
	3.3.1 Impact of mHealth	42	3.13	A Focus on Lowering Barriers to Data Access for Cancer Research	48
3.4	Data Access	43		3.13.1 Informed Consent and Consent-Derived Access	48
3.5	Translational Research	44		3.13.2 Easy-to-Use Data Repositories	48
3.6	Capturing the Patient Experience Across the Continuum of Care	46		3.13.3 Data Altruism and Citizen Contributions	48
3.7	Empowering the Patient as a Full Participant in Research	46	3.14	Precision Medicine Drivers	49
3.8	Building a National Learning Health Care System for Cancer	46		List of Acronyms and Abbreviations	51
3.9	Incentives for Data Sharing	46		References	51
	3.9.1 Standardization of Common Data Elements	47			
	3.9.2 Meaningful Use of Common Data Elements	47			

3.1 DRIVERS

The value of information about cancer care, treatment, and outcomes and the importance of data sharing for maximizing the effectiveness and dissemination of care have become clear in the cancer research community. These realizations are transformational and it is clear that access to data and analytics is no longer just the purview of biostatisticians, computer scientists, and biomedical informaticians. The 2014 debate over "net neutrality" highlighted the pervasive recognition that democratized access to information is a valuable underpinning of our systems of commerce and government. There is an increased recognition of the utility and value of data.

B. Hesse, D. Ahern & E. Beckjord: Oncology Informatics.
DOI: http://dx.doi.org/10.1016/B978-0-12-802115-6.00003-3

However, there is also a fundamental schism with the thinking divided into two camps—those who believe that data are precompetitive (and should be openly shared to the extent possible under our current legal and ethical frameworks) and those who view data as competitive and therefore a potentially monetized asset. In this chapter, we make the argument from a public good standpoint, that health care data, including data required for process improvement, are critical for improving health outcomes and should be precompetitive.

3.2 DATA LIQUIDITY

The phrase "data liquidity" emphasizes the fluid nature of data. For the impact and value of health care data to be fully realized, data will need to be available, timely, accurate, complete, consistent, and well-annotated. Data liquidity enables data quality [1] and promotes data reuse [2–7]. This approach is very much aligned with Open Data initiatives and the Future of Research Communications and e-Scholarship (Force11) discussions around the FAIR Guiding Principles—Findable, Accessible, Interoperable, Reusable [8,9] and groups implementing infrastructure necessary to support FAIR [10,11] (Fig. 3.1).

Regarding the issues of consent, patient privacy, and patients' rights, Denmark and Scotland have made the availability of population-level health care data for quality improvement and research use feasible without requiring consent by every participant. Every patient in both countries by virtue of using national health insurance coverage consents to receive treatment and contribute their data for approved research purposes. Access to data is viewed separately from patient engagement in research studies directly involving the patient, which require informed consent. Principles of privacy are maintained and enforced. Attempts to identify individuals or actions that disclose identity or reduce privacy are illegal and subject to prosecution [12–14]. An overview of national registries and policies is available from the Organization for Economic Co-operation and Development [15]. A current treatment of biobanking is also available [16]. Another resource is an overview of registries and legal strictures used in Denmark [17].

Looking at the sensitivity and secondary use of data, it is an increasingly debated topic and groups like the Global Alliance for Genomics and Healthcare [18] are very engaged in understanding and promoting the precompetitive use of genomics and health care data. The National Institutes of Health (NIH) released in January 2015 a Genomic Data Sharing Policy, in which genomic data generated with NIH funding is required to be deposited in an openly available repository, subject to data access approval for controlled access data (typically clinical data) [19].

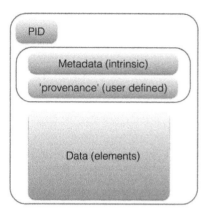

FIGURE 3.1 A schematic of data packet that supports the use of FAIR. It has a primary ID, which may be linked to a Digital Object Identifier, or be a universally unique ID. The packet can be of arbitrary size, but has defined metadata and user defined attributes that enable machine-readable parsing and computation on the packet. The data encapsulated in the packet can be small, such as a single triple in an RDF store, or be derived from a single observation, a single image, a series of images, or encompass a complete data set, such as a complete submission to a database like dbGaP. For a large packet with multiple types of data, ideally it would consist of a set of packets, each describing one type of data, or describing information about one point in a time series.

3.3 DATA SCIENCE

The ability to convert data into information and then into knowledge is a distinct area of expertise and a scientific domain, called "data science." Fundamental shifts are occurring in our ability to organize, manage, annotate, and learn from data. The most visible of these shifts is an increasing emphasis on big data and the concomitant transformation of each person in our society from being a data consumer to being a data provider. These data and access by consumers to their own data as well as performance data across health care providers and various types of providers will be a disruptive force in health care. Other sectors of the economy have gone through this transformation and it can profoundly disrupt the relationship between service providers and consumers. For example, Kodak and the development of the digital camera is a cautionary tale [20]. The availability of movies through on-demand streaming has transformed the movie industry, with some companies like Netflix effectively making the transition from physical media to streaming [21] and other streaming devices such as Hulu are being created [22]. The transition from CDs to mp3s and later streaming has had a similar impact on the music industry [23–26]. Likewise, consumer access to data in health care will inevitably have a similar transformative impact.

3.3.1 Impact of mHealth

Smartphones, wearables, and other sensor- and Internet-enabled devices are revolutionizing our world and our experiences, and have the potential to revolutionize cancer prevention, care, control, and survivorship. The ability of these devices to create so-called "frictionless data" is enormous and our ability to use them to improve health is only at the anecdotal stage now. Collectively, the application of these devices to health care is referred to as "mHealth." An ecosystem of precompetitive (open data) organizations is emerging to develop the standards and mechanisms for sharing the kind of data these devices generate [27–30]. Data sets are also becoming more available [31]. Frictionless has also been applied to "low friction" dynamic consent [32] and health care organization interactions using mobile devices [33].

It is important to realize that one of the reasons that sensor data are so powerful is because they are annotated with substantial metadata that can provide rich context and provenance for the data, enabling significant inferences about the meaning of the data. Such metadata can include geolocation data, accelerometer data, battery data, global positioning system (GPS) information (beyond geolocation), and other device usage information. The way we usually aggregate data in research and in health care removes these primary annotations, even for lab data. Valuable information about the devices used to generate lab data, validates runs and normalizes instrumentation. And how the subsequent data are handled is often only present in the lab information system or the instrument itself. This has profound impact later on our ability to utilize big data approaches to analyze clinical data. Raw sensor data are incredibly informative but are not currently available to the health care enterprise or for broader analysis nationally or internationally.

In the biomedical research space and health care arena, there has been a fundamental shift in perception regarding the role of data. Data, information, and computing were previously considered "infrastructure" (where expenditures are to be carefully managed and minimized), are now understood as a strategic asset, for which expenditures and activities need to be carefully coordinated with the strategic and operational priorities of the organization. These changes extend into our thinking about delivering care and practicing evidence-based medicine. The acquisition of data, the liquidity of information, and the conversion of information into knowledge are impacting clinical care in fundamental ways. For instance, there has been an increasing turn toward "evidence-based medicine" [34] where the strength of the data supporting specific therapies and clinical decision making is dependent on clear research data and clinical evidence. Precision medicine itself is predicated on translating the presentation of the patient in the clinic, including labs, imaging, diagnostics, and genomics to provide targeted prevention and therapeutic strategies

[35]. Data warehousing has moved beyond improved reporting and financial analysis to improved analytics and quality improvement, and is more than just a reflection of the electronic medical record (EMR). Data warehousing aggregates data from many sources to support discovery, data mining, analytics, and visualization [36]. Patient access to the EMR has also changed with health care organizations viewing shared access as a way to better interact with patients [37,38].

Nonetheless, the patient is and will remain the center of a care encounter. However, there is a growing recognition that the diagnosis and course should be informed by the experience and outcome of prior patients across an organization and across the nation, and be informed by but not limited to the personal experiences of the care team. The 2007 Institute of Medicine (IOM) report, "The Learning Healthcare System" laid the ground work for this view [39]. The 2011 IOM report on precision medicine further highlighted the need [40]. This call was extended and amplified in the 2013 IOM report, "Delivering High-Quality Cancer Care: Charting a New Course for a System in Crisis." [41] To realize the vision laid out in these reports, we must overcome several fundamental challenges involving data, information, and knowledge:

- *Lowering barriers* to *data access* for cancer research;
- *Integrating data* and learning from basic and clinical research across the continuum of cancer care (translational research);
- *Capturing the patient experience* across the continuum of care, including patient-reported outcomes (PROs), with consistent, interpretable annotations to enable inter-patient learning, analytics, and data science; and
- *Empowering the patient as a full participant in research.*

Each of these challenges should be considered in terms of drivers and implications.

3.4 DATA ACCESS

Currently, it is very difficult to share data across projects, across care encounters, across organizations, and across providers. This difficulty encumbers learning, whether that learning is focused on quality improvement, understanding the patient experience, or identifying opportunities for improvement in detection, care delivery, acute care episodes, or long-term care or survivorship. It is also particularly frustrating for patients who are trying to move information about their own health history between care providers, clinics, and specialists. In research, it is also hard for patients to donate their information in meaningful ways. Some of this is technical, for example, the US Veterans Affairs' patient health portal called *MyHealtheVet* that uses the Blue Button feature [42]; and some is regulatory (the Health Insurance Portability and Accountability Act of 1996 (HIPAA) and the Federal Policy for the Protection of Human Subjects (Common Rule)) raising barriers of liability and legal constraints. While there are many barriers, the consent, legal, and regulatory constraints disappear when the patient is directly involved. Looking forward, providing patients with easy means to obtain and share their health data for care and research is paramount. Creating an independent patient-controlled repository for sharing data has met with limited success (HealthVault, Google Health), due in part to patients' (consumers) privacy concerns and the inability of existing health care providers and systems to provide a sufficiently easy mechanism for transmitting and sharing data to create a personal health record [43].

Creating the necessary exchange structure such as Blue Button for instance, and providing universal import and export methods for patients is perhaps the most viable avenue for meaningful data sharing focused on the patient. To turn this into reality will require a significant uptake in the use of the Blue Button specification by electronic health record (EHR) vendors for both export and import. Patient empowerment must allow patients to access, curate their own data, and provide corrections back to the source for empowerment to be meaningful and transformative. This meshes well with observations from the crowd sourcing and citizen science experience—lowering the barriers for accessing data is critical for broad review and engagement. Practicing medicine in the 21st century will require 21st-century approaches. Wikipedia has shown that the wisdom of crowds is real and scalable for curation of large data sets [44,45].

For data to be made available for curation and meaningfully exchanged, it must be annotated with known, shared, and discoverable semantics. We need to make clinical and biomedical research vocabularies, terminologies, and ontologies more discoverable and accessible, and we need to make it easier to integrate their use into existing workflows. There are other barriers to the meaningful sharing of data including differences in the way patients are consented for different studies, institutional sensitivities, and regulated data. Data are seldom accessible across an organization or between research projects unless they share a single institutional review board (IRB) approval. The National Cancer Institute (NCI)-supported Surveillance, Epidemiology, and End Results (SEER) registries are an example of overcoming some of these barriers, providing a virtual pooled repository that offers access to a large amount of population-based cancer data with a single request. We need to both harmonize data access requirements and consents across classes of projects and provide innovative mechanisms for making these data available in larger "buckets." This

is one of the keys to enabling new big data analytic approaches.

Another thing to consider about these barriers is that most data scientists cannot access clinical cancer data (imaging, laboratory data, and high-throughput clinical data) and often turn to social media for data. The current status quo in 2015 for data scientists is they typically do not work in the medical field and have little knowledge of the regulations and approval processes necessary to gain access to these data, and they are not part of a clinical research team. Confounding this issue is that access must be obtained project by project, institution by institution. Gaining access to these data sets, and enough of them to enable big data approaches to these data sets is exceptionally daunting, and limits the scope and audacity of innovation. These barriers have driven many members of the data science community to eschew clinical data and instead focus on publicly available data sets such as Twitter feeds to perform interesting big data analyses. These analyses are everything from identifying "top influencers" [46], which are directly relevant for uncovering "driver mutations" from cancer patients' next gen sequencing data [47–52], to emotional content analysis and geospatial analysis of tweets to identify accidents and other significant events.

The use of social media as a social sensor is possible because of the open nature of the data. Currently, it is relatively difficult to apply these same techniques to cancer data because it is much less accessible and much more project- and institution-focused and controlled. This stymies the wishes of many patients to make their data widely available to solve important issues in cancer care and confounds most researchers who would like to work on these issues. Currently, the workaround is to create large research registries, cohort studies, and population-based trials, but these approaches are expensive and even the largest efforts are only a subset of all patients with a disease.

3.5 TRANSLATIONAL RESEARCH

A second challenge is to integrate data and learning from basic and clinical research with cancer care in a way that enables predictive models and patient-specific simulations to be created, which in turn will make it easier for sophisticated decision-support tools to improve patient outcomes.

This issue is much more complicated than data access, since it requires well-annotated data in all aspects of research and care, and a level of ontological consistency that would enable machine-computable comparisons. In the big data community, there is a lot of emphasis on discoverability and automated, semantics-free discovery and analysis. These approaches work well for certain types of carefully selected questions for which changes in pattern or flow are important, but understanding the inherent meaning is not necessary. A good example of this in the financial industry is looking for fraud in credit card transactions. Conversely, Netflix and their recommender system, Cinematch, is based on a deep understanding of customers and content, availability, and trending, including past history, to make accurate suggestions. Because it is costly to obtain large data sets, presently there is a paucity of appropriate large data sets to generate predictive models that are relevant in model systems research and human care settings and are sufficiently informative to be relevant for predictions based on individual presentations.

One approach to combining model systems research is the Monarch Initiative [53], which is starting to show the tremendous power of combining findings from model systems with clinical data. The approach in the Monarch Initiative is to identify semantically similar phenotypes across different organisms, described by different research communities (Fig. 3.2).

This is done by a process called "logical decomposition" as described by Mungall et al. [54]. An example of this process listed in their paper allows us to infer that the human phenotype ontology (HP) term craniosynostosis (HP:0001363) is equivalent to the mammalian phenotype ontology (MP) term premature suture closure (MP:0000081). These methodologies and predictive models are in turn informing how we run clinical trials. For instance, adaptive clinical trials such as the NCI-Molecular Analysis for Therapy Choice (NCI-MATCH) Trial, where the diagnosis, lab values, and genetic features identified as clinical actionable mutations are used to assign a patient to a specific treatment arm, where evidence can come from model systems [55] (Fig. 3.3).

These approaches, even without broad sharing of clinical data, are dramatically enhancing our ability to apply model system data and observations to patients in the clinic, bridging preclinical models with the clinic. Expanding our understanding of cancer biology and mechanisms of resistance using preclinical models is one

of the pillars of the NCI Precision Medicine Initiative—Oncology [56,57]. The other two pillars are expanding access to genetically informed clinical trials, such as NCI-MATCH and Pediatric MATCH. The third pillar is

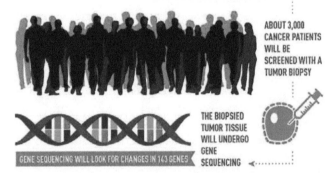

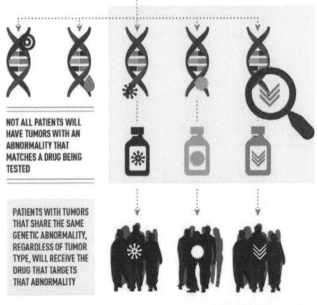

FIGURE 3.3 The NCI-Molecular Analysis for Therapy Choice (NCI-MATCH) Trial, where the diagnosis, lab values, and genetic features identified as clinical actionable mutations are used to assign a patient to a specific treatment arm, where evidence can come from model systems.

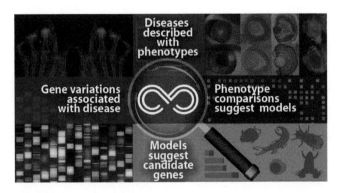

FIGURE 3.2 Monarch Initiative.

the informatics necessary to build the knowledge system necessary to capture, learn, and apply the findings from the first two pillars.

3.6 CAPTURING THE PATIENT EXPERIENCE ACROSS THE CONTINUUM OF CARE

There are several sides to this challenge—broadly speaking; this includes accurately capturing the patient experiences over time during various kinds of health care encounters, as well as outside a care encounter—diet, exercise, family, friends, and the workplace. The contribution of lifestyle to cancer risk and cancer recovery is poorly understood, but poor nutrition, sleep, and exercise patterns clearly contribute to risk of cancer and other diseases [58]. PRO measures can apply in care and home settings, and can be used to assess subtle and not-so-subtle changes in quality of life, cognition, mobility, and many other domains. The Patient Reported Outcomes Measurement Information System (PROMIS) [59], the Quality of Life in Neurological Disorders (Neuro-QoL) [60], the NIH Toolbox for the Assessment of Neurological and Behavioral Functions (NIH Toolbox) [61], and the Patient Reported Outcomes Version of the Common Terminology Criteria for Adverse Effects (PRO-CTCAE) [62] platforms are all examples of large, open source, well validated instruments for use in PROs. Many of these instruments are also available as computer adaptive tests from resources such as the Assessment Center and this dramatically lowers the burden experienced by the patient and improves quality of life for all involved [63]. The availability of these instruments on smartphones and tablets also opens up additional sensor information for use in novel instruments and measures. One example of such an application is the use of accelerometers in smartphones to measure the steadiness of a gait versus the much more difficult analysis of a video [64].

The proper annotation of the data flowing into the EHR and associated systems in a way that promotes data reuse is critical for learning from the experience and outcomes of every cancer patient. A barrier to meaningful data liquidity in EHRs is the loss of detailed instrument information (one type of metadata) [65]. From a data science standpoint, the detailed knowledge of instrument specifics is critical for big data analytics as are many other types of metadata that inform the context of the data captured in the EHR [66]. The NIH Big Data to Knowledge (BD2K) activities is one venue for addressing some of these deficiencies [67,68].

3.7 EMPOWERING THE PATIENT AS A FULL PARTICIPANT IN RESEARCH

The current research infrastructure is set up to treat the patient's involvement in clinical research as a point in time, and in particular the patient's ability to consent and provide active input in research is often limited to a single encounter. This undermines our ability to more actively engage cancer patients in research and makes it much more difficult to improve data sharing consistent with the wishes of the patient [69]. Moving into a more active consent mode, such as data sharing authorization using Facebook, could take a passive process and put the patient truly in the center of the research data sharing process, recognizing that any particular model for consent and patient engagement will not appeal universally. Dynamic consent modes should be the standard to fully empower patients as research participants. The project Consent to Research [70] hosted at Sage Bionetworks has developed the Participant-Centered Consent (PCC) toolkit [71]. Providing not just milestones but also real information about the meaning and value emerging from research will create an engaged, supportive public. The information needs to be accurate, well-constructed, understandable to an appropriate audience, and informative. These should be attributes we strive toward for all our research outcomes.

3.8 BUILDING A NATIONAL LEARNING HEALTH CARE SYSTEM FOR CANCER

The breadth of the above points can easily lead to considering the problem so massive that it requires an effort akin to "boiling the ocean," which is unlikely to succeed. Instead we need to focus on some specific, actionable projects that provide real value in understanding cancer, improving care for tomorrow's cancer patient, and start to create a national learning health care system for cancer. Our ability to build and sustain a national learning health care system is predicated on several transformations that are already underway.

3.9 INCENTIVES FOR DATA SHARING

The implementation of the NIH Genomics Data Sharing Policy (GDS) [19] is an important first step which starts to set the expectation that all genomic data will be shared and shareable. At the same time the NIH GDS does *not* directly change the existing values of professional recognition or value in promotion. However, the NIH GDS makes explicit an acknowledgment of the critical contribution that data sharing, software sharing, and creating interoperable, portable data play in advancing science and fundamental discovery. We need to advocate as data consumers, data producers, and patient advocates to create the reward system necessary to make data sharing and associated components recognized as critical to realizing the full potential of cancer research, particularly in precision medicine. An important part of that reward system will be the use of micro-attribution and the tracking of not just publications and citations, but the use of software, data sets, and even annotations of data sets into derived works. Being able to see the usage and redistribution of software, data, and other information artifacts will be critical in building a meaningful open science ecosystem that rewards data sharing and software sharing. The NIH BD2K-funded Data Discovery Index [72] is one step in creating this infrastructure. Digital Object Identifiers such as provided by DataCite [73] and distributed micro tracking mechanisms like block chain [74] have the potential to contribute substantially to this evolving data sharing incentive ecosystem as well.

3.9.1 Standardization of Common Data Elements

Building on standardized common data elements will enable knowledge sharing and embed knowledge along many different axes, with a focus on discoverability, portability, and interoperability (see Chapter 1: "Creating a Learning Healthcare System in Oncology"). In all these activities, the focus must remain on utility, usability, and flexibility. Overarching domain models and monolithic information models are too difficult and costly to maintain. To try and harmonize the many models available in cancer research, the Biomedical Research Integrated Domain Group (BRIDG) model was created in 2003 [75]. It is a joint effort of NCI, the Clinical Data Interchange Standards Consortium (CDISC), the US Food and Drug Administration (FDA), and Health Level Seven (HL7). The recent acceptance of the BRIDG model as an International Organization for Standardization (ISO) standard (see [76,77]) will allow BRIDG to accept by reference other ISO health care standard information models [78]. This brings in the CDISC data elements as well as many parts of the NCI metathesaurus. BRIDG is the reference model behind the CDISC SHARE metadata repository.

3.9.2 Meaningful Use of Common Data Elements

Meaningful use stage 1 and stage 2 were designed to implement a level of conformance for EHRs. However, meaningful use did not include interoperability and test the ability of systems to meaningfully exchange and use the data exchanged. Taking meaningful use to that next level where it is possible to build an open interface that works with multiple EHR vendors is underway with projects like SMART on FHIR [79]. An additional step in the value chain for research will be to capture clinical information in EHRs and make clinical data accessible and relevant for research. Conversely, there are fundamental parts of clinical research, such as disease progression and cancer recurrence, which need to be coded in the EHR and made accessible for both improved care and clinical research. While EHRs are unlikely to directly enable comparative analysis, cohort identification, or many other secondary uses for clinical data, data warehousing and data marts layered on top of EHRs and associated systems can and should support clinical process improvement, quality assurance, and research questions whenever feasible [4].

3.10 ADAPTIVE INSTRUMENTS

Adaptive instruments have been developed for PROs in a number of psychosocial, cognitive and functional domains through PROMIS [59], Neuro-QoL [60], and the NIH Toolbox [61]. These instruments are efficient to deliver, are highly validated in many populations, and are accurate over a large range of values while requiring a small number of questions. They are therefore ideal for decreasing patient/participant burden and can be delivered through a variety of devices. Many of the instruments are available through the Assessment Center [63]. A small number of assessments are also available as iOS Apps [80].

3.11 ONTOLOGIES AND WORKFLOW SYSTEMS

Ontologies and workflow systems that are designed to capture information about data collection, temporal representation of healthcare-related events, and enable data discovery and automated reasoning are an important part of the research ecosystem. The National Center for Biomedical Ontology (NCBO) Bioportal for example provides a SPARQL Protocol and RDF Query Language (SPARQL) endpoint to query over [81] and several tools for using natural language processing to connect ontology terms with occurrences in unstructured (or structured) text [82–85]. These approaches have been used in cancer pharmacogenomics [86], interpretation of copy number variation and clinical phenotype [87], and anatomical cross-species classification [88].

3.12 CONNECTED HEALTH AND MOBILE TECHNOLOGIES

Mobile devices and embedded devices are bringing information to the individual and enabling automatic data collection and functional determination with little intervention. Dynamic consent, sophisticated sensors, and many other innovations change the possibilities of what we can learn about our patients while minimizing manual data collection.

Some additional drivers include:

Dropping cost of molecular testing, "-omics," and imaging—coupled to a concomitant decrease in invasiveness of the techniques and technologies. These tests are critical to precision medicine and will serve to improve diagnostics, prognostic indicators, and enhance clinical decision support.

Modeling of cancer biology to understand outcomes. It is increasingly clear that there are numerous molecular, tumor microenvironment, and microbiota changes as well as histological markers that are highly informative and lead to subclassification of patients and cancer in a way that informs treatment and targeting of the underlying abnormal pathways in specific patients. This is the foundation of precision medicine and it will require us to have multiscalar, temporally rich data about cancer so we can more fully understand the complex set of interactions that contribute to cancer, protect us from cancer, and promote cancer initiation, progression, and metastasis.

3.13 A FOCUS ON LOWERING BARRIERS TO DATA ACCESS FOR CANCER RESEARCH

As previously noted, there are substantial barriers to data access. There are a few aspects of lowering barriers to data sharing that are amenable to information systems and data science approaches. We need to continually maintain a focus on how we lower barriers to cancer data so we can maximize the utility of those data to forward both fundamental and applied understanding of mechanisms of cancer, effective prevention, optimized treatment, and maximized health during survivorship. As previously mentioned, the ability to exchange meaningful patient data through mechanisms like Blue Button is crucial to both interoperability and to empowering patients to access, review, and control their data.

3.13.1 Informed Consent and Consent-Derived Access

We need a consistent, shareable, highly vetted approach to informed consent and associated training resources. One aspect of consent was already discussed in the need for dynamic "E Consent" as described here [70]. The project includes a "participant-centered consent toolkit" [71] that provides a framework for involving patients in consented research studies. The focus is to provide research participants an easy to consume view of what they are consenting to and a way to revisit that consent and participate in related studies. The current NIH Genomic Data Sharing Policy is another source of well vetted guidance and documentation on participation and consent [19,89]. The National Center for Advancing Translational Sciences (NCATS)-funded Clinical and Translational Science Awards (CTSA) Program community and the NCI-funded Cancer Centers have also been working through consent. The Informed Consent Ontology is one product of that effort [90,91].

Training in informed consent needs to be at multiple levels for the research team, for the IRB, for the patient/research participant and family, and for the data scientist making use of derived data. We also need data release policies that enable a "library card" access model, where projects making use of a unified consent form require a single access control point, so access to primary data is simplified. The NCI SEER Registry uses this model for access to the SEER data [92,93]. The NIH is moving toward this model, and Database of Genotypes and Phenotypes (dbGAP) now has "consent group" policies [94].

3.13.2 Easy-to-Use Data Repositories

We need to have easy-to-use methods for annotating deposited data with discoverable/machine-readable semantics. ArrayExpress at the European Bioinformatics Institute (EBI) is an example of a flexible mechanism for depositing microarray data that encourages annotation of data elements with open biomedical ontologies as well as clinical standards [95]. The use of natural language processing methodologies for enhancing annotation using controlled vocabularies and ontologies is also important [83]. For cancer genomic data, the NCI Genomic Data Commons (GDC) will be the preferred and recommended location to store cancer data that includes genomic information [96].

3.13.3 Data Altruism and Citizen Contributions

The ability for individuals to contribute their data (data altruism) and participate in research measuring side effects (including standardized adverse events and toxicity classification) offer opportunities for access and analysis of the data. Access and analysis of research data by the public has been dubbed "citizen science" and has been exemplified by projects such as Zooniverse, where participants can learn how to classify galaxies and then review hundreds of thousands of astronomy pictures. Extending this into the cancer realm, providing tools that enable patients to capture the natural history of their disease and the impact of treatment on their life will enable citizen science for cancer. The NCI's PRO-CTCAE project, for instance, is a pilot to bring "experiential" adverse event reporting directly to clinical trial participants [62]. Internet connectivity and mobile devices reach ever more deeply into the fabric of our society. In 2016, the current projection (summer 2015) are for nearly 200 million smartphones to be in use in the United States alone [97], and according to an October 2014 Pew report [98] 64% of American adults own a smartphone, 32% own an e-reader, and 42% own a tablet computer. From the US Census report in 2013, 84% of households have a computer, with 78% having a desktop or laptop computer, and 64% having a handheld computer [99]. This easy accessibility and expected connectivity is changing the way Americans interact with health care and clinical research, and enables a new level of active participation—citizen science [100].

As a complement to citizen science, the ability of patients to be "data donors" lays the foundation of a new kind of participation in clinical research—data altruism, where the patient contributes his or her clinical data either broadly (broad consent) or to specific projects. As mentioned earlier, the E Consent movement seeks to provide members of the public with a much more granular and informative way to consent to research, and have developed a participant-centered consent toolbox to enable research projects to include this type of consent. A part of the vision behind the NCI GDC is to enable direct donation of genomic and clinical data to the repository, creating a class of "cancer information donors" to contribute to the learning health system envisioned in the 2011 IOM (now National Academy of Medicine) report. To make this a reality, standards for exchanging genomic data as well as clinical information need to be developed. The Global Alliance for Genomics and Health (GA4GH) is developing the genomic data exchange standards and exploring existing methods like the Blue Button to exchange clinical information [18]. As previously mentioned, the Blue Button is designed to allow the exchange of data from EHRs (eg, lab values, patient history, imaging). Creating a useful ecosystem does rely on EHR vendors supporting the Blue Button. Currently, most EHRs support data downloads to the patient as PDFs and other document-centric formats including the HL7 Consolidated-Clinical Document

Architecture (C-CDA) format [101]. Documents formats, even C-CDA, make it difficult to aggregate data and exchange interoperable, computable data. For patient and family health history, there is a freely available tool in English and Spanish called the Surgeon General's Family Health Portrait [102,103]. The Family Health History tool includes mappings to existing standards and features the Systemized Nomenclature of Medicine (SNOMED) terminology when available, allows for detailed family pedigree collection, and promotes sharing among family members. Validation studies with the tool have been done [104,105]. The source code for this tool is also freely available [106]. These data are fundamental for understanding genetic and genomic data from a familial standpoint and will be critical for unraveling complex disease relationships, risk factors, responses to therapy, pharmacogenomics, and outcomes for individuals. There is active interest in taking the Family Health History tool and incorporating it into existing EHRs [107–110] as well as patient cohort studies [111,112]. Having a single, shared representation for data collected across many different populations and diseases is critical for understanding rare diseases and rare cancer subtypes.

In addition to the Family Health Portrait tool, there has been a lot of interest and growing usage of PROMIS, Neuro-QoL, NIH Toolbox, and PRO-CTCAE. These tools, like the Family Health History tool, allow the structured and shareable capture of a diverse set of PROs and functional measures across a wide set of neuro-psycho-social measures [113]. These shared measures are critical for understanding the complex interplay between inherited, environmental, and psycho-social factors that impact prevention, treatment, and survivorship in cancer.

The ability to share these data along with complex lab data, including genomic sequencing, is truly critical. As mentioned earlier, the NCI is creating the Cancer GDC. The GDC is envisioned as a place where all cancer-related data (including genomic information) can be stored and shared. An important part of the design of the GDC is to enable the Cancer Information Donor, where individuals can deposit their data to contribute to our knowledge of cancer. The GDC will include privacy protections and the ability for many organizations as well as individual citizens to share genomic, health, family, and disease measures responsibly.

3.14 PRECISION MEDICINE DRIVERS

Cancer research, cancer prevention, cancer treatment, cancer control, and patient outcomes will all benefit from the focus on precision medicine. Dr Douglas R. Lowy, in 2015 as the Acting Director of NCI, gave this definition, based on the 2011 National Academy report

Toward Precision Medicine: Building a Knowledge Network for Biomedical Research and a New Taxonomy of Disease: "Interventions to prevent, diagnose, or treat cancer, based on a molecular and/or mechanistic understanding of the causes, pathogenesis, and/or pathology of the disease. Where the individual characteristics of the patient are sufficiently distinct, interventions can be concentrated on those who will benefit, sparing expense and side effects for those who will not."

Our ability to gather and integrate evidence from preclinical models, from patients in the clinic, and from clinical trials is critical to the success of precision medicine for cancer. We need to build multiscale, predictive models of cancer that are based on fundamental understanding of biology, and can integrate clinical findings, including imaging, pathology, family history, lab data, and of course molecular analyses including sequencing and mass spectrometry. Each of these domains has an important role to play in building meaningful predictive models for cancer. Existing NCI investments in imaging, common data elements (and the necessary semantics and vocabularies), tools for patient data entry (CTCAE-PRO, Family Health History, the PROMIS/Neuro-QoL/NIH Toolbox instruments), and understanding genomic and microenvironment contributions to cancer are critical assets. The Cancer Genome Atlas (TCGA) [114], the Therapeutically Applicable Research to Generate Effective Treatments (TARGET) [115], the Cancer Genome Characterization Initiative (CGCI) [116], and the Cancer Target Discovery and Development project (CTD²) [117], among others, all contribute to fundamental components necessary for precision oncology.

The world of cancer science and cancer care is changing and will continue to change. Clinical genomics and deep sequencing are now commonplace in many cancer care organizations for cancer types shown to be amenable to and informed by these approaches. These data will enable us to understand the prevalence of germline and somatic variants, their association with risk (germline variants), and their contribution to outcomes in a given disease and therapy. We also have an opportunity to carefully examine treatment response to look for early indications of response (or lack of response) to therapy using patient-reported data. These can include fairly subtle responses (eg, fatigue, nociception, sleep patterns, neuropathy, hair loss, nail discoloration, cognition, equilibrioception, proprioception, kinesthesia, edema, depression, and lymphedema). Also, more carefully capturing and delineating these responses will be very helpful for research and for patients. The lack of information on symptom prevalence, severity, and disease staging and progression creates anxiety for patients and is an area of blindness in our understanding of subtle differences between therapies. We need to be able to incorporate these data into predictive models. For us to realize the value of these approaches we need to create mechanisms for engaging patients to capture these data broadly and uniformly, and in turn enable sharing these data, models, and simulations to allow both the creation of analyses and validation of the models.

There are multiple projects currently under consideration or in active development that will inform and start to create this capacity. The American Society of Clinical Oncologists (ASCO) [118] is creating the Cancer Learning Intelligence Network for Quality (CancerLinQ) [119] for sharing some of these data for quality purposes across any and all oncology clinics, from individual oncologist practices to large continuum of care providers. The Clinical Sequencing Exploratory Research program, funded by the National Human Genome Research Institute, was started in 2010 to fund the ethical, legal, and psychosocial research required to integrate sequencing into the clinic [120]. ClinVar is a repository run by the National Center for Biotechnology Information (NCBI) that seeks to aggregate data on mutations and phenotypes including supporting evidence, providing evidence behind the actionability of specific mutations in a disease context [121]. The Clinical Genome Resource (ClinGen) [122] is an NIH-funded (as of mid 2015, cofunded by the National Human Genome Research Institute, the Eunice Kennedy Shriver National Institute of Child Health and Human Development, and NCI) to build an annotation and curation framework for capturing evidence for both germline and somatic mutations. It uses ClinVar as the repository of that evidence, but includes more guidelines and restrictions on what constitutes evidence by disease and datatype. The Global Alliance for Genomics and Health (GA4GH) [18] is defining data structures, policies, and best practices to enable sharing of the molecular, clinical, and other attributes that are critical for understanding the genomic context of disease and health, and defining the conditions under which these data can be shared at a global scale. Cancer is a global disease and will require global participation to effectively address it.

In summary, we need to use data to inform and enhance our understanding of fundamental cancer biology as well as build predictive models for cancer risk, cancer prevention, and cancer therapy. Our ability to effectively address prevention, treatment, control, and survivorship will require fundamental shifts in data liquidity (making cancer data findable, accessible, interoperable, and reusable) and effectively engage the public and cancer patients in cancer research as citizen scientists and data donors (data altruists).

LIST OF ACRONYMS AND ABBREVIATIONS

ASCO American Society of Clinical Oncology
BD2K Big Data to Knowledge
BRIDG Biomedical Research Integrated Domain Group
CancerLinQ Cancer Learning Intelligence Network for Quality
C-CDA Consolidated-Clinical Document Architecture
CDISC Clinical Data Interchange Standards Consortium
CGCI Cancer Genome Characterization Initiative
ClinGen Clinical Genome Resource
CTD² Cancer Target Discovery and Development
CTSA Clinical and Translational Science Awards
dbGAP Database of Genotypes and Phenotypes
EBI European Bioinformatics Institute
EHR Electronic health record
EMR Electronic medical record
FAIR Findable, Accessible, Interoperable, Reusable
FDA Food and Drug Administration
FHIR Fast Health Interoperability Resources
GA4GH Global Alliance for Genomics and Health
GDC Genomic Data Commons
GDS Genomics Data Sharing Policy
GPS Global positioning system
HIPAA Health Insurance Portability and Accountability Act
HL7 Health Level Seven
HP Human phenotype ontology
IOM Institute of Medicine
IRB Institutional review board
ISO International Organization for Standardization
MP Mammalian phenotype ontology
NCATS National Center for Advancing Translational Sciences
NCBI National Center for Biotechnology Information
NCBO National Center for Biomedical Ontology
NCI National Cancer Institute
NCI-MATCH NCI-Molecular Analysis for Therapy Choice
Neuro-QoL Quality of Life in Neurological Disorders
NIH National Institutes of Health
NIH Toolbox NIH Toolbox for the Assessment of Neurological and Behavioral Functions
PCC Participant-Centered Consent
PRO Patient-reported outcome
PRO-CTCAE Patient Reported Outcomes Version of the Common Terminology Criteria for Adverse Effects
PROMIS Patient Reported Outcomes Measurement Information System
RDF Resource Description Framework
SEER Surveillance, Epidemiology, and End Results
SHARE Shared Health and Clinical Research Electronic library
SMART Sustainable Medical Applications and Reusable Technologies
SNOMED Systemized Nomenclature of Medicine
SPARQL SPARQL Protocol and RDF Query Language
TARGET Therapeutically Applicable Research to Generate Effective Treatments
TCGA The Cancer Genome Atlas

References

[1] ISO 8000; 2015 [November 16, 2015]. Available from: <https://en.wikipedia.org/wiki/ISO_8000>.

[2] Cimino J. Collect once, use many: enabling the reuse of clinical data through controlled terminologies. J Am Health Inf Manage Assoc 2007;78(2):24–9.

[3] Safran C. Reuse of clinical data. Yearb Med Inform 2014;9:52–4.

[4] Kahn MG, Brown JS, Chun AT, Davidson BN, Meeker D, Ryan PB, et al. Transparent reporting of data quality in distributed data networks. eGEMs 2015;3(1):1052.

[5] Dentler K, Teije AT, de Keizer NF, Corner R. Barriers to the reuse of routinely recorded clinical data: a field report. Stud Health Technol Inform 2013;192:313–7.

[6] Weiskopf NG, Weng C. Methods and dimensions of electronic health record data quality assessment: enabling reuse for clinical research. J Am Med Inform Assoc 2013;20(1):144–51.

[7] Helton E. CDISC standards: enabling reuse without rework. Appl Clin Trials 2006.

[8] Force 11. The FAIR Data Principles-For comment. [November 16, 2015]. Available from: <https://www.force11.org/group/fairgroup/fairprinciples>.

[9] Force 11. Guiding Principles for Findable, Accessible, Interoperable and Re-usable Data Publishing. [November 16, 2015]; Version B1.0. Available from: <https://www.force11.org/node/6062>.

[10] FAIRDOM. [November 16, 2015]. Available from: <http://fairdom.org/>.

[11] Data FAIRport Find, Access, Interoperate, and Re-Use Data. [November 16, 2015]. Available from: <http://datafairport.org/>.

[12] Selinger C. The right to consent: is it absolute? Br J Med Pract 2009;2(2):50–4.

[13] Department of Health. Confidentiality: NHS Code of Practice. London; 2003.

[14] NHS Scotland, NHS Code of Practice on Protecting Patient Confidentiality; 2003.

[15] OECD Strengthening health information infrastructure for health care quality governance. OECD health policy studies. Paris: OECD Publishing; 2013.

[16] Hofmann S, Solbakk JH, Hofmann B, editors. The ethics of research biobanking. US: Springer; 2009.

[17] Nys H, Goffin T, Stultiens L, Borry P, Dierickx K. Patient rights in the EU-Denmark. European Ethical-Legal Papers. Leuven; 2007.

[18] Global Alliance for Genomics and Health. [November 16, 2015]. Available from: <http://genomicsandhealth.org/>.

[19] National Institutes of Health. Genomic Data Sharing. [November 16, 2015]. Available from: <https://gds.nih.gov/>.

[20] Mui C. How Kodak Failed; 2012 [November 16, 2015]. Available from: <http://www.forbes.com/sites/chunkamui/2012/01/18/how-kodak-failed/>.

[21] Global entertainment and media outlook; 2015–2019 [November 16, 2015]. Available from: <http://www.pwc.com/us/em/outlook>.

[22] McCormick R. Video streaming services could make more money than the US box office by 2017; 2014 [November 16, 2015]. Available from: <http://www.theverge.com/2014/6/4/5781104/netflix-and-peers-will-make-more-money-than-box-office-by-2017>.

[23] Ben-Ameh C. The impact of music streaming on the music industry (Economic and Management): a case study of spotify: Northumbria University; 2014.

[24] PBS Newshour. Can the music industry survive the streaming revolution? 2015.

[25] Arthur C. Streaming: the future of the music industry, or its nightmare? The Guardian; 2015.

[26] Haworth Video/Audio Team. Streaming services impact on the music industry in Haworth blog; 2015.

[27] Open Knowledge Foundation. Our goal is a world of frictionless data. [November 16, 2015]. Available from: <http://data.okfn.org/>.

[28] Pollock R. Frictionless data: making it radically easier to get stuff done with data. Open Knowledge blog; 2013.

[29] Open Knowledge Foundation. A frictionless data ecosystem. [November 16, 2015]. Available from: <http://data.okfn.org/vision>.

[30] Thompson M. Frictionless health: the top 5 reasons the future of healthcare will be mobile. Huffington Post; 2013.

[31] Wang T. Top 10 datasets for health hackers. Rock Health; 2014.

[32] Hayden EC. Open-data project aims to ease the way for genomic research. Nature 2012.

[33] Wicklund E. mHealth Masters: Joe Kvedar's quest to personalize health; 2014 [November 16, 2015]. Available from: <http://www.mhealthnews.com/news/mhealth-masters-joe-kvedars-quest-personalize-health>.

[34] Evidence-based medicine. [November 16, 2015]. Available from: <https://en.wikipedia.org/wiki/Evidence-based_medicine>.

[35] Collins FS, Varmus H. A new initiative on precision medicine. N Engl J Med 2015;372(9):793–5.

[36] Terry K. New healthcare data warehousing model gains favor. Information Week; 2013.

[37] Patient portal adoption: baby boomers vs. millennials infographic. HIT Consultant; 2014.

[38] Viewing patients as partners: patient portal implementation and adoption. Meaningful Use Case Studies; 2012 [November 16, 2015]. Available from: <https://www.healthit.gov/providers-professionals/patients-first-health-care-case-study>.

[39] Institute of Medicine Olsen L.Aisner D, McGinnis JM, editors. The learning healthcare system: workshop summary (IOM Roundtable on Evidence-Based Medicine), 374. Washington, DC: The National Academies Press; 2007.

[40] National Research Council Toward precision medicine: building a knowledge network for biomedical research and a new taxonomy of disease. Washington, DC: The National Academies Press; 2011, p. 142.

[41] Institute of Medicine Levit L, editor. Delivering high-quality cancer care: charting a new course for a system in crisis, 412. Washington, DC: The National Academies Press; 2013.

[42] Turvey C, Woods S. Blue button use by patients to access and share health record information using the department of veterans affairs' online patient portal. J Am Med Inform Assoc 2014;21(4):657–63.

[43] Spil T, Klein R. Personal health records success: why Google health failed and what does that mean for Microsoft Healthvault? In: 47th Hawaii international conference on system sciences (HICSS); 2014.

[44] Ohlig J. Establishing Wikidata as the central hub for linked open life science data. Wikimedia Deutschland blog; 2014.

[45] Khare R, Good BM, Leaman R, Su AI, Lu Z, et al. Crowdsourcing in biomedicine: challenges and opportunities. Brief Bioinform 2016;17(1):23–32.

[46] Northwestern University. Most influential tweeters of all? Depends on the topic. Science Daily; 2010.

[47] TCGA Pan-Cancer Analysis. [November 16, 2015]. Available from: <http://www.nature.com/tcga/>.

[48] Schwartzentruber J, Korshunov A, Liu XY, Jones DT, Pfaff E, Jacob K, et al. Driver mutations in histone H3.3 and chromatin remodelling genes in paediatric glioblastoma. Nature 2012;482(7384):226–31.

[49] The Cancer Genome Atlas Research Network Weinstein JN, Collisson EA, Mills GB, Mills Shaw KR, Ozenberger BA, et al. The cancer genome atlas pan-cancer analysis project. Nat Genet 2013;45(10):1113–20.

[50] Kandoth C, McLellan MD, Vandin F, Ye K, Niu B, Lu C, et al. Mutational landscape and significance across 12 major cancer types. Nature 2013;502(7471):333–9.

[51] Lawrence MS, Stojanov P, Mermel CH, Robinson JT, Garraway LA, Golub TR, et al. Discovery and saturation analysis of cancer genes across 21 tumour types. Nature 2014;505(7484):495–501.

[52] Leiserson MDM, Vandin F, Wu HT, Dobson JR, Eldridge JV, Thomas JL, et al. Pan-cancer network analysis identifies combinations of rare somatic mutations across pathways and protein complexes. Nat Genet 2015;47(2):106–14.

[53] The Monarch Initiative. [November 16, 2015]. Available from: <http://monarchinitiative.org/>.

[54] Mungall CJ, Gkoutos GV, Smith CL, Haendel MA, Lewis SE, Ashburner M. Integrating phenotype ontologies across multiple species. Genome Biol 2010;11(1):R2.

[55] National Institutes of Health. NCI-MATCH trial will link targeted cancer drugs to gene abnormalities; 2015 [November 16, 2015]. Available from: <http://www.nih.gov/news-events/news-releases/nci-match-trial-will-link-targeted-cancer-drugs-gene-abnormalities>.

[56] Varmus H. Precision medicine initiative and cancer research. Cancer Currents blog; 2015.

[57] National Cancer Institute. NCI and the precision medicine initiative; 2015 [November 16, 2015]. Available from: <http://www.cancer.gov/research/key-initiatives/precision-medicine>.

[58] Weiderpass E. Lifestyle and cancer risk. J Prev Med Public Health 2010;43(6):459–71.

[59] PROMIS. Dynamic tools to measure health outcomes from the patient perspective. [November 16, 2015]. Available from: <http://www.nihpromis.org/default#5>.

[60] Neuro-QoL. Quality of life in neurological disorders. [November 16, 2015]. Available from: <http://www.neuroqol.org/Pages/default.aspx>.

[61] NIH Toolbox. [November 16, 2015]. Available from: <http://www.nihtoolbox.org/Pages/default.aspx>.

[62] National Cancer Institute. Patient-Reported Outcomes Version of the Common Terminology Criteria for Adverse Events (PRO-CTCAE); 2015 [November 16, 2015]. Available from: <http://healthcaredelivery.cancer.gov/pro-ctcae/>.

[63] Assessment Center. What is assessment center? [November 16, 2015]. Available from: <https://www.assessmentcenter.net/>.

[64] Juen J, Cheng Q, Prieto-Centurion V, Krishnan JA, Schatz B. Health monitors for chronic disease by gait analysis with mobile phones. Telemed J e-Health 2014;20(11):1035–41.

[65] Metadata. 2015 [November 16, 2015]. Available from: <https://en.wikipedia.org/wiki/Metadata>.

[66] Scudellari M. Biobank managers bemoan underuse of collected samples. Nat Med 2013;19(3):253.

[67] National Institutes of Health. All BD2K events; 2015 [November 16, 2015]. Available from: <https://datascience.nih.gov/bd2k/all-events>.

[68] Stanford Medicine Center for expanded data annotation and retrieval. [November 16, 2015]. Available from: <http://med.stanford.edu/cedar.html>.

[69] Kaye J, Curren L, Anderson N, Edwards K, Fullerton SM, Kanellopoulou N, et al. From patients to partners: participant-centric initiatives in biomedical research. Nat Rev Genet 2012;13(5):371–6.

[70] Sage Bionetworks. E Consent. [November 16, 2015]. Available from: <http://sagebase.org/e-consent/>.

[71] Sage Bionetworks. Participant-Centered Consent Toolkit. [November 16, 2015]. Available from: <http://sagebase.org/pcc/participant-centered-consent-toolkit/>.

[72] BioCADDIE. Biomedical and healthcare data discovery index ecosystem. [November 16, 2015]. Available from: <https://biocaddie.org/>.

[73] DataCite. Frequently asked questions. [November 16, 2015]. Available from: <https://www.datacite.org/faq>.

[74] Block Chain Database; 2015 [November 16, 2015]. Available from: <https://en.wikipedia.org/wiki/Block_chain_(database)>.

[75] BRIDG: Biomedical Research Integrated Domain Group; 2015 [November 16, 2015]. Available from: <http://bridgmodel.org/>.

[76] Vadakin A. CDISC. CDISC announces BRIDG model for research as final ISO standard; 2015.

[77] BRIDG: Biomedical Research Integrated Domain Group. BRIDG and ISO; 2015 [November 16, 2015]. Available from: <http://bridgmodel.nci.nih.gov/news-folder/bridg-and-iso>.

[78] ISO Standards Catalogue. IT applications in health care technology. [November 16, 2015]. Available from: <http://www.iso.org/iso/home/store/catalogue_ics/catalogue_ics_browse.htm?ICS1=35&ICS2=240&ICS3=80&>.

[79] SMART. Tech stack for health apps. [November 16, 2015]. Available from: <http://docs.smarthealthit.org/>.

[80] Resource material for the NIH Toolbox iPad application. [November 16, 2015]. Available from: <http://www.nihtoolbox.org/Resources/NIHToolboxiPadapp/Pages/default.aspx>.

[81] BioPortal SPARQL examples. [November 17, 2015]. Available from: <http://sparql.bioontology.org/examples>.

[82] Annotator web service; 2012 [November 16, 2015]. Available from: <http://www.bioontology.org/wiki/index.php/Annotator_Web_service>.

[83] Jonquet C, Shah N, Musen M. The open biomedical annotator. Summit Transl Bioinform 2009;2009:56–60.

[84] Whetzel PL. NCBO technology: powering semantically aware applications. J Biomed Semant 2013(4 Suppl. 1):S8.

[85] BioPortal Annotator. [November 17, 2015]. Available from: <https://bioportal.bioontology.org/annotator>.

[86] Wang L, Liu H, Chute CG, Zhu Q. Cancer based pharmacogenomics network supported with scientific evidences: from the view of drug repurposing. BioData Mining 2015;8:9.

[87] Köhler S, Schoenberg U, Czeschik JC, Doelken SC, Hehir-Kwa JY, Ibn-Salem J, et al. Clinical interpretation of CNVs with cross-species phenotype data. J Med Genet 2014;51(11):766–72.

[88] Mungall CJ, Torniai C, Gkoutos GV, Lewis SE, Haendel MA. Uberon, an integrative multi-species anatomy ontology. Genome Biol 2012;13(1):R5.

[89] National Institutes of Health. Genomic Data Sharing: frequently asked questions. [November 16, 2015]. Available from: <https://gds.nih.gov/13faqs_gds.html#h1>.

[90] ICO-Ontology. [November 16, 2015]. Available from: <https://code.google.com/p/ico-ontology/>.

[91] Lin Y, Harris M, Manion F, Eisenhauer E, Zhao B, Shi W, et al. Development of a BFO-based Informed Consent Ontology (ICO). In: International conference on biomedical ontology; 2014.

[92] National Cancer Institute. About the SEER Registries. [November 16, 2015]. Available from: <http://seer.cancer.gov/registries/>.

[93] National Cancer Institute. SEER-Medicare: Overview of the process for obtaining data; 2015 [November 16, 2015]. Available from: <http://healthcaredelivery.cancer.gov/seermedicare/obtain/>.

[94] Tryka KA, Hao L, Sturcke A, Jin Y, Kimura M, Wang ZY, et al. The database of genotypes and phenotypes (dbGaP) and PheGenI The NCBI Handbook [Internet]. Bethesda, MD: National Center for Biotechnology Information (US); 2013.

[95] ArrayExpress-functional genomics data. [November 16, 2015]. Available from: <https://www.ebi.ac.uk/arrayexpress/>.

[96] National Cancer Institute. NCI establishes genomic data commons to facilitate identification of molecular subtypes of cancer and potential drug targets. National Cancer Institute; 2014.

[97] Number of smartphone users in the United States from 2010 to 2018; 2015 [November 16, 2015]. Available from: <http://www.statista.com/statistics/201182/forecast-of-smartphone-users-in-the-us/>.

[98] Pew Research Center. Mobile technology fact sheet; 2014 [November 16, 2015]. Available from: <http://www.pewinternet.org/fact-sheets/mobile-technology-fact-sheet/>.

[99] File T, Ryan C. Computer and Internet use in the United States: 2013. In: American Community Survey Reports. Washington, DC: US Census Bureau; 2014.

[100] List of citizen science projects; 2015 [November 16, 2015]. Available from: <https://en.wikipedia.org/wiki/List_of_citizen_science_projects>.

[101] Consolidated CDA overview; 2014 [November 16, 2015]. Available from: <https://www.healthit.gov/policy-researchers-implementers/consolidated-cda-overview>.

[102] My Family Health Portrait. [November 16, 2015]. Available from: <https://familyhistory.hhs.gov/FHH/html/index.html>.

[103] Online Version of 'My Family Health Portrait' Available in English and Spanish. FDA Consum 2006;40(3):16–7.

[104] Feero WG, Facio FM, Glogowski EA, Hampel HL, Stopfer JE, Eidem H, et al. Preliminary validation of a consumer-oriented colorectal cancer risk assessment tool compatible with the US surgeon general's my family health portrait. Genet Med 2015;17(9):753–6.

[105] Facio FM, Feero WG, Linn A, Oden N, Manickam K, Biesecker LG. Validation of my family health portrait for six common heritable conditions. Genet Med 2010;12(6):370–5.

[106] Repository for the HTML5 Version of the Family Health History Tool. [November 16, 2015]. Available from: <https://github.com/CBIIT/FHH>.

[107] Owens KM, Marvin ML, Gelehrter TD, Ruffin MT, Uhlmann WR. Clinical use of the surgeon general's "My Family Health Portrait" (MFHP) tool: opinions of future health care providers. J Genet Couns 2011;20(5):510–25.

[108] Berger KA, Lynch J, Prows CA, Siegel RM, Myers MF. Mothers' perceptions of family health history and an online, Parent-generated family health history tool. Clin Pediatr (Phila) 2013;52(1):74–81.

[109] Widmer C, DeShazo JP, Bodurtha J, Quillin J, Creswick H, et al. Genetic counselors' current use of personal health records-based family histories in genetic clinics and considerations for their future adoption. J Genet Couns 2013;22(3):384–92.

[110] Giovanni MA, Murray MF. The application of computer-based tools in obtaining the genetic family history. Curr Protoc Hum Genet 2010 Chapter 9: p. Unit 9.21.

[111] Newcomb P, Canclini S, Cauble D, Raudonis B, Golden P, et al. Pilot trial of an electronic family medical history in US faith-based communities. J Prim Care Community Health 2014;5(3):198–201.

[112] Pettey CM, McSweeney JC, Stewart KE, Price ET, Cleves MA, Heo S, et al. Perceptions of family history and genetic testing and feasibility of pedigree development among african americans with hypertension. Eur J Cardiovasc Nurs 2015;14(1):8–15.

[113] Institute of Medicine Capturing social and behavioral domains and measures in electronic health records: phase 2. Washington, DC: The National Academies Press; 2014, p. 374.

[114] The Cancer Genome Atlas. [November 16, 2015]. Available from: <http://cancergenome.nih.gov/>.

[115] National Cancer Institute. TARGET: Therapeutically Applicable Research to Generate Effective Treatments; 2015 [November 16, 2015]. Available from: <https://ocg.cancer.gov/programs/target>.

[116] National Cancer Institute. CGCI: Cancer Genome Characterization Initiative; 2015 [November 16, 2015]. Available from: <https://ocg.cancer.gov/programs/cgci>.

[117] National Cancer Institute. CTD^2: Cancer Target Discovery and Development; 2015 [November 16, 2015]. Available from: <https://ocg.cancer.gov/programs/ctd2>.

[118] ASCO: American Society of Clinical Oncology. [November 16, 2015]. Available from: <http://www.asco.org/>.

[119] ASCO Cancer LINQ. [November 16, 2015]. Available from: <http://cancerlinq.org/>.

[120] National Human Genome Research Institute. Clinical Sequencing Exploratory Research (CSER); 2015 [November 16, 2015]. Available from: <http://www.genome.gov/27546194/>.

[121] What is ClinVar? [November 16, 2015]. Available from: <http://www.ncbi.nlm.nih.gov/clinvar/intro/>.

[122] ClinGen: Clinical Genome Resource; 2015 [November 16, 2015]. Available from: <https://www.clinicalgenome.org/>.

I. AN EXTRAORDINARY OPPORTUNITY

4

Engaging Patients in Primary and Specialty Care

Alex H. Krist MD, MPH[1], Donald E. Nease MD, MPH[2],
Gary L. Kreps PhD[3], Linda Overholser MD, MPH[4]
and Marc McKenzie BS, MBA[5]

[1]Department of Family Medicine and Population Health, Virginia Commonwealth University, Richmond, VA, United States [2]Department of Family Medicine, University of Colorado, Denver, CO, United States [3]Center for Health and Risk Communication, Department of Communication, George Mason University, Fairfax, VA, United States [4]Department of General Internal Medicine, University of Colorado, Denver, CO, United States [5]Retired Computer Industry Senior Executive, Survivor of Cancer and Stem-Cell Transplant, Windsor, CO, United States

OUTLINE

4.1 Introduction	56	
4.1.1 The Value of Patient Engagement Across the Cancer Control Continuum	56	
4.1.2 Primary, Specialty, Hospital, and Community Care Delivery Systems	57	
4.2 Overview of HIT Tools to Engage Patients	61	
4.2.1 Electronic Health Records	61	
4.2.2 Patient Portals and Personal Health Records	61	
4.2.3 Patient e-Health Tools	62	
4.2.4 A National Strategy to Promote HIT for Patient Engagement	62	
4.2.5 General Limitations of Current Systems	63	
4.2.6 A Model for Making HIT More Patient-Centered	63	
4.3 Key Patient Engagement Activities	66	
4.3.1 Empowering Patients With Health Information	66	

4.3.2 Gathering Patient-Reported Information	67
4.3.3 Engaging Patients in Medical Decision Making	68
4.3.4 Patient Engagement to Manage Transitions of Care	71
4.3.5 Engaging Patients and Caregivers for Survivorship Planning	72
4.4 HIT Implementation to Promote Patient Engagement	73
4.5 Conclusions	77
List of Acronyms and Abbreviations	77
References	77

B. Hesse, D. Ahern & E. Beckjord: Oncology Informatics.
DOI: http://dx.doi.org/10.1016/B978-0-12-802115-6.00004-5

4.1 INTRODUCTION

Leonard Kish famously declared engaged patients to be "the blockbuster drug of the century" in a 2012 post on the HL7Standards Blog. Kish cites as evidence in his blog post the impressive numbers tallied by several studies examining outcomes for coordinated chronic care, implying that engaging patients as partners in their care will improve outcomes at a level far beyond that of pharmaceuticals. In his subsequent post, Kish goes on to describe specifics of how technology that gathers and tracks personal health data may provide a driving factor for patient engagement.

This chapter will address the topic of patient engagement directly as it relates to health information technology (HIT) in the context of cancer prevention, detection, treatment, and survivorship. There are many ways to define patient engagement, but we align with that used by Carmen, "We define patient and family engagement as patients, families, their representatives, and health professionals working in active partnership at various levels across the health care system—direct care, organizational design and governance, and policy making—to improve health and health care" [1]. The emphasis is on an active partnership, and for our purposes we will focus on the direct care aspects and how HIT can facilitate engagement.

4.1.1 The Value of Patient Engagement Across the Cancer Control Continuum

Why is patient engagement important in health care? What evidence is there that supports a focus on engaging patients and their families? Why is patient engagement an important aspect of HIT as applied to cancer prevention, diagnosis, treatment, and survivorship? The rationale for actively partnering with patients in their care becomes obvious when viewed from the perspective of time spent by patients actually in health care facilities versus time spent in other settings. A striking example of this comes from an analysis of the value of patient time involved in colonoscopy-based screening for colorectal cancer. The mean total time to complete screening was 81.5 hours, including dietary modification, prep completion, actual dedicated time (travel to the screening site, undergoing the colonoscopy, and travel back home), and time to return to routine activities [2]. At any point in the chain of events prior to actually undergoing screening, if patients are not able to complete the requirements of dietary changes and prep completion, the process breaks down.

In 2011 the Commonwealth Fund conducted an international survey of patients with "complex health needs" spanning 11 industrialized countries and focusing on the relationship between engagement and health care quality. While there were substantial differences among countries in the level of engagement experienced by respondents, there was a consistent relationship across countries—between higher levels of engagement and higher perceptions of quality of care, lower medical error rates, and higher perceptions of the local health systems [3]. A recent paper highlighting four case studies in diverse countries and health care settings further shows the importance of engaging patients and the resulting improvements in health care quality and outcomes [4].

Coulter, in a review of proven strategies to enhance patient engagement, provides a useful delineation of focus areas for engagement: improving health literacy, helping patients make appropriate health decisions, and improving quality of care processes [5]. Within each area there are important ways that HIT can be brought to bear. For example, personalized health information is proven to enhance engagement, and the delivery of health information tailored to specific patient needs can be greatly facilitated through access to electronic problem and medication lists. Shared decision-making (SDM) tools can be employed in an electronic format and delivered both within health care settings and at home, and greatly enhance patient's engagement in decisions about their care. Cancer prevention, diagnosis, treatment, and survivorship present unique challenges and opportunities for patient engagement and application of HIT. Often multiple settings, specialties, and systems are involved. The decisions are often complex and require evaluation of not only health data but also personal preferences and values. Treatment regimens, their side effects, and caregiving needs are also complex and may span long periods of time.

There is a growing literature on how patient engagement impacts outcomes in the cancer arena. In breast cancer prevention, *BRCA 1* and *BRCA 2* genetic counseling and testing is important for managing hereditary breast and ovarian cancer risks. Testing and counseling remains disproportionately low among Black women at risk, and recent data suggests that medical mistrust plays an important role [6]. Survey data from cancer survivors with leukemia, colorectal, or bladder cancer demonstrates how increasing survivors' participation self-efficacy results in an increased perceptions of personal control, increased level of trust, and decreased feeling of uncertainty. Both of these pathways were important in improving survivor's psychosocial outcomes as measured by the SF-36 Mental Health Component Summary scale [7]. In a qualitative interview study of Latina women's breast and cervical cancer screening behaviors, health care clinician communication styles were identified as important [8]. Specifically, "good" communication was identified as a sense of not feeling rushed, feeling like their clinician understood them and having access to a qualified interpreter when needed. Poor communication involved feeling rushed, seeing too many different clinicians, not being understood, and a lack of trust and privacy when using interpreters. Interpersonal characteristics that are modifiable through engagement efforts have been identified to predict surveillance participation in cancer survivors [9]. Survivors of pediatric cancer identified as being self-controlling or worried versus collaborative resulted in significantly different rates of bone density, echocardiogram, and mammography testing.

When considering the ways that patient engagement techniques and strategies can be implemented in cancer care, it is useful to consider the entire spectrum. While a minority of patients may agree to whatever screening is recommended by a clinician, when the follow through becomes complex and confusing even these patients may fail to complete recommended screening procedures unless they are fully engaged in the decision-making process. Whether identified as a result of screening or presentation with symptoms, a cancer diagnosis and referral process is one that also demands application of SDM tools and techniques including provision and navigation of vast repositories of information that patients often access on their own when they first consider a possible cancer diagnosis. Treatment regimens may be dictated by tissue diagnoses and staging. However, adherence to these often complex and burdensome regimens and managing associated side effects demands the enlistment of patients, family, and caregivers as full partners in the treatment process. Finally, completion of treatment, remission, reconnection with primary care, and survivorship support again require patients to navigate among different specialists, primary care, the community, and sources of information. Failure to fully engage with patients in the survivorship stages may put them at increased risk for recurrence and complications (see Part II, Chapter 9, "Survivorship" by Beckjord et al.).

Dr Neeraj Arora, a cancer researcher, formerly at the National Cancer Institute and now at the Patient-Centered Outcomes Research Institute (PCORI), and a cancer survivor, provides an insightful perspective on how technology has impacted his ability to access information and participate in decisions over 20 years as a survivor of Non-Hodgkin's lymphoma [10]. Specifically, he describes how in the 1990s he used print media, face-to-face interaction with clinicians, and e-mail-based support groups. In 2007, he was diagnosed with congestive heart failure as a complication of his cancer treatment, and took advantage of vastly improved access to health information online, e-mail interaction with clinicians, online support group message boards, chat rooms, and even a remote monitoring system for his Implantable Cardioverter Defibrillator. Dr Arora cites all of these

electronic modalities as being helpful to him as a survivor. However, he also acknowledges the potential for multiple sources of information to create anxiety and confusion, highlighting the continued importance of being able to communicate with a trusted clinician to help sort through and process the information.

In summary, patient engagement is a critically important dimension of high-quality cancer care, whether it be screening, diagnosis, treatment, or survivorship. This chapter will provide insights on how HIT can be successfully employed to promote and enhance the level and quality of patient engagement across the cancer control continuum.

4.1.2 Primary, Specialty, Hospital, and Community Care Delivery Systems

A spectrum of settings, resources, expertise, and information is required to support each domain of the cancer control spectrum in engaging patients. Care includes multiple patient–clinician relationships that may change in relative importance as patients go through the cancer trajectory. Patient resource needs and support also change over time. To create a connected seamless system of care for patients, clinicians from different settings must work together in a complementary manner throughout the cancer control spectrum. Each setting—primary care, specialty care, hospital, and community setting—has a unique role and value in supporting patients and caregivers.

4.1.2.1 Primary Care Setting

Primary care includes family medicine, general internal medicine, pediatrics, and general obstetrical and gynecology practices. The Institute of Medicine (IOM) defines primary care as "the provision of *integrated, accessible health care services* by clinicians who are *accountable* for addressing a large *majority of personal health needs*, developing a *sustained partnership* with *patients*, and practicing in the *context of family and community*" [11]. The IOM identifies seven key attributes that characterize primary care stating that primary care is (1) accessible, (2) coordinated, (3) sustained, (4) comprehensive, (5) a partnership with patients, (6) person-centered, and (7) integrated. Central to primary care is the patient–clinician relationship, family and community for context, and an integrated delivery system as a means for extending and improving delivery of care (see Fig. 4.1).

The IOM makes the assertion that "primary care is the logical foundation of an effective health care system because it can address the large majority of health problems in the population." Evidence clearly demonstrates that primary care is good for health within countries and internationally [12]. Health is better in areas with

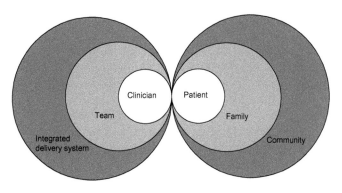

FIGURE 4.1 The Institute of Medicine's visual representation of primary care demonstrates the interdependence of primary care components including (1) the centrality of the patient–clinician relationship, (2) how family and community provide context to understand and assist patients and clinicians with care, and (3) the team of health care professionals and integrated delivery systems as a means to extend and improve care. These same principles can also be extended to the cancer care delivery system. *Source: Adapted from the Institute of Medicine report, Primary Care (Donaldson MS, Yordy KD, Lohr KN, Vanselow NA. Primary care: America's health in a new era. Washington, DC: National Academy Press; 1996).*

more primary care physicians; people who receive care from primary care physicians are healthier, and the characteristics of primary care are associated with better health. Primary care extends life span, reduces morbidity, increases patient satisfaction, reduces disparities, and is highly cost-effective. It is also consistently and frequently where the majority of people receive their care [13].

In 2004, a new model or philosophy for organizing, delivering, and improving primary care emerged—the Patient-Centered Medical Home (PCMH). The model has been adopted and endorsed by the American Academy of Pediatrics, American Academy of Family Physicians, and the American College of Physicians. The PCMH model was designed in response to a growing recognition of the unsustainable increased costs of health care and gaps in quality of care, with the goal of improving primary care access, quality, value, and efficiency. PCMH principles include a team approach to care, use of quality improvement methodology to continuously assess and improve care processes, provision of care that is patient-centered and comprehensive, population-based approaches to care, and adoption of HIT to facilitate these principles [14]. The PCMH is ideally suited to improving all domains of the cancer control continuum by encouraging a proactive and anticipatory approach to care.

Some key primary care roles in the cancer control continuum include delivery of preventive care (eg, health behavior counseling, screening, immunizations, and chemoprevention); initial diagnosis and management of cancer; ensuring continuity of care and whole person care during cancer treatment; long-term surveillance

after cancer treatment; and end-of-life planning. Ideally, patients establish a relationship with a primary care clinician when healthy. This trusting relationship allows the primary care clinician to influence unhealthy behaviors to prevent cancer; promote screening to identify cancer at an earlier stage when it is easier to treat; participate in selection and referral to a specialist as well as selection of initial treatment; and even initiate end-of-life planning—ideally prior to development of life-threatening conditions. Given their breadth of knowledge, when screening tests return abnormal or patients present with new symptoms, primary care clinicians are uniquely positioned to determine the next steps and initiate referrals for care once a diagnosis is made. With their whole person focus to care, primary care clinicians can play a vital role in coordinating care during cancer treatment, addressing treatment complications, and managing unrelated chronic conditions and new issues. Finally, because of their longitudinal approach to care, primary care clinicians are well suited to resume care after cancer treatment ends, which includes monitoring for long-term side effects from treatment, watching for cancer recurrence, promoting health activities, and screening for new primary cancers.

Historically, primary care clinicians have not been as involved in care during active cancer treatment or in the immediate survivorship phase. While the focus of care to meet the patient's immediate needs when diagnosed with cancer should often shift to the specialty setting, not continuing the relationship with the primary care clinician can create a fragmented and siloed care delivery experience for patients [15]. During this time, patients may miss out on the support that the relationship with their primary care clinician can provide.

4.1.2.2 Specialty and Hospital Setting

As medical knowledge has evolved and treatments become more sophisticated, varied, and targeted to specific conditions, the skills required to assess and deliver care have also evolved. For cancer patients, oncologists frequently play the major role in making a diagnosis, deciding on a treatment plan, delivering and monitoring treatment, and making initial surveillance for treatment success and cancer recurrence (initial can be defined as the first 5 years after treatment). Given the wide variety of cancer treatments available, there are many types of oncologists that could become involved in care, including surgical oncologists, medical oncologists, and radiation oncologists. Sometimes nononcology providers will direct treatment and surveillance for cancer, such as an endocrinologist for thyroid cancer, urologist for prostate cancer, or gastroenterologist and/or surgeon for early stage colon cancers. In short, multimodal therapy with a team of specialists has become more the standard of care for patients with cancer rather than the exception.

When a patient is diagnosed with cancer, he or she may not only have a shift in the main care delivery team from primary care to cancer specialists, but there may also be a shift from ambulatory-based to hospital-based care. This may never occur, it may happen once, or it can be a repeated event depending on the nature of treatment and the complications a patient experiences. Some treatments (eg, major surgery or some chemotherapy regiments) mandate hospital-based care. Likewise some complications (eg, neutropenic fever) are better managed in the hospital. If hospital care is required, hospital specialists may be called upon for consultation or comanagement. This further adds to the team of treating clinicians. It also triggers two transitions in care—from ambulatory to hospital care and then a return to ambulatory care.

A unique challenge faced by cancer specialists, compared to primary care clinicians is that they generally do not have a background familiarity or relationship with a patient when initially consulted about a potential cancer diagnosis—The exception being for patients with a prior cancer history. This is particularly difficult given that being confronted with a cancer diagnosis is a momentous and scary event for patients. As a result, it is essential for cancer specialists to rapidly establish a trusting relationship to partner with and engage patients in their care.

Once a cancer diagnosis is made, the relationship between patients and their cancer team can quickly become quite strong. Patients look to their cancer specialist as an expert who is hopefully providing a life-saving treatment—a treatment that may also have some real potential for significant adverse risks and harms. Patients and their loved ones look to their cancer team for guidance, reassurance, hope, and answers to difficult questions about their diagnosis, treatment, and prognosis. Accordingly, cancer care must provide many of the same attributes as primary care and be accessible, coordinated, sustained, comprehensive, a partnership, person-centered, and integrated. Furthermore, the cancer care setting must be organized similar to the PCMH for cancer patients. The centrality of the patient–clinician relationship, understanding of family and community context, and coordination within an integrated delivery system to extend and improve care, as depicted in Fig. 4.1, all apply to cancer care. The main distinctions from primary care are that cancer care (1) is structured around an episode of care—cancer diagnosis, treatment, and initial surveillance—although not infrequently this episode can be for an extended time period (eg, 5 plus years) and (2) is focused on cancer and the associated issues related to cancer and its treatment. However, some have proposed the concept of a medical oncology home for cancer patients that would provide the full range of patient services [16].

The processes of care to support cancer treatment and surveillance goals in a specialty or hospital setting do have some important differences from the primary care setting. This has implications for the HIT needs of cancer specialists and patients receiving cancer care. However, not unlike primary care, good cancer treatment is dependent on having reliable and accurate diagnostic and treatment information. The documentation needs during cancer care, in terms of diagnosis and treatment, are both very detailed and very specific. Details about a diagnosis are increasingly complex and include cancer type; pathology information; cancer stage and progression; receptor status (eg, estrogen-receptor status for breast cancer); and genetic information. To complicate matters, information about diagnosis can change over time for patients (eg, stage progression for patients failing treatment). Additionally, our knowledge and understanding as a field, in terms of information about diagnosis, is evolving as we learn about new prognostic and treatment markers. This may make it important to add diagnostic information to patient's documentation and clarify gaps in a patient's record when diagnosed prior to knowledge of new markers.

Treatment protocols, particularly when involving chemotherapy, are similarly complex. Protocols need to be both standardized based on the evidence and tailored to an individual patient's needs. This is complex in terms of documenting a patient's progression through a treatment protocol and any adjustments that have been made to the treatment protocol. In some cases, clinicians need to be able to identify experimental treatment protocols for patients with more rare cancers or who have failed standard therapies. This is often done in the context of participating in national trials to both potentially help the patient and advance knowledge about treatment regimens. Throughout standard or experimental protocols, mechanisms need to be in place to help alert clinicians to and identify adverse reactions and treatment failures. Identifying adverse reactions and treatment failures may be based on quantitative information (eg, laboratory results or radiographic studies) or qualitative information (eg, patient symptoms such as pain or fevers). Given how important it is for clinicians to follow a patient's progression through treatment and know when a patient is experiencing an adverse reaction or treatment failure, helping patients understand this information to partner in their care is paramount.

Once treatment is completed, an added challenge is ensuring that the patient and future care team members, including the patient's primary care clinician, know all necessary information about the diagnosis, treatment, prognosis, and long-term surveillance plans. One solution is to provide cancer treatment summaries and survivorship care plans (TS/SCPs) [15,17]. While these are discussed in greater detail later in the chapter, here are some current challenges with TS/SCPs to note: there are multiple accepted TS/SCP formats; there is limited evidence empirically demonstrating the value of TS/SCPs; the processing time and personnel required to prepare TS/SCPs is intense and often not reimbursable; and the best way to store, share, and update TS/SCPs is unknown [18]. However, given the importance of this type of information for a patient's future care and follow-up care, beginning in 2015, the American College of Surgeons Commission on Cancer has begun to require that all accredited institutions have in place a strategy for the provision of TS/SCPs to all patients completing cancer treatment. HIT could play a prominent role in creating TS/SCPs, integrating TS/SCPs into a patient's standard health information, and translating content into lay language to better inform and engage patients as partners in their long-term care.

4.1.2.3 Community Setting

Patients, even those with cancer, spend a small fraction of their lives interacting with the clinical care delivery system. Accordingly, the community where patients live, work, play, and learn is critically important in terms of understanding contextual factors that influence health and thinking about how the community can be part of the clinical care delivery and support system for patients (see Part I, Chapter 2, "Reducing Cancer Disparities Through Community Engagement: The Promise of Informatics" by Oh et al.). Many blue-ribbon panels, such as IOM, have advocated for better integration of the community and clinical care delivery systems [19–21]. Integration is consistent with the PCMH model and our national goal of improving population health. Integration could be beneficial across the cancer control spectrum, from the prevention and early detection of cancer to the treatment and surveillance of cancer patients.

Contextual factors and socioeconomic determinants of health have a tremendous impact on health outcomes. It has been estimated that a combination of environmental exposures, social circumstances, and behavioral patterns contribute more to premature mortality in the United States than genetic predispositions and direct health care combined [22]. These factors would also influence responses to cancer treatments. Yet, we have limited understanding of how to improve these social and environmental influences on health. Overall, our clinical care system needs to do a better job of supporting public health and community-led health solutions. The concept of the community championing health is not new, but it has received increased attention through the "communities of solution" movement [23]. Community organizations know their local needs and resources. They are well positioned to partner with community members, public health entities, hospitals, clinicians, and other stakeholders to identify, plan, and address population health needs. Community strategies may be similar to clinical strategies such as funding community health workers, providing health education, or addressing access to clinical care. However, community strategies may also focus on other issues like education, employment, housing, or crime. When addressed, these factors may actually improve health more than traditional clinical interventions.

For its part, the clinical care system also needs the community to support its interests. Most clinicians and practices, primary or specialty care, are stressed and struggle to meet all of the needs of their patients. Many interventions are best delivered in the community and not in the clinical setting. Examples include health behavior counseling support for a patient trying to quit smoking or emotional and logistical support for a patient facing a new cancer diagnosis and undergoing cancer treatment. Community members can help to translate new research and disseminate established evidence-based practices in a way that is relevant, tailored, and meaningful to the community [24]. Community members can help identify health care priorities and feasible interventions. This is exemplified by the use of Boot Camp Translation (BCT) methodology to develop a community intervention to promote colon cancer screening [25].

HIT solutions are needed to integrate community and clinical care. Data-sharing strategies that allow linkages at the patient, practice, and community level to coordinate care and facilitate communication have been identified as one of the "grand challenges" that can help to shape the future of patient and community centered care [23].

4.1.2.4 Rethinking the Care Delivery System

A common need across the cancer control continuum is the need for seamless communication and coordination of care across settings, clinicians, and caregivers. This is particularly important for cancer care. For patients and caregivers, this can improve satisfaction and health outcomes. For clinicians and practices, this can make the stresses of delivering care easier and it can align care activities and goals. Nationally, this can improve public health and reduce health care expenditures. For all of these reasons, it is worth continuing to explore and test new paradigms of care delivery.

Much like the PCMH model, the Accountable Care Organization (ACO) model strives to incentivize the triple aim of improved health, improved care delivery, and reduced cost by creating collective accountability for ACO participants to achieve quality and cost goals [26]. While rooted in primary care, ACO's focus is on coordinating care and managing transitions. An additional focus is preventing illness and managing the sickest patients who have the highest costs and worst outcomes. Accordingly, preventing and treating cancer will be essential ACO tasks. The success of the ACO model will likely rely on effective health information exchange among participants, which could pose logistical challenges for nonintegrated care delivery systems. While some ACO models have been proven to be successful for preventive care and management of common chronic conditions [27], whether the ACO model will be successful for cancer care, particularly acute treatment, remains unproven. What is known is that engaging patients as partners in their care will be essential for any ACO-like model of care. What role patients and communities will play in shaping ACO initiatives beyond proposed quality metrics of patient satisfaction, is unclear.

4.2 OVERVIEW OF HIT TOOLS TO ENGAGE PATIENTS

Effective HIT, appropriately implemented and used, is critically needed to better engage patients in care. HIT has a prominent role in both the PCMH and ACO models of care. It needs to move beyond simply documenting care to promote patient activation through health information sharing, patient education, and self-management tools; communication between patients and care teams; and population management including proactive outreach and reminders for patients and clinicians. The general HIT tools to engage patients are electronic health records (EHRs), patient health records (PHRs) or patient portals, and patient e-health tools. These tools can support a wide range of engagement activities and are fundamentally changing the ways patients and clinicians interact.

4.2.1 Electronic Health Records

While originally functioning as a mere digital version of a patient's paper chart, EHRs now go beyond storing patient data and are an informatics pillar for engaging patients in care. For their part, hospitals, health systems, and ambulatory practices have embraced EHRs and are working to implement and use EHRs to their full potential. Fully 80% of hospitals, over half of ambulatory practices, and two-thirds of primary care practices have adopted an EHR [28]. At its core, an EHR provides a place to create and manage a patient's health information in a standardized format. Since the information is digital, it can be shared with other health care organizations, clinicians, and patients. This can allow for the aggregation of all pertinent patient information from multiple sources for both clinicians and patients.

By having and sharing information, the EHR serves as a rich clinical data repository for patients to access (described below) and to drive practice and clinician patient engagement activities. For example, as part of

Meaningful Use—a $27 billion incentive program for practices and hospitals to adopt EHRs—clinicians are expected to give patients a clinical summary after office visits that includes basic clinical information such as care provided, old and new medications, upcoming appointments, and patient instructions. If done well, clinical summaries can raise awareness of what occurred during the office visit, activate patients, and assist in care coordination. EHRs can also have embedded patient educational material both linked to and tailored by the patient's clinical information. Alerts and reminders can use information in the EHR to prompt clinicians to engage with patients in certain ways and at certain times, such as prompting a motivational interviewing session during a teachable moment.

The EHR can be a key platform to coordinate team activities that support and engage patients. This can occur within and across care settings when EHR functionality is interconnected. The simplest example of how an EHR can coordinate team activities is sharing records, such as encounter notes or clinical summaries that list and detail engagement activities. More robust systems can allow for the tasking of care team members and documenting completed steps. Further, the clinical information in the EHR is ideally suited to support population health management activities. This can allow practices to proactively identify and reach out to patients in need of care as well as track population health, adjusted for illness severity, and nationally and regionally benchmarked.

4.2.2 Patient Portals and Personal Health Records

Patient portals and PHRs serve as a focal point of entry for patients to access, manage, and act on their health information. Two distinct options are available: (1) stand-alone PHRs offered by industry, health insurance plans, or others; and (2) integrated PHRs, often referred to as patient portals, that function more as an extension of a practice's or health system's EHR for patients. There is some debate as to which model will benefit patients more [29]. Both can be linked to existing patient clinical data and both can provide similar functionality. A distinct advantage of integrated PHRs is that they can allow for more patient–clinician interaction. Conversely, integrated PHRs may lack key health information if the clinician's EHR is not integrated into a broader health information network. To a large extent, Meaningful Use is driving clinicians to rapidly adopt and promote integrated PHRs. In some cases, this results in patients having multiple PHRs with multiple clinicians to access and maintain. In the future, the distinction between these two types of PHRs may become blurred as PHR functionality becomes more standardized, health information is more broadly exchanged, and systems become more interoperable and integrated.

Another aspect of PHRs is that they are a central tool for engaging patients. One function that patients have widely adopted is the provision of secure email messaging. This gives patients increased access to their health care team, supports asynchronous care, and streamlines the workflow within practices. Secure messaging has been shown to improve quality outcomes, patient satisfaction, self-management, and care delivery [30,31]. Secure messaging is a core functionality for most integrated PHRs and is among one of the more highly used PHR functions [32,33]. While clinicians initially feared secure messaging would add to their busy workload, on the whole this fear has not been realized. In fact, clinicians often report reduced workload through easier communication. This can make tasks, like informing patients of laboratory results, faster and easier. The second core functionality of PHRs is sharing health information with patients. This can be as simple as showing a list of medications, diagnoses, and allergies. Or it can be more robust and include laboratory and radiology results, clinical summaries, and even office notes. How much information is shared is determined by what information is accessible, the configured PHR's functionality, and what practices and health systems chose to show patients. Having access to this information has been shown to help patients feel better prepared for clinical encounters, know more about their health care, increase medication adherence, and generally be more engaged in care [34].

More advanced PHRs go beyond the basic patient engagement functions of secure messaging and sharing clinical information. Patient educational material can be linked to clinical information in PHRs such as diagnoses and medications, effectively directing patients to trusted sources of tailored information. This process is being put into place nationally with the MedlinePlus Connect initiative. Educational material can even be tailored to a patient's specific clinical profile [31]. While highly useful and valuable for patients, this is more complicated to create and maintain. PHRs can also show patients a status of where they are at with receiving recommended care and alert them as they become overdue for services. The PHR can serve as a mechanism for patients to share patient-reported information with their care team. This may include (1) important elements of the health history such as family history, health behaviors, and mental health symptoms; (2) patient values, goals, and preferences needed to make clinical decisions; (3) patient priorities to guide care; (4) specific complaints and symptoms; or (5) even patient-reported outcomes (PROs) that can be used to assess and measure the quality of care. Further, the PHR can be a place where patients receive asynchronous care, beyond secure messaging, such as virtual encounters through clinician–patient video.

PHRs of the future could even provide patients personalized health information about their community, home and work environments, and occupational hazards and opportunities.

4.2.3 Patient e-Health Tools

Patient e-health tools are a broad category of electronic tools and services that are patient oriented such as personal monitoring devices, mobile health applications, and Internet resources [35]. Target users can include patients, families, and caregivers. While patient e-health tools represent a rapidly expanding market, the current use of these tools and their impact on health is not fully understood and their potential to improve health has also not been fully realized.

More than 80% of US Internet users have searched for health information online. Devices and applications to track and monitor health are widely available for patients to use. The technology to support patients passively monitoring everything from daily exercise to sleep quality to exposure to local environmental health hazards (eg, air quality) is rapidly advancing. Additionally, these tools have unprecedented capacity to instantly access massive amounts of data to help inform patients (eg, nutritional information from food barcodes). While evidence is emerging that using patient e-health tools improve health, a major limitation with many of these tools is that they are not integrated into the health care delivery system. Patients often have no way of sharing information from these tools with their care team.

4.2.4 A National Strategy to Promote HIT for Patient Engagement

In the United States, the Office of the National Coordinator (ONC) has developed a strategy to advance the use of patient engagement through HIT called the "Three A's" strategy [35]. The first A, and what ONC has the greatest ability to control, is to increase patient *access* to HIT. Access is being promoted through Meaningful Use. In addition to promoting HIT adoption, Meaningful Use includes EHR/PHR functionality and use mandates that engage patients like secure messaging, clinical summaries, patient reminders, patient educational material, and basic patient-reported information (eg, family history and advanced directives). Access is also being promoted through the Blue Button Pledge program, which can allow patients to download their health information from data holders via a standardized "Blue Button" and can allow sharing of health information via Direct (a standardized way of pushing data to where it is needed).

The second A stands for enabling *action*. ONC is committed to supporting developers who enable e-health tools. This includes supporting ongoing initiatives like the Blue Button Pledge program and periodic "challenges" and pilot programs to fund new and innovative patient engagement activities that can be nationally disseminated. The final A is for efforts to shift patient and clinician *attitudes* toward patient engagement through HIT. This includes fostering trust in privacy and security, supporting patients' rights to access health information, and using the power of storytelling to share examples of how patient engagement is improving health outcomes.

4.2.5 General Limitations of Current Systems

Despite the potential for HIT to engage patients in their care, clinicians and patients alike are quick to complain about the current state of HIT. Many clinicians' lives revolve around their EHR. It is common for a clinician to simultaneously access, view, and enter information in his or her EHR throughout a patient encounter. Many clinicians spend personal time in front of their computers completing tasks and messaging patients. As a result, many clinicians express frustration with their EHRs. Clinicians state that their EHRs have limited functionality and this aspect creates extra work as clerical and data entry tasks are added to their already overburdened workloads [36]. They also find that taking a computer into the exam room can detract from clinician–patient communication and relationship building. Additionally, while documentation of structured clinical data may be improving, the importance of patient narrative is increasingly ignored [37].

Many have questioned whether HIT and the Meaningful Use objectives directing their design support health care delivery models such as ACOs, the PCMH, and even primary and ambulatory care more broadly [38–40]. EHRs and PHRs remain disease-focused rather than whole-person focused. Critical health influences are often not included such as personal risk factors, health behaviors, family structure and dynamics, social determinants of health, and occupational and environmental influences. Recently, five national primary care organizations developed consensus recommendations that identify additional HIT functionality that clinicians need to provide care to and engage patients; key functionality needs included:

1. Human factors design to ensure that technology supports users' needs;
2. Enhanced extraction, interpretation prioritization, and presentation of critical health information for individual patients at the point of care and for a clinician's patient panel;
3. Advanced information exchange to coordinate care across clinicians and settings;
4. Greater patient engagement tools and supports;

5. Population management innovations, including predictive analytics, to proactively deliver care outside of traditional office visits;
6. Environmental and community information such as local resources and social determinants of health;
7. Reduced documentation burden; and
8. Integration of care across settings—particularly between the health care setting and community [40].

From a patient perspective, a major obstacle to increased use of HIT is lack of access to tools, not a lack of interest. When given the opportunity to access and review their health information online or communicate with their clinician electronically, the vast majority of patients do so [34]. Despite concerns about the "digital divide," age, education, race, ethnicity, and income are poor indicators of which patients will use HIT. In fact, HIT may prove to be a valuable tool for reducing health disparities [41]. Notwithstanding interest, patients do worry about their medical records going digital, expressing fears about whether their privacy and confidentiality can be truly maintained in an era when access to patients' health information has such value [42].

4.2.6 A Model for Making HIT More Patient-Centered

In 2011, Krist and Woolf identified five levels of functionality for well-designed patient-centered HIT systems—collecting patient-reported information, collecting existing clinical information from multiple sources, translating information into lay language, making recommendations by applying information to guidelines, and facilitating informed patient action (see Fig. 4.2) [43]. Depending on the purpose of the HIT tool, some or all of these functionalities will be important. This model is particularly applicable when applied to PHRs.

Overall, patient-centered HIT tools must be relevant, helpful, and easy for patients to access and use [44]. Ideally, they will also be interactive so as to provide patients with relevant feedback about questions or concerns they may have. The best systems can match the unique health information needs and orientations of individual patients to be personally relevant, informative, and useful. Particularly important for oncology care, patient-centered HIT systems should also be sensitive to the emotional states of users, provide sensitive and caring responses, and reinforce the development of a trusting clinician–patient relationship. Key questions that can help guide the design of patient-centered systems include:

- *How interactive is the HIT system?* Does the system enable patients to ask questions and receive relevant answers? Can patients provide feedback about their care and about use of the system? Can the system be designed to elicit information from patients?

Level   Functionality

Level	Functionality
1	Collect patient information, such as self-reported demographic and risk factor information (health behaviors, symptoms, diagnoses, and medications)
2	Integrate patient information with clinical information through links to the electronic medical record and/or claims data
3	Interpret clinical information for the patient by translating clinical findings into lay language and delivering health information via a user-friendly interface
4	Provide individualized clinical recommendations to the patient, such as screening reminders, based on the patient's risk profile and on evidence-based guidelines
5	Facilitate informed patient action integrated with primary and specialty care through the provision of vetted health information resources, decision aids, risk calculators, personalized motivational messages, and logistical support for appointments and follow-up

FIGURE 4.2   Five levels of functionality to help make HIT more patient-centered. *Source: Adapted from Krist AH, Woolf SH. A vision for patient-centered health information systems. JAMA 2011;305(3):300–1.*

- *Is the HIT system designed to capture audience attention?* Is the system interesting, relevant, and enjoyable for patients to use? If not, patients may be reluctant to use health information systems.
- *Does the HIT system communicate health information clearly?* Is the information easy for patients to understand, apply to their own health situations, and use to make informed health decisions?
- *Does the HIT system communicate health information compellingly?* Do messages encourage patients to participate in decision making, motivate them to engage in care, and persuade them to follow medical recommendations?
- *Does the HIT system communicate humanely and sensitively?* Is the system relationally-sensitive, providing the patient empathy, social support, and encouragement to build their personal resilience and well-being?
- *Will the system adapt to unique user communication orientations?* Can the system accommodate the

patient's preferred language, education level, literacy and numeracy level, and personal interests in a culturally sensitive manner?
- *Does the HIT system provide patients with health content information that is relevant to their specific health conditions, concerns, and information needs?* Can the system match information provided to patients with their unique health history, health risk profile, and treatment and prevention schedule?
- *Will the HIT system promote immediacy?* Immediacy refers to communication that is engaging, personally involving, and dramatic so as to encourage feelings of interest, closeness, and excitement. Communicating with high levels of immediacy enhances attention, learning, cooperation, and satisfaction [45].

If clinical information is required to support a patient-centered HIT tool, it should be accessed from existing sources whenever possible. Patients cannot be expected to remember, or even to have to keep track of details such as diagnoses, laboratory dates and results, pathology reports, complex chemotherapy, or radiation treatments, etc. Likewise, for many patient-centered HIT tools, mere clinical information is not enough. Information only known by patients, such as how they think or feel or what they want, must be provided by the patient. Patient-centered HIT can bring together information to share with the care team and uniquely activate and engage patients (Level 1 and Level 2 functionality).

Presenting clinical content in lay or plain language is another critical element of patient-centered HIT. Some systems confuse rather than inform patients. This is especially true for patients with lower health literacy. Medical records are notoriously difficult for most patients to understand. Merely showing existing clinical content presents a health literacy challenge for almost any patient. This is more complicated when people are sick and may not think as clearly as usual and when they are concerned and even fearful about their health conditions. They may be cognitively impaired by medications, pain, nausea, fatigue, and a whole host of conditions that further interfere with communication. It is not surprising that patients who are confronting serious health problems such as cancer often experience difficulties understanding complex health information.

Beyond merely aggregating and showing patients their health information, higher functioning patient-centered systems can render clinical advice. This can be automated through applied logic grounded on evidence-based guidelines and standards of care. Alternatively, the system can allow for members of the patient's health care team to define displayed clinical advice. There are challenges with both automated and clinician defined advice. Providing clinician defined advice is more time-consuming and may not be timely. It may also at times depart from evidence-based guidelines. Automated advice can help to reinforce guideline-based care, but it may be spurious or too generic advice—correct for the general population, but wrong for an individual patient. In either scenario, there may be multiple guidelines or standards of care, deciding which an HIT system will follow needs justification.

Most critical to engaging patients in their care is the fifth level of functionality, helping patients to take action. This level of functionality is often necessary to improve both care delivery and health outcomes. This can be done through personalizing information to increase its relevance to patients, motivating patients through persuasive and tailored content, supporting self-management, and even providing logistical support and follow-up. Ideally, this would all be done in coordination with the patient's care team.

Regrettably, most HIT programs do not live up to these patient-centered communication standards. Many HIT systems are overly complex, formal, technical, and difficult to use. The information they provide is often just the basic medical facts, presented in relatively dispassionate, boring, and unimaginative ways. Even worse, the health promotion messages provided on many of these HIT systems can sometimes actually be insulting and disempowering to patients. Advice and content to promote action can be overly directive and prescriptive or presented as inflexible, static one-way messages, with minimal interaction and opportunities for patient involvement. Much of the design emphasis to date has needed to focus on technical issues rather than on making the system effective at patient communication. This is a limitation given that health promoting communication is an intricate, interactive process that depends on the quality of relevant adaptive messages that are exchanged over time.

4.2.6.1 MyPreventiveCare: A Patient-Centered Design Success

One successful patient-centered design story is the MyPreventiveCare application to promote US Preventive Services Task Force (USPSTF) recommendations, which is generically called an interactive preventive health record (IPHR). Details of the MyPreventiveCare IPHR design have been previously published and sample content is available online [31,46]. In brief, the MyPreventiveCare IPHR functions as an application integrated into a clinician's EHR and integrated PHR. A patient can log into their clinician's PHR and click on the MyPreventiveCare icon. Using existing single sign on solutions patient credentials are passed to the MyPreventiveCare IPHR, which extracts hundreds of clinical data elements from the EHR database. Patients also complete a health risk assessment (HRA) and enter needed clinical information not extractable from the EHR.

The IPHR applies programmed logic, based on the USPSTF recommendations and dozens of additional chronic care recommendations, to generate a personally tailored list of prevention and chronic care recommendations. The interface offers patients hyperlinks to detailed personal messages that explain each preventive service or chronic care need and its rationale. The messages reference relevant details in the patient's history (eg, prior laboratory test values and dates), includes links to evidence-based educational material and decision aids, summarizes next steps, and provides action buttons so patients to initiate and follow through on care recommendations. Message content is modeled after Healthfinder, but personalized to each patient's profile. Patients are further able to use this content to prepare for visits that includes an opportunity for the patient to update his/her medical record, review needed care that will be discussed at the visit, SDM tools (described in detail below), prioritization exercises, and an opportunity for the patient to share his/her confidence with making health behavior changes or improving uncontrolled chronic conditions. After the patient uses the MyPreventiveCare IPHR, the system automatically forwards a summary to the EHR inbox of the patient's clinician, which can be used for proactive identification of care needs outside of visits and serve as standing orders for care team members to initiate care.

A unique element of the MyPreventiveCare IPHR design is that it was built using principles promoted by the PCORI in their methodology report. Throughout the design, implementation, and evaluation process, clinicians and patients were engaged as codevelopers and coinvestigators. This results in a design that patients and clinicians valued, met their needs, and could be integrated into the primary care practice workflow. As a result of this process, participants developed a nationally disseminated implementation guide [47]. Nearly 200 clinicians and more than 70,000 patients routinely use the system. Additionally, in a randomized controlled trial, MyPreventiveCare IPHR users were twice as likely as nonusers to be up-to-date on all indicated preventive services postintervention and screening rates increased by 9–23% for colorectal, breast, and cervical cancer screening among users [31]. Practices also successfully incorporated the IPHR into their workflow—using it to prepare patients for visits, augment health behavior counseling discussions, explain test results, issue automatic patient reminders for overdue services, prompt clinicians about services patients need during encounters, and formulate personalized prevention plans.

4.3 KEY PATIENT ENGAGEMENT ACTIVITIES

4.3.1 Empowering Patients With Health Information

Relevant, timely, and accurate health information is arguably the most important resource for empowering patients to enable them to participate fully in making important health care decisions and directing their care. This is especially relevant for cancer care, where there are often so many factors to consider when making the best health care choices [48]. Cancer is a complex array of health challenges, with many different sites, stages, causes, screening strategies, treatment strategies, and prognoses. Patients need an overwhelming amount of specific and detailed information to understand and manage their health. To add to this complex information environment, active programs of cancer research are rapidly generating new knowledge about the biological mechanisms underlying different forms of cancer, new screening and diagnostic techniques, and new forms of treatment and care for different cancers.

It is very difficult for patients to find and navigate useful evidence-based information [49]. Adding to the complexity of the process, cancer is an emotionally charged topic, because it is both common and life-threatening. Receiving a diagnosis of cancer can be a major shock to most patients. Accordingly, cancer communication HIT programs need to not only address information needs but also psychological and socioemotional needs. Care must be taken to provide patients information without confusing or upsetting them. These patient information needs are clearly articulated in Jessie Grumman's book, "AfterShock: What to do when the doctor gives you—or someone you love—a devastating diagnosis." Patient education and engagement are central to coping with cancer and HIT is viewed as a powerful tool to promote these ideals [50].

4.3.1.1 Three Ways HIT Can Inform and Educate Patients

Patients' most basic information need is to have access to their own personal health information. This concept is echoed in e-Patient Dave's constant mantra, "Gimme my damn data!" Although patients have the legal right to their information, access has been constrained culturally and technically. Meaningful Use (stage 2) is beginning to tackle this problem by mandating the provision of clinical summaries to patients after 50% of office visits and providing patients summaries for 65% of care transitions including up-to-date problem, medication, and allergy lists. Similarly, PHRs are increasingly giving patients increased on demand access to view their most up-to-date health information. PHRs are serving as a platform to electronically share clinical summaries and care transition plans. The OpenNotes movement is pushing patient access to health information even further by advocating for giving patients access to their entire health record, including clinician notes. Some clinicians have expressed concerns with giving patients full access to all of their health information fearing that it will lead to confusion and worry, while creating extra work for clinicians to explain information and address unfounded patient concerns. These fears have largely been unrealized. Multiple OpenNotes studies have demonstrated that sharing this information results in increased patient preparation for visits, greater understanding of conditions, better care plan recall, improved treatment adherence, and feeling more in control of health. Clinicians largely do not report extra work. Most patients did not contact their clinician in response to reviewing notes and the ones who did largely wanted to know more about their health issues, medications, and results, representing an opportunity for increased patient understanding and partnership [51].

Another major way that HIT can help inform patients is to increase access to educational material. Most patients are already online searching for health information and there is an overwhelming amount of information available to patients today. Some information is of questionable value and the volume of information can make it difficult for patients to find the information that their clinician would want them to review. To cope with these challenges, patients may use trusted sources of information such as www.cancer.gov, www.cancer.org, www.mayoclinic.org, www.webmd.com. Patients may also use their clinician's PHR as an entry point to access educational material endorsed by their clinician. Meaningful Use (stage 2) mandates the provision of patient-specific education resources for 10% of patient encounters. Some EHRs have partnered with educational companies (eg, HealthWise and Up-to-Date) to incorporate educational material into the EHR. Through the EHR's computerized physician order entry system, clinicians can "order" educational material to be printed or emailed to their patient. An alternative solution has been to link educational material to diagnoses, medications, and laboratory tests within a PHR. This can be accomplished through tools like MedlinePlus Connect, a free service provided by the National Library of Medicine that directs patients to educational materials and videos. Another example is the MyPreventiveCare IPHR described above that linked patients to tailored educational material, calculators, planning tools, and logistical support for preventive and chronic care based on their clinical profile and national guidelines. Many studies have clearly demonstrated that the provision of patient educational material can benefit a range of cancer issues such as screening, health behaviors, decision making, treatment adherence, management of treatment complications, and pain management.

HIT can also support patient education by linking patients with experts and other patients to share firsthand knowledge and personal experiences. HIT can allow patients to connect virtually as individuals or groups as well as anonymously or identifiably. One example is the social network site PatientsLikeMe, described in more detail in Chapter 16. These connections can help patients learn how to address psychosocial needs, learn about uncommon conditions, and normalize experiences.

Many challenges remain with providing patients information to promote patient engagement in care. Patient health information may be stored in multiple information silos. PHRs that only access some information silos will be incomplete. Much of the documentation created as part of care is designed for clinicians. It contains technical language and is not formatted for patients, suggesting a need to reengineer antiquated clinical notes, diagnosis lists, and other clinical data elements to be more patient-centered. Overall, to be beneficial patients need the right educational material at the right time. Yet the workflow to provide information

largely depends on patients finding information on their initiative or clinicians identifying information for patients. Smart mechanisms to anticipate and automate patient information needs are needed.

4.3.2 Gathering Patient-Reported Information

Another promising way that HIT can engage patients in their care is to facilitate the collection of patient-reported information. There is a range of patient-reported activities that can include (1) review and update of health information; (2) share health behaviors; (3) complete mental health screen; (4) identify goals, preferences, and priorities; (5) report symptoms and narrative; (6) share self-monitoring metrics; and (7) provide PROs. Patient-reported information is a powerful tool that can inject the patient's voice into the medical record informing and guiding care. It can occur in an unstructured manner as exemplified by a patient initiating a secure message to the clinician. Or it can occur in a structured manner at key touch points in the care delivery process as when a patient is asked to complete a Patient Health Questionnaire-2 to screen for depression prior to a visit and responses are stored as part of the standard data architecture.

Giving patients access to their medical record will result in their identifying inaccuracies. Inaccuracies may be the result of outdated information, care delivered, and changes made in other settings, or patient–clinician misperceptions. In the MyPreventiveCare IPHR study previously described, 59% of patients identified and updated their preventive and chronic care information after reviewing their record and almost universally, clinicians accepted these changes and incorporated them into the patient's record [31]. HIT solutions that facilitate the patient identification and correction of information can not only improve documentation but also reduce clinician workload. For example, avatars have been successfully used to automate medication reconciliation during discharge planning. Some patients even preferred interacting with the avatar than a clinician [52].

A cornerstone of any encounter is eliciting the patient's story. This is fundamental to making a diagnosis, guiding treatment, identifying and preventing health risks, and monitoring for illness recurrence. HIT is increasingly used as a tool to initially collect history of the present illness or symptoms as exemplified by tools like Instant Medical History. HIT is also increasingly used by patients to self-monitor their health and some of these tools even allow patients to share this information with their clinician. Initiating the exchange of basic information prior to encounters and giving patients a chance to think through the issues they want to discuss with their clinician can make encounters more focused and productive.

While clinicians agree that knowing about patient's health behaviors and mental health is an important part of caring for patients, routinely collecting this information among all the other competing clinical demands is difficult. This applies to both the primary care setting for the provision of preventive care and the specialty setting for the provision of cancer care. Unhealthy behaviors and mental health needs are ubiquitous and lead to increased morbidity and mortality in all patients. To encourage the routine collection of this information, the Centers for Medicare & Medicaid Services (CMS) has mandated the routine provision of patient-centered HRAs, also known as a health risk assessment plus (HRA Plus), as part of an Annual Wellness Visit. An HRA Plus systematically screens for health behavior and mental health risks, allows patients to prioritize concerns, provides immediate feedback, supports goal setting, alerts clinicians to patients' concerns, provides follow-up activities, and monitors progress toward achieving improvement goals [53].

The final domain of patient-reported information is the collection of PROs. PROs include any patient-reported health status for physical, mental, and social well-being. PROs are increasingly used as outcomes in research studies, tools to understand the patient experience when receiving clinical care, and measures of the quality of care being provided. The power of PROs is that the information collected cannot be found in traditional clinical measures. The National Institutes of Health has funded the development and widespread adoption of a set of PROs that can be used across a wide variety of conditions and patient populations called the Patient Reported Outcomes Measurement Information System (PROMIS) tools.

One challenge with collecting patient-reported information is integrating the process into the existing care workflow. A critical consideration is ensuring that the patient is queried at the right time and that the responses reach the clinician at the right time. The simplest workflow is to have the patient report information prior to an encounter and deliver the information to the clinician during the encounter as this is an easy time to act on the information. Querying patients outside of encounters can more proactively identify issues, but this requires a mechanism to decide what patient-reported information should be assessed and a mechanism to alert the right care team member when response to the information is needed. Building upon a clinician's EHR/PHR infrastructure can facilitate this process.

While patient-reported information is often directly collected by clinicians and practice personal during patient interactions, HIT can facilitate a more effective and less labor intensive process. The My Own Health Report (MOHR) study highlights the value of HIT for collecting patient-reported information. In this cluster-randomized pragmatic trial, nine diverse pairs of primary care practices were asked to field the MOHR HRA Plus, which addressed diet, exercise, smoking, alcohol, drug use, stress, depression, anxiety, and sleep. Prior to wellness and chronic care visits patients were invited to complete MOHR and a summary of responses were sent electronically to clinicians for review with patients during the encounter. MOHR included questions to assess behaviors and mental health; classification of responses as to no, some, or high concern; motivational feedback for patients including initial improvement steps and a space to create SMART goals (specific, measurable, achievable, realistic, and timely); and an opportunity to define which risks patients wanted to change and discuss with the clinician. Study outcomes included whether this process was feasible in primary care, the frequency and prioritization of patient health risks, and the influence of the process on goal setting, health behaviors, and mental health. Collectively, the results told an interesting story. It was feasible to field an HRA Plus in primary care—1782 of 3591 approached patients completed MOHR. Fielding the HRA Plus was labor intensive, adding nearly 23 minutes to already busy encounters, but highly valuable, identifying an average of 5.8 unhealthy behaviors and mental health concerns among respondents and increasing the number of patients who reported they made a goal to make changes and actually made an improvement [54,55].

Several needs remain in order for HIT to more fully support the process of patient-reported information. Agreement is needed as to the best domains and specific questions to solicit patient-reported information. The PROMIS measures are working to standardize PROs. A recent IOM committee started the process of standardizing social and behavioral domains [56]. Further, data standards are needed for the storage and exchange of patient-reported information. Cultural changes from patients and clinicians are needed to set the expectation that patients will report information and clinicians will review and access patient-reported information. Collectively, HIT can provide the much needed infrastructure to support all of these needed activities.

4.3.3 Engaging Patients in Medical Decision Making

Across the cancer control continuum, clinicians and patients face a range of medical decisions. Decisions might include, but are not limited to, whether to make a health behavior change, when to start or how to get screened, how to prioritize competing needs, which treatment option to start, or when to change or stop a treatment. Some decisions are straightforward, with one clear ideal choice. However, many decisions have multiple options, each with a different profile of advantages and disadvantages. Some decisions are best made on clinical grounds, based on the nature of the condition, the patient's personal risks, comorbidities, or contraindications. Other decisions must be made based on the patient's values, preferences, and life circumstances. These decisions benefit from patient engagement and participation in the decision-making process.

There is growing emphasis on shifting the traditional paternalistic health care delivery model, in which clinicians make choices for patients, to one in which clinicians serve as navigators and not pilots, and patients make their medical decisions. Engaging patients in medical decision making can be recommended for a number of reasons. From an ethical perspective, it supports patient autonomy and self-determination. Interpersonally, an engaged decision-making process promotes confidence and trust in the clinician–patient relationship. Educationally, it improves knowledge, sets reasonable expectations about benefits and harms, and reduces decision conflict. Ultimately, the consequences of a patient's choice cannot be shared with anyone else and the patient must suffer or enjoy the outcomes associated with medical decisions.

4.3.3.1 Examples of Decisions That Require Patient Engagement

Four examples highlight the range of cancer control continuum decisions benefiting from patient engagement: (1) whether to make a health behavior change, (2) whether, when, and how to get cancer screening, (3) which cancer treatment to receive, and (4) when to stop a treatment. Quitting smoking is one of the best decisions a patient can make. Clinicians often tell patients to quit smoking, but ultimately the patient must agree and choose to make a change. This decision often occurs over time in the primary care, specialty, community, and home setting, with multiple clinicians repeating and reinforcing the recommendations over time until the patient is ready to change. Even once a patient decides to quit, further details must be decided. When to quit? How to quit? What additional supports are needed (eg, smoking cessation medications, nicotine replacement, or behavioral counseling)?

For many cancer screening services there are decisions that require patient engagement [57]. These decisions typically occur in primary care settings and may be part of a wellness, acute care, or chronic care visit—frequently with limited time for making a fully informed decision. One example is the age to start breast cancer screening. There is a close balance of benefits and harms with starting mammograms before the age of 50. As a result, whether a woman in her forties should get a mammogram depends on her personal risks, values, and preferences. Similarly prostate cancer screening may have limited or no benefit, yet many men want to be

screened. Even colon cancer screening, which is clearly beneficial, has several screening options (eg, colonoscopy or stool testing).

Once diagnosed with cancer, patients may face several equally effective treatment options with different benefits and harms. Making a treatment decision often requires inputs and discussions with multiple members of the care team (eg, primary care clinician, oncologist, or surgeon). Since these are viewed as "bigger" decisions, patients and clinicians often schedule one or more office visits dedicated just to making a treatment decision. Two classic examples include whether to have a radical prostatectomy versus watchful waiting for men with prostate cancer and whether to have a modified radical mastectomy or lumpectomy with radiation for women with early stage breast cancer. In both examples, the first treatment is more aggressive and may be valued by those concerned about spread or recurrence while the second treatment spares the prostate or breast and may be valued by those who want less invasive treatment. In both examples, each treatment has similar long-term survival and recurrence rates and are acceptable choices.

When to stop cancer treatment is another difficult decision faced by patients whose cancer treatment is not going well. This can be an abrupt decision if a patient is experiencing complications from treatments or rapid cancer progression. Ideally, this type of decision can be made over a longer period of time, starting when a patient considers end-of-life planning even prior to being diagnosed with cancer (see Section 4.3.5). This complex decision involves multiple family members in addition to the patient. In some cases, the patient may not be capable of making the decision. Given these issues, accurate information about patient wishes and documentation are critically important.

4.3.3.2 Decision-Making Models

There is a large body of evidence about how best to support patients with medical decisions that addresses decision-making models, the decision-making process, and aids to support decisions. Two decision-making models that are often used interchangeably include *shared decision making* and *informed decision making*. SDM is broadly defined as a process in which patients are engaged as active partners with their clinician in clarifying medical options and choosing a preferred course of care. The USPSTF believes a shared decision is one in which (1) the patient understands the risk and seriousness of the condition being addressed; (2) understands the service including the risks, benefits, alternatives, and uncertainties; (3) has weighed his or her values regarding potential benefits and harms of the service; and (4) is engaged in the decision at the desired level [58].

Some consider informed decision making as a broader process that also encompasses SDM and can occur in the health care setting or community with the intention of informing an individual's decision [59]. The emphasis of informed decision making is more about the end result of the patient's knowledge about the decision, while SDM focuses more on the process of how a decision is made. Informed decision making parallels the idea of informed consent for research participation. In fact, undergoing a formal informed consent process may be warranted for big decisions, like surgery. Some even advocate formal informed consent for decisions like cancer screening, although practically implementing such a policy would be time-consuming and difficult.

Decision aids are a well-established tool for engaging patients in decisions [60]. Decision aids may be pamphlets, videos, or web-based tools. They are designed to make the decision explicit, describe the options and their associated benefits and harms, and help patients consider options from a personal perspective. To date, decision aids have been demonstrated to increase patient knowledge, lower decisional conflict related to feeling uninformed about options, increase the proportion of patients actively involved with decision making, improve satisfaction with the decision and decision-making process, increase the proportion choosing not to get screened with tests that have a close balance of benefits and harms, and reduce the proportion choosing more invasive treatments. There is mixed evidence suggesting that using a decision aid may be more burdensome for clinicians, requiring more time during visits. Decision aids that demonstrate probabilities and explicitly help patients weigh values in a patient-centered manner seem to be more effective in engaging patients.

Another strategy to engage patients in decision making is to incorporate other members of the care team in the process (eg, nurses) or even create new positions dedicated solely to helping patients make decisions (eg, decision coaches) [61]. This is consistent with the PCMH and ACO models in which all team members function at their highest level and it is not dependent on busy clinicians to accomplish every task.

While the logic for engaging patients in medical decision making is clear, it is often carried out in practice poorly. Clinicians are too busy for long discussions; few can quote accurate data or separate themselves from their own biases; and many lack the training, aptitude, or incentives to apply patient preferences, values, and life circumstances to decisions. Patients themselves may not understand that there are multiple options and a decision to make; if they recognize that there is a choice, it may be difficult to understand the evidence of benefits and harms to participate in decision making; and many may fear the consequences of making a decision. Decision aids, while beneficial, are infrequently used in practice and few practices have nonclinician staff helping patients make decisions [62].

4.3.3.3 *Using HIT for Decision Making*

HIT can provide a solution to help clinicians and patients by facilitating information sharing; helping patients to understand information; personalizing estimates of risks and benefits; standardizing presentation of information; promoting both automation and person-to-person exchanges of information; and facilitating the decision-making process over time, distance, and decision-making participants.

Patients are frequently unaware that they have a choice to make and clinicians spend much of their limited time conveying basic information. As defined by the HealthIT. gov National Learning Consortium, well-designed HIT systems can anticipate when patients will face a care choice, invite patients to participate in decisions, present options, provide information about benefits and risks, and guide patients through evaluating options. All of this can occur prior to or outside of visits allowing clinicians to focus on higher level tasks like answering patient questions, ensuring patients understand the information, facilitating the decision, and assisting patients with following through on a decision. Automating this process whenever possible, rather than relying on clinician or staff initiation, will ensure routine and systematic implementation. This is easier for simple recurring decisions (eg, whether to be screened), but will require innovative informatics and workflow solutions for less common decisions.

To convey information in an objective, evidence-based manner, patient portals can direct patients to existing decision aids. High-quality aids are available at no cost from the Mayo Clinic and Ottawa Hospital Research Institute. Because expecting patients to identify the specific aid they need is a barrier, portals need embedded logic and easy navigational tools to direct patients to the right aid at the right time.

The next generation of patient educational material and decisions aids will focus on personalizing information to fully support precision medicine [43]. Using existing evidence, modeling, and predictive analytics, generic information can be transformed to present personalized risks and benefits. This will require careful integration of decision aids with clinical information as well as ensuring that models and analytics do not overstep evidence and misestimate an individual's risks [63]. How information is presented to patients is also critically important. Technology allows for sharing of video and interactive media that is more engaging and easy to understand. Information such as the number needed to treat (or screen) and the number needed to harm, may be of value to patients and clinicians (available from www.thennt. com). Yet, both clinicians and patients have difficulty understanding information about risks and benefits and novel patient-centered methods of presenting quantitative health information are critically needed—both in terms of content and technical advances [64,65].

To close the loop, decision aids can share patient-reported information with clinicians prior to visits. Important information includes where the patient is at with making a decision, additional information needs, comprehension of information, fears and worries, desired next steps, etc.

4.3.4 Patient Engagement to Manage Transitions of Care

Transitions in care occur for many medical conditions, but perhaps no other diagnosis has the potential to incur as many transitions as cancer [66]. Transitions include, but are not limited to, primary care clinician to diagnostic testing, primary care clinician to oncologist, oncologist to other needed specialists, outpatient care to hospital care for cancer treatment (and back to outpatient care), outpatient care to hospital care for management of treatment complications (and back to outpatient care), oncologist to primary care clinician for management of other chronic conditions (and back to the oncologist for cancer care), and oncologist to primary care clinician for long-term survivorship care. Each of these transitions is a handoff when errors may occur, overarching care goals can become confused, and patients can get lost in the process. Each setting and each care team has related but distinct patient care roles, priorities, and competing demands. Each setting may have its own informatics infrastructure, which may or may not have some level of integration. Throughout transitions, patients and their caregivers need support. Poor information transfer between clinicians during care transitions has been identified as a major problem and multiple interventions have focused on improving communication between clinicians [67]. Given that the patient is the one constant across all transitions, robust patient engagement is another approach to manage transitions and help ensure continuity of care.

Findings from a 2011 systematic review of interventions to improve cancer care continuity and outcomes during transitions highlight the challenges [68]. Fifty-one studies tested case management strategies, shared care models, interdisciplinary teams, patient-held records, telephone follow-up, tele-health communication, enhanced medical records, and care protocols. None of the tested interventions improved continuity or the transition process. An added complexity is that patients receiving care from multiple clinicians often report not knowing who to contact for specific issues [67]. Patients may even feel intimidated about sharing concerns or symptoms out of fear of being perceived as complaining or questioning treatment; and patients may perceive that symptoms are just a part of what is to be expected, assuming that their symptoms may not be worth bringing up [69]. Clinicians need to create a safe and receptive environment that allows patients and caregivers to share information; and there needs to be clear designations as to who the patient should report information as well as an easy mechanism for the information to be routed to the appropriate clinician.

In the United States, CMS is focused on improving the care transition process through payment reform and Meaningful Use requirements. To incent hospitals to do better discharge planning, payments are increasingly denied for "avoidable" readmissions. Stage 2 Meaningful Use is targeting all transitions in care by mandating the provision of care summaries for 65% of care transitions. Care summaries must include up-to-date problem, medication, and allergy lists. The application of patient-centered design to the electronic discharge process is beginning to show some benefits in terms of patient satisfaction and the quality of discharge materials patients receive when leaving the hospital [70]. Whether these benefits will translate into reduced readmissions or improved health outcomes remains to be seen.

4.3.4.1 Engaging Patients to Manage Care Transitions

Patient navigation is one evidence-based strategy being applied to help manage care transitions across the cancer control continuum. Patient navigators were originally employed to help patients overcome socio-economic barriers and get cancer screening and have been shown to reduce health disparities [71]. Patient navigators can guide patients through the complexities of the health care system to ensure patients get what they need when they need it and can even link patients to community resources. While mainly studied as a tool to promote screening, the American Cancer Society and Patient-Reported Outcomes Working Group cite the navigator concept as having promise for guiding patients through cancer treatment, symptom management, managing late and long-term treatment effects, overcoming barriers to adopt healthy behaviors, and reducing caregiver burden [72,73].

Promoting patient self-management is another strategy to support transitions in care. Self-management is one of six elements of the Chronic Care Model, a proven framework to guide quality improvement for a number of chronic conditions [74]. Cancer can also be viewed as a chronic illness and cancer care occurs in a continuum that stretches from prevention to the end of life. A review of self-management interventions designed to enable patients and caregivers to manage their cancer care identified benefits such as increased knowledge, symptom improvement, and better quality of life [75]. Notably, the authors point out that patient goals and willingness to participate in self-management may change over time. During active cancer treatment the focus is on reporting and managing symptoms, but once active cancer treatment is complete prevention, health behaviors, and regaining or maintaining functional status become priorities. Group visits may also prove useful in providing patient education, skills training, and support for groups of patients preparing for care transitions. Group visits have been used successfully for other conditions such as pregnancy, asthma, diabetes, and rheumatoid arthritis. More recently, group visits have been shown to be useful in preparing patients for discharge after being newly diagnosed with breast cancer or in supporting survivorship planning for patients who have completed active treatment of their cancer [76,77].

All of the above strategies for supporting care transitions—providing patients clinical summaries, improving clinician–clinician communication, access to patient navigators, supporting self-management, and group visits—need HIT support for success. The creation of clinical summaries is currently a part of any certified EHR, but the next generation of patient-centered summaries to provide more robust support is still being developed. Clinician–clinician communication needs informatics infrastructure to allow easy and seamless transfer for relevant clinical information and governance to ensure that clinicians and patients are on the same page about what information is shared and when it is shared. Some have advocated for a unique "Wiki" style approach to information sharing, in which multiple users in different settings can contribute to and benefit from information in a medical record system over time. This model would allow for real-time data sharing, links to outside resources, and a dynamic communication system of communication that can be adapted to different settings [78]. The benefits of patient navigators and group visits will be severely attenuated if activities and decisions are not shared with the care team. HIT can support this communication as well as connect navigators to patients and bring groups of like patients together. HIT can even automate the provision of self-management resources to patients, track patient success with self-management, and alert the care team when self-management is not working or has identified concerning findings.

4.3.5 Engaging Patients and Caregivers for Survivorship Planning

A major cancer care activity that has received significant attention is survivorship planning. While this topic is detailed in Part II, Chapter 9, "Survivorship," it is reviewed here in the context of patient engagement. The IOM and others recommend that all patients who have completed long-term active treatment receive a TS/SCP [15]. A treatment summary (TS) is a document that details information about diagnosis, including pathology, tumor markers, and other relevant testing; and contains comprehensive treatment information,

including cumulative dosages, treatment dates, complications, and care team members. The survivorship care plan (SCP) is a document focused on recommendations for cancer recurrence surveillance, strategies to maintain health, and resources for psychosocial and practical support [15]. A good TS/SCP can both inform and engage the patient as well as serve as living documentation and communication to future clinicians involved in a patient's care.

Barriers to the implementation and delivery of TS/SCPs have been well documented [18,79,80]. Not surprisingly, TS/SCPs are not widely used. Studies have consistently documented that both cancer survivors and primary care clinicians infrequently receive them [81–83]. When patients receive a TS/SCP, they report having more survivorship discussions with their clinicians and when primary care clinicians report receiving a TS/SCP from an oncologist they report engaging their patients more in survivorship care [82,84].

4.3.5.1 What Do Patients Want From Survivorship Care Planning?

As the best practices for the design and implementation of TS/SCPs are still being developed, there is an opportunity to learn how to make survivorship truly patient-centered. Cancer survivors want their TS/SCP to include terminology that is easy to understand and minimizes the use of technical terms. They want recommendations and detailed educational content that takes into account their specific cultural factors, local context, and the social influences of family roles and their faith community [83]. Patients and caregivers identify psychosocial concerns as a significant challenge and one of their highest priorities, yet experience inadequate support in these domains during survivorship care [85].

There is some uncertainty and disagreement as to who is best suited to provider survivorship care to cancer patients—oncologists or primary care clinicians [86–88]. The treating oncologist may have the most detailed information about the patient's cancer and may have established a strong relationship with the patient during treatment. However, many patient's long-term health issues are not related to cancer, but rather other chronic conditions, psychosocial issues, and health behaviors, all of which are more in the purview of the primary care clinician. One systematic review found that many survivors desire a proactive approach from their primary care clinician and concluded that "the type of support that survivors want from their general practitioner covers a large part of their health care needs" [85]. If a primary care clinician assumes the long-term care of a cancer survivor, it begs the question of who should take ownership of the TS/SCP—the oncologist who treated the patient or the primary care clinician who will continue to care for the patient. The oncologist may know the most about the diagnosis and treatment, but the primary care clinician will need to do what is outlined. Patients perceive both groups of clinicians as capable of developing TS/SCPs.

4.3.5.2 The Role of the Caregivers and the Community in Survivorship

While much of the emphasis of improving cancer survivorship care is centered on answering the use of TS/SCPs in the specialty and primary care settings, it is worth remembering that a static document is insufficient to close the gaps in cancer survivorship care. Patients' clinical history evolves over time and influences outside of the medical setting have a tremendous impact on patients' health and well-being. Community and caregiver involvement can be an important source of support. Several community-based interventions demonstrate the importance of community in survivorship planning.

One such example is Caring for My Caregivers (*Cuidando a mis Cuidadores*), an intervention developed by a community-based organization to help improve quality of life for Latina breast cancer survivors and their families [89]. The intervention consists of a series of eight group sessions to engage survivors and caregivers using the culturally important principles of personalismo, the "expectation to develop warm relationships," and familismo, the "social valuing of the family unit over the individual interests." Using true community-based participatory research (CBPR) principles, the community-based organization and academic researchers have partnered to design a randomized controlled trial to evaluate the effect of the intervention. Together the teams are identifying important PROs to assess (eg, quality of life and satisfaction with and adherence) and define how standardized the intervention needs to be versus responsive to local and participant needs. Though the final results of the intervention are not yet available, the paper presented by Rush et al. demonstrates the importance of not only patient engagement but engagement of community and the importance of the caregiver in interventions that help support cancer patients in survivorship.

Another CBPR collaboration between academic researchers, rural community cancer coalitions, and hospitals in New York and Pennsylvania describes the development of community plans to respond to the needs of colon cancer survivors in rural communities [90]. Participants identified that cancer survivors in rural areas primarily rely on local resources for support, like primary care and local public health, but local resources may be limited in many of these communities. Teams conducted community needs assessments in 14 communities. Commonly identified barriers to care included lack of knowledge about or access to existing community resources, limited psychosocial support, poor transportation to care, poor access to treatment related care, and limited primary care. Linking survivors to primary care and to existing resources was an important solution. An effort in Tennessee used similar CBPR methods as part of an informative planning process to develop an online "survivorship community" that would help cancer survivors, raise community awareness, bring professional organizations together, and promote collaboration and communication—all to ensure that cancer survivors in Nashville had one of the strongest support networks in the nation [91]. Identified online needs included a focus on the entire continuum of cancer care; connections between medical providers and community services; educational opportunities for community members including live chats with experts, speakers bureaus, and information about ongoing research; financial and employment services for patients; and emotional and psychosocial support for cancer patients and caregivers.

4.4 HIT IMPLEMENTATION TO PROMOTE PATIENT ENGAGEMENT

In the final section of this chapter, we will consider the implementation challenges associated with applying HIT to patient engagement across the cancer control spectrum. All too often patient portals, SDM tools, and patient e-health tools are implemented with a "Field of Dreams" mentality, "If we build it, they will come." In reality this is rarely the case. In fact, as will be discussed below, it is best to involve end-users—patients and clinicians—in the actual design of HIT systems. Additionally, we will draw from specific examples discussed earlier in the chapter to describe practical strategies to enhance implementation. Patients know best what they need and can be powerful allies in designing and implementing HIT. This is clearly highlighted by one patient's story detailed in Box. 4.1.

To gain perspective on how patients perceive the health care system, it is useful to review what has been termed the "ecology of medical care" (see Fig. 4.3). This ecology framework describes the degree to which a population interacts with different domains of the health care system. During any given month, out of a population of 1000 persons, only 217 actually take on the role of patient by visiting a clinician's office, only 8 become hospitalized, and only 1 is seen at an academic medical center. Patients that engage with the health care system are entering an unfamiliar and potentially frightening world, especially if confronting a new cancer diagnosis. Additionally, much of the research in terms of new cancer trials, new HIT design, and HIT implementation occurs in more academic centers. Yet findings from these settings may not be very generalizable, highlighting a need to extend research more broadly into the community.

BOX 4.1

MY CANCER INFORMATION JOURNEY

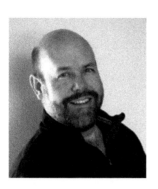

A personal note from Marc McKenzie
Windsor, CO, USA

Before cancer abruptly landed on my doorstep, I must admit to maintaining a comfortable distance from and even ignorance about cancer. With no family history and no one close to me going through cancer, it was an enigma to me. Why did families make such a big deal about it? Little did I know that I would soon learn how cancer puts every aspect of your life through a chipper-shredder—changing my belief in what my life has been about and who I am. I was unprepared to learn every detail about how my body works and to see my loved ones deal with the terror of my mortality. Should I even try?

Now I know the importance of information as an oncology patient—everything from information about screening, diagnosis, treatment, and the management of the neverending after-effects of cancer treatment.

My journey began May 2013. My health had been deteriorating for several years and despite my efforts to unravel the cause, I was getting worse. Because I felt rotten, I had to close my successful executive management consulting firm and quit my chairmanship of an industry consortia. Then I had great luck—and it was luck—to pass a kidney stone. This led to an ER visit where I got a CT scan. The good news was I passed the stone. The bad news was I had metastatic cancer. The ER doctor wept. He almost couldn't get through telling my wife and me about the findings. He was confused that we were elated. We finally knew why my health had been so bad. We had actionable information.

My luck continued. A few days later I got dual pulmonary emboli, putting me back in the hospital. While unconscious, an outstanding hospitalist seized control and got me the best pulmonologist and oncologist in Northern Colorado. I also got life-saving biopsies, PET scans, surgeries, thoracenteses, blood work, bone biopsies, and a medication port. When I was sent home, I had a diagnosis—diffuse, large B-Cell Non-Hodgkins

Lymphoma, stage IV and very aggressive. Further luck—it had not crossed the blood–brain barrier and I did not have leukemia.

My education began. Many doctors groan about the Internet as a source of information, but medicine only has itself to blame. We are in the information age and patients need information. Medicine controls information like a dark age guild. Why does our health care system make information so hard to get? Patients are capable of objective thought and research. I have gone to stupid lengths to access journals, data, and medical discussions related to my condition. It is the rare patient who can pay for journals, has research staff to find information, or even knows what information is important.

My research led me to find and get enrolled in a phase III trial. I received treatment 24 hours a day for 1 of 3 weeks for 5 months. My care transferred to the trial's principal investigator. My engagement, knowledge, and personal tenacity helped him to get me enrolled in the trial. No one will fight harder for a patient than the patient. To me, owning my care, owning my healing vision was everything.

When I started the trial, my body was riddled with 15 pounds of tumors. My nurses could literally watch the tumors disappear with treatment. Getting through all six treatment cycles was hell. I went into remission for 3 months until a solitary tumor appeared in my sigmoid colon. Now my care transitioned to a radiation oncologist. After 25 rounds of radiation, the tumor was gone. To ensure the success of my second remission, I received a dual infant chord stem-cell transplant. I received chemo and total body irradiation titered to almost kill me, followed by a small bag of stem cells. It took almost 3 weeks for the graft to take and longer to begin making my own blood. The stem-cell transplant made all the other treatments look like nothing—the transplant was real hell. My fantastic doctors, nurses, family, friends, church, and most especially my wife kept me alive. Cancer is a team sport and a positive attitude kept me going.

As I write this I am in the early phases of recovery. Today, I am battling graft versus host disease. No fun, but the cancer is gone. Now I am in a position to share what patients' need to be engaged in their care:

- Medical data is about me. It is mine. *Period.* You have the privilege of creating it, seeing it, and using it. I can read it unedited. I don't need you to gently, cautiously unveil facts or impressions.
- I am more engaged and more aware of my body's nuances than you are. Use my awareness to help guide you.

- Please keep my health information up-to-date. When I review my medication list in your EHR, it is usually wrong. That is not right.
- Help me to find the information I need and learn how to use it.
- The transplant section of my portal is stubbed-out, but not populated with anything and made me wonder if something was missing. Hide sections from patients which are not used as part of your medical process.
- Show me everything in my record—all of my notes, results, tests, and consultations. I should not have to ask, cajole, beg, or threaten to see my information.
- Don't make me wait to see my information. This slows down my treatment and creates unnecessary risk and anxiety.
- Show me my information visually. Help me to quickly understand what my information means with graphs, charts, tables, and other innovative displays.
- Find a way of making it easier to communicate with my doctors through e-mail and instant messaging. I don't want to annoy my doctor, but truly there are more efficient ways than always forcing face-to-face consultations.
- Help me get care without having to come to the office. When I am sick, it is hard to come to you, and I don't want to expose myself to the pathogens in your office, or even use precious energy.
- I have never been shown my care goals or my treatment progress—wouldn't that be something!

It is clear to me that policies, processes, and social change within health care is where the real work is needed. Companies like Apple, Fitbit, and Microsoft will continue to make handy devices like my web-connected scale, but it is how these tools are used that will make the difference for patients.

One last thing I want to comment on is the role of solid primary care continuity versus the armada of oncology specialists who obviously have to be the primary drivers of healing. My family doc is a fantastic, solid, and bright all around physician. He knows me. He remembers what I was like when I was well (before cancer), what my behaviors were like and my disciplined commitment to healthy diet, exercise, and mental health. An important thing for me was that through all the long phases of difficult treatment, with all the flavors of doctors involved, I made sure to keep consultations with my family doc three to four times a year. Not only did I want to keep him up to speed, but he has been an anchor. My medical oncologist who is also fantastic recently told me that contrary to the Hippocratic oath, that oncologists "first do harm." The treatments available right now are destructive, full of risk and horrible to experience. It's just the truth.

Oncologists appropriately get very focused on getting to the "cure." My family doc never gives up on keeping me a whole person. It's a natural tension that should be encouraged, and the information linkages should really make the best of this.

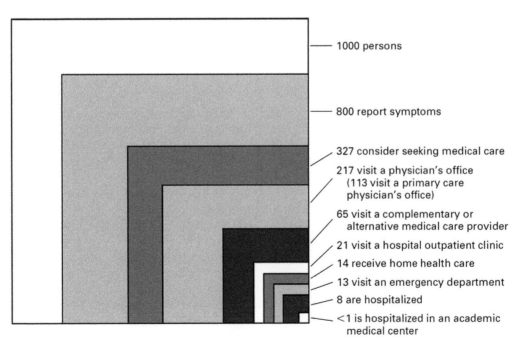

FIGURE 4.3 The monthly prevalence of illness in the community and the roles of various sources of health care. *Source: Adapted from Green LA, Fryer Jr GE, Yawn BP, Lanier D, Dovey SM. The ecology of medical care revisited. N Engl J Med 2001;344(26):2021–5.*

Implementation begins with design. A major flaw in the development and implementation of some patient-centered HIT programs has been that the intended beneficiaries of these programs may not be closely involved in the design process. The experience gap between "expert designers" and "patient users" is often too great for designers to create systems that will meet the needs of users without their input. Fortunately, participatory design techniques can improve the design and implementation of patient-centered HIT systems. Active involvement of users in the design and implementation of HIT can ensure these systems are communicatively appropriate, usable, and relevant [92].

Participatory design, also called user-centered design, is a powerful way to utilize the expertise of users in designing and continuously revising patient-centered HIT programs [93]. Participatory design has been defined as an approach to the assessment, design, and development of technological and organizational systems that places a premium on the active involvement of potential or current users. These design approaches originated in the 1970s in the fields of architecture, engineering, computer science, and other sociotechnical fields, and are now being adopted in health and social sciences—and particularly in health communication. This approach consists of interconnected "feedback loops" of defining issues and developing and testing solutions, called "build and evaluate loops" [94].

In HIT systems, user-centered design methods consist of a variety of approaches to iteratively engage the intended audience members in defining issues and cocreating messages, functionality, and distribution strategies. Specific methods for informing participatory design can include the use of focus groups, in-depth interviews, usability testing, observations, surveys, and other means of gathering input from patients throughout the development and evaluation of the system. For example, *usability testing* refers to a broad range of structured methods that engage users in designing systems such as in-person cognitive interviews and observations of individual patients using a system [95]. Multiple rounds of usability tests and resulting revisions can help identify specific design problems and ensure that the final system and content will appeal to key needs, workflows, beliefs, attitudes, and values of targeted audience members as well as use familiar and accepted language, engaging images, and examples to illustrate key points.

This kind of participatory testing can be used after the audience analysis is conducted, communication objectives are set, and draft content is developed. For example, in an initiative to develop health information and monitoring tools for people with Crohn's disease, participatory design methods helped develop highly sophisticated mobile applications. In this case, even though patients identified their perceived needs at the outset of the planning phase of designing these digital information systems, participatory techniques continued to identify ever-finer preferences and suggestions for improvement over time [93]. This process is particularly valuable to inform design for low literacy users and users with disabilities. Involvement of end-users in designing HIT systems also bears benefits for clinician engagement. A recent paper highlights how clinician involvement in design and buy-in for HIT delivered clinical decision support minimizes alert fatigue [96].

Practically speaking, how should patients be engaged as partners in design and implementation of HIT solutions? User-centered design principles provide one way of gaining input into the design of systems, but this may prove impractical at the individual practice level. Another, perhaps more practical strategy that has proven effective in engaging local stakeholders at the community or practice level is BCT. BCT was initially developed through work in the High Plains Research Network and its Community Advisory Council to create patient and community relevant messaging and strategies to promote colorectal cancer screening. It has been shown to increase both awareness and screening rates in rural communities [25]. BCT involves a series of in-person and brief 30-minute telephone meetings conducted typically over a 6–9 month period around a focused topic. Participants are steeped in the evidence around the topic area, and through facilitated conversations develop a local approach around what to communicate about the topic and how to get the word out. BCT is now being used to translate generic tools and messages about self-management to locally relevant tools that are being implemented in primary care practices.

Another strategy to support local implementation is patient advisory groups. Successful patient advisory groups are built on trusting relationships. The Centers for Disease Control and Prevention has developed the Partnership Trust Tool Survey that covers key aspects of building trusting relationships with community members. The concepts of good/clear communication and mutual benefit apply equally well to working with patients as advisors on implementation of clinical processes and HIT. Throughout any iterative design and implementation process, patient and community advisors need to be treated as coequals and compensated adequately without assuming their efforts are "volunteer work."

In summary, implementation of HIT tools and systems to foster patient engagement should be viewed as a process that values, seeks, and listens to input from patients and clinicians alike. Setting a stage for engagement during implementation and even earlier—during conception and design—will pay off with patients and clinicians that continue to collaborate using the systems they have helped fashion.

4.5 CONCLUSIONS

Effectively engaging patients takes effort for clinicians, but it improves the care delivery experience and health outcomes. Patient engagement promotes patient autonomy, a central ethical principle that recognizes the patient as an independent and rational decision maker capable of self-determination. HIT is an effective tool to help engage patients in their care across the cancer control continuum. Among many patient engagement activities, HIT can be used to inform and educate patients, gather patient-reported information, support medical decision making, promote self-management, encourage healthy behaviors, manage transitions in care, and promote survivorship planning. Further attention to patient-centered design will ensure that systems continue to meet the needs of end-users.

LIST OF ACRONYMS AND ABBREVIATIONS

ACO Accountable Care Organization
CBPR Community based participatory research
CMS Centers for Medicare & Medicaid Services
HRA Health risk assessment
PCMH Patient-Centered Medical Home
PROs Patient-reported outcomes
SDM Shared decision making
TS/SCPs Treatment summaries and survivorship care plans
USPSTF US Preventive Services Task Force

References

[1] Carman KL, Dardess P, Maurer M, Sofaer S, Adams K, Bechtel C, et al. Patient and family engagement: a framework for understanding the elements and developing interventions and policies. Health Aff (Millwood) 2013;32(2):223–31.

[2] Jonas DE, Russell LB, Sandler RS, Chou J, Pignone M. Value of patient time invested in the colonoscopy screening process: time requirements for colonoscopy study. Med Decis Making 2008;28(1):56–65.

[3] Osborn R, Squires D. International perspectives on patient engagement: results from the 2011 Commonwealth Fund Survey. J Ambul Care Manage 2012;35(2):118–28.

[4] Laurance J, Henderson S, Howitt PJ, Matar M, Al Kuwari H, Edgman-Levitan S, et al. Patient engagement: four case studies that highlight the potential for improved health outcomes and reduced costs. Health Aff (Millwood) 2014;33(9):1627–34.

[5] Coulter A. Patient engagement–what works? J Ambul Care Manage 2012;35(2):80–9.

[6] Sheppard VB, Mays D, LaVeist T, Tercyak KP. Medical mistrust influences black women's level of engagement in BRCA1/2 genetic counseling and testing. J Natl Med Assoc 2013;105(1):17–22.

[7] Arora NK, Weaver KE, Clayman ML, Oakley-Girvan I, Potosky AL. Physicians' decision-making style and psychosocial outcomes among cancer survivors. Patient Educ Couns 2009;77(3):404–12.

[8] Torres E, Erwin DO, Trevino M, Jandorf L. Understanding factors influencing Latina women's screening behavior: a qualitative approach. Health Educ Res 2013;28(5):772–83.

[9] Cox CL, Zhu L, Hudson MM, Steen BD, Robison LL, Oeffinger KC. Survivor typologies predict medical surveillance participation: the childhood cancer survivor study. Psychooncology 2013;22(7):1534–42.

[10] Arora NK. Patient engagement in a rapidly changing communication environment: reflections of a cancer survivor. J Natl Cancer Inst Monogr 2013;2013(47):231–2.

[11] Donaldson MS, Yordy KD, Lohr KN, Vanselow NA. Primary care: America's health in a new era. Washington, DC: National Academy Press; 1996.

[12] Starfield B, Shi L, Macinko J. Contribution of primary care to health systems and health. Milbank Q 2005;83(3):457–502.

[13] Green LA, Fryer Jr. GE, Yawn BP, Lanier D, Dovey SM. The ecology of medical care revisited. N Engl J Med 2001;344(26):2021–5.

[14] Wender RC, Altshuler M. Can the medical home reduce cancer morbidity and mortality? Prim Care 2009;36(4):845–58.

[15] Hewitt MS, Greenfield S, Stovall E. From cancer patient to cancer survivor: lost in transition. Washington, DC: National Academies Press; 2005.

[16] Sprandio JD. Oncology patient-centered medical home. Am J Manag Care 2012;18(4 Spec No.):SP191–2.

[17] Earle CC. Failing to plan is planning to fail: improving the quality of care with survivorship care plans. J Clin Oncol 2006;24(32):5112–6.

[18] Stricker CT, Jacobs LA, Risendal B, Jones A, Panzer S, Ganz PA, et al. Survivorship care planning after the institute of medicine recommendations: how are we faring? J Cancer Surviv 2011;5(4):358–70.

[19] IOM (Institute of Medicine) Primary care and public health: exploring integration to improve population health. Washington, DC: The National Academies Press; 2012.

[20] Krist AH, Shenson D, Woolf SH, Bradley C, Liaw WR, Rothemich SF, et al. Clinical and community delivery systems for preventive care: an integration framework. Am J Prev Med 2013;45(4):508–16.

[21] Taplin SH, Anhang Price R, Edwards HM, Foster MK, Breslau ES, Chollette V, et al. Introduction: understanding and influencing multilevel factors across the cancer care continuum. J Natl Cancer Inst Monogr 2012;2012(44):2–10.

[22] Schroeder SA. Shattuck Lecture. We can do better–improving the health of the American people. N Engl J Med 2007;357(12):1221–8.

[23] The Folsom Group. Communities of solution: the Folsom Report revisited. Ann Fam Med 2012;10(3):250–60.

[24] Westfall JM, Mold J, Fagnan L. Practice-based research—"Blue Highways" on the NIH roadmap. JAMA 2007;297(4):403–6.

[25] Norman N, Bennett C, Cowart S, Felzien M, Flores M, Flores R, et al. Boot camp translation: a method for building a community of solution. J Am Board Fam Med 2013;26(3):254–63.

[26] Collins LG, Wender R, Altshuler M. An opportunity for coordinated cancer care: intersection of health care reform, primary care providers, and cancer patients. Cancer J 2010;16(6):593–9.

[27] Bodenheimer T, West D. Low-cost lessons from Grand Junction, Colorado. N Engl J Med 2010;363(15):1391–3.

[28] Schoen C, Osborn R, Squires D, Doty M, Rasmussen P, Pierson R, et al. A survey of primary care doctors in ten countries shows progress in use of health information technology, less in other areas. Health Aff (Millwood) 2012;31(12):2805–16.

[29] Tang PC, Lee TH. Your doctor's office or the Internet? Two paths to personal health records. N Engl J Med 2009;360(13):1276–8.

[30] Goldzweig CL, Orshansky G, Paige NM, Towfigh AA, Haggstrom DA, Miake-Lye I, et al. Electronic patient portals: evidence on health outcomes, satisfaction, efficiency, and attitudes: a systematic review. Ann Intern Med 2013;159(10):677–87.

[31] Krist AH, Woolf SH, Rothemich SF, Johnson RE, Peele JE, Cunningham TD, et al. Interactive preventive health record to enhance delivery of recommended care: a randomized trial. Ann Fam Med 2012;10(4):312–9.

[32] Ralston JD, Coleman K, Reid RJ, Handley MR, Larson EB. Patient experience should be part of meaningful-use criteria. Health Aff (Millwood) 2010;29(4):607–13.

[33] Silvestre AL, Sue VM, Allen JY. If you build it, will they come? The Kaiser Permanente model of online health care. Health Aff (Millwood) 2009;28(2):334–44.

[34] Delbanco T, Walker J, Bell SK, Darer JD, Elmore JG, Farag N, et al. Inviting patients to read their doctors' notes: a quasi-experimental study and a look ahead. Ann Intern Med 2012;157(7):461–70.

[35] Ricciardi L, Mostashari F, Murphy J, Daniel JG, Siminerio EP. A national action plan to support consumer engagement via e-health. Health Aff (Millwood) 2013;32(2):376–84.

[36] McDonald CJ, Callaghan FM, Weissman A, Goodwin RM, Mundkur M, Kuhn T. Use of internist's free time by ambulatory care Electronic Medical Record Systems. JAMA Intern Med 2014;174(11):1860–3.

[37] Nguyen L, Bellucci E, Nguyen LT. Electronic health records implementation: an evaluation of information system impact and contingency factors. Int J Med Inform 2014.

[38] Bitton A, Flier LA, Jha AK. Health information technology in the era of care delivery reform: to what end? JAMA 2012;307(24):2593–4.

[39] Palfrey JS, Sofis LA, Davidson EJ, Liu J, Freeman L, Ganz ML. The Pediatric Alliance for Coordinated Care: evaluation of a medical home model. Pediatrics 2004;113(5 Suppl.):1507–16.

[40] Krist AH, Beasley JW, Crosson JC, Kibbe DC, Klinkman MS, Lehmann CU, et al. Electronic health record functionality needed to better support primary care. J Am Med Inform Assoc 2014.

[41] Turner-Lee N, Smedley BD, Miller J. Minorities, mobile broadband and the management of chronic diseases. Washington, DC: Joint Center for Political and Economic Studies; 2012.

[42] Vodicka E, Mejilla R, Leveille SG, Ralston JD, Darer JD, Delbanco T, et al. Online access to doctors' notes: patient concerns about privacy. J Med Internet Res 2013;15(9):e208.

[43] Krist AH, Woolf SH. A vision for patient-centered health information systems. JAMA 2011;305(3):300–1.

[44] Kreps GL. Achieving the promise of digital health information systems. J Public Health Res 2014;3(3):471.

[45] Kreps GL, Neuhauser L. Artificial intelligence and immediacy: designing health communication to personally engage consumers and providers. Patient Educ Couns 2013;92(2):205–10.

[46] Krist AH, Peele E, Woolf SH, Rothemich SF, Loomis JF, Longo DR, et al. Designing a patient-centered personal health record to promote preventive care. BMC Med Inf Decis Making 2011;11:73.

[47] Department of Family Medicine. Virginia Commonwealth University. A how-to guide for using patient-centered personal health records to promote prevention. Rockville, MD: Agency for Healthcare Research and Quality; 2012.

[48] O'Hair HD, Kreps GL, Sparks L. Handbook of communication and cancer care. Cresskill, NJ: Hampton Press; 2007.

[49] Neuhauser L, Kreps GL. Online cancer communication: meeting the literacy, cultural and linguistic needs of diverse audiences. Patient Educ Couns 2008;71(3):365–77.

[50] Gruman JC. Making health information technology sing for people with chronic conditions. Am J Prev Med 2011;40(5 Suppl. 2):S238–40.

[51] Nazi KM, Turvey CL, Klein DM, Hogan TP, Woods SS. VA OpenNotes: exploring the experiences of early patient adopters with access to clinical notes. J Am Med Inform Assoc 2014.

[52] Jack B, Greenwald J, Forsythe S, O'Donnell J, Johnson A, Schipelliti L, et al. Developing the tools to administer a comprehensive hospital discharge program: The ReEngineered Discharge (RED) Program Henriksen K, Battles JB, Keyes MA,

Grady ML, editors. Advances in patient safety: new directions and alternative approaches (vol. 3: Performance and tools). Rockville, MD: Agency for Healthcare Research and Quality; 2008.

[53] Goetzel RZ, Staley P, Ogden L, Stange P, Fox J, Spangler J, et al. A framework for patient-centered health risk assessments—providing health promotion and disease prevention services to Medicare beneficiaries. Atlanta, GA: US Department of Health and Human Services, Centeres for Disease Control and Prevention; 2011.

[54] Krist AH, Phillips SM, Sabo RT, Balasubramanian BA, Heurtin-Roberts S, Ory MG, et al. Adoption, reach, implementation, and maintenance of a behavioral and mental health assessment in primary care. Ann Fam Med 2014;12(6):525–33.

[55] Phillips SM, Glasgow RE, Bello G, Ory MG, Glenn BA, Sheinfeld-Gorin SN, et al. Frequency and prioritization of patient health risks from a structured health risk assessment. Ann Fam Med 2014;12(6):505–13.

[56] Capturing social and behavioral domains and measures in electronic health records: phase 2. Washington (DC); 2015.

[57] U.S. Preventive Services Task Force. Preventive Services. 2014.

[58] Sheridan SL, Harris RP, Woolf SH. Shared decision making about screening and chemoprevention. A suggested approach from the U.S. Preventive Services Task Force. Am J Prev Med 2004;26(1):56–66.

[59] Briss P, Rimer B, Reilley B, Coates RC, Lee NC, Mullen P, et al. Promoting informed decisions about cancer screening in communities and healthcare systems. Am J Prev Med 2004;26(1):67–80.

[60] Stacey D, Legare F, Col NF, Bennett CL, Barry MJ, Eden KB, et al. Decision aids for people facing health treatment or screening decisions. Cochrane Database Syst Rev 2014;1 CD001431.

[61] Woolf SH, Chan EC, Harris R, Sheridan SL, Braddock III CH, Kaplan RM, et al. Promoting informed choice: transforming health care to dispense knowledge for decision making. Ann Intern Med 2005;143(4):293–300.

[62] Wyatt KD, Branda ME, Anderson RT, Pencille LJ, Montori VM, Hess EP, et al. Peering into the black box: a meta-analysis of how clinicians use decision aids during clinical encounters. Implement Sci 2014;9:26.

[63] Amir E, Freedman OC, Seruga B, Evans DG. Assessing women at high risk of breast cancer: a review of risk assessment models. J Natl Cancer Inst 2010;102(10):680–91.

[64] Ancker JS, Kaufman D. Rethinking health numeracy: a multidisciplinary literature review. J Am Med Inform Assoc 2007;14(6):713–21.

[65] Iyengar S. The art of choosing, 1st ed. New York, NY: Twelve; 2010.

[66] Beckjord EB, Rechis R, Nutt S, Shulman L, Hesse BW. What do people affected by cancer think about electronic health information exchange? Results from the 2010 LIVESTRONG Electronic Health Information Exchange Survey and the 2008 Health Information National Trends Survey. J Oncol Pract 2011;7(4):237–41.

[67] Prouty C, Mazor K, Greene S, Roblin D, Firneno C, Lemay C, et al. Providers' perceptions of communication breakdowns in cancer care. J Gen Intern Med 2014;29(8):1122–30.

[68] Aubin M, Giguère A, Martin M, Verreault R, Fitch MI, Kazanjian A, et al. Interventions to improve continuity of care in the follow-up of patients with cancer. Cochrane Database Syst Rev 2012;7. Available from: <http://onlinelibrary.wiley.com/doi/10.1002/14651858.CD007672.pub2/abstract;jsessionid=B1A89E23F98E2AB7A38CDD588809DAD2.f04t04>.

[69] Lubberding S, van Uden-Kraan CF, Te Velde EA, Cuijpers P, Leemans CR, Verdonck-de Leeuw IM. Improving access to supportive cancer care through an eHealth application: a qualitative needs assessment among cancer survivors. J Clin Nurs 2015;24(9–10):1367–79.

[70] Buckler LT, Teasdale C, Turner M, Schadler A, Schwieterman TM, Campbell CL. The patient-centered discharge-an electronic discharge process is associated with improvements in quality and patient satisfaction. J Healthc Qual 2014. Available from: <http://www.ncbi.nlm.nih.gov/pubmed/?term=Buckler+LT+AND+the+patient-centered+discharge>.

[71] Freeman H, Muth B, Kerner J. Expanding access to cancer screening and clinical follow-up among medically underserved. Cancer Pract 1995;3(1):19–30.

[72] Pratt-Chapman M, Simon MA, Patterson AK, Risendal BC, Patierno S. Survivorship navigation outcome measures. Cancer 2011;117(S15):3573–82.

[73] Fiscella K, Ransom S, Jean-Pierre P, Cella D, Stein K, Bauer JE, et al. Patient-reported outcome measures suitable to assessment of patient navigation. Cancer 2011;117(S15):3601–15.

[74] Wagner EH. Chronic disease management: what will it take to improve care for chronic illness? Eff Clin Pract 1998;1(1):2–4.

[75] McCorkle R, Ercolano E, Lazenby M, Schulman-Green D, Schilling LS, Lorig K, et al. Self-management: enabling and empowering patients living with cancer as a chronic illness. CA: A Cancer J Clin 2011;61(1):50–62.

[76] Trotter K, Frazier A, Hendricks C, Scarsella H. Innovation in survivor care: group visits. Clin J Oncol Nurs 2011;15(2):E24–33.

[77] Thompson J, Coleman R, Colwell B, Freeman J, Greenfield D, Holmes K, et al. Preparing breast cancer patients for survivorship (PREP)—a pilot study of a patient-centred supportive group visit intervention. Eur J Oncol Nurs 2014;18(1):10–16.

[78] Naik AD, Singh H. Electronic health records to coordinate decision making for complex patients: what can we learn from wiki? Med Decis Making 2010;30(6):722–31.

[79] Brennan ME, Gormally JF, Butow P, Boyle FM, Spillane AJ. Survivorship care plans in cancer: a systematic review of care plan outcomes. Br J Cancer 2014;111(10):1899–908.

[80] Mayer DK, Birken SA, Check DK, Chen RC. Summing it up: an integrative review of studies of cancer survivorship care plans (2006–2013). Cancer 2015;121(7):978–96.

[81] Forsythe LP, Parry C, Alfano CM, Kent EE, Leach CR, Haggstrom DA, et al. Use of survivorship care plans in the United States: associations with survivorship care. J Natl Cancer Inst 2013;105(20):1579–87.

[82] Blanch-Hartigan D, Forsythe LP, Alfano CM, Smith T, Nekhlyudov L, Ganz PA, et al. Provision and discussion of survivorship care plans among cancer survivors: results of a nationally representative survey of oncologists and primary care physicians. J Clin Oncol 2014;32(15):1578–85.

[83] Keesing S, McNamara B, Rosenwax L. Cancer survivors' experiences of using survivorship care plans: a systematic review of qualitative studies. J Cancer Surviv 2014;9:1–9.

[84] Dulko D, Pace CM, Dittus KL, Sprague BL, Pollack LA, Hawkins NA, et al. Barriers and facilitators to implementing cancer survivorship care plans. Oncol Nurs Forum 2013;40(6):575–80.

[85] Hoekstra R, Heins M, Korevaar J. Health care needs of cancer survivors in general practice: a systematic review. BMC Fam Pract 2014;15:94.

[86] Potosky AL, Han PKJ, Rowland J, Klabunde CN, Smith T, Aziz N, et al. Differences between primary care physicians' and oncologists' knowledge, attitudes and practices regarding the care of cancer survivors. J Gen Intern Med 2011;26(12):1403–10.

[87] Cheung WY, Neville BA, Cameron DB, Cook EF, Earle CC. Comparisons of patient and physician expectations for cancer survivorship care. J Clin Oncol 2009;27(15):2489–95.

[88] Klabunde C, Han P, Earle CC, Smith T, Ayanian JZ, Lee R, et al. Physician roles in the cancer-related follow-up care of cancer survivors. Fam Med 2013;45(7):463–74.

[89] Rush C, Darling M, Elliott M, Febus-Sampayo I, Kuo C, Muñoz J, et al. Engaging Latina cancer survivors, their caregivers, and community partners in a randomized controlled trial: Nueva Vida intervention. Qual Life Res 2014:1–12.

[90] Lengerich EJ, Kluhsman BC, Bencivenga M, Allen R, Miele MB, Farace E. Development of community plans to enhance survivorship from colorectal cancer: community-based participatory research in rural communities. J Cancer Surviv 2007;1(3):205–11.

[91] Weiss JB, Lorenzi NM. Building a shared vision for an online cancer survivorship community. AMIA Annu Symp Proc 2009;2009:690–4.

[92] Neuhauser L, Kreps GL. Integrating design science theory and methods to improve the development and evaluation of health communication programs. J Health Commun 2014;19(12):1460–71.

[93] Neuhauser L, Kreps GL, Syme SL. Community participatory design of health communication interventions Kim DK, Singhal A, Kreps GL, editors. Health communication: strategies for developing global health programs. New York, NY: Peter Lang Publishers; 2013. p. 227–43.

[94] Markus ML, Majchrzak A, Gasser LA. Design theory for systems that support emergent knowledge processes. Manag Inf Syst Q 2002;26:179–212.

[95] Nielsen J. Designing web usability. Idianapolis, IN: New Riders Publishing; 2000.

[96] Green LA, Nease Jr. RF, Klinkman MS. Clinical reminders designed and implemented using cognitive and organizational science principles do not produce reminder fatigue: a longitudinal cohort study. J Am Board Fam Med 2015;28(3):351–9.

5

Coordination at the Point of Need

Katherine K. Kim PhD, MPH, MBA, Janice F. Bell PhD, MPH, MN, Sarah C. Reed MSW, MPH and Robin Whitney RN

Betty Irene Moore School of Nursing, University of California Davis, Sacramento, CA, United States

OUTLINE

5.1 Introduction   81

5.2 Frameworks for Care Coordination   83
    5.2.1 Definitions of Care Coordination   83
    5.2.2 Elements of Care Coordination   83
    5.2.3 Chronic Care Model   84
    5.2.4 Integrated Patient Care   84
    5.2.5 Community-Wide Care Coordination   86

5.3 HIT Functions for Care Coordination   88
    5.3.1 Person-Centered Coordination   89
    5.3.2 Shared Care Planning   89
    5.3.3 Within and Across Health Care Teams   89
    5.3.4 Across Multiple Teams   90

5.4 Current Efforts in Informatics and Coordination at the Point of Need   90
    5.4.1 Within and Across Health Care Teams   90
    5.4.2 Within Person and Family Teams   91
    5.4.3 Across Person and Health Care Teams   91
    5.4.4 Across Multiple Teams   92
    5.4.5 Shared Care Plans   94

5.5 Opportunities for Oncology Informatics at the Point of Need   96

List of Acronyms and Abbreviations   97

References   97

5.1 INTRODUCTION

Globally, for individuals with chronic or prolonged conditions such as cancer, care is complicated, fragmented, and poorly coordinated [1]. It is not unusual for individuals with cancer to experience transitions from home to physician office, clinic, outpatient service, emergency department, inpatient hospital, and community-based settings attended by different practitioners and numerous specialists at each. The challenges faced by individuals and their family members are many. For instance, specialty oncology care—involving surgery, chemotherapy, radiotherapy, and other treatment modalities—occurs in cancer centers which may be geographically distant from patients' homes. Oncology specialists involved in an individual's care may not be in close communication with a patients' primary care provider. For others, particularly older adults, care may occur in the absence of family or community support. Cancer care problems are compounded when care is provided in fragmented and disconnected systems and providers do not have adequate access to information about the care received by patients in other settings. The burden then falls on the patient to try and coordinate across the many members of their care "team."

Many individuals with cancer also have multiple comorbidities that further complicates the delivery of coordinated and effective care. Health-related activity

B. Hesse, D. Ahern & E. Beckjord: Oncology Informatics.
DOI: http://dx.doi.org/10.1016/B978-0-12-802115-6.00005-7

81

over the life span is both dynamic and diverse. Over time, individuals experience some times when health care services are needed and at other times there is little interaction with the health care system. Accordingly, persons with cancer are likely to benefit from care coordination interventions. However, recent national reports criticize the current state of cancer care for inadequate coordination of care transitions, for not being patient-centered, and for not basing care decisions on the latest scientific evidence [2]. Moreover, no large-scale studies have focused on outcomes of care coordination interventions in oncology patient populations. Such studies are needed at all stages of the cancer care continuum—from prevention and screening to diagnosis and treatment through survivorship and end of life—to understand the ways in which care coordination might uniquely benefit patients with cancer. The challenge of care coordination is depicted in Fig. 5.1.

Recent national reports criticize care for not being person-centered, not making care decisions on the latest scientific evidence, and not adequately coordinating transitions [2–4]. As further evidence of the changing perspective on care coordination is the move by the Centers for Medicare & Medicaid Services (CMS) to implement a new payment and care delivery model for cancer called the Oncology Care Model [5]. The new program aims to improve quality of care and population health while lowering costs. To this end, CMS will fund physician-led oncology practices to implement innovative approaches to delivering chemotherapy, where reimbursement is based on the quality of the outcomes achieved, rather than on the volume of services provided [6]. The three key areas of focus are (1) linking payment to quality, (2) improving and innovating in care delivery, and (3) sharing information broadly to support and improve decision making. Application of health information technology (HIT) is an explicit requirement of participation in the program, and there will be many opportunities for technology to support quality improvement in this model [7]. For example, participating providers must employ an electronic health record (EHR) that fulfills federal criteria for demonstration of meaningful use, provide 24/7 patient access to clinicians who have real-time access to relevant medical records, and implement a data-driven continuous improvement process [7].

The Oncology Care Model has met with some criticism for its continued reliance on a payment model that, while reformed, is still viewed by some as essentially fee-for-service [8]. In 2014, the American Society of Clinical Oncology proposed more extensive payment reforms to

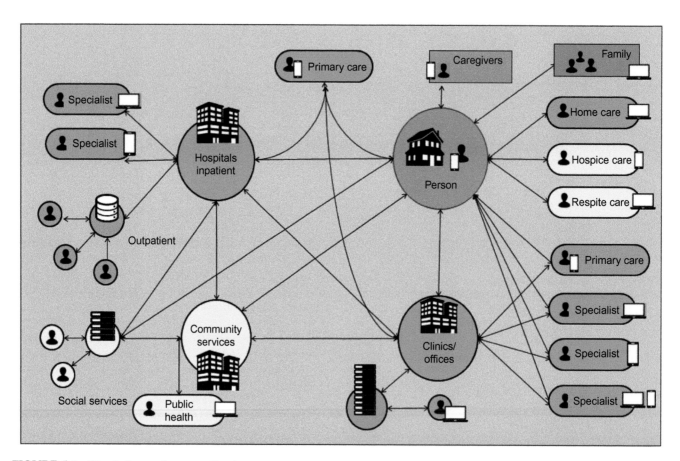

FIGURE 5.1 The challenge of care coordination.

support patient-centered oncology care [9]. These recommendations included a major shift away from fee-for-service payment models (ie, billing for office visits and chemotherapy administration), and instead toward payment models that would support telephone or e-mail visits, care planning, and care coordination [9].

Despite criticisms, the Oncology Care Model marks the beginning of important changes in the delivery of oncology care. The US Department of Health and Human Services has declared its intention for 85% of fee-for-service payments to be linked with quality by 2016 [10]. Care coordination plays a central role in these efforts including, potentially, new forms of payment for care coordination for individuals with chronic diseases [10]. Cancer will be the first chronic disease specifically targeted for these payment model reform efforts. Therefore, the Oncology Care Model serves as an important first step in demonstrating whether these innovative approaches to care coordination and novel applications of HIT can improve quality and reduce costs.

These national efforts highlight that the coordination of care must extend beyond traditional points of care which refer to the time and place where health care services are delivered, typically in hospital and ambulatory settings. Central to the major premise of this chapter, coordination must also occur at the "point of need," or all the times and places when health-related conversations occur and health choices and decisions are made among individuals, their family and caregivers, clinicians and health care teams, and community resource providers. One example of a point of need is when individuals experience nausea related to chemotherapy at home and seek resources or advice on how to manage their symptoms. Another example is the transition from active treatment to survivorship when the oncology team communicates and plans with the individual, family, and primary care provider about monitoring and following up needs.

5.2 FRAMEWORKS FOR CARE COORDINATION

5.2.1 Definitions of Care Coordination

No consensus definition exists for the term care coordination, which has evolved to refer to many interrelated concepts including care management, case management, disease management, and shared care. In a recent systematic review more than 40 different definitions were identified for the term, which the authors synthesized as follows:

> Care coordination is the deliberate organization of patient care activities between two or more participants (including the patient) involved in a patient's care to facilitate the appropriate

delivery of health care services. Organizing care involves the marshalling of personnel and other resources needed to carry out all required patient care activities and is often managed by the exchange of information among participants responsible for different aspects of care [3].

Among patients with chronic conditions, including cancer, effective care coordination is increasingly viewed as a promising approach to achieving the triple aim outcomes of improved patient experiences of care (including quality and satisfaction); improved population health; and reduced per capita cost of care [11,12]. Indeed, a recent Institute of Medicine (IOM) report suggests that care coordination could result in $240 billion in annual health care savings [13]. Mechanisms through which care coordination is believed to lead to triple aim outcomes include improved treatment adherence; increased provider use of evidence-based guidelines; improved communication within and across care teams; improved care transitions with reduced fragmentation of care; improved symptom monitoring; and improved access to needed services [14]. Importantly, effective care coordination interventions are expected to reduce potentially preventable health service use including costly emergency department visits and inpatient readmissions. Successful care coordination models have demonstrated reduced hospital admissions and expenditures across a variety of chronic conditions [15–23].

5.2.2 Elements of Care Coordination

Care coordination activities involve assessment, planning, implementation, and evaluation and are typically supported by evidence-based guidelines and protocols [24]. The activities are organized by the care coordinator with the participation of other care team members, including the patient, caregiver/family members, and health care providers. The care coordination process promotes the active engagement of the patient (and caregiver) in his/her health care through self-management and ongoing encouragement, direction, and reinforcement.

Comprehensive assessment is required to understand the health care needs, goals of care, and resources available to patients with complex chronic conditions such as cancer. Usually this assessment occurs face-to-face, often over several meetings, and data are collected across multiple domains (eg, physical, social, psychological, cognitive, lifestyle, cultural, developmental, spiritual, demographic, financial, environmental, functional, social support, resources, and health service use). Assessment data are collected systematically, often using standardized instruments, and are used to understand patients' identified values and preferences for care. Assessment results include documentation of the patients' perspectives on the most difficult aspects of managing their illness, their fears, their baseline knowledge of their conditions, and their goals for care. This information informs the development of care plans that include goals shared by the patient and care coordinator [24].

Care Planning includes collaborative activities toward developing a plan of care with participation of the patient, family, and health care team. Patients participate in this process by setting their goals for care and assisting the team to personalize and prioritize care plan recommendations. Through the care planning process, a comprehensive, evidence-based plan of care is developed to address all of the patient's health-related needs in the context of the patient's values, requirements, and preferences.

Implementation activities include identifying barriers to the achievement of the agreed upon action plan, with the patient and care team engaging in problem solving to reduce such barriers. In this phase, the care coordinator may be involved in teaching about disease processes, medications, and evidence-based self-management strategies; health coaching to reinforce positive steps taken by the patient; and making referrals to appropriate health and community services and supports. Above all, implementation activities involve coordination of health and community services, including efforts to synchronize communication between all of those who provide care for the patient—including specialist physicians; hospital and emergency staff; rehabilitation therapists; mental health professionals; home care providers; social workers; and community-based agencies (eg, exercise programs, faith-based organizations, and other support groups). This coordination is especially important during transitions between hospitals and other sites of follow-up care.

Evaluation involves proactive monitoring, with documenting patient progress toward care goals, performing a reassessment at each contact (especially following emergency department visits or hospital admissions), and revising the goals and/or plan of care accordingly.

Several frameworks have emerged for understanding care coordination as the organization of care, complementary to the delivery of care, and for highlighting the importance of informatics. In the following section, we introduce three complementary frameworks: chronic care model (CCM), integrated patient care (IPC) framework, and community-wide care coordination (CWCC). The CCM provides a theory of how chronic care operates, the attendant elements of high-quality care, and suggests best practices in the realms of the model. The IPC framework focuses on measurement of the elements of integration which is prerequisite to evaluating interventions. And, CWCC expands the scope of coordination to encompass points of need in relevant communities.

5.2.3 Chronic Care Model

One of the foundational frameworks underlying care coordination is the CCM that explicates the relationships among structures, participants, services, interactions, that lead to high-quality health care and health outcomes [25]. A related review of randomized clinical trials (RCTs) and observational studies, successful interventions, and chronic care programs yielded identification of common elements of high-quality chronic illness care to provide effective and appropriate care of chronically ill patients, as well as strategies for the individuals and families to cope with illness and its therapies [26]. The identified elements fall into the following categories: (1) use of plans and protocols; (2) reorganization of the practice to meet needs of patients; (3) attention to information and behavior change needs; (4) ready access to clinical expertise; and (5) supportive information systems. This model has been widely applied to inform comprehensive consideration of infrastructure and intervention aspects of approaches to chronic disease management.

Recent work applying the model to care coordination focuses on the goal of smooth handling of referrals and transitions (http://www.improvingchroniccare.org/index.php?p=Change_Package&s=354). This led to an updated model adding two elements: (6) building relationships and agreements among providers (including community agencies) with shared expectations for communication and care; and (7) developing connectivity via electronic or other information pathways that encourage timely and effective information flow between providers and community agencies. The elements are listed in Table 5.1 in a side-by-side comparison with the two frameworks described below. The table compares how each of the frameworks describe components related to concepts of person, plan, technology, within team, across team, and time.

5.2.4 Integrated Patient Care

In the IPC framework, Singer et al. propose that integration or coordination as a process is distinct from the object of integration, which may be organizational structure, activities, or alternatively, patient care [27]. This distinction suggests that an integrated delivery structure is not equivalent to IPC as they are two different targets. For example, accomplishing the structural components of a patient-centered medical home such as availability of a patient portal for requesting appointments and offering visit summaries is not necessarily evidence of accomplishing the outcome of patient-centered coordinated care. The authors also operationalize a definition of IPC as "coordinated across professionals, facilities, and support systems; continuous over time and between visits; tailored to the patients' needs and preferences;

TABLE 5.1 Comparison of Care Coordination Frameworks

Category	Elements of high-quality chronic care related to chronic care model (CCM)	Domains of integrated patient care (IPC)	Domains of community-wide care coordination (CWCC)
1. Person	*Patient self-management and behavioral change support*: Systematic attention to the information and behavioral change needs of patients	*Patient centered*: Care team members design care to meet patients' (also family members and other informal caregivers') needs and preferences; processes enhance patients' engagement in self-management	*Person-centered coordination:* Empowers individuals to exercise autonomy, collaborate in decision making, and optimize coordination. Supports development and delivery of coordination activities that respond to individuals' values, needs, and preferences. Individuals are patients at some points, but not at all points
2. Plan	*Explicit plans and protocols*: Use of a protocol or plan that provides an explicit statement of what needs to be done for patients, at what intervals, and by whom. Use of evidence-based guidelines	*Shared responsibility*: Both the patient and his or her family and care team members are responsible for the provision of care, maintenance of good health, and management of financial resources	*Shared care planning*: An inclusive process of comprehensive assessment, goal-setting and planning, implementation, and evaluation of an individuals' course of health over the life span. The resulting documentation, an evolving shared care plan, may have greater detail on shorter time periods when intensive focus is necessary
3. Technology	*Supportive information systems for population health and panel management*: Information about patients, their care, and their outcomes, tracking for population health, and panel management *Developing connectivity via electronic or other information pathways* that encourage timely and effective information flow between providers and community agencies		*Health information technology enablement*: Helps individuals to fulfill CWCC activities with the information and tools to achieve health outcomes. Helps teams to support individuals' health goals, efficiently manage groups they serve, and contribute to population health goals. Enables coordination at points of need
			Point of need for coordination
4. Within team	*Clinical expertise*: Ready access to necessary expertise *Practice redesign*: Reorganization of the practice to meet the needs of patients who require more time, a broad array of resources, and closer follow-up. This includes the organization of the practice team and the allocation of tasks among them, the management of patient contact (appointments, follow-up), and the use of a variety of health care professionals	*Coordinated within care team*: The individual providers (which may include physicians, nurses, other clinicians, support staff, and administrative personnel who routinely work together to provide medical care for a specified group of patients, "care team") deliver consistent and informed patient care and administrative services for individual patients, regardless of the care team member providing them	*Within teams*: There are three types of teams: family teams, health care teams, and community teams. Within the team, there are certain roles and responsibilities, specific activities that regularly occur, particular information that is helpful, and unique workflows to address
5. Across team	*Building relationships and agreements* among providers and community agencies with shared expectations for communication and care	*Coordinated across care teams*: All care teams that interact with patients, including specialists, hospital personnel, and pharmacies and deliver consistent and informed patient care and administrative services, regardless of the care team providing them Coordinated between care teams and community resources: Care teams consider and coordinate support for patients by other teams offered in the community (eg, Meals on Wheels)	*Across teams*: The person, family teams, health care teams, and community teams interact with each other. Teams may also have intense interaction as is the case when multiple providers are simultaneously delivering health care services. Communication must occur between those health care teams, individuals, and family teams to coordinate appointments, reconcile medications, and assure that treatments are not in conflict

(Continued)

TABLE 5.1   Comparison of Care Coordination Frameworks *Continued*

Category	Elements of high-quality chronic care related to chronic care model (CCM)	Domains of integrated patient care (IPC)	Domains of community-wide care coordination (CWCC)
6. Time		*Continuous familiarity with patient across time*: Clinical care team members are familiar with the patient's past medical condition and treatments; administrative care team members are familiar with patient's payment history and needs *Continuous proactive and responsive action between visits*: Care team members reach out and respond to patients between visits; patients can access care and information 24/7	*Over time*: Conventionally, care coordination occurs in the context of one health care service such as a hospitalization with 30 days of follow-up after discharge. In contrast, the CWCC perspective on time is over the continuum of care, and the life span of a person. Different teams are active at different times, and the level of participation also varies

and based on shared responsibility between patient and caregivers for optimizing health." This operationalization highlights the patient-centeredness of the IPC framework and supports measure development for the components of coordination.

5.2.5 Community-Wide Care Coordination

A conceptual framework for person-centered, CWCC builds on the previous two models and emphasizes the dynamic relationships and workflows between and among players and defines a new concept of "point of need" for coordination [28]. A point of need is any time and place when health-related conversations occur and health choices and decisions are made among individuals, their family and caregiver teams, clinicians and health care teams, and community resource teams. While members of teams may not identify themselves as such, we describe them as teams because they are known to each other and their activities supporting health of an individual are codependent.

The person with whom health is being coordinated is the person or individual. Family teams include patients and those close to them such as family members, friends, and other informal caregivers who are involved in their health. Health care teams are made up of clinical, ancillary, or administrative personnel and may be discipline- or setting-specific. There are also community teams that offer resources such as preventive health screenings, health outreach, and education; instrumental support services such as meals, transportation, and respite care; or social support via online patient communities and in-person groups.

The person, family teams, health care teams, and community teams interact with each other. They may have minimal interaction as is the case when a referral is made, with one team handing off a request for a service to another. For example, an individual might receive a flyer from a community organization advertising free blood pressure screenings at a health fair. This community team member might suggest the individual follow up with a primary care provider. An example of a more involved case is a care coordinator on a health care team who refers individuals to a transportation service to help them attend their appointments. The individual and family team might coordinate multiple trips over a period of time, involving ongoing coordination with that community service.

The shared care planning process includes individuals, family teams, health care teams, and community teams as appropriate. In alignment with person-centeredness, the inclusion of participants in the process should be driven by the individual. Thus, care is coordinated dynamically across teams and over time, but the person is always engaged.

The point of need for care coordination, that is, when health-related conversations occur and health choices and decisions are made, can occur for an individual, within teams, across teams, and change over time.

To illustrate the relevance of this framework to individuals, lung cancer survivor Janet Freeman-Daily offers a personal account of the story of her care coordination over 4 years of lung cancer treatment in Box 5.1 (used with permission).

Below is an illustration of the CWCC framework and its dynamic nature applied to the cancer continuum (Fig. 5.2). The top frame shows that the person is the center and involved in every phase of the continuum and care coordination. The second frame shows the teams that might be involved during the prevention and screening phase of the continuum of an individual's health. The three types of teams are represented by circles: family teams are gray circles, health care teams are dark gray, and community teams are light gray. The intersections between teams (where circles overlap) are points of need where a component of care coordination is required, for example, data collection, planning, decision making,

---

BOX 5.1

JANET FREEMAN-DAILY'S CARE COORDINATION STORY

Being in treatment for advanced lung cancer over the past 4 years, I've experienced many issues with care coordination.

Person-Centered Coordination: I like to share decision making with my health care team. When I was nearing the end of my postdiagnosis hospital stay, I was surprised to hear "you're being discharged in an hour"—no one had asked what questions I had about my follow-up care, or even whether I had a ride home. I was given a piece of paper with contact information for only *one* of the four specialists on my new health care team, and told I had prescriptions waiting at a pharmacy. I wasn't sure how to go about gathering the rest of the information I needed. This system was evidently efficient for the hospital, but not for me, the patient.

Shared Care Planning: Even when a facility has exceptionally good teamwork, patients can still be uncertain how to proceed when an issue arises. For instance, when I develop severe shortness of breath after a chemo session, should I contact my oncologist or my pulmonologist? When I developed intense chest pain upon swallowing during concurrent chemo and radiation, who do I contact for pain medicine: the radiation oncology nurse, or the oncology nurse?

Across Health Care Teams Coordination: When I travel away from my home care team for a second opinion or a clinical trial, the only way to transfer my data between facilities is via fax or hand carry because EHR systems cannot yet share data. I keep a stack of radiology image CDs along with pathology, radiology, and other vital reports in a three-foot-deep file drawer at home because facilities often cannot fill records requests on short notice. When I was discharged after a 10-day hospital stay, I was told a contractor would contact me to train me and provide supplies for daily peripherally inserted central catheter (PICC) line care and maintenance. No one asked me about the distance to the contractor from my home—after a couple of weeks, I accidentally discovered I could have my weekly PICC line flush at a clinic four miles away instead of driving 20 miles to the contractor's site.

Across Health Care Team and Family Team Coordination: The patient as well as family members and other caregivers may share responsibility for the patient's well-being. Having multiple caregivers involved increases the risk of miscommunications and inaccurate data. During my hospitalization after my cancer diagnosis, several family members visited me in the hospital. No one (including me) was present for every update from the health care team. This led to miscommunication and different interpretations of my status. For example, my sister (who had talked to the surgeon alone while I was in recovery) left the hospital convinced I was dying. However, I as the patient (who talked to the oncologist while I was alone) heard I might be curable. The opportunity for miscommunication is compounded for patients whose condition requires the coordination of data collection and medication among multiple caregivers. No effective tools exist to coordinate data, communication, and status updates between the health care team and caregivers/family members who tend the patient at different times of day.

Across Time Coordination: When I developed a pulmonary embolism on a clinical trial, the trial facility had no record of another blood clot I'd had over 2 years earlier at my home facility (good thing my chemobrain remembered). EHR systems evolve over time too, creating additional issues—a software upgrade scrambled my insurance data in the billing system, and suddenly I was billed thousands of dollars for my periodic scans and clinic appointment that my insurance had covered for years. Chronically ill patients spend more time unraveling insurance snafus than healthy patients, just when they need fewer things to worry about. My care facilities provide an online patient portal, but appointment scheduling and e-mail messages sent via the EHR system seem to vanish in the ether. Fortunately, most of my providers respond to e-mails and voicemails promptly. However, most of my health care data is not accessible via the online portal, and I am only able to correct errors in the records if I stumble upon a person with the correct authority, time, and savvy.

---

information sharing, tracking and monitoring, communication, or logistics. Some individuals have family members or friends who are involved in their health but others do not. We do assume that a family team is available for everyone. The person, family team if there is one, and primary health care team may be involved. If the individual receives a result that suggests referral to specialists for diagnosis and treatment, a patient navigator program (one type of community team) might assist with that transition.

The third frame shows the diagnosis and treatment phase. The roles of teams, who they interact with, and the intensity of effort (depicted by the size of the circle), differs over time. In this phase, many additional health

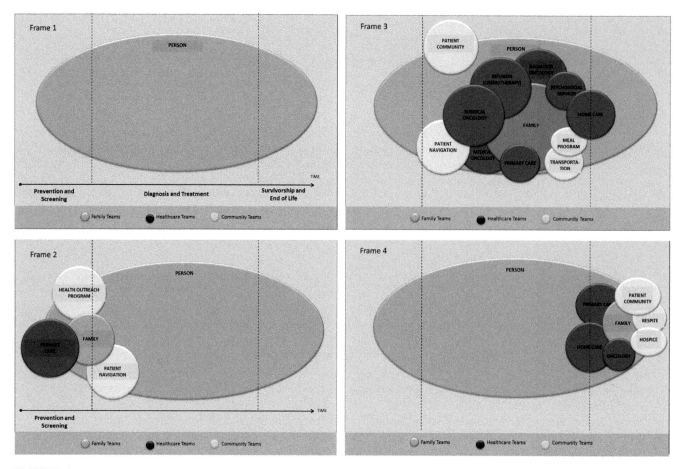

FIGURE 5.2   Community-wide care coordination over the cancer care continuum.

care teams representing specialists are involved and likely have a greater role in coordinating with the person and their family team. For many individuals who receive a diagnosis, one of the first things they do is look for patient groups (a community team) who can provide information and support.

In the fourth frame, treatment is ending, and the individual enters a survivorship phase in which they try to regain health and are vigilant regarding potential reoccurrence. A primary health care team likely becomes more involved again, but specialty health care teams may interact periodically for check-ups. The continuum is not simply linear: an individual may experience alternating periods of survivorship and diagnosis/treatment and continue prevention/screening activities throughout. Over the continuum, there are different combinations of participants and teams, changing points of need, as well as varying requirements.

All three frameworks address the concepts of person, plan, and the coordination within and among teams. CCM and CWCC explicitly address the need for HIT to support care coordination while IPC and CWCC expound on the importance of time and longitudinal coordination. Finally, CWCC highlights the central role

of teams including the person/family team and the community team. CWCC also defines the point of need as well as the dynamic nature of the relationships among the teams over the life span. The life span perspective, in contrast to time between visits with providers, is particularly important for cancer survivorship.

5.3 HIT FUNCTIONS FOR CARE COORDINATION

While EHRs are necessary they may not be sufficient to enable a learning health care system for cancer envisioned by the IOM, which recommends infrastructure and "real-time analysis of data from cancer patients in a variety of care settings" [29]. Several authors have described HIT functions necessary for both general care coordination and cancer care coordination. The compilation below, organized by the coordination concepts from Table 5.1, illustrates the breadth and depth of requirements. Requirements described in this section are followed by examples of projects and studies that have implemented some of these functions in the next section.

5.3.1 Person-Centered Coordination

Patient- or person-centered care coordination is responsive to the needs, values, and preferences of the individual. Individual access to comprehensive and actionable health data for the individual and their family and caregivers is a first step in achieving person-centeredness. A comprehensive data set is important to allow individuals to fully participate in their care. This includes the information in the EHR, clinician notes, care plans, tests, and results [30]. To make this information actionable, educational materials and decision tools should also be offered that are relevant to the individual's health status at opportune moments [31]. Both of these requirements suggest that infrastructure must be in place to understand when and where those opportune moments occur such that those tools can be targeted appropriately. In addition, information about the individual's situation and preferences, such as self-management capability and family or caregiver resources; observations of daily living and patient-reported health status such as side effects, and experiences; and preferred contact, should be in the EHR so that the care team can be responsive to the individual [32,33]. A longitudinal patient health record (PHR) owned by the individual and populated by interoperable monitoring devices and EHRs is one possibility for enabling infrastructure.

5.3.2 Shared Care Planning

Shared care planning is a process that involves collaboration among patients, family and caregivers, health care teams, and others to develop a shared understanding of both the goals and interventions that make up the trajectory of care. During planning, tools for assessing risk are helpful in identifying those patients who may require more intensive coordination. These tools may be in the form of scoring algorithms applied to clinical indicators in the EHR or data collected from interviews or other patient-generated data. Availability of relevant literature and evidence-based guidelines for treatment planning and ongoing tracking of care plan items are equally important [31]. The documentation of the outcomes of this planning process, referred to as a shared care plan, should be accessible to all relevant parties, editable, and revised as care progresses. The shared care plan may also become the basis for a transition of care summary that serves to communicate fundamental information to the family and other health care and community teams.

The Office of the National Coordinator for Health Information Technology sponsored the Standards and Interoperability Transitions of Care Initiative to define an interoperable longitudinal care plan to improve coordination across transitions of care involving acute and long-term providers, home health agencies, rehabilitation, and social and other support services [34]. The components of this care plan are detailed health concerns; patient and clinical goals; interventions and instructions; and health status evaluation populated with computable, standardized data. One study suggests that a transition of care summary should also include rationale and communication elements such as: name and contact information for all clinicians and who to contact with questions; advance directives; medications and reason for medication; management of high-risk medications; patient's ability to comprehend, remember, and capacity to consent to treatment; any impairments; patient likes and dislikes, problems, goals and expectations, and self-management plan; and patient instructions [35]. One exemplar of a longitudinal care plan specific to oncology is the survivorship care plan. The survivorship care plan offers a summary of the patient's treatment course, recommendations for follow-up care of symptoms and problems, ongoing cancer surveillance, and health promotion that may be helpful both to the patient and to future health care teams [36]. Both the process and documentation of shared care planning could be collected, analyzed, communicated, and updated through HIT.

5.3.3 Within and Across Health Care Teams

The primary HIT system used by health care teams is the EHR. For coordination with the health care team, a robust EHR should support not only the aggregation of data, but also the analytical and workflow needs that are critical to effective care coordination. A recent review of HIT functions and chronic care management process and clinical outcomes found several positive relationships: data in or connected to an EHR, reports of guideline adherence and unfinished care plan elements, and specialized chronic care order entry systems with disease-specific checks and order templates, referrals to a specialist or nurse care manager, and team member role-specific orders [37]. Other key functions for health care teams include: electronic access to guidelines/decision support; structured problem; allergies; medication lists; tracking of tasks against care plan; trends over time about complications and deterioration; roles and contacts of health care team members; and comprehensive care plan for all conditions [32]. The coordination across health care teams that may practice in different specialties, locations, or organizations requires additional capabilities for sharing of records/health information exchange, follow-up on referrals and reporting back of findings or patient disposition, and cross-organizational tracking of care plan activities [31,32].

5.3.4 Across Multiple Teams

Collaboration between health care teams and person/family teams share requirements with those described in patient-centeredness and shared care planning as those are domains in which much of the activity is collaborative. There are other requirements specific to the collaborations between these teams for which the full loop of communication and follow through are critical [29,31,32]. This loop begins with easy scheduling of appointments perhaps through a portal or PHR that streamlines the process for health care sites and improves accessibility for patients. Electronic downloadable visit summaries and patient education materials allow the person/family team to recall what occurred at the visit and the intended plan of care, and to follow up on their responsibilities. The loop continues with tracking of orders for labs and radiology not only to confirm fulfillment but also to assure that results, interpretation, and additional instructions have been provided to both the health care team and patient. Secure messaging and up-to-date contact information for the health care and person/family teams must be available to facilitate these communications.

Medication reconciliation is another function that relies on active engagement of person/family and health care teams in order to prevent adverse drug events and to achieve clinical goals. Reconciliation requires performing a comprehensive inventory of all prescribed and over-the-counter medications including name, dosage, frequency, and route; identifying the medications the person is actively taking and not taking; and identifying the source of medication orders/prescriptions. With this information, teams can prevent adverse drug interactions, make timely therapeutic changes as appropriate, and develop tactics to enhance adherence. The data for medication reconciliation may be sourced from EHRs and/or pharmacy management systems and patient self-report, and are needed at initial reconciliation and on an ongoing basis as changes are made. Medication reconciliation requires one type of patient-generated data related to medication adherence, but there are numerous others. Data such as physical activity and food consumption may serve primarily self-management purposes. Other data such as signs and symptoms may benefit from clinical input to self-management and be relevant to timely care coordination intervention or patient reported outcomes. Strategies for identifying, reviewing, and responding to patient-generated data are also needed.

Little attention has been paid to the elicitation of HIT functions or enabling technical infrastructure needed for care coordination within person/family teams and community teams, or across multiple, diverse teams whether family, community, or health care. In addition, coordination over the life span has received almost no attention.

5.4 CURRENT EFFORTS IN INFORMATICS AND COORDINATION AT THE POINT OF NEED

There have been a number of studies of HIT and care coordination in chronic disease management that demonstrate potential for improving outcomes including early intervention based on remote reporting of signs and symptoms via a handheld device [38], communication with care coordinators via videophones and messaging [39], and patient reporting by telephone [23]. There are still serious implementation challenges, however [40], and persistent health disparities when using HIT for care coordination [41]. Most coordination interventions still use low-level interactive technologies, such as telephone and fax, and so far no interventions have tackled the challenges of coordinating care across multiple teams, multiple settings, and over time [35]. Projects that have addressed the challenges of coordinating care in oncology are fewer, and have focused primarily on health care teams or their limited interaction with patients. These are described below.

5.4.1 Within and Across Health Care Teams

Health care teams enjoy the most comprehensive features for care coordination, particularly with robust EHRs. Galligioni et al. developed an electronic oncological patient record and highlighted the ability of "total" management of patients with cancer. Their data also revealed that providers felt it was "additional work" and had a "negative impact on doctor–patient relationships" [42]. While the authors reported their system was developed applying a user-centered design approach, the user-centered focus was on providers and did not include patients. Although EHRs and the variety of functions they may include (eg, decision support tools, electronic ordering of chemotherapy) offer many solutions to address the complex needs of cancer patients, significant barriers remain in their widespread acceptance and use [43].

An additional challenge of HIT-enabled care coordination is significant overlap of activities that may seem distinct; for example, and perhaps most noticeably, communication, workflow, and symptom management. Communication tasks could include items such as appointment reminders and patient-provider e-mail/messaging but it also may include notification about symptom management concerns of patient-reported symptoms via electronic questionnaire. Further, this notification on symptom management concerns could trigger further communication and workflow needs.

5.4.2 Within Person and Family Teams

There are several social networks that support care coordination among family teams. These online communities primarily focus on coordination of instrumental support for activities of daily living. Social networks that allow for both within family team and community team collaboration can have a significant impact on health care throughout the cancer continuum [44]. While very promising in the opportunity to provide connections and support, concerns remain about inaccurate information, lack of professional oversight, and overall misuse [44].

One example, while not exclusive to oncology populations, is CaringBridge. CaringBridge, founded in 1997, serves approximately 500,000 people a day. Anderson et al. evaluated connection and social support among CaringBridge users during a health care event and identified four key benefits: "providing information, receiving encouragement from messages, convenience, and psychological support" [45].

Lotsa Helping Hands is another patient support social network founded in 2005. While there is no published literature identified evaluating care coordination activities using this site among an oncology population, the need for community involvement and support is clearly described by Mangurian who wrote of her personal experience navigating system complexities as a parent of a pediatric oncology patient [8]. Among those with cancer, few studies evaluate the engagement of family members and caregivers of patients' use of technology to support communication and workflow [46,47].

5.4.3 Across Person and Health Care Teams

Cancer care across the continuum often involves complex treatment choices and decisions. Technology-enabled decisional support and aids, including prevention efforts in cancer care via educational modules and guided web-based interventions, may offer great promise in supporting patients, family members, and caregivers. However, within the limited research that has been conducted, almost all literature is focused on the development and testing of tools and interventions, with little known about how to overcome significant implementation barriers [48–51].

While much of the literature on care coordination among health care teams focuses on workflow support and communication, symptom management is almost inextricably linked to communication, as most of the reported outcomes examine patient-provider communication. Examples include appointment reminders, including text messaging [52–54], provider order entry [55], electronic messaging [56], and unique studies examining the communication between providers and insurance companies [57] and patients' reviews of provider documentation of medical appointments [58,59].

Research examining technology-assisted, self-report assessments for symptom management, quality of life concerns, self-care support for improved patient-provider communication, and patient distress in oncology have been widely published; although, many of these studies have evaluated the acceptability and/or use of technology, not specific health outcomes [60–63]. In a review of the use and possibilities of electronic patient-reported outcome systems (ePROs) in oncology clinical practice, Bennett et al. identify areas across the cancer continuum that "support multiple clinical activities, including assessment of symptoms and toxicities related to chemotherapy and radiation, postoperative surveillance, and symptom management during palliative care and hospice" [64].

In 2009, Abernethy et al. published results from a longitudinal pilot study of 66 metastatic breast cancer patients using eTablets over a 6-month period [60]. Patients completed electronic surveys on symptoms and quality of life. They examined the feasibility and acceptability of the "Patient Care Monitor" (PCM) and found that most patients found it easy to use, read, and navigate, with 74% indicating the PCM would help them remember symptoms to report to their clinician. Bausch reported that patients with cancer were able to use a web interface during chemotherapy to report treatment toxicity symptoms during an 8-week period [65]. In later studies, Bausch examined the feasibility of advanced cancer patients reporting toxicity symptoms and found that while satisfaction with the symptom reporting was 91%, only 51% of patients felt communication with their care team was improved [61,62]. Relatedly, Bausch evaluated the nurses' use of the symptom reporting data and identified that "only one of the seven nurses discussed reports with patients frequently, with insufficient time being the most common barrier to discussions" [62]. Finally, Snyder et al. evaluated the use, usefulness, and acceptability of PatientViewpoint among prostate and breast cancer patients and their providers [66]. PatientViewpoint is a web-based tool that allows providers to assign symptom questionnaires/surveys to patients, which upon completion may be linked to their EHRs. Similar to other studies, results show that most patients (92%) found the system easy to use, and 70% of patients found the system "useful" and helped them to remember symptoms to discuss with their provider. Additionally, only 49% of patients reported that it helped improve communication with their provider and surprisingly, only 39% identified improved quality of care [66]. Among providers, 79% reported using the symptom data and among a median score of three patient-identified concerns only one was reviewed during the patient's appointment [66].

Additionally, some literature reports on the use, feasibility, and validity of specific technology-enabled instruments and surveys [67,68]. Fann et al. evaluated the feasibility and the construct validity of the Patient Health Questionnaire-9 (PHQ-9) depression screening among a diverse group of cancer patients using a web-based touchscreen survey format [67]. Feasibility was measured with completion of the survey (96%) and the time (mean) it took to complete the survey (2 minutes). Taenzer evaluated an electronically administered quality of life survey (European Organization for Research and Treatment of Cancer (EORTC) QLQ-C30) versus the same paper-based survey among lung cancer patients [68]. Outcome measures included patient satisfaction, patient and provider discussion of concerns identified by the survey, and provider documentation. While patients in both groups reported high satisfaction, patients completing the electronic EORTC QLQ-C30 identified more quality of life concerns, with more concerns discussed during the patient's appointment.

More recently, intervention studies have examined the effectiveness of technology-enabled symptom reporting and symptom management on patient-reported outcomes. Kroenke et al. conducted an RCT over a 12-month period, comparing the effectiveness of telecare management on pain and depression, along with automated home-based symptom monitoring by interactive voice recording or Internet, in patients with cancer among 16 community-based oncology practices, both urban and rural [69]. A nurse and physicians specialist team led the telecare management. Overall, the authors found greater improved pain and depression outcomes among those receiving the intervention [69].

Additionally, Berry et al. conducted a multisite RCT of 660 patients with various cancer diagnoses and stages [70]. They evaluated the effect of the Electronic Self-Report Assessment-Cancer (ESRA-C) on patient-provider discussions of patient-reported symptoms and quality of life issues. Patients completed assessments on touchscreen notebook computers and provider teams received a graphical summary report prior to the patient appointment. Berry and colleagues found increased discussion of patient symptoms in the intervention group. In a related RCT of 752 cancer patients recruited from two comprehensive cancer centers, traditional symptom and quality of life assessment combined screening with "targeted education, communication coaching and the opportunity to track/graph symptoms and quality of life over time" [71]. Berry et al. conclude that education, support, and coaching when added to symptom and quality of life screening reduces distress, particularly among those older than 50 years.

To address the symptom management concerns of oncology patients, studies are beginning to evaluate technology-enabled symptom management tools and online interventions [7]. Grimmett et al. have begun an exploratory RCT of 125 posttreatment cancer survivors to address fatigue using online self-management intervention compared with paper leaflets [7].

5.4.4 Across Multiple Teams

Online social support (virtual support groups, discussion groups, etc.) facilitates care across person/family teams and community teams when the support is provided from those outside the family team. In a recent review by Bouma et al., Internet-based support programs were evaluated and summarized into three categories: "social support groups, online therapy groups for psychosocial/physical symptoms, and online systems integrating information, support, and coaching services" [72]. They reported improved effects on both quality of life and social support in each category [72]. The Young Adult Program at the Dana-Farber Cancer Institute in Boston, Massachusetts created an institution-specific website to "meet the supportive and emotional needs of young adults (18–39 years old)" [73]. The website includes social networking and has demonstrated increased connectedness among those who participate [73]. Caregivers may also benefit from online support communities, although research is more limited [74,75]. While the majority of the online social support literature is focused on diagnosis and active treatment, interventions across the cancer continuum show promise, including screening [5,76].

One area where considerable work has been done is patient navigation, which represents an area that engages the person and multiple teams. In cancer care, patient navigation has long been used to facilitate patient access to timely and appropriate care [77]. Rooted in a community-centered approach to care coordination, the original goal of patient navigation was to reduce disparities in cancer outcomes by targeting efforts in the prevention and screening phases of the cancer continuum [77]. Since its inception, patient navigation has been shown to improve follow-up time between abnormal screening and diagnosis in a variety of other settings and populations, including in cervical, colorectal, and prostate cancers [77]. The concept of patient navigation has expanded to encompass many navigator roles and interventions across the cancer care continuum from prevention through survivorship and end-of-life care [77]. A 2011 review of patient navigation studies noted the increasing heterogeneity of patient navigator backgrounds. While navigators are still most commonly trained lay people from the target community, nurses, or private independent practitioners (http://www.medsavvyhealthadvocates.com), navigation programs have now been implemented with case managers, social workers, tumor registrars, and even peer cancer patients serving in these roles [78]. The majority of studies on the efficacy of patient navigation have examined cancer screening rates as outcomes. Nine out of ten efficacy studies published between 2007 and 2010 found statistically significant effects of patient navigation interventions on screening rates or improved stage at diagnosis. For example, one patient navigation intervention achieved a 55% mammography rescreening rate compared to 1.5% in a control group, and another achieved a 27% colorectal cancer screening rate compared to 12% in the control group [78].

Patient navigation interventions have not been as consistently successful in other phases of the cancer continuum. A 2011 systematic review found that only two of seven identified studies on the efficacy of patient navigation interventions for patients in active treatment demonstrated significant differences in outcomes between groups receiving patient navigation and controls [79]. Individuals who received patient navigation during treatment for head and neck cancers reported improved satisfaction with care and emotional quality of life, and also had significantly fewer hospitalizations compared with those who did not receive patient navigation [79]. Among patients undergoing radiation therapy for cancer, those with patient navigators experienced significantly fewer treatment interruptions compared to those without navigators (3 fewer interrupted days, on average) [79]. In more recent work, patient navigation interventions in the active treatment phase have been reported to help patients address financial and communication barriers as well as transportation difficulties [80], and to increase the proportion of patients receiving recommended adjuvant therapy for breast cancer [81].

Differences in outcomes might, in part, be explained by differences in the groups targeted for patient navigation, and by the person in the role of navigator. For example, many studies of patient navigation in the active treatment phase of care use clinical navigators, such as nurses or case managers. Using clinical navigators who are part of the system of care may not be as effective as using lay navigators who are part of the patients' community. The use of community-based navigators has been a critical element of many successful patient navigation programs, and may help promote trust between patients and care providers in some communities [82]. In addition, patient navigation interventions may be most appropriate when targeted at groups who are likely to have problems accessing needed care or understanding treatment options [83]. One study, for example, found that having a clinical navigator reduced time between diagnosis and oncologist consultation significantly for elderly patients, but made no difference for younger patients [84]. Similarly, many successful navigator interventions have been implemented in communities with

historically low rates of participation in recommended screening and follow-up care, whether due to access, transportation, or other cultural barriers to receiving care [85,86]. Perhaps not surprisingly, then, studies of patient navigation interventions in groups that are not targeted based on their need for assistance overcoming barriers have not demonstrated the same substantial benefits [87]. A meta-analysis of patient navigation studies conducted between 2007 and 2011 determined that patient navigation did have a moderate effect in reducing treatment delays. However, these effects were not seen immediately, but only after the first 90 days of care [79,88]. In addition, the greatest benefit was seen in centers that had the most substantial delays in follow-up care preimplementation [89].

While the best approaches to implementing patient navigation programs and the most appropriate measures of their success are still under discussion, their potential to benefit care coordination and clinical outcomes is now widely accepted. Since 2011 the American College of Surgeons Commission on Cancer has required a patient navigation process for the accreditation of cancer programs [90]. As these programs develop, the potential of patient navigation to improve a variety of outcomes across the cancer continuum will become more clear.

Looking at HIT, there are many ways in which it could enhance and improve patient navigation programs. Evaluation of navigators' activities reveals that patient navigators generally spend a great deal of time gathering or documenting information in patients' electronic medical records, and work with a variety of individuals to plan care, including the patient, family and caregivers, community support services, and clinical providers [91]. HIT tailored to the needs of patient navigation programs would not only support navigators in performing their job duties, but also allow for large-scale data collection and analysis of the outcomes of such programs. Several such programs exist, such as OncoNav [92], NurseNav [93], and Cordata Oncology [94]. Most software offers some level of integration with commonly used EHR systems and, perhaps because of this integration, is designed primarily for clinical nurse navigators. However, some programs offer communication with patients and other care team members through web-based portals. Others offer "community navigation" features that can assist in implementing patient navigation programs and tracking community-wide outcomes across a system of care [93]. While few technology solutions have been developed specifically for community-based lay navigation programs, the Harold P. Freeman Patient Navigation Institute offers online training for lay navigators as well as mobile learning apps [95].

Outside of patient navigation there are only a few studies of care coordination across teams, particular those that engage family and community teams with health care teams. One such study, an RCT, used technology supported communication "to assess the effects of an online symptom reporting system on caregiver preparedness, physical burden and negative mood" [96]. Metastatic or advanced breast, lung, and prostate cancer patients and their caregivers were recruited from five US cancer centers to participate in the Comprehensive Health Enhancement Support System (CHESS), an online symptom reporting and education tool. Both groups had access to the tool with one group having the additional Clinician Report (CR), which offers an alert function to clinicians about certain electronic patient-reported outcomes. Patients and caregivers in the CHESS+ CR group reported "less negative mood," which the authors conclude may suggest that they "experience less emotional distress due to the CR's timely communication of caregiving needs in symptom management to clinicians" [96]. This area is addressed more substantively in Chapter 10, "Advanced Cancer: Palliative, End of Life, and Bereavement Care."

Another study in progress involves an RCT of a Personal Health Network (PHN) which aims to demonstrate and evaluate a comprehensive platform for coordinating care during chemotherapy [97]. The PHN is a social networking platform delivered through either a tablet application or website to patients undergoing chemotherapy, their family members, nurse care coordinators, extended health care team, and community resources. The PHN includes the following functions:

- Health care, family, and community team members invited into an individual's PHN.
- Patient self-report assessment instruments and outcomes reported online. This and other instruments used at visits and in-between visits to monitor symptoms.
- Nurse care coordinator performed evidence-based protocols appropriate to the needs, symptoms, and requests of the patient.
- A shared care plan published to all members of the PHN.
- Care plan activities scheduled, assigned to members of the PHN, and tracked.
- Nurse care coordinator monitored care plan, with communication to physicians and other care team members as needed.
- Patient education materials, instructions, and plans delivered to individual and family team through the PHN library, with notification by voice/text message that resources are available.
- Communication among individual, health care, family, and community teams using voice/text messaging, audio/video calls within PHN, and reminders are pushed to participants.

Fig. 5.3 shows screenshots of the tablet application.

5.4.5 Shared Care Plans

A critical component of a care coordination program is a collaborative, accessible, and well-monitored shared care plan. Shared care plans have evolved as an approach to promote coordinated care for individuals with chronic diseases who have multiple providers involved in their care. Ideally, shared care plans should facilitate communication between health care and patient teams, across health care teams, and across time. Since the shared care plan is, as its name implies, meant to be used by multiple groups, its purpose is not only to provide traditional, clinical care planning, but also to promote self-management and patient engagement.

Despite its potential, shared care planning has not been extensively implemented or studied. A 2007 Cochrane review of shared care interventions found limited evidence that such interventions improved outcomes other than medication management [98]. Reviewers noted that relatively weak study designs and scant descriptions of the "usual care" received by control groups limited the ability to detect potentially important benefits of the interventions [98]. Major limitations of the reviewed studies included a lack of patient involvement (ie, care was shared between health care teams but not between health care and patient teams), and underuse of potentially helpful HIT support [98]. The Institute for Healthcare Improvement and Agency for Healthcare Quality and Research both provide links to shared care plans on their websites (http://www.ihi.org/resources/Pages/Tools/MySharedCarePlan.aspx, http://www.orau.gov/ahrq/sms_tool_06.asp?p=sms_home). In both instances, the care plans are patient-led. Although intended for use by all health care team members, these shared care plans are currently not integrated as part of the medical record, placing the responsibility for initiating and coordinating these documents on the patient. Research that tests the effectiveness of web-based shared care plans that have some level of interoperability with commonly used EHRs will provide important insight into the feasibility of using shared care plans to enhance care coordination for individuals with chronic diseases.

In cancer care, the survivorship care plan, a form of shared care plan, has been recommended as a specific approach to shared care planning to help improve the transition from active treatment back to long-term surveillance and survivorship care [99]. Survivorship care plans are addressed in greater detail by Beckjord et al. in Chapter 9 "Survivorship." However, there is still no consensus on the best way to implement these care plans. As with shared care plans in other chronic disease settings, HIT is both a current barrier and a potential future solution for effective implementation of cancer survivorship care plans. With a multitude of EHRs currently on the market, finding a survivorship care planning template

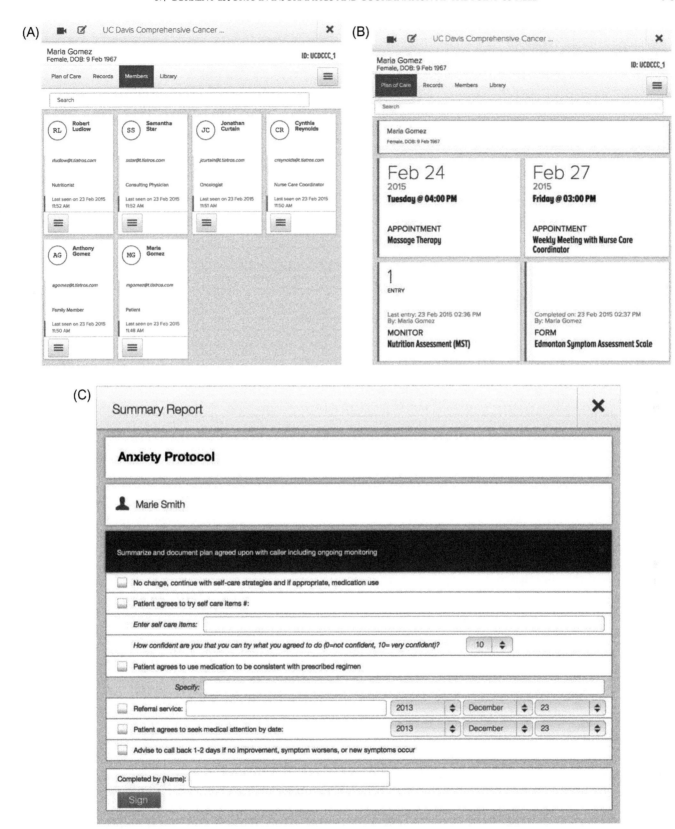

FIGURE 5.3 Personal Health Network for chemotherapy care coordination. (A) Members of the individual's Personal Health Network, (B) task view of shared care plan, (C) nurse care coordination symptom management protocol, (D) patient self-report instrument, and (E) self-management library.

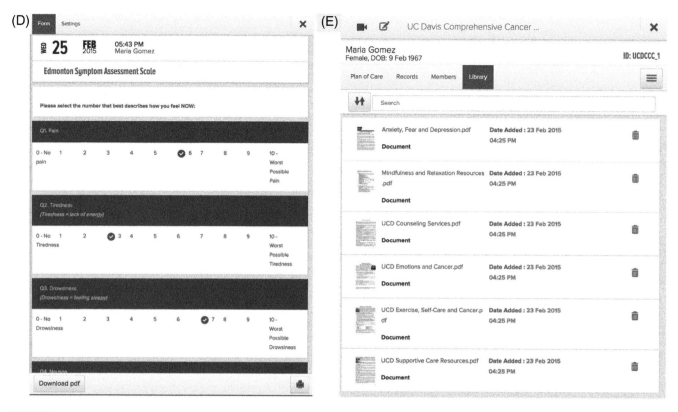

FIGURE 5.3 Continued

that not only works for the oncology practice, but also allows for patient interaction and communication with other specialists and primary care providers who may use different EHR systems is a major challenge with no immediate solution [100]. However, promising pilot studies demonstrate that cancer survivorship care plans can be successfully implemented, at least in settings where providers and patients all have access to the same EHR system [101]. Integrating the survivorship care plan into an oncology practice's EHR allows for some information to be automatically populated, rather than manually documented by the oncologist, saving valuable time. Patients in the pilot studies generally felt the care plans were useful and easy to access. However, missing information about care that was received from providers outside the system was problematic [101]. Substantial resources are needed to implement survivorship care plans. Future research is critical, not only to demonstrate whether or not the benefits of survivorship care planning justify the use of these resources, but also to evaluate approaches that make their implementation more feasible [102].

5.5 OPPORTUNITIES FOR ONCOLOGY INFORMATICS AT THE POINT OF NEED

There are numerous opportunities to contribute to the improvement of oncology care coordination through

HIT. First, there is a need for a comprehensive elicitation of HIT requirements for care coordination. There is a large gap in the understanding of the requirements for within person/family teams beyond instrumental support for activities of daily living. While most of the work has focused on the health care team and the EHR, we must move beyond the health care team and consider the requirements across multiple teams including the interactions among health care, family, and community teams as they interact around coordination of care for individuals. In considering these teams as a complete community around the individual, the multiple points of need become apparent as does the criticality of systems for organizing the varied and complex workflows across them all. This comprehensive view of care coordination would set the foundation for shared accountability in which patients are empowered and central to decision making throughout their life span.

HIT for integrated care coordination across a community is emerging, however, there are few comprehensive platforms that can support care coordination across the diversity of participants. An informal search led by one of the authors aimed at identifying and assessing commercial platforms involved companies known to the authors, an extensive web search, phone interviews, and system demonstrations (Kim, Lindeman, unpublished). Among the 25 systems reviewed, none provided adequate capabilities such as those described in this chapter. Most were able to address health care team coordination with limited functions for patients such as a portal for results delivery and appointment scheduling requests. All were lacking functions for deeper person-centered engagement and coordination across multiple teams, which limits the potential to accomplish shared decision making and accountability. The findings from this informal assessment of commercial platforms is not surprising given the preponderance of published literature that addresses only the early stages of design and feasibility.

Perhaps a function of the nascency of the field, there is little evidence of efficacy of HIT-enabled care coordination. However, the field would be enhanced if studies paid attention to effectiveness of implementation even when conducting early stage investigations. Without effective implementation of a technology-enabled care coordination program, the potential efficacy of the intervention may never be realized. This would suggest the greater use of user-centered design of both HIT and the intervention itself including all potential participants, and the measurement of implementation and care coordination variables.

HIT is a critical enabler of emerging care models such as the Oncology Care Model and the Learning Healthcare System for Cancer that depend upon effective care coordination to improve health care, cost, quality, and ultimately population health. There is great opportunity for informatics to collaborate with clinicians, patients, and all individuals who participate in the complex and complicated processes of coordination to design, implement, and evaluate HIT solutions to address the challenges we face in aiming for those outcomes.

LIST OF ACRONYMS AND ABBREVIATIONS

CCM Chronic care model
CHESS Comprehensive Health Enhancement Support System
CMS Centers for Medicare and Medicaid Services
CR Clinician Report
CWCC Community-wide care coordination
EHR Electronic health record
EORTC European Organization for Research and Treatment of Cancer
ePRO Electronic patient-reported outcome system
ESRA-C Electronic Self-Report Assessment-Cancer
HIT Health information technology
IOM Institute of Medicine
IPC Integrated patient care
PCM Patient Care Monitor
PHN Personal Health Network
PHQ-9 Patient Health Questionnaire-9
PHR Patient health record
PICC Peripherally inserted central catheter
QLQ-C30 Quality of Life Questionnaire-Core 30
RCT Randomized clinical trial

References

[1] Schoen C, Osborn R, Squires D, Doty M, Pierson R, Applebaum S. New 2011 survey of patients with complex care needs in eleven countries finds that care is often poorly coordinated. Health Aff (Millwood) 2011;30(12):2437–48.

[2] Smith TJ, Hillner BE. Bending the cost curve in cancer care. N Engl J Med 2011;364(21):2060–5.

[3] McDonald KM, Sundaram V, Bravata DM, Lewis R, Lin N, Kraft SA, et al. AHRQ technical reviews. Closing the quality gap: a critical analysis of quality improvement strategies (Vol. 7: Care Coordination). Rockville, MD: Agency for Healthcare Research and Quality (US); 2007.

[4] Chen A, Brown R, Archibald N, Aliotta S, Fox PD. Best practices in coordinated care. 2000.

[5] Hwang KO, Ottenbacher AJ, Graham AL, Thomas EJ, Street Jr. RL, Vernon SW. Online narratives and peer support for colorectal cancer screening: a pilot randomized trial. Am J Prev Med 2013;45(1):98–107.

[6] Xavier AJ, d'Orsi E, Wardle J, Demakakos P, Smith SG, von Wagner C. Internet use and cancer-preventive behaviors in older adults: findings from a longitudinal cohort study. Cancer Epidemiol Biomarkers Prev 2013;22(11):2066–74.

[7] Grimmett C, Armes J, Breckons M, Calman L, Corner J, Fenlon D, et al. RESTORE: an exploratory trial of an online intervention to enhance self-efficacy to manage problems associated with cancer-related fatigue following primary cancer treatment: study protocol for a randomized controlled trial. Trials 2013;14:184.

[8] Mangurian C, Cowan MJ. The missing vital sign. BMJ 2013;347:f4163.

[9] Noar SM, Ribisl KM, Althouse BM, Willoughby JF, Ayers JW. Using digital surveillance to examine the impact of public figure pancreatic cancer announcements on media and search query outcomes. J Natl Cancer Inst Monogr 2013;2013(47):188–94.

[10] Burwell SM. Setting value-based payment goals—HHS efforts to improve U.S. health care. N Engl J Med 2015;372(10):897–9.

[11] Carroll AE, Frakt AB. New evidence supports, challenges, and informs the ambitions of health reform. JAMA 2013;309(24):2600–1.

[12] Kocher RP, Adashi EY. Hospital readmissions and the Affordable Care Act: paying for coordinated quality care. JAMA 2011;306(16):1794–5.

[13] IOM Roundtable on value & science-driven health care: the healthcare imperative: lowering costs and improving outcomes: workshop serious summary. Washington, DC: National Academies Press; 2010.

[14] Brown RS, Ghosh A, Schraeder C, Shelton P. Promising practices in acute/primary care Schraeder C, Shelton P, editors. Comprehensive care coordination for chronically ill adults. New York, NY: John Wiley & Sons, Inc.; 2011.

[15] Wagner EH, Davis C, Schaefer J, Von Korff M, Austin B. A survey of leading chronic disease management programs: are they consistent with the literature? Manag Care Q 1999;7(3):56–66.

[16] Bodenheimer T, Berry-Millett R. Follow the money—controlling expenditures by improving care for patients needing costly services. N Engl J Med 2009;361(16):1521–3.

[17] Naylor MD, Brooten D, Campbell R, Jacobsen BS, Mezey MD, Pauly MV, et al. Comprehensive discharge planning and home follow-up of hospitalized elders: a randomized clinical trial. JAMA 1999;281(7):613–20.

[18] Naylor MD, Brooten DA, Campbell RL, Maislin G, McCauley KM, Schwartz JS. Transitional care of older adults hospitalized with heart failure: a randomized, controlled trial. J Am Geriatr Soc 2004;52(5):675–84.

[19] Coleman EA, Parry C, Chalmers S, Min SJ. The care transitions intervention: results of a randomized controlled trial. Arch Intern Med 2006;166(17):1822–8.

[20] Boult C, Boult LB, Morishita L, Dowd B, Kane RL, Urdangarin CF. A randomized clinical trial of outpatient geriatric evaluation and management. J Am Geriatr Soc 2001;49(4):351–9.

[21] Brown R, Peikes D, Peterson G, Schore J. The promise of care coordination: models that decrease hospitalizations and improve outcomes for Medicare beneficiaries with chronic illness. Mathematica Policy Research Inc.; 2009. Available from: <http://www.mathematica-mpr.com/~/media/publications/pdfs/health/care_coordination_models.pdf>.

[22] Brown RS, Peikes D, Peterson G, Schore J, Razafindrakoto CM. Six features of Medicare coordinated care demonstration programs that cut hospital admissions of high-risk patients. Health Aff (Millwood) 2012;31(6):1156–66.

[23] Peikes D, Chen A, Schore J, Brown R. Effects of care coordination on hospitalization, quality of care, and health care expenditures among Medicare beneficiaries: 15 randomized trials. JAMA 2009;301(6):603–18.

[24] Schraeder C, Brunker CP, Hess I, Hale BA, Berger C, Waldschmidt V. Intervention components Schraeder C, Shelton P, editors. Comprehensive care coordination for chronically ill adults. New York, NY: John Wiley & Sons, Inc.; 2011.

[25] Wagner EH. Chronic disease management: what will it take to improve care for chronic illness? Eff Clin Pract 1998;1(1):2–4.

[26] Wagner EH, Austin BT, Von Korff M. Organizing care for patients with chronic illness. Milbank Q 1996;74(4):511–44.

[27] Singer SJ, Burgers J, Friedberg M, Rosenthal MB, Leape L, Schneider E. Defining and measuring integrated patient care: promoting the next frontier in health care delivery. Med Care Res Rev 2011;68(1):112–27.

[28] Kim KK, Bell JF, Boicey C, Freeman-Daily J, Hull S, McCollister-Slipp A, Joseph JG. A framework for person-centered, community-wide care coordination. American Medical Informatics Association 2015 Annual Symposium; San Francisco, CA; 2015.

[29] Levit L, Balogh E, Nass S, Ganz PA. A learning health care information technology system for cancer Delivering high-quality cancer care: charting a new course for a system in crisis: National Academies Press; Washington, DC; 2013.262.

[30] Walker J, Leveille SG, Ngo L, Vodicka E, Darer JD, Dhanireddy S, et al. Inviting patients to read their doctors' notes: patients and doctors look ahead: patient and physician surveys. Ann Intern Med 2011;155(12):811–9.

[31] Hesse BW, Hanna C, Massett HA, Hesse NK. Outside the box: will information technology be a viable intervention to improve the quality of cancer care? JNCI Monogr 2010;2010(40):81–9.

[32] Samal L, Hasan O, Venkatesh AK, Volk LA, Bates DW. Health information technology to support care coordination and care transitions: data needs, capabilities, technical and organizational barriers, and approaches to improvement. Washington, DC: National Quality Forum; 2012.

[33] Cheng C, Stokes TH, Wang MD, editors. caREMOTE: the design of a cancer reporting and monitoring telemedicine system for domestic care. In: Annual International Conference of the IEEE Engineering in Medicine and Biology Society, EMBC, 2011. IEEE; 2011.

[34] Standards & Interoperability Framework Longitudinal coordination of care: interoperable care plan exchange use case v2.0. Washington, DC: Office of the National Coordinator for Health Information; 2014.

[35] Samal L, Dykes P, Greenberg J, Hasan O, Venkatesh A, Volk L, et al. Environmental analysis of health information technology to support care coordination and care transitions. Washington, DC; 2012.

[36] Ganz PA, Hahn EE. Implementing a survivorship care plan for patients with breast cancer. J Clin Oncol 2008;26(5):759–67.

[37] Dorr D, Bonner LM, Cohen AN, Shoai RS, Perrin R, Chaney E, et al. Informatics systems to promote improved care for chronic illness: a literature review. J Am Med Inform Assoc 2007;14(2):156–63.

[38] Baker LC, Johnson SJ, Macaulay D, Birnbaum H. Integrated telehealth and care management program for Medicare beneficiaries with chronic disease linked to savings. Health Aff 2011;30(9):1689–97.

[39] Darkins A, Ryan P, Kobb R, Foster L, Edmonson E, Wakefield B, et al. Care coordination/home telehealth: the systematic implementation of health informatics, home telehealth, and disease management to support the care of veteran patients with chronic conditions. Telemed e-Health 2008;14(10):1118–26.

[40] Cumming J. Integrated care in New Zealand. Int J Integr Care 2011;11(Special 10th Anniversary Edition):e138.

[41] Weinstock RS, Teresi JA, Goland R, Izquierdo R, Palmas W, Eimicke JP, et al. Glycemic control and health disparities in older ethnically diverse underserved adults with diabetes: five-year results from the Informatics for Diabetes Education and Telemedicine (IDEATel) study. Diabetes Care 2011;34(2):274–9.

[42] Galligioni E, Berloffa F, Caffo O, Tonazzolli G, Ambrosini G, Valduga F, et al. Development and daily use of an electronic oncological patient record for the total management of cancer patients: 7 years' experience. Ann Oncol 2009;20(2):349–52.

[43] Warner J, Hochberg E. Where is the EHR in oncology? J Natl Compr Cancer Netw 2012;10(5):584–8.

[44] Masic I, Sivic S, Toromanovic S, Borojevic T, Pandza H. Social networks in improvement of health care. Mater Sociomed 2012;24(1):48–53.

[45] Anderson IK. The uses and gratifications of online care pages: a study of CaringBridge. Health Commun 2011;26(6):546–59.

[46] Maddock C, Lewis I, Ahmad K, Sullivan R. Online information needs of cancer patients and their organizations. Ecancermedicalscience 2011;5:235.

[47] Kinnane NA, Milne DJ. The role of the Internet in supporting and informing carers of people with cancer: a literature review. Support Care Cancer 2010;18(9):1123–36.

[48] Basch E, Abernethy AP. Supporting clinical practice decisions with real-time patient-reported outcomes. J Clin Oncol 2011;29(8):954–6.

[49] Berry DL, Halpenny B, Wolpin S, Davison BJ, Ellis WJ, Lober WB, et al. Development and evaluation of the personal patient profile-prostate (P3P), a Web-based decision support system for men newly diagnosed with localized prostate cancer. J Med Internet Res 2010;12(4):e67.

[50] DuBenske LL, Gustafson DH, Shaw BR, Cleary JF. Web-based cancer communication and decision making systems: connecting patients, caregivers, and clinicians for improved health outcomes. Med Decis Making 2010;30(6):732–44.

[51] Watts KJ, Meiser B, Wakefield CE, Barratt AL, Howard K, Cheah BC, et al. Online prostate cancer screening decision aid for at-risk men: a randomized trial. Health Psychol 2014;33(9):986–97.

[52] Nease Jr. DE, Ruffin MT, Klinkman MS, Jimbo M, Braun TM, Underwood JM. Impact of a generalizable reminder system on colorectal cancer screening in diverse primary care practices: a report from the prompting and reminding at encounters for prevention project. Med Care 2008;46(9 Suppl. 1):S68–73.

[53] de Jongh T, Gurol-Urganci I, Vodopivec-Jamsek V, Car J, Atun R. Mobile phone messaging for facilitating self-management of long-term illnesses. Cochrane Database Syst Rev 2012;12 Cd007459.

[54] Vodopivec-Jamsek V, de Jongh T, Gurol-Urganci I, Atun R, Car J. Mobile phone messaging for preventive health care. Cochrane Database Syst Rev 2012;12 Cd007457.

[55] Gillaizeau F, Chan E, Trinquart L, Colombet I, Walton RT, Rege-Walther M, et al. Computerized advice on drug dosage to improve prescribing practice. Cochrane Database Syst Rev 2013;11 Cd002894.

[56] Wallwiener M, Wallwiener CW, Kansy JK, Seeger H, Rajab TK. Impact of electronic messaging on the patient-physician interaction. J Telemed Telecare 2009;15(5):243–50.

[57] Casalino LP, Nicholson S, Gans DN, Hammons T, Morra D, Karrison T, et al. What does it cost physician practices to interact with health insurance plans? Health Aff (Project Hope) 2009;28(4):w533–43.

[58] Delbanco T, Walker J, Bell SK, Darer JD, Elmore JG, Farag N, et al. Inviting patients to read their doctors' notes: a quasi-experimental study and a look ahead. Ann Intern Med 2012;157(7):461–70.

[59] Feeley TW, Shine KI. Access to the medical record for patients and involved providers: transparency through electronic tools. Ann Intern Med 2011;155(12):853–4.

[60] Abernethy AP, Herndon II JE, Wheeler JL, Day JM, Hood L, Patwardhan M, et al. Feasibility and acceptability to patients of a longitudinal system for evaluating cancer-related symptoms and quality of life: pilot study of an e/Tablet data-collection system in academic oncology. J Pain Symptom Manage 2009;37(6):1027–38.

[61] Basch E, Artz D, Iasonos A, Speakman J, Shannon K, Lin K, et al. Evaluation of an online platform for cancer patient self-reporting of chemotherapy toxicities. J Am Med Inform Assoc 2007;14(3):264–8.

[62] Basch E, Iasonos A, Barz A, Culkin A, Kris MG, Artz D, et al. Long-term toxicity monitoring via electronic patient-reported outcomes in patients receiving chemotherapy. J Clin Oncol 2007;25(34):5374–80.

[63] Tariman JD, Berry DL, Halpenny B, Wolpin S, Schepp K. Validation and testing of the Acceptability E-scale for web-based patient-reported outcomes in cancer care. Appl Nurs Res 2011;24(1):53–8.

[64] Bennett AV, Jensen RE, Basch E. Electronic patient-reported outcome systems in oncology clinical practice. CA Cancer J Clin 2012;62(5):337–47.

[65] Basch E, Artz D, Dulko D, Scher K, Sabbatini P, Hensley M, et al. Patient online self-reporting of toxicity symptoms during chemotherapy. J Clin Oncol 2005;23(15):3552–61.

[66] Snyder CF, Blackford AL, Wolff AC, Carducci MA, Herman JM, Wu AW, et al. Feasibility and value of PatientViewpoint: a web system for patient-reported outcomes assessment in clinical practice. Psychooncology 2013;22(4):895–901.

[67] Fann JR, Berry DL, Wolpin S, Austin-Seymour M, Bush N, Halpenny B, et al. Depression screening using the Patient Health Questionnaire-9 administered on a touch screen computer. Psychooncology 2009;18(1):14–22.

[68] Taenzer P, Bultz BD, Carlson LE, Speca M, DeGagne T, Olson K, et al. Impact of computerized quality of life screening on physician behaviour and patient satisfaction in lung cancer outpatients. Psychooncology 2000;9(3):203–13.

[69] Kroenke K, Theobald D, Wu J, Norton K, Morrison G, Carpenter J, et al. Effect of telecare management on pain and depression in patients with cancer: a randomized trial. JAMA 2010;304(2):163–71.

[70] Berry DL, Wang Q, Halpenny B, Hong F. Decision preparation, satisfaction and regret in a multi-center sample of men with newly diagnosed localized prostate cancer. Patient Educ Couns 2012;88(2):262–7.

[71] Berry DL, Hong F, Halpenny B, Partridge AH, Fann JR, Wolpin S, et al. Electronic self-report assessment for cancer and self-care support: results of a multicenter randomized trial. J Clin Oncol 2014;32(3):199–205.

[72] Bouma G, Admiraal JM, de Vries EG, Schroder CP, Walenkamp AM, Reyners AK. Internet-based support programs to alleviate psychosocial and physical symptoms in cancer patients: a literature analysis. Crit Rev Oncol Hematol 2015;95(1):26–37.

[73] Fasciano KM, Souza PM, Braun I, Trevino K. An innovative website in the United States for meeting the emotional and supportive care needs of young adults with cancer. J Adolesc Young Adult Oncol 2015;4(1):44–9.

[74] Dolce MC. The internet as a source of health information: experiences of cancer survivors and caregivers with healthcare providers. Oncol Nurs Forum 2011;38(3):353–9.

[75] Klemm P, Wheeler E. Cancer caregivers online: hope, emotional roller coaster, and physical/emotional/psychological responses. Comput Inform Nurs 2005;23(1):38–45.

[76] Obadina ET, Dubenske LL, McDowell HE, Atwood AK, Mayer DK, Woods RW, et al. Online support: impact on anxiety in women who experience an abnormal screening mammogram. Breast (Edinburgh, Scotland) 2014;23(6):743–8.

[77] Freeman HP. The origin, evolution, and principles of patient navigation. Cancer Epidemiol Biomarkers Prev 2012;21(10):1614–7.

[78] Paskett ED, Harrop J, Wells KJ. Patient navigation: an update on the state of the science. CA Cancer J Clin 2011;61(4):237–49.

[79] Paskett ED, Katz ML, Post DM, Pennell ML, Young GS, Seiber EE, et al. The Ohio Patient Navigation Research Program: does the American Cancer Society patient navigation model improve time to resolution in patients with abnormal screening tests? Cancer Epidemiol Biomarkers Prev 2012;21(10):1620–8.

[80] Madore S, Kilbourn K, Valverde P, Borrayo E, Raich P. Feasibility of a psychosocial and patient navigation intervention to improve access to treatment among underserved breast cancer patients. Support Care Cancer 2014;22(8):2085–93.

[81] Ko NY, Darnell JS, Calhoun E, Freund KM, Wells KJ, Shapiro CL, et al. Can patient navigation improve receipt of recommended breast cancer care? Evidence from the National Patient Navigation Research Program. J Clin Oncol 2014;32(25):2758–64.

[82] Battaglia TA, Bak SM, Heeren T, Chen CA, Kalish R, Tringale S, et al. Boston Patient Navigation Research Program: the impact of navigation on time to diagnostic resolution after abnormal cancer screening. Cancer Epidemiol Biomarkers Prev 2012;21(10):1645–54.

[83] Byers T. Assessing the value of patient navigation for completing cancer screening. Cancer Epidemiol Biomarkers Prev 2012;21(10):1618–9.

[84] Basu M, Linebarger J, Gabram SG, Patterson SG, Amin M, Ward KC. The effect of nurse navigation on timeliness of breast cancer care at an academic comprehensive cancer center. Cancer 2013;119(14):2524–31.

[85] Allen JD, Perez JE, Tom L, Leyva B, Diaz D, Idali Torres M. A pilot test of a church-based intervention to promote multiple cancer-screening behaviors among Latinas. J Cancer Educ 2014;29(1):136–43.

[86] Raich PC, Whitley EM, Thorland W, Valverde P, Fairclough D, Denver Patient Navigation Research Program Patient navigation improves cancer diagnostic resolution: an individually randomized clinical trial in an underserved population. Cancer Epidemiol Biomarkers Prev 2012;21(10):1629–38.

[87] Fiscella K, Whitley E, Hendren S, Raich P, Humiston S, Winters P, et al. Patient navigation for breast and colorectal cancer treatment: a randomized trial. Cancer Epidemiol Biomarkers Prev 2012;21(10):1673–81.

[88] Lee JH, Fulp W, Wells KJ, Meade CD, Calcano E, Roetzheim R. Patient navigation and time to diagnostic resolution: results for a cluster randomized trial evaluating the efficacy of patient navigation among patients with breast cancer screening abnormalities, Tampa, FL. PLoS One 2013;8(9):e74542.

[89] Freund KM, Battaglia TA, Calhoun E, Darnell JS, Dudley DJ, Fiscella K, et al. Impact of patient navigation on timely cancer care: the Patient Navigation Research Program. J Natl Cancer Inst 2014;106(6) dju115.

[90] Langton JM, Pesa N, Rushton S, Ward RL, Pearson SA. Uptake of a web-based oncology protocol system: how do cancer clinicians use eviQ cancer treatments online? BMC Cancer 2013;13:112.

[91] Clark JA, Parker VA, Battaglia TA, Freund KM. Patterns of task and network actions performed by navigators to facilitate cancer care. Health Care Manage Rev 2014;39(2):90–101.

[92] OncoNav [cited March 4, 2015]. Available from: <http://www.onco-nav.com/?cid=53>.

[93] NurseNav [cited March 4, 2015]. Available from: <http://www.nursenav.com/>.

[94] Cordata Oncology [cited March 4, 2015]. Available from: <http://www.cordatahealth.com/oncology>.

[95] Harold P. Freeman Patient Navigation Institute [cited March 4, 2015]. Available from: <http://www.hpfreemanpni.org/the-program/mobile-learning-apps.php>.

[96] Chih MY, DuBenske LL, Hawkins RP, Brown RL, Dinauer SK, Cleary JF, et al. Communicating advanced cancer patients' symptoms via the Internet: a pooled analysis of two randomized trials examining caregiver preparedness, physical burden, and negative mood. Palliat Med 2013;27(6):533–43.

[97] Kim KK, Bell J, Reed S, Joseph JG, Bold R, Cerrone KL, et al., A novel personal health network for patient-centered chemotherapy care coordination. In: 2014 International Conference on Collaboration Technologies and Systems (CTS); pp. 449-456. IEEE, 2014.

[98] Smith SM, Allwright S, O'Dowd T. Effectiveness of shared care across the interface between primary and specialty care in chronic disease management. Cochrane Database Syst Rev 2007(3) Cd004910.

[99] Stovall E, Greenfield S, Hewitt M. From cancer patient to cancer survivor: lost in transition. National Academies Press; Washington; DC, 2005.

[100] Zabora JR, Bolte S, Brethwaite D, Weller S, Friedman C. The challenges of the integration of cancer survivorship care plans with electronic medical records. Semin Oncol Nurs 2015;31(1):73–8.

[101] Tevaarwerk AJ, Wisinski KB, Buhr KA, Njiaju UO, Tun M, Donohue S, et al. Leveraging electronic health record systems to create and provide electronic cancer survivorship care plans: a pilot study. J Oncol Pract 2014;10(3):e150–9.

[102] Stricker CT, Jacobs LA, Risendal B, Jones A, Panzer S, Ganz PA, et al. Survivorship care planning after the institute of medicine recommendations: how are we faring? J Cancer Surviv 2011;5(4):358–70.

PART II

SUPPORT ACROSS THE CONTINUUM

6

Prevention, Information Technology, and Cancer

Glen D. Morgan PhD[1] and Michael C. Fiore MD, MPH, MBA[2]

[1]Tobacco Control Research Branch, Behavioral Research Program, Division of Cancer Control and Population Sciences, National Cancer Institute, Rockville, MD, United States [2]Center for Tobacco Research and Intervention, University of Wisconsin School of Medicine and Public Health, Madison, WI, United States

OUTLINE

6.1 Overview	104	
6.1.1 Cancer Epidemiology	104	
6.1.2 Cancer Prevention	104	
6.2 Key Behaviors of Interest for the Prevention of Cancer	104	
6.2.1 Challenges of Maintaining Behavioral Change	104	
6.2.2 Smoking and Other Tobacco Use	105	
6.2.3 Overweight and Obesity	106	
6.2.4 Physical Inactivity	106	
6.2.5 Poor Nutrition	106	
6.2.6 Alcohol Consumption	107	
6.2.7 Sun Damage	107	
6.2.8 Viral Infection	107	
6.3 Current Use of Information Technology for Cancer Prevention	107	
6.3.1 Example of IT Use: Skin Cancer Prevention	108	
6.4 Electronic Health Records	108	
6.4.1 EHRs and Tobacco Cessation	108	
6.4.2 Using Lung Cancer Screening Visits to Provide Smoking Cessation Interventions	111	
6.4.3 Linking Patients to Their State Tobacco Quitlines and Closed-Loop Functionality	112	
6.4.4 Engaging Physicians to Improve Patients' Health	112	
6.4.5 Patient Registries as a Means of Promoting Cancer Prevention	113	
6.4.6 Challenges of EHRs	113	
6.4.7 The Changing Regulatory and Policy Environment	114	
6.5 Mobile, Web, and Wearable Applications	115	
6.5.1 mHealth and Cancer Prevention	115	
6.5.2 Tobacco and Smoking Behaviors	116	
6.5.3 Nutrition and Physical Activity	116	
6.5.4 Alcohol Consumption	117	
6.5.5 Sun Protection	117	
6.5.6 mHealth Research Gaps and Opportunities	117	
6.6 Summary and Future Directions	118	
List of Acronyms and Abbreviations	119	
Acknowledgments	119	
References	119	

6.1 OVERVIEW

Preventing cancer can serve as a powerful component of a comprehensive effort to decrease the burden of cancer on our society. Increasing cancer prevention efforts in clinical oncology, primary care, and other health care settings provides a substantial and largely untapped potential to reduce morbidity and mortality. This chapter reviews cancer risk factors that are amenable to preventive interventions and outlines how current and future technology-supported protocols can be used to strategically extend and improve cancer prevention efforts.

6.1.1 Cancer Epidemiology

In the United States in 2015, an estimated 1,665,370 people will be diagnosed with cancer, and an estimated 589,430 people will die of it [1]. Cancer of the lung and bronchus and cancer of the colon and rectum were among the top three sites for both men and women across races. Death rates and incidence rates for the four most common cancers (prostate, breast, lung, and colorectal), as well as for all cancers combined, are declining [2]. Despite this progress, much work remains to be done as some cancer incidence rates remain stable and others continue to rise. For example, incidence rates for melanoma are still rising, and lung cancer incidence rates in women also continue to rise. Of significant concern is that many subpopulations demonstrate elevated risk for cancer, and people with low socioeconomic status have the highest rates of both new cancers and cancer deaths. Also worrisome is that younger cancer survivors are smoking more than cancer survivors in the general population (Table 6.1).

6.1.2 Cancer Prevention

Cancer prevention encompasses behavioral risk factor modification, vaccination, chemoprevention, and screening and detection. This chapter focuses on the identification, assessment, documentation, and modification of behavioral factors associated with increased cancer risk, usually referred to as "primary prevention." Screening and detection (secondary prevention) will be covered in detail in the next chapter, but screening will be touched on here as an opportunity to intervene with cancer risk behaviors.

A recent National Cancer Institute (NCI) report [3] noted that cancer prevention, particularly the prevention of lung cancer that is primarily caused by tobacco use or exposure, has the potential to save more lives than treatment. It has been estimated that most cancer mortality in the United States can be attributed to behaviors such as tobacco use, physical inactivity, excessive alcohol consumption, overexposure to sunlight, and other factors such as obesity and poor nutrition. About 30% of cancer mortality is due to tobacco use [4]. Poor nutrition, sedentary behavior or physical inactivity, and obesity combined account for another 35% of the cancer burden.

6.2 KEY BEHAVIORS OF INTEREST FOR THE PREVENTION OF CANCER

Patterns of behavioral risk factors for cancer illustrate both progress and areas of critical need. Though the decrease in smoking in the last half century has been hailed as a major public health victory, tobacco use remains the largest single preventable cause of cancer [3]. Nutritional and dietary factors are also of concern: alcohol consumption has risen slightly since the mid-1990s; fruit and vegetable intake is not increasing; and red meat and fat consumption is not decreasing. All of these factors have been cited as possible links to increased risk of cancer [2]. As the number of Americans who are becoming either overweight or obese climbs, the connection between cancer and obesity is receiving more attention.

The behavioral risk factors that are the principal focus of this chapter have multiple determinants, from biological to behavioral to economic to social. This has been most extensively reviewed regarding tobacco use, where initiation by youth has been linked to social influences (both family members and peers) as well as to media marketing. Biological factors implicated in tobacco use include differences in uptake and dependence linked to individual variation in nicotine metabolism, which in turn has been linked to gene variation [5]. The influence of economic and policy factors is reflected by the substantial reductions in smoking prevalence rates observed following increases in cigarette excise tax rates and implementation of clean indoor air ordinances.

Similar to tobacco, high caloric and high fat food products that are associated with obesity are heavily marketed in the United States. Moreover, increasing portion sizes, and consumption of high caloric beverages and restaurant meals are contributing to excess weight [6]. Taking a page from health policy efforts designed to reduce tobacco use, there have been initiatives to control trans fats, restrict caloric drink access and size, and tax high fructose beverages.

6.2.1 Challenges of Maintaining Behavioral Change

Sustaining the behavioral change necessary for health risk reduction is challenging both for patients and practitioners. This is generally characterized in the research literature as either maintenance of behavioral change or, alternatively adherence to medical recommendations.

TABLE 6.1 Top 10 Cancer Sites: 2011, United States—All Races

	Male		Female	
Rank	All races site	All races rate (per 100,000)	All races site	All races rate (per 100,000)
1	Prostate	128.3	Female breast	122
2	Lung and bronchus	73	Lung and bronchus	52
3	Colon and rectum	46.1	Colon and rectum	34.9
4	Urinary bladder	35.1	Corpus and uterus, NOS	25.4
5	Melanomas of the skin	25.3	Thyroid	20.5
6	Non-Hodgkin lymphoma	22.6	Melanomas of the skin	15.6
7	Kidney and renal pelvis	21	Non-Hodgkin lymphoma	15.5
8	Oral cavity and pharynx	17	Ovary	11.3
9	Leukemias	16.5	Kidney and renal pelvis	11
10	Pancreas	13.8	Pancreas	10.7

US Cancer Statistics Working Group. United States Cancer Statistics: 1999–2011 incidence and mortality web-based report. Atlanta, GA: US Department of Health and Human Services, Centers for Disease Control and Prevention and National Cancer Institute; 2014. Available at: www.cdc.gov/uscs.

A return to the original behavior, condition, or status is usually described as relapse, slip, or failure.

The relapsing pattern of tobacco use among smokers who try to quit led to the characterization of tobacco use or dependence as a chronic condition or chronic disease. In 2000, the Surgeon General's report *Reducing Tobacco Use* [7] concluded that

> tobacco dependence is best viewed as a chronic disease with remission and relapse. Even though both minimal and intensive interventions increase smoking cessation, most people who quit smoking with the aid of such interventions will eventually relapse and may require repeated attempts before achieving long-term abstinence.

The US Public Health Service's (USPHS) Clinical Practice Guideline *Treating Tobacco Use and Dependence* [8] has consistently framed tobacco use in the same terms, stating in the 2008 update, "Tobacco dependence is a chronic disease that often requires repeated intervention and multiple attempts to quit." It might be conceptually useful to medical clinicians to similarly characterize weight loss, physical activity, diet, and nutrition as behavioral patterns that fluctuate and vary, and that require sustained effort by the patient and attention and prompting by the medical provider to achieve long-term desired outcomes.

6.2.2 Smoking and Other Tobacco Use

More than 6.5 million Americans have died from smoking-related cancers (and 20 million from all smoking-related diseases) since 1964 [9]. Smoking causes about 30% of all US deaths from cancer. Types of cancer implicated in smoking include those of the lung, esophagus, larynx, mouth, throat, kidney, bladder, pancreas, stomach, and cervix [10]. Though the overall prevalence of smoking among adults is now less than half of what it was in the 1960s, those declines have not been equal across all sociodemographic strata. Smoking-related cancer risk disparities are evident among smokers who are in lower income brackets, are less educated, and have a history of psychiatric and/or substance abuse diagnoses. Avoiding tobacco use is the single most important step Americans can take to reduce the cancer burden in this country [2]. If smoking persists at the current rate among young adults in this country, 5.6 million of today's Americans younger than 18 years old are projected to die prematurely from a smoking-related illness [9].

Cigar consumption is growing in the United States, and cigar smokers have increased risk for lung, pancreas, and bladder cancers [11]. Smokeless tobacco use is more popular among men than women and is associated with elevated risks of oral, esophageal, and pancreatic cancers [12]. Emerging tobacco products such as e-cigarettes and hookahs are quickly gaining popularity among adolescents [13]. Though the health effects of e-cigarettes remain to be established, there is concern that they will induce youth to try cigarettes and other tobacco products that have established cancer risks.

Comprehensively addressing smoking in clinical practice requires the committed involvement of all staff (eg, medical assistants or roomers, nurses, physicians, and other primary clinicians) as well as modifications in practice workflows. Integrating tobacco use assessment, documenting tobacco use status in electronic health records (EHRs), and prompting of the delivery of interventions during all electronic and personal (face-to-face) encounters is critical to increasing treatment delivery, acceptance, and effectiveness. Repeated prompts to quit smoking optimize patient engagement in changing behavior.

The effectiveness of counseling and pharmacologic interventions in increasing smoking cessation rates among patients is supported by extensive research [8]. Brief smoking cessation interventions that are integrated into routine clinical care during a medical visit have been shown to be effective. Tobacco cessation advice and support should be provided by the whole health professional team, including both physicians and other nonphysician clinicians (eg, nurse practitioners, physician's assistants, nurses, pharmacists, community workers, and social workers). Brief advice appears to work by triggering increased numbers of quit attempts and increasing the chances of success of quit attempts. The USPHS's Clinical Practice Guideline [8] states that "minimal interventions lasting less than 3 minutes increase overall tobacco abstinence rates." For those not ready to quit at this time, counseling can boost the motivation to quit by personalizing the costs and risks of the patient's tobacco use (eg, tying it to the patient's health, economic status, and family situation). Counseling also provides an opportunity to warn the patient about obstacles or hurdles to quitting and to encourage the patient to use coping strategies to avoid and resist temptations or urges to smoke [14].

Medications such as nicotine replacement therapy (NRT), bupropion, and varenicline have also been found to be effective treatments for smoking cessation. NRT has been shown to be effective in both health care and over-the-counter-like settings without additional counseling [8,15], but the absolute quit rates are higher when pharmacological and behavioral treatments are combined. An international review of the cost-effectiveness of pharmaceutical products for cessation by Cornuz and colleagues found that these therapies compared favorably with other preventive interventions [16]. An excellent resource for the practitioner and the health care system is the previously mentioned USPHS's Clinical Practice Guideline [8], which was comprehensively updated in 2008.

6.2.3 Overweight and Obesity

Although rates of overweight have stabilized, prevalence of adult obesity is increasing in the United States [2]. In 2009–10, 33% of adults were overweight and 36% were obese. Excess body weight, both overweight and obesity, are implicated in 20–30% of certain cancers, such as colon, postmenopausal breast, uterine, esophageal, and renal cell. Evidence is highly suggestive that obesity also

increases risk for cancers of the pancreas, gallbladder, thyroid, ovary, and cervix, and for multiple myeloma, Hodgkin lymphoma, and aggressive prostate cancer [6]. In the United States, excess body weight contributes to 14–20% of all cancer-related mortality. Weight control, physical activity, and nutrition are key factors in cancer prevention and are the most important modifiable cancer risk determinants for Americans who do not smoke.

6.2.4 Physical Inactivity

Approximately one-third of adults report getting no physical activity during their leisure time [2]. Sedentary individuals have higher rates of cancer and poorer cancer outcomes [17]. Physical activity at work or during leisure time is linked to a 30% lower risk for colon cancer. Both vigorous and moderate levels of physical activity appear to reduce cancer risk. Physical activity is also associated with lower risk of breast cancer and possibly lung and endometrial cancers. Studies continue to examine whether physical activity has a role in reducing the risk of other cancers.

Several national groups have recommended that people engage in regular physical activity. The US Department of Health and Human Services' (HHS) *2008 Physical Activity Guidelines for Americans* [18] recommended at least 1 hour of physical activity every day for children and adolescents and 2.5 hours of moderately intense aerobic activity or 1.25 hours of vigorous activity for adults each week. This was a slight departure from former recommendations, which focused on a daily routine rather than a cumulative weekly total for adults, recommending at least 30 minutes per day of moderate physical activity for 5 or more days each week.

6.2.5 Poor Nutrition

Fruit, vegetables, and components of plant foods such as fiber have long been associated with reducing cancer risk. Cancers specifically linked to low rates of fruit and vegetable consumption include cancers of the mouth, pharynx, larynx, esophagus, stomach, and lung [2]. The Greek European Prospective Investigation into Cancer and Nutrition (EPIC) cohort study reported a significant reduction in total cancer risk associated with high consumption of both fruit and vegetables [19]. In the EPIC study from 10 European countries, there was a weak inverse association between high consumption and total cancer risk [20].

High intake of red and processed meat is associated with significant increased risk of colorectal, colon, and rectal cancers. The overall evidence from prospective studies supports limiting red and processed meat consumption as one of the dietary recommendations for the prevention of colorectal cancer [21].

6.2.6 Alcohol Consumption

Drinking alcohol increases the risk of cancers of the mouth, esophagus, pharynx, larynx, and liver in men and women, and of breast cancer in women [4]. In general, these risks increase after about one daily drink for women and two daily drinks for men. These levels of alcohol consumption are defined as "moderate" according to the 2010 Dietary Guidelines for Americans [22]. Alcohol intake limits were exceeded by 22% of men ages 31–50 years, and by 12% of women ages 51–70 years [23].

The chances of getting liver cancer increase markedly with five or more drinks per day [6]. Heavy alcohol use may increase the risk of colorectal cancer and increases the risk for most alcohol-related cancers. The earlier an individual begins heavy, sustained alcohol use, the greater his or her cancer risk. Combining alcohol and tobacco increases the risk of some cancers far more than the independent effects of either drinking or smoking alone. Regular consumption of even a few drinks per week is associated with an increased risk of breast cancer in women—a risk that is particularly high in women who do not ingest enough folate.

6.2.7 Sun Damage

New cases of melanoma skin cancer increased markedly between 1975 and 2009, with a projected number of 76,100 new cases in 2014 [24]. More than 2 million people in the United States were diagnosed in 2006 with basal cell or squamous cell (nonmelanoma) skin cancer, the two most common types of skin cancer in the country, and 40–50% of Americans who live to age 65 will have nonmelanoma skin cancer at least once.

Most skin cancers—including melanoma, the deadliest form of skin cancer—can be prevented. Studies suggest that reducing unprotected exposure to the sun and avoiding artificial ultraviolet (UV) light from indoor tanning beds, tanning booths, and sun lamps can lower the risk of skin cancer [2].

Only about two-thirds of US adults report that they protect themselves from the sun [2]. The percentage of adults who report being sunburned has increased since 2005. Although use of one or more sun protective measures has changed little over the last few decades, the newly defined Healthy People 2020 measure shows some recent promise: during 2005–10, 70% of adults reported that they protected themselves from the sun [25].

6.2.8 Viral Infection

Infection with human papillomavirus (HPV) is the established cause of most cervical cancers [26]. The direct medical costs of HPV in the United States are estimated at $5 billion a year [27]. In the United States,

25% of females ages 14–19, 45% of women ages 20–24, and 27% of women ages 25–29 are infected with HPV [28]. The Centers for Disease Control and Prevention (CDC) recommends that all boys and girls begin the three-shot HPV vaccination regimen at age 11 or 12 [29]. Catch-up vaccinations are also recommended for males through age 21 and for females through age 26, if they did not receive the vaccination when they were younger. However, only 49% of adolescent females have begun the vaccination series, and only 32% have received all three doses required for full immunization [30]. Given that adolescent HPV immunization rates are suboptimal, it has been suggested that EHR systems prompt providers to remind young people to become vaccinated. As vaccines are developed for other viruses related to cancer (eg, Epstein-Barr and Hepatitis C), EHRs can be used to promote adherence to recommended vaccination schedules. A recent study [31], however, failed to demonstrate improved adolescent immunization rates associated with such provider prompts. This suggests that more research is necessary to understand how to improve the effectiveness of provider prompts to address this important cancer prevention objective.

6.3 CURRENT USE OF INFORMATION TECHNOLOGY FOR CANCER PREVENTION

Information technology (IT) provides new means of informing both patients and the general public about effective cancer prevention strategies. By more efficiently linking individuals and clinicians with cancer prevention opportunities, these new methods hold promise for reducing the more than 500,000 cancer deaths in the United States per year.

In a review of IT and cancer prevention, Jimbo and colleagues [32] defined IT as

> any equipment, interconnected system, or subsystem of equipment used in the automatic acquisition, storage, manipulation, management, movement, control, display, switching, interchange, transmission, or reception of technology. Information technology includes computers, ancillary equipment, software, firmware and similar procedures, services (including support services), and related resources.

The authors' review focused on the impact of IT on the delivery of cancer preventive services in primary care offices [32]. Conducted before the wide-scale adoption of certified EHR technology, or meaningful use, the review evaluated 30 studies that assessed cancer prevention and IT. The authors reported that early IT efforts were primarily focused on the prevention of breast, cervical, and colorectal cancers, with about half of the 30 studies focused exclusively on providers and the rest on the patient. In almost all instances, the technology innovation was limited to some type of reminder system directed at either the patient or the provider, with the goal of increasing engagement in a cancer prevention activity (eg, mammography screening, pap testing, breast examination, and sigmoidoscopy). The authors concluded that IT systems that automatically prompted users, provided specific recommendations rather than assessments, and provided support at the time of decision making were most successful. Their overall conclusion was that the impact of the tested reminder systems on increasing cancer screening was "modest at best" [32].

In light of these modest findings, the authors emphasized the importance of moving from the limited early interventions described in their review (primarily computer-generated letters to patients and provider reminders) to more technologically advanced interventions involving computer-generated audits, feedback, and report cards as well as more sophisticated EHR innovations and applications [32]. As a framework for possible IT advances for cancer prevention, Jimbo and colleagues adapted the 2008 USPHS's Tobacco Use and Dependence treatment algorithm [8], developing a modified "5 A's" approach that identified potential cancer prevention IT interventions that could be tied to a clinic visit (eg, before the clinic visit "Assess" status regarding cancer screening interventions and "Advise" patient prior to the visit regarding necessary testing) (Fig. 6.1).

6.3.1 Example of IT Use: Skin Cancer Prevention

Skin cancer prevention is a clinical intervention for which a number of IT strategies have been attempted. In one example, Hornung and colleagues [33] developed a multimedia computer program for the primary prevention of skin cancer among children and piloted it in an elementary school in rural North Carolina. Seven months after the intervention, students who received the multimedia training had significantly improved their knowledge and attitudes about skin cancer and sun tanning risks compared with students who received a standard teacher-led training intervention, although the differences in actual behaviors did not reach statistical significance. In another effort to use IT to promote skin cancer prevention, Barysch and colleagues [34] developed an Internet-based campaign against skin cancer in Switzerland that included education, instruction for self-assessment, and evaluation of skin lesions to be conducted online by expert dermatologists (see Chapter 7: "Early Detection in the Age of Information Technology"). The website attracted many users, including middle-aged males, who often under participate in such programs. The process led to identification of 494 at-risk lesions. Of these, the team of expert dermatologists determined that

28.5% were "suspicious for skin cancer." Lastly, Gerbert and colleagues [35] assessed the effectiveness of an Internet-based tutorial in improving the skin cancer triage skills of primary care physicians (PCPs). Physicians who received this training demonstrated significantly better skin cancer diagnosis and evaluation compared to control physicians.

6.4 ELECTRONIC HEALTH RECORDS

Many features of EHR technology make it particularly applicable to cancer prevention and screening interventions, including:

- Prompts that can be programmed to alert clinicians and/or patients to take cancer prevention actions based on established criteria (eg, presence of a risk factor, age, time since last screening test).
- Evidence-based algorithms that assist clinicians in efficiently delivering cancer prevention interventions (eg, smoking cessation counseling and/or medication guides, photos to help discern the pathology of skin lesions).
- Communication tools that share the outcomes of a cancer prevention intervention in a Health Insurance Portability and Accountability Act (HIPAA) compliant way with the patient, selected clinicians, and other individuals within and outside the health care system.
- Closed-loop functionality that can refer patients to outside entities for cancer prevention interventions (eg, a state-based tobacco cessation quitline) and then allow the outcome of that referral to be added to the patient's EHR while complying with HIPAA rules; for example, for a telephone quitline, a referral that includes the patient's quit date, as well as information on smoking medication (start and end dates, dose) mailed to the patient from the quitline.
- Patient registries that allow clinics and health systems to sort patients based on risk factors, demographics, and test results for selective cancer prevention interventions.

6.4.1 EHRs and Tobacco Cessation

Among the many uses of EHR technology for cancer screening and prevention, tobacco use intervention may be the application that has received the most research attention. The most recent Cochrane Review on this topic (2014) identified 16 studies that tested the use of an EHR to improve documentation and/or treatment of tobacco use [36]. Most of these studies evaluated the impact of EHR changes on rates of identification of tobacco users

Timing	5 A's	

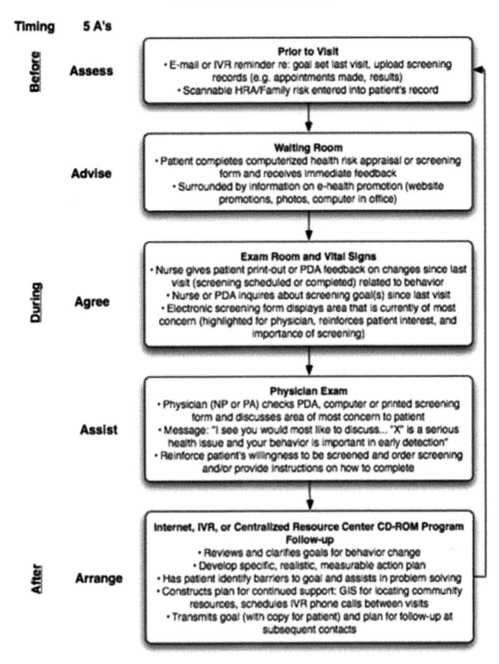

Before — **Assess**

Prior to Visit
- E-mail or IVR reminder re: goal set last visit, upload screening records (e.g. appointments made, results)
- Scannable HRA/Family risk entered into patient's record

Advise

Waiting Room
- Patient completes computerized health risk appraisal or screening form and receives immediate feedback
- Surrounded by information on e-health promotion (website promotions, photos, computer in office)

During — **Agree**

Exam Room and Vital Signs
- Nurse gives patient print-out or PDA feedback on changes since last visit (screening scheduled or completed) related to behavior
- Nurse or PDA inquires about screening goal(s) since last visit
- Electronic screening form displays area that is currently of most concern (highlighted for physician, reinforces patient interest, and importance of screening)

Assist

Physician Exam
- Physician (NP or PA) checks PDA, computer or printed screening form and discusses area of most concern to patient
- Message: "I see you would most like to discuss... 'X' is a serious health issue and your behavior is important in early detection"
- Reinforce patient's willingness to be screened and order screening and/or provide instructions on how to complete

After — **Arrange**

Internet, IVR, or Centralized Resource Center CD-ROM Program Follow-up
- Reviews and clarifies goals for behavior change
- Develop specific, realistic, measurable action plan
- Has patient identify barriers to goal and assists in problem solving
- Constructs plan for continued support: GIS for locating community resources, schedules IVR phone calls between visits
- Transmits goal (with copy for patient) and plan for follow-up at subsequent contacts

FIGURE 6.1 5 A's Framework—details the five major steps to interventions: Ask, Advise, Assess, Assist, and Arrange; and includes examples from steps prior to a visit through follow-up.

and delivery of cessation treatment such as electronic prescribing of cessation medication, rather than on cessation rates themselves. In most instances, use of EHR was associated with improvements in both identification and delivery of treatment, results that were consistent with the recommendations in the USPHS's 2008 update of the Clinical Practice Guideline *Treating Tobacco Use and Dependence* [8].

The 16 studies identified for the Cochrane review [36] included 6 group-randomized trials, 1 patient-randomized study, and 9 nonrandomized observation studies.

The review found that these 16 studies were of fair to good quality; none directly assessed patient quit rates. Key findings from the studies addressed some of the "5 A's" clinical interventions recommended by USPHS's 2008 update of the Clinical Practice Guideline, as follows [8].

6.4.1.1 Ask Smoker Identification

Two studies [37,38] identified smokers at significantly higher rates when the EHR was used to prompt clinic staff to complete this prevention intervention. However,

Rindal and colleagues [39] found no increase in the already very high levels of smoking status documentation (97.5%) by dental care providers in his study. This high level of documentation is evidence of a cancer prevention success story that resulted, in part, from advances in IT. Tobacco cessation clinical practice guideline recommendations [8], meaningful use requirements, and early calls to include smoking status in vital signs [40] have collectively contributed to a new clinical standard of care: in the United States today, smoking status is obtained and documented for virtually all inpatients and outpatients at the time of their clinic visit or hospital admission [41].

6.4.1.2 Advise All Smokers to Quit and Assess Interest in Quitting

One study [38] reported that clinics where an EHR promoted clinical intervention had higher rates of advising patients to quit smoking and assessing interest in quitting than control clinics (advising patients to quit: 71.6% in intervention clinics vs 52.7% in control clinics; assessing interest in quitting: 65.6% in intervention clinics vs 40.1% in control clinics). Another study [39] reported only postintervention data for 15 dental clinics that were randomly assigned to: (1) an EHR-based dental record intervention that prompted providers to ask about and discuss smoking and interest in quitting; or (2) a usual-care control condition. Measured outcomes included a comparison in rates of asking about tobacco use, discussing quitting, and referring patients who used tobacco to a telephone quitline. Overall, providers in the intervention clinics (relative to those in the control clinics) were more likely to ask about interest in quitting (87% vs 70%), and to discuss strategies for quitting smoking (47% vs 26%).

6.4.1.3 Assist With Cessation

The Cochrane review [36] identified a number of studies that assessed whether EHR prompts increased clinicians' rates of assisting smokers by directly offering cessation counseling or by providing medications or a referral to additional counseling (eg, a telephone quitline) during a medical visit. For example, Linder and colleagues [37] found that EHR prompts in intervention clinics (vs control clinics without such prompts) resulted in higher rates of connecting smokers to external cessation counselors (3.9% vs 0.3%, $p<0.001$), but not higher rates of prescribing a cessation medication. Bentz and colleagues [38] showed higher rates of providing and documenting counseling (20.1% vs 10.5% among control clinics without EHR prompts, $p<0.001$), but not higher rates of referral to a telephone quitline. Two additional studies by Vidrine and colleagues [42,43] documented significantly higher proportions of smokers enrolling in treatment with a quitline in clinical settings with electronic-based prompts for quitline linkages compared to settings without such prompts.

The Cochrane review [36] also identified four observational studies that documented that EHR system changes increase the rate of assistance provided to smokers visiting various health care settings. In one of the larger studies, which examined the hospital records of more than 17,000 patients in a Boston hospital, Koplan and colleagues [44] used a pre–post design to examine the impact of adding a "tobacco order set" (that included orders for a cessation consultation and cessation medications) to the admission screens of a hospital's computerized order-entry system. After this EHR-based order set was implemented, the authors found a statistically significant increase in the proportion of admitted smokers referred for cessation counseling and in physician orders for cessation medications.

6.4.1.4 Additional Studies

Other studies, not included in the Cochrane report, have assessed the impact of EHR modifications on smoking cessation interventions. For example, Kruse and colleagues [45] studied how PCPs viewed the feasibility and acceptability of a one-click EHR function to refer smokers to a centralized tobacco treatment coordinator who called the smokers, provided brief counseling, connected them to ongoing treatment, and gave feedback to the PCPs. Clinicians were rewarded for participation as part of the pay-for-performance reimbursement that was tied to utilization of the new technology. Over 18 months, involving 36 PCPs and 2894 smokers from two community health centers (CHCs), the authors reported that 81% of the PCPs used the EHR capability more than once, generating 466 referrals. Overall, about 15% of the known smokers visiting the clinics were referred to evidence-based treatment during the study period. While these results were impressive, the Cochrane group elected to exclude this study because the impact of the EHR changes could not be separated from the impact of the pay-for-performance changes.

Finally, EHR modifications have been used to intervene with some populations that have particularly high rates of smoking, including lower income individuals. For example, the New York City Department of Health and Mental Hygiene established the Health eQuits program [46,47], funded by the CDC. Health eQuits targeted CHCs that had already implemented EHR technology to determine whether they could use that technology to increase the delivery of smoking cessation intervention. Specifically, Health eQuits challenged 19 CHCs with EHR functionality to demonstrate higher rates of smoking status documentation and cessation intervention, providing financial incentives if rates of documentation and intervention exceeded baseline levels. The EHR modifications were extensive and represent a model of the broad capacity of this technology to enhance cancer prevention interventions. These modifications included: (1) automated quarterly reports on clinician and clinic performance on the Health eQuit program (reports gave rates of documentation of smoking status, smoking prevalence, and proportion of current smokers who received at least one cessation intervention); (2) a tally of incentive payments earned based on intervention rates with smokers; (3) use of a clinical decision support tool; and (4) a patient registry to identify smokers within the EHR and alert the clinician to address smoking with that patient at that visit.

At baseline, across the 19 New York City CHCs, the mean rate of delivery of at least one cessation intervention to smokers (counseling, cessation medication, or referral to the New York State quitline) was 23% among documented smokers (range across clinics: 0–54%). At the end of the program, 18 months later, the rate of intervention had increased markedly, with 54% of documented smokers having received at least one cessation intervention (range across clinics: 12–91%). During the 18-month intervention, 36,572 smokers received at least one cessation intervention, compared with only 6515 smokers during the 12-month baseline period (Fig. 6.2).

6.4.2 Using Lung Cancer Screening Visits to Provide Smoking Cessation Interventions

In a 2013 review of the scientific evidence, the US Preventive Services Task Force (USPSTF) concluded that low-dose computed tomography (LDCT) cancer screening of the lungs can significantly reduce mortality from lung cancer among heavy current and former smokers. Based on this finding, the USPSTF recommended that:

> Asymptomatic adults aged 55 to 80 who have a 30 pack-year smoking history and currently smoke or have quit within the last 15 years should be screened annually for lung cancer with low-dose computed tomography, and that screening should continue until the patient has not smoked for 15 years.

This new lung cancer screening recommendation has led insurers, including Medicare, to now pay for LDCT screening, and the availability and use of this test have increased substantially. This increase in LDCT lung cancer screening provides an opportunity for an additional technology-prompted cancer prevention intervention: providing smoking cessation treatment at the time of the LDCT lung cancer screening. One important reason to consider linking these two cancer interventions is the concern that lower smoking cessation rates might result among current smokers who received negative LDCT screening results, as a result of these smokers believing they are no longer at risk (the "health certificate effect") [48].

To assess this possibility, the USPSTF reviewed studies that assessed this potential unintended consequence. This review yielded mixed results. For example, Ashraf and colleagues [49] examined the effects of LDCT screening for lung cancer on smoking rates in 4104 Danish participants, half of whom received annual LDCT lung

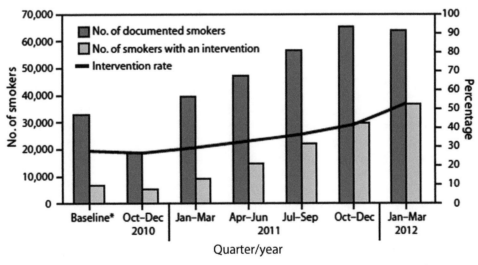

* Baseline data were collected during October 2009–September 2010.

FIGURE 6.2 Number of documented smokers, number of smokers with an intervention, and intervention rate, by quarter—19 community health centers, New York, City, October 2010–March 2012—A bar chart showing the number of documented smokers, number of smokers with an intervention, and intervention rate by quarter, among 19 community health centers in New York City during October 2010–March 2012. At baseline, 23% of identified smokers had received counseling, cessation medications, or both, with a range of 0–54% and a median of 16% among the CHCs. At the end of the program, 54% of smokers had received at least one cessation intervention, with a range of 12–91% and a median of 58%. As rates of documentation of smoking status improved, intervention rates also increased.

cancer screening tests and half of whom received no screening test. One year after the initial screening period, the biochemically confirmed quit rate among individuals who were smokers at baseline was essentially identical both in the LDCT group (11.9%) and the no-screening control group (11.8%). All participants received minimal (<5 minutes) smoking cessation counseling. Relapse rates also were similar across the two groups—10.0% in the LDCT group and 10.5% in the control group. In another European study [50], 1284 Dutch male smokers were randomized to LDCT lung cancer screening or no screening. Two years after the baseline screening period, prolonged smoking abstinence rates of 13.7% were observed in the LDCT group compared to 14.9% in the no-screening group ($p = 0.35$). In this study, all participants received a smoking cessation brochure or a questionnaire through which people could ask for tailored, computerized cessation support.

A Minnesota study [51] involving 926 current smokers assessed the impact of three annual LDCT screens for lung cancer on both health outcomes and smoking cessation. Most of the smokers at baseline did not receive smoking cessation assistance, and the study did not include a comparison group that did not undergo LDCT lung cancer screening. A statistically significant increase was found in the likelihood of self-reported smoking cessation among individuals who were told they had abnormal LDCT lung scans. In a similar study, Styn and colleagues [52] assessed quitting behavior among 2094 baseline active smokers who underwent LDCT lung cancer screening, comparing those who received a physician referral for an abnormal CT finding with those who did not. At 1 year, these investigators found a statistically significant increase in smoking cessation rates among individuals who received a referral because of an abnormal CT result.

Lastly, a 2014 study by Tammemagi and colleagues [53] evaluated the impact of lung cancer screening results on short- and long-term smoking cessation rates among the 15,489 baseline current smokers included in the NCI-funded National Lung Screening Trial. These researchers found that for participants who were smokers at baseline, the type of screening result was an important and statistically significant predictor of continued smoking; those with negative lung cancer screening results had lower rates of cessation over 7 years of follow-up compared to individuals with abnormal LDCT screening findings. The authors interpreted their results as suggesting that the "health certificate effect" was not a major effect in their study, but acknowledged that they did not test this effect definitively.

Collectively, these studies highlight the potential of the lung cancer screening test as an opportunity for smoking cessation intervention, and the potential for EHR-based technology to link these two interventions and prompt tobacco cessation treatment.

6.4.3 Linking Patients to Their State Tobacco Quitlines and Closed-Loop Functionality

Among its many capabilities, the EHR can refer patients with cancer risk factors to external entities that can provide cancer prevention interventions. Specifically, the ability to refer smokers visiting primary care settings to a state-based telephone tobacco cessation quitline has been extensively evaluated. Vidrine and colleagues [42] randomly assigned 10 family practice clinics in Houston to two conditions. In the intervention clinics, smokers were linked electronically to their state tobacco cessation quitline using an expanded EHR capacity. In the control clinics, smokers were given a quitline referral card and encouraged to call the quitline on their own. Among smokers connected electronically to the quitline via the EHR, 7.8% enrolled in quitline treatment, compared to 0.6% of those given a referral card and encouraged to call—a 13-fold increase in the proportion of smokers enrolled in treatment.

In an expansion of referral functionality, Adsit and colleagues [54] evaluated the potential of an EHR's "closed-loop" capability. In this study, the authors assessed the ability of the EHR to electronically refer smokers to a telephone tobacco cessation quitline. Then, in a significant innovation, the quitline and EHR vendors (two independent entities) developed coordinated technical programming to allow for the results of the quitline referral to be electronically inputted into the patient's EHR. In this demonstration project, 14% of smokers visiting two primary care clinics were referred to the state quitline using the new EHR functionality versus only 0.3% using the previous method of referral (paper fax). The closed-loop component of this new functionality worked effectively; for every referred patient, the quitline was able to send back outcome data on whether the patient was successfully contacted, if the patient set a tobacco cessation quit date, and what medications were prescribed by the quitline (typically over-the-counter nicotine replacement medications), directly populating the individual patient's EHR in a HIPAA-compliant way.

6.4.4 Engaging Physicians to Improve Patients' Health

EHR technology can be utilized in a number of ways to engage clinicians in interventions that can reduce cancer risk. One means of achieving this outcome is to use the EHR in a surveillance function and to communicate to clinicians findings regarding that surveillance. Cowburn and colleagues [55] used this EHR functionality when they assessed the association between insurance status and cervical cancer screening in community health settings in Oregon and California. They showed that the absence of insurance coverage was negatively associated with the likelihood of receiving a Pap test, identifying a high-risk population for intervention within these settings. White and Kenton [56] used the EHR for a training function, developing three EHR-based tools to educate providers on cervical cancer screening guidelines. Implementing the training program with additional electronic medical record prompts improved compliance with cervical cytology guidelines, including improved targeting of the screening test toward high-risk individuals.

6.4.5 Patient Registries as a Means of Promoting Cancer Prevention

One EHR feature that can be applied to cancer prevention interventions is the patient registry capability: EHR technology that can systematically sort patients based on a variety of clinical, demographic, and physiologic parameters. One of the most common clinical applications of this feature has been the development of a diabetes registry that sorts patients based on a variety of possible parameters: prior elevated blood glucose or hemoglobin A1C level; body mass index; use of a diabetes medication in the last 1–5 years; and/or the inclusion of a diagnosis of diabetes in the problem list. Use of such criteria can help select patients with either a diagnosis or a risk of diabetes. Then, by targeting such selected patients, EHR technology can prompt the patient, clinician, or health care system to undertake certain preventive, diagnostic, or treatment interventions. For example, the EHR might scan the records of each diabetic patient and prompt him or her to schedule and complete a podiatry exam if warranted. Similarly, if a diabetic patient has not undergone a check of his or her hemoglobin A1C in the past 6 months (a test that should be completed every 3 months), a series of escalating prompts may signal to the patient the importance of regularly undergoing this test [57].

Similarly, patient registries may be used for cancer prevention activities. In one innovative application of patient registries, Womble and colleagues [58] used EHR technology to establish a registry of males with newly diagnosed, but low-risk, prostate cancer, in an effort to manage these patients with active surveillance—periodic Prostate-Specific Antigen (PSA) testing. The authors used EHR technology to ensure that these PSA tests took place on schedule as needed; 49% of the patients fulfilled criteria and could be followed successfully under this active surveillance model. This cancer prevention innovation successfully helped prevent overtreatment of indolent prostate cancer and the unnecessary surgery, radiation, and hormonal therapy that expose these individuals to substantial risks and high costs. In an accompanying editorial, Cooperberg [59] highlighted the power of this patient registry as an innovative tool to provide quality care to these individuals, stating "the registry truly serves as the surging tide raising all boats."

EHR-based patient registries have also been used to identify and target tobacco users for intervention. In one such study, Sherman and colleagues [60] established a system to sort smokers in 10 primary care clinics and target them for referral to telephone-based cessation counseling. These results were compared to findings from eight comparison clinics. Over a 1-year intervention period, almost 3000 smokers were identified from the intervention clinics; almost one-half of them were then successfully connected to a telephone cessation quitline, and 11% of them had quit smoking 6 months later. The authors concluded that the use of such EHR-based patient registries for targeted tobacco cessation intervention can have substantial impact on clinic-wide smoking rates.

6.4.6 Challenges of EHRs

The widespread adoption of EHR technology in health care settings offers tremendous opportunity to coordinate cancer prevention treatment in a manner that is consistent, efficient, and sustained over time. Although the use of EHR and IT offers extraordinary potential for cancer prevention, the response to these innovations by clinicians, health systems, and the public has been mixed. That mixed response has resulted in large part from concerns about clinical workflow, added burden, and efficiency.

In an effort to better understand challenges to the adoption of EHR and meaningful use, Heisey-Grove and colleagues [61] assessed more than 140,000 providers in 2012. The authors conceptualized these challenges as falling into four categories: (1) practice issues (eg, workflow adoption, provider engagement, training, vendor selection); (2) vendor issues (eg, upgrade needs; delays in implementation, installation, certification; inadequate training or support materials); (3) attestation process issues (eg, calculating patient volume, lack of an operational Medicaid program, Medicaid or Medicare technical or administrative challenges); and (4) meaningful use measures (eg, achieving core quality measures). Their surveillance highlighted the myriad of organizational and implementation challenges to widespread EHR adoption.

Pizziferri and colleagues [62] performed a time–motion study in five primary care clinics involving 20 physicians to assess physician time utilization before and after implementation of EHRs as well as physicians' perceptions of EHR. Postimplementation, the mean overall time spent per patient during clinic sessions decreased by 0.5 minutes (from 27.55 to 27.05 minutes per patient). A majority of survey respondents believed that EHR use resulted in quality improvements, yet only 29% reported that EHR documentation took the same amount of time or less compared to paper-based health record systems. While the EHR did not require more time for physicians during a clinic session, the authors recommended further studies to assess the EHR's potential impact on nonclinic time.

While many have evaluated the response of physicians to the widescale implementation of EHR technology, little is known about patients' response to this technological innovation. Kim and colleagues [63] attempted to evaluate challenges to using an electronic personal health record (ePHR) by a low-income elderly population. While 70 individuals were initially identified for the evaluation, only 44 used the technology, and only 14 of these completed the survey. While their data available for interpretation were limited, the authors found that use of the ePHR was hindered by the participants' poor computer and Internet skills, technophobia, low health literacy, and limited physical and/or cognitive abilities. They concluded that "those who can benefit most from an ePHR system may be the least able to use it" and that "disparities in access to and use of computers, the Internet, and ePHRs may exacerbate health care inequality in the future" [63]. An in-depth discussion of user-centered design can be found in Chapter 11: "Data Visualization Tools for Investigating Health Services Utilization Among Cancer Patients" in this book.

6.4.7 The Changing Regulatory and Policy Environment

The regulatory and policy environment has evolved markedly to encourage and/or mandate that health systems use EHR technology more broadly and more effectively. While these regulatory and policy changes create a powerful incentive to adopt such technology, the science base regarding how to most effectively utilize EHR technology to promote cancer prevention interventions is both new and modest.

6.4.7.1 Meaningful Use: A Federal Incentive Program to Encourage Adoption and Use of EHR Technology

In 2009, the Health Information Technology for Economic and Clinical Health (HITECH) Act [64] was passed and signed into law. HITECH is designed to encourage clinicians and health systems to adopt EHR technology and use it to achieve certain benchmarks on a variety of evidence-based health care goals ("meaningful use" requirements). The HITECH Act provides financial incentives to both physicians and hospitals that adopt and demonstrate the meaningful use of EHR systems.

HITECH has been a remarkably powerful piece of legislation because it is not just an investment in technology but was designed to reward the meaningful

use of that technology. As described by the first director of the Office of the National Coordinator for Health Information Technology (ONC), David Blumenthal, "By focusing on the efficient use of EHRs with certain capabilities, the HITECH Act makes clear that the adoption of records is not a sufficient purpose: it is the use of EHRs to achieve health and efficiency goals that matters" [64]. He described the four goals of HITECH as: "define meaningful use, encourage and support the attainment of meaningful use through incentives and grant programs, bolster public trust in electronic information systems by ensuring their privacy and security, and foster continued health information technology (HIT) innovation" [64]. Blumenthal highlighted the importance of these goals: "Information is the lifeblood of modern medicine. HIT is destined to be its circulatory system" [64].

The impact of this legislation was remarkable, rapidly transforming health records in the United States from paper records to electronic health (eHealth) systems. From 2008 to 2013, the proportion of US physicians who report using EHRs increased from 17% to 78% [65]. By June of 2014, more than 400,000 clinicians (75% of the nation's eligible clinicians) and more than 4500 hospitals (92% of eligible hospitals) had adopted EHR systems required for meaningful use payments (Fig. 6.3).

6.4.7.2 The Affordable Care Act and Guidance on Treating Tobacco Dependence

A core component of the Affordable Care Act (ACA, or "Obamacare") was its provisions regarding clinical preventive services. Specifically, the ACA mandates that health insurers must cover, without cost-sharing requirements, clinical preventive health services that have an A or B rating in the current recommendations of the USPSTF, including smoking cessation treatment that has a USPSTF A rating. While providing such general guidance, the ACA legislative language did not specify what constitutes ACA-compliant smoking cessation treatment.

In May 2014, a guidance document describing in detail what constitutes ACA-compatible cessation coverage was released by the HHS, the US Department of the Treasury, and the US Department of Labor. This guidance specified that all covered individuals are eligible for two courses of smoking cessation treatment per year with each course of treatment including:

- four tobacco-cessation counseling sessions (telephone, group, or individual) with each session lasting a minimum of 10 minutes; and
- a 90-day course of any tobacco-cessation medications approved by the US Food and Drug Administration (FDA) (prescription or over-the-counter) that are prescribed by a health care provider [66].

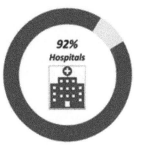
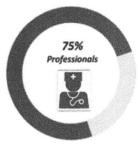

❖ As of June 2014, more than 403,000 professionals, representing 75% of the nation's eligible professionals, have received incentive payments through the EHR Incentive Programs.

❖ Over 4500 hospitals, representing 92% of eligible hospitals, including Critical Access Hospitals, have received incentive payments through this program to date.

FIGURE 6.3 Eligible hospitals and professionals paid under the EHR Meaningful Use Incentive Programs—Two donut graphs displaying eligible hospitals and professionals paid under the EHR Incentive Programs. As of June 2014, more than 403,000 professionals, representing 75% of the nation's eligible professionals, have received incentive payments through the EHR Incentive Programs. More than 4500 hospitals, representing 92% of eligible hospitals, including Critical Access Hospitals, have received incentive payments through this program to date. *Source: CMS EHR Incentive Program data, June 2014.*

6.5 MOBILE, WEB, AND WEARABLE APPLICATIONS

Today HIT has the potential to reach almost 3 billion Internet users and 7 billion people with mobile-cellular subscriptions worldwide [67]. Because of technological advances and widespread adoption of new technologies, eHealth has expanded into mobile health, or mHealth, which harnesses the power of portable technology to efficiently transmit and receive data and information to enhance health outcomes. mHealth can operate through numerous devices, including smartphones, personal digital assistants (PDAs), tablets, standard cellphones, wearable devices, game consoles, and more. These devices' capabilities for short message service (SMS), multimedia message service (MMS), Internet access, direct calls, and other mobile applications (apps) are widely used and studied for health and medical purposes [68].

SMS, MMS, and other mobile applications partially account for the ease and utility of mobile devices. SMS allows for brief interactions or exchanges of text information; MMS performs a similar function for video and images; and apps are used with or without the Internet as a platform for data collection and information sharing. Each media tool can produce customized messages for patients, which can lead to improved health outcomes. Personalization is enhanced by the real-time continuous data collection that is made possible by device mobility. With greater quantities of accurate data, mHealth can lead to better health management and reduced burden of disease.

The widespread use of mobile devices opens mHealth projects to numerous target populations, such as patients, doctors, nurses, underserved or low-income populations, and the general public. mHealth is particularly beneficial in improving the process of care in low-resource areas [69]. mHealth also has the potential to reduce health disparities and health care costs because of the widespread penetration of mobile devices across sociodemographic strata and the extraordinarily low costs associated with providing health information, including cancer prevention information, on a large scale.

Along with the ubiquity of smartphones and other mobile devices, there has been a multitude of mobile applications that take medical readings, monitor health, and prompt health behavior change. These include calorie counters, wearable sensors that monitor heart rate or track physical activity, and apps to help people lose weight, stop smoking, and sleep better. As of 2012, roughly 19% of smartphone owners had downloaded at least one app to manage or track their health, the most commonly downloaded apps being exercise, diet, and weight management apps [70]. The FDA notes that 500 million smartphone users worldwide will be using a health care application by 2015, and by 2018, 50% of the more than 3.4 billion smartphone and tablet users will have downloaded mHealth applications [71].

There is a growing body of mHealth research addressing health behavior interventions, including: smoking cessation and tobacco use, physical activity, diet, alcohol consumption, and sun protection. While there is limited research on the effectiveness of smartphone apps in promoting behavior change, research utilizing SMS is widespread among clinical trials, pilot studies, and new study designs.

6.5.1 mHealth and Cancer Prevention

Research has shown that using mHealth tools significantly improves adherence to medicine regimens and affects sunscreen use and smoking quit rates [72]. SMS, MMS, automated voice services, and the Internet have been the main vehicles used in successful eHealth and mHealth cancer prevention projects.

Although mHealth has the capacity to promote primary cancer prevention, little research has studied the efficacy of most of the apps that are currently available. Bender and colleagues [73] found 295 smartphone apps related to cancer, yet no research addressing their effectiveness and impact exists. A total of 46% of the available apps pertained to cancer in general, while other apps focused on awareness, educational information, early detection, fundraising, and social support. While these apps might facilitate cancer prevention, research findings are currently lacking to estimate their effects.

6.5.2 Tobacco and Smoking Behaviors

There is growing research support of the efficacy and utility of mHealth applications for smoking cessation. A recent Cochrane review [74] acknowledged the benefit of mobile phone-based smoking cessation interventions but noted that positive outcomes tended to be associated with text messaging applications. The Community Preventive Task Force [75] concluded that there was sufficient evidence to support recommending mobile phone-based interventions for tobacco cessation. In the years following up to the recommendation and since then, numerous meta-analyses have been conducted to determine the effectiveness of mHealth interventions.

A review by Whittaker and colleagues [74] found that SMS, Internet programs, and interactive voice response service (IVRS) all showed positive effects for self-reported, short-term quitting. IVRS provided voice recordings with time-specific information on the health effects of cessation. It ensured user engagement by motivating participants to seek more information and visit the web page of the day. A subsequent review by Whittaker and colleagues [76] found that SMS, Internet programs, and video messaging had positive effects, leading to cessation that lasted at least 6 months (relative risk (RR) = 1.71, 95% confidence interval (CI) = [1.49, 1.99]).

Spohr and colleagues [77] found that SMS interventions were associated with an increase in smoking cessation rates at the 3- and 6-month follow-ups when compared to the control condition (odds ratio (OR) = 1.35, 95% CI = [1.23, 1.48]). Similarly, Free and colleagues [78] found short-term, self-reported abstinence rates were significantly higher for pooled SMS programs (RR = 2.18, 95% CI = [1.80, 2.70]). In both studies, automated SMS interventions varied in design, but often contained messages providing quit advice, motivational messages, interactive polls and quizzes, information on NRT, links to helplines, and information about social support. These results were affirmed for long-term, self-reported, and biochemically tested quit rates using mHealth strategies.

Analogous to previous research, Stop Smoking with Mobile Phones (STOMP) used SMS to provide cessation tips, trivia, polls, quizzes, buddies, and on-demand help. The success of the STOMP trials led to its implementation nationally in New Zealand, and expansion to studies in the United Kingdom. In initial trials, cessation success was noted at 6 weeks, and verified cessation abstinence at 6 months was significantly increased among participants who received the text messaging intervention (RR 2.20, 95% CI = [1.80–2.68]) [79]. Based on the available evidence for SMS interventions on smoking cessation, these techniques may offer benefits when incorporated into standard health care services.

Given the enormous penetrance and reach of web and mobile devices, it is important to evaluate the real-world effectiveness of such interventions and to widely disseminate interventions found to be effective at the population level. The NCI smokefree.gov represents one of the world's largest smoking cessation and health behavior change mHealth-based intervention services. Initially launched as a single website in 2003, the program now encompasses 5 websites, 15 text message programs, 4 smartphone apps, and a dozen social media platforms targeted to a variety of populations. In 2013, more than 5 million users interacted with smokefree.gov resources. The smokefree.gov website and related mHealth platforms include resources designed to motivate people to quit; they provide information and behavioral skills training to smokers to improve quit success and help sustain abstinence. Additional intervention support is also provided for related health behaviors such as mood management, diet, and physical activity. In a test of five different population-based treatments, the NCI smokefree.gov website was shown to be an effective population-based smoking cessation intervention [80].

While findings are promising for SMS and MMS-based interventions for tobacco cessation, less research has been published concerning mobile apps for smoking (and other tobacco) cessation. Abroms [81] reviewed 47 publicly available iPhone apps related to smoking cessation and found that only 11% of these aligned with one of the USPHS's 2008 Clinical Practice Guideline for treating tobacco dependence [8]. Few of these 47 apps provided smokers with proven tobacco cessation treatments: only 4.3% connected smokers to quitlines, and 8.5% provided intratreatment social support. As with the research on apps related to cancer, findings on tobacco cessation apps suggest that more research is necessary before recommending these as evidence-based interventions.

6.5.3 Nutrition and Physical Activity

To address the increased cancer risk and rising health costs associated with obesity and overweight, mHealth technologies have been developed to encourage patients to reach and maintain a healthy weight, increase physical activity, and improve diet. Systematic reviews have addressed the topic of mHealth as it relates to diet, nutrition, and physical activity. These reviews include numerous studies that used a range of technologies. Results have been mixed, and these results have been influenced by the type of technology used and the healthy weight behavior targeted.

6.5.3.1 Support for Weight Loss

Research suggests that self-monitoring and social support are effective contributors to successful weight loss. mHealth makes it possible for people to track their behavior related to losing weight using either an online journal or mobile diary application, and provides social support via the Internet or mobile phone. Three studies have assessed the use of PDAs, mobile apps, and websites to support weight loss compared with traditional paper-and-pencil tracking methods. All studies found that greater adherence to self-monitoring helped participants achieve greater weight loss [82–84]. Khaylis and colleagues [85], reviewing the use of online journals, pedometers, and PDAs, also found that when participants were held accountable, the technology was effective in improving weight loss.

6.5.3.2 Increased Physical Activity for Weight Loss

mHealth interventions provide a system for individuals to be held accountable for their physical activity. Systematic reviews looked at web-based interventions [86], pedometer usage [87], PDAs, mobile phone applications [87,88], and SMS technology [89]. Findings for using these tools to increase physical activity and lose weight are mixed. Pedometer usage and mobile phone apps were consistently successful in increasing activity, while PDAs had inconsistent results and require more research [87,88]. Web-based interventions had a less significant impact on increased physical activity than other methods, and again, findings were mixed.

Wearable devices such as Fitbit, classified as accelerometers, are becoming increasingly popular [89]. Researchers have not evaluated the effectiveness of accelerometers with online data access to assess and increase physical activity.

6.5.4 Alcohol Consumption

Mobile technology may be a successful strategy for reaching the 85% of problem drinkers who never come into contact with professional help [90]. A large number of mobile applications focus on alcohol use, but few have been scientifically reviewed. A needs assessment by Cohn and colleagues [90] found 567 alcohol-related mobile apps, but only 29% were related to alcohol cessation. Of those, 90% used empirically based treatment methods: motivational counseling, self-control training, and social support. Weaver and colleagues

[91] conducted a similar review of the top 250 alcohol-related apps from iTunes and Google Play. Only 11% of those studied were related to health promotion or reduced consumption. Both of these reviews noted that the majority of alcohol-related apps facilitate alcohol use and are for entertainment purposes only. Although there are apps focused on controlling alcohol use, to date no research has been conducted to determine their efficacy.

Web-based interventions have been studied but were found to have limited effectiveness. Bewick and colleagues [92] reviewed the literature and found that participants had positive attitudes toward web-based interventions, but results were inconsistent, with some interventions increasing alcohol consumption instead of reducing it.

6.5.5 Sun Protection

While most people know the benefits of sunscreen and reducing UV light exposure, this knowledge often does not translate to behavior change. Few SMS programs and apps have been developed to promote and reinforce the necessary behavior change. One study found that individuals who received daily SMS reminders to apply sunscreen and notices about the daily local weather applied sunscreen 56% of the time compared to the control group who applied sunscreen only 30% of the time [93]. Other mHealth methods to reduce UV exposure include phone applications, but as of 2012, there were only 19 sun behavior health apps [94].

The results of UV reduction and sunscreen application apps are mixed. One study found that individuals using the SolarCell app in the United States spent more time in the shade, but application of sunscreen decreased compared to those in control groups [95]. The SunSmart app, a component of a larger public health campaign in Australia to reduce UV exposure, has also had mixed results. The app had been downloaded more than 80,000 times, but only 40% of adults reported using UV alerts or sun protection information to make decisions about time spent in the sun. Of individuals who used the app, 90% stated that it was important to them and recommended the app to others [68]. The efficacy of mHealth tools for promoting healthy sun behavior needs further evaluation.

6.5.6 mHealth Research Gaps and Opportunities

mHealth applications have clearly engaged consumers. As a result, they offer great promise for reducing behavioral cancer risk factors. A key concern and research imperative is the empirical demonstration of treatment effectiveness among application users. This is especially true about demonstrating acceptability and impact in low- and middle-income countries, since the majority of studies have been conducted in high-income countries. Future research development should address the need for grounding in strong health behavior theory. Results of a systematic review of Internet interventions promoting health behavior change indicated that interventions varied in their use of theory, but those with a stronger theory base were generally associated with a larger effect size [96].

Research concerning mHealth may be enhanced by utilizing optimized study designs, data capture and analysis methods, and infrastructure. One methodological approach to consider before beginning mHealth trials is the use of a multiphase optimization strategy (MOST), a highly efficient application of engineering principals to prescreen and detect potentially viable intervention components [97]. MOST methods allow for the efficient identification of "active" intervention components. Randomized control trials are generally viewed as a best research practice, but because of their long lag time that often includes lumping of a number of intervention components, they might be less effective for the evaluation of quickly evolving technology [98,99].

Other innovative designs, incorporating the continuous evaluation of evolving interventions (CEEI), can take technological upgrades into account and thereby serve as a more efficient evaluation approach than other study designs. As a trial progresses, CEEI makes it possible to assess new versions of the interventions against previous versions. For data aggregation, statistical analysis, and sophisticated algorithms, researchers recommend drawing techniques from computer and engineering science because of the real-time data and within-person variance that is captured by mHealth tools. Lastly, it is important that the proper infrastructure is in place within clinics and hospitals, specifically for use of common measures and public sharing [100]. For this field to thrive, health care settings must promote innovation and encourage collaboration among professionals with differing expertise.

With the surge of medical mobile apps, the FDA has mapped out guidelines regarding its intentions for monitoring and regulating mobile device apps. The FDA's approach aligns with the risk-based approach the agency uses to ensure safety and effectiveness for other medical devices. The FDA plans to provide general guidance for apps that make decisions or behavioral suggestions or that individuals will use to log, record, track, or evaluate information related to developing or maintaining general fitness, health, or wellness [71].

Use of mHealth is a relatively novel practice, which calls for unique considerations apart from assessments of effectiveness. Confidentiality, privacy, and legal and ethical issues are highly sensitive topics because of the virtual network of mHealth data. This is particularly true if mobile devices are lost or stolen, as they can contain highly personal health and lifestyle information [100].

6.6 SUMMARY AND FUTURE DIRECTIONS

IT innovations that focus on cancer prevention represent an enormous opportunity to reduce cancer morbidity and mortality in the United States. While the reduction in smoking prevalence over the last half century has been appropriately heralded as a great public health accomplishment, half of physicians in the United States still neglect to advise smokers to quit during routine medical visits. High rates of physical inactivity and excess body weight represent other important modifiable cancer risk factors that could be integrated into regular clinical care practice protocols. In addition to targeting clinicians and their patients in the health care setting, applications of cancer prevention IT (eg, mHealth) can directly target the patient or consumer, thereby expanding the reach, and potential impact, of such innovations.

There is growing empirical literature that can guide adoption of such cancer prevention interventions. The successful implementation of these interventions by health care systems, however, will require a great degree of sensitivity to critical front line clinical issues including: workflow, an increasingly complex regulatory environment, and overburdened providers already dealing with frequent technology advances. The way forward may lie in strategically leveraging IT-supported protocols. EHR systems offer the possibility of practice surveillance, provider prompts and order sets that potentially can integrate and streamline assessing patient risk factors and engaging them in behavioral change action plans designed to reduce cancer risk. In addition, mHealth applications via tablets and smartphones that already have the advantage of near universal adoption, can facilitate education and support and can provide targeted guidance that is portable and available 100% of the time.

Though the pace of technology has accelerated far ahead of empirical evidence on efficacy and effectiveness, it is clear that the potential impact of these changes is enormous and, perhaps will be transformative in terms of reducing the burden of cancer illness and death. In addition to science documenting efficacy, the most urgent research and development needs are to advance EHRs beyond their current limited role serving as data repositories and providing clinician reminders to the richer potential of turning outward, targeting patients, clinicians, and possibly others to engage them in evidence-based cancer prevention activities. This evolution may be facilitated by EHR developers and vendors engaging patients in early design activities. Moving from automating cancer prevention interventions that use generic interventions based on outcome algorithms, to individualized interventions based on patient characteristics may have the added advantage of increasing patient satisfaction and heightening the likelihood that they will engage in cancer prevention behaviors. Development of organized, efficient, evidence-based IT innovations holds great potential for enhancing cancer prevention.

LIST OF ACRONYMS AND ABBREVIATIONS

ACA Affordable Care Act
APP Application
CDC Centers for Disease Control and Prevention
CEEI Continuous evaluation of evolving interventions
CHCs Community health centers
eHealth Electronic health
EHR Electronic health record
ePHR Electronic personal health record
EPIC European Prospective Investigation into Cancer and Nutrition
FDA US Food and Drug Administration
HHS US Department of Health and Human Services
HIPAA Health Insurance Portability and Accountability Act
HIT Health information technology
HITECH Health Information Technology for Economic and Clinical Health
HPV Human papillomavirus
IT Information technology
IVRS Interactive voice response service
LDCT Low-dose computed tomography
mHealth Mobile health
MMS Multimedia message service
NCI National Cancer Institute
NRT Nicotine replacement therapy
PCPs Primary care physicians
PDA Personal digital assistant
PSA Prostate-specific antigen
SMS Short message service
STOMP Stop Smoking with Mobile Phones
USPSTF US Preventive Services Task Force
UV Ultraviolet

Acknowledgments

The authors are grateful to Dana Chomenko, Alexandra Stern, and Amanda Huffman for their valued contributions.

References

[1] American Cancer Society Cancer facts & figures 2015. Atlanta, GA: American Cancer Society; 2015.

[2] National Cancer Institute Cancer trends progress report—2011/2012 update. Bethesda, MD: U.S. Department of Health and Human Services, National Cancer Institute; 2012. Available from: <http://progressreport.cancer.gov/sites/default/files/archive/report2011.pdf>.

[3] National Cancer Institute Building on opportunities in cancer research: an annual plan and budget proposal for fiscal year 2016. Bethesda, MD: National Cancer Institute; 2014.

[4] American Cancer Society Cancer facts & figures 2014. Atlanta, GA: American Cancer Society; 2014.

[5] Pianezza ML, Sellers EM, Tyndale RF. Nicotine metabolism defect reduces smoking. Nature 1998;393(6687):750.

[6] Kushi LH, Byers T, Doyle C, Bandera EV, McCullough M, McTiernan A, et al. American Cancer Society guidelines on nutrition and physical activity for cancer prevention: reducing the risk of cancer with healthy food choices and physical activity. CA Cancer J Clin 2012;62(1):30–67.

[7] U.S. Department of Health and Human Services Reducing tobacco use: a report of the Surgeon General. Atlanta, GA: U.S. Department of Health and Human Services, Centers for Disease Control and Prevention, National Center for Chronic Disease Prevention and Health Promotion, Office on Smoking and Health; 2000.

[8] Fiore MC, Jaen CR, Baker TB, Bailey WC, Benowitz N, Curry SJ, et al. Treating tobacco use and dependence: 2008 update. Clinical practice guideline. Rockville, MD: U.S. Department of Health and Human Services, Public Health Service; 2008.

[9] U.S. Department of Health and Human Services The health consequences of smoking—50 years of progress: a report of the Surgeon General. Atlanta, GA: U.S. Department of Health and Human Services, Public Health Service, Office of the Surgeon General; 2014.

[10] U.S. Department of Health and Human Services How tobacco smoke causes disease: the biology and behavioral basis for smoking-attributable disease: a report of the Surgeon General. Atlanta, GA: U.S. Department of Health and Human Services, Centers for Disease Control and Prevention, National Center for Chronic Disease Prevention and Health Promotion, Office on Smoking and Health; 2010.

[11] Chen J, Kettermann A, Rostron BL, Day HR. Biomarkers of exposure among U.S. cigar smokers: an analysis of 1999–2012 National Health and Nutrition Examination Survey (NHANES) data. Cancer Epidemiol Biomarkers Prev 2014;23(12):2906–15.

[12] Boffetta P, Hecht S, Gray N, Gupta P, Straif K. Smokeless tobacco and cancer. Lancet Oncol 2008;9(7):667–75.

[13] Centers for Disease Control and Prevention Electronic cigarette use among middle and high school students—United States, 2011–2012. Morb Mortal Wkly Rep 2013;62:729–30.

[14] Fiore MC, Baker TB. Clinical practice. Treating smokers in the health care setting. N Engl J Med 2011;365(13):1222–31.

[15] Hughes JR, Shiffman S, Callas P, Zhang J. A meta-analysis of the efficacy of over-the-counter nicotine replacement. Tob Control 2003;12(1):21–7.

[16] Cornuz J, Gilbert A, Pinget C, McDonald P, Slama K, Salto E, et al. Cost-effectiveness of pharmacotherapies for nicotine dependence in primary care settings: a multinational comparison. Tob Control 2006;15(3):152–9.

[17] Winzer BM, Whiteman DC, Reeves MM, Paratz JD. Physical activity and cancer prevention: a systematic review of clinical trials. Cancer Causes Control 2011;22(6):811–26.

[18] U.S. Department of Health and Human Services 2008 physical activity guidelines for Americans. Washington, DC: U.S. Department of Health and Human Services; 2008.

[19] Benetou V, Orfanos P, Lagiou P, Trichopoulos D, Boffetta P, Trichopoulou A. Vegetables and fruits in relation to cancer risk: evidence from the Greek EPIC cohort study. Cancer Epidemiol Biomarkers Prev 2008;17(2):387–92.

[20] Boffetta P, Couto E, Wichmann J, Ferrari P, Trichopoulos D, Bueno-de-Mesquita HB, et al. Fruit and vegetable intake and overall cancer risk in the European Prospective Investigation into Cancer and Nutrition (EPIC). J Natl Cancer Inst 2010;102(8):529–37.

[21] Chan DS, Lau R, Aune D, Vieira R, Greenwood DC, Kampman E, et al. Red and processed meat and colorectal cancer incidence: meta-analysis of prospective studies. PLoS One 2011;6(6):e20456.

[22] Dietary Guidelines Advisory Committee Report of the dietary guidelines advisory committee on the dietary guidelines for Americans, 2010. Washington, DC: U.S. Department of Agriculture, Agricultural Research Service; 2010.

[23] National Center for Health Statistics, Centers for Disease Control and Prevention. About the National Health and Nutrition Examination Survey. NHANES website. Hyattsville, MD: National Center for Health Statistics; [updated February 3, 2014]. Available from: <http://www.cdc.gov/nchs/nhanes/about_nhanes.htm>.

[24] National Cancer Insitute SEER Stat fact sheets: melanoma of the skin. Surveillance epidemiology and end results program. Bethesda, MD: National Cancer Institute; 2014. Available from: <http://seer.cancer.gov/statfacts/html/melan.html>.

[25] Office of Disease Prevention and Health Promotion Healthy people 2020. Washington, DC: U.S. Department of Health and Human Services; 2015. Available from: <https://www.healthy-people.gov/>.

[26] Small SL, Sampselle CM, Martyn KK, Dempsey AF. Modifiable influences on female HPV vaccine uptake at the clinic encounter level: a literature review. J Am Assoc Nurse Pract 2014;26(9):519–25.

[27] Insinga RP, Dasbach EJ, Elbasha EH. Assessing the annual economic burden of preventing and treating anogenital human papillomavirus-related disease in the US: analytic framework and review of the literature. Pharmacoeconomics 2005;23(11):1107–22.

[28] Dunne EF, Unger ER, Sternberg M, McQuillan G, Swan DC, Patel SS, et al. Prevalence of HPV infection among females in the United States. JAMA 2007;297(8):813–9.

[29] Markowitz LE, Dunne EF, Saraiya M, Chesson HW, Curtis CR, Gee J, et al. Human papillomavirus vaccination: recommendations of the Advisory Committee on Immunization Practices (ACIP). MMWR Recomm Rep 2014;63(RR-05):1–30.

[30] Centers for Disease Control and Prevention National and state vaccination coverage among adolescents aged 13 through 17 years—United States, 2010. MMWR Morb Mortal Wkly Rep 2011;60(33):1117–23.

[31] Szilagyi PG, Serwint JR, Humiston SG, Rand CM, Schaffer S, Vincelli P, et al. Effect of provider prompts on adolescent immunization rates: a randomized trial. Acad Pediatr 2015;15(2):149–57.

[32] Jimbo M, Nease Jr DE, Ruffin MT, Rana GK. Information technology and cancer prevention. CA Cancer J Clin 2006;56(1):26–36.

[33] Hornung RL, Lennon PA, Garrett JM, DeVellis RF, Weinberg PD, Strecher VJ. Interactive computer technology for skin cancer prevention targeting children. Am J Prev Med 2000;18(1):69–76.

[34] Barysch MJ, Cozzio A, Kolm I, Hrdlicka SR, Brand C, Hunger R, et al. Internet based health promotion campaign against skin cancer—results of www.skincheck.ch in Switzerland. Eur J Dermatol 2010;20(1):109–14.

[35] Gerbert B, Bronstone A, Maurer T, Berger T, McPhee SJ, Caspers N. The effectiveness of an Internet-based tutorial in improving primary care physicians' skin cancer triage skills. J Cancer Educ 2002;17(1):7–11.

[36] Boyle R, Solberg L, Fiore M. Use of electronic health records to support smoking cessation. Cochrane Database Syst Rev 2014;12 CD008743.

[37] Linder JA, Rigotti NA, Schneider LI, Kelley JH, Brawarsky P, Haas JS. An electronic health record-based intervention to improve tobacco treatment in primary care: a cluster-randomized controlled trial. Arch Internal Med 2009;169(8):781–7.

[38] Bentz CJ, Bayley BK, Bonin KE, Fleming L, Hollis JF, Hunt JS, et al. Provider feedback to improve 5A's tobacco cessation in primary care: a cluster randomized clinical trial. Nicotine Tob Res 2007;9(3):341–9.

[39] Rindal DB, Rush WA, Schleyer TK, Kirshner M, Boyle RG, Thoele MJ, et al. Computer-assisted guidance for dental office tobacco-cessation counseling: a randomized controlled trial. Am J Prev Med 2013;44(3):260–4.

[40] Fiore MC. The new vital sign. Assessing and documenting smoking status. JAMA 1991;266(22):3183–4.

[41] Centers for Medicare & Medicaid Services. EHR incentive programs: the official web site of the Medicare and Medicaid electronic health records (EHR) incentive programs. Baltimore: MD Centers for Medicare & Medicaid Services; [updated March 24, 2015]. Available from: <http://www.cms.gov/Regulations-and-Guidance/Legislation/EHRIncentivePrograms/index.html?redirect=/ehrincentiveprograms/>.

[42] Vidrine JI, Shete S, Cao Y, Greisinger A, Harmonson P, Sharp B, et al. Ask-advise-connect: a new approach to smoking treatment delivery in health care settings. JAMA Intern Med 2013;173(6):458–64.

[43] Vidrine JI, Shete S, Li Y, Cao Y, Alford MH, Galindo-Talton M, et al. The ask-advise-connect approach for smokers in a safety net healthcare system: a group-randomized trial. Am J Prev Med 2013;45(6):737–41.

[44] Koplan KE, Regan S, Goldszer RC, Schneider LI, Rigotti NA. A computerized aid to support smoking cessation treatment for hospital patients. J Gen Intern Med 2008;23(8):1214–7.

[45] Kruse GR, Chang Y, Kelley JH, Linder JA, Einbinder JS, Rigotti NA. Healthcare system effects of pay-for-performance for smoking status documentation. Am J Manag Care 2013;19(7):554–61.

[46] Duquaine D, Farley SM, Sacks R, Mandel-Ricci J, Silfen SL, Shih SC. Designing a quality improvement program with electronic health records: New York City's Health eQuits. Am J Med Qual 2015;30(2):141–8.

[47] Silfen SL, Farley SM, Shih SC, Duquaine DC, Ricci JM, Kansagra SM, et al. Increases in smoking cessation interventions after a feedback and improvement initiative using electronic health records—19 community health centers, New York City, October 2010–March 2012. MMWR Morb Mortal Wkly Rep 2014;63(41):921–4.

[48] van der Aalst CM, van Klaveren RJ, de Koning HJ. Does participation to screening unintentionally influence lifestyle behaviour and thus lifestyle-related morbidity? Best Pract Res Clin Gastroenterol 2010;24(4):465–78.

[49] Ashraf H, Tonnesen P, Holst Pedersen J, Dirksen A, Thorsen H, Dossing M. Effect of CT screening on smoking habits at 1-year follow-up in the Danish Lung Cancer Screening Trial (DLCST). Thorax 2009;64(5):388–92.

[50] van der Aalst CM, van den Bergh KA, Willemsen MC, de Koning HJ, van Klaveren RJ. Lung cancer screening and smoking abstinence: 2 year follow-up data from the Dutch-Belgian randomised controlled lung cancer screening trial. Thorax 2010;65(7):600–5.

[51] Townsend CO, Clark MM, Jett JR, Patten CA, Schroeder DR, Nirelli LM, et al. Relation between smoking cessation and receiving results from three annual spiral chest computed tomography scans for lung carcinoma screening. Cancer 2005;103(10):2154–62.

[52] Styn MA, Land SR, Perkins KA, Wilson DO, Romkes M, Weissfeld JL. Smoking behavior 1 year after computed tomography screening for lung cancer: effect of physician referral for abnormal CT findings. Cancer Epidemiol Biomarkers Prev 2009;18(12):3484–9.

[53] Tammemagi MC, Berg CD, Riley TL, Cunningham CR, Taylor KL. Impact of lung cancer screening results on smoking cessation. J Natl Cancer Inst 2014;106(6) dju084.

[54] Adsit RT, Fox BM, Tsiolis T, Ogland C, Simerson M, Vind LM, et al. Using the electronic health record to connect primary care patients to evidence-based telephonic tobacco quitline services: a closed-loop demonstration project. Transl Behav Med 2014;4(3):324–32.

[55] Cowburn S, Carlson MJ, Lapidus JA, DeVoe JE. The association between insurance status and cervical cancer screening in community health centers: exploring the potential of electronic health

records for population-level surveillance, 2008–2010. Prev Chron Dis 2013;10:E173.

[56] White P, Kenton K. Use of electronic medical record-based tools to improve compliance with cervical cancer screening guidelines: effect of an educational intervention on physicians' practice patterns. J Low Genit Tract Dis 2013;17(2):175–81.

[57] Weber V, Bloom F, Pierdon S, Wood C. Employing the electronic health record to improve diabetes care: a multifaceted intervention in an integrated delivery system. J Gen Intern Med 2008;23(4):379–82.

[58] Womble PR, Montie JE, Ye Z, Linsell SM, Lane BR, Miller DC, et al. Contemporary use of initial active surveillance among men in Michigan with low-risk prostate cancer. Eur Urol 2015;67(1):44–50.

[59] Cooperberg MR. Progress in management of low-risk prostate cancer: how registries may change the world. Eur Urol 2015;67(1):51–2.

[60] Sherman SE, Takahashi N, Kalra P, Gifford E, Finney JW, Canfield J, et al. Care coordination to increase referrals to smoking cessation telephone counseling: a demonstration project. Am J Manag Care 2008;14(3):141–8.

[61] Heisey-Grove D, Danehy LN, Consolazio M, Lynch K, Mostashari F. A national study of challenges to electronic health record adoption and meaningful use. Med Care 2014;52(2):144–8.

[62] Pizziferri L, Kittler AF, Volk LA, Honour MM, Gupta S, Wang S, et al. Primary care physician time utilization before and after implementation of an electronic health record: a time-motion study. J Biomed Inform 2005;38(3):176–88.

[63] Kim EH, Stolyar A, Lober WB, Herbaugh AL, Shinstrom SE, Zierler BK, et al. Challenges to using an electronic personal health record by a low-income elderly population. J Med Internet Res 2009;11(4):e44.

[64] Blumenthal D. Launching HITECH. N Engl J Med 2010; 362(5):382–5.

[65] Hsiao C-J, Hing E. Use and characteristics of electronic health record systems among office-based physician practices: United States, 2001–2013, NCHS Data Brief No. 143. Hyattsville, MD: U.S. Department of Health and Human Services, Centers for Disease Control and Prevention, National Center for Health Statistics; 2014.

[66] McAfee T, Babb S, McNabb S, Fiore MC. Helping smokers quit—opportunities created by the Affordable Care Act. N Engl J Med 2015;372(1):5–7.

[67] International Telecommunication Union The world in 2014: ICT facts and figures. Geneva: International Telecommunication Union; 2014.

[68] Adibi S, editor. mHealth multidisciplinary verticals. Boca Raton, FL: CRC Press, Taylor & Francis Group; 2015.

[69] Holeman I, Evans J, Kane D, Grant L, Pagliari C, Weller D. Mobile health for cancer in low to middle income countries: priorities for research and development. Eur J Cancer Care (Engl) 2014;23(6):750–6.

[70] Fox S, Duggan M. Mobile health 2012. Washington, DC: Pew Research Center; 2012.

[71] Food and Drug Administration Mobile medical applications: guidance for industry and Food and Drug Administration Staff. Silver Spring, MD: U.S. Department of Health and Human Services, Food and Drug Administration; 2015.

[72] Davis SW, Oakley-Girvan I. mHealth education applications along the cancer continuum. J Cancer Educ 2015;30(2):388–94.

[73] Bender JL, Yue RY, To MJ, Deacken L, Jadad AR. A lot of action, but not in the right direction: systematic review and content analysis of smartphone applications for the prevention, detection, and management of cancer. J Med Internet Res 2013;15(12):e287.

[74] Whittaker R, Borland R, Bullen C, Lin RB, McRobbie H, Rodgers A. Mobile phone-based interventions for smoking cessation. Cochrane Database Syst Rev 2009(4) CD006611.

[75] The Community Guide. Reducing tobacco use and secondhand smoke exposure: mobile phone-based cessation interventions. [Updated December 2011] Available from: <www.thecommunityguide.org/tobacco/index.html>.

[76] Whittaker R, McRobbie H, Bullen C, Borland R, Rodgers A, Gu Y. Mobile phone-based interventions for smoking cessation. Cochrane Database Syst Rev 2012;11 CD006611.

[77] Spohr SA, Nandy R, Gandhiraj D, Vemulapalli A, Anne S, Walters ST. Efficacy of SMS text message interventions for smoking cessation: a meta-analysis. J Subst Abuse Treat 2015;56:1–10.

[78] Free C, Phillips G, Galli L, Watson L, Felix L, Edwards P, et al. The effectiveness of mobile-health technology-based health behaviour change or disease management interventions for health care consumers: a systematic review. PLoS Med 2013;10(1) e1001362.

[79] Free C, Knight R, Robertson S, Whittaker R, Edwards P, Zhou W, et al. Smoking cessation support delivered via mobile phone text messaging (txt2stop): a single-blind, randomised trial. Lancet 2011;378(9785):49–55.

[80] Fraser D, Kobinsky K, Smith SS, Kramer J, Theobald WE, Baker TB. Five population-based interventions for smoking cessation: a MOST trial. Transl Behav Med 2014;4(4):382–90.

[81] Abroms LC, Padmanabhan N, Thaweethai L, Phillips T. iPhone apps for smoking cessation: a content analysis. Am J Prev Med 2011;40(3):279–85.

[82] Turner-McGrievy GM, Beets MW, Moore JB, Kaczynski AT, Barr-Anderson DJ, Tate DF. Comparison of traditional versus mobile app self-monitoring of physical activity and dietary intake among overweight adults participating in an mHealth weight loss program. J Am Med Inform Assoc 2013;20(3):513–8.

[83] Burke LE, Styn MA, Sereika SM, Conroy MB, Ye L, Glanz K, et al. Using mHealth technology to enhance self-monitoring for weight loss: a randomized trial. Am J Prev Med 2012;43(1):20–6.

[84] Acharya SD, Elci OU, Sereika SM, Styn MA, Burke LE. Using a personal digital assistant for self-monitoring influences diet quality in comparison to a standard paper record among overweight/obese adults. J Am Diet Assoc 2011;111(4):583–8.

[85] Khaylis A, Yiaslas T, Bergstrom J, Gore-Felton C. A review of efficacious technology-based weight-loss interventions: five key components. Telemed J E Health 2010;16(9):931–8.

[86] Kuijpers W, Groen WG, Aaronson NK, van Harten WH. A systematic review of web-based interventions for patient empowerment and physical activity in chronic diseases: relevance for cancer survivors. J Med Internet Res 2013;15(2):e37.

[87] Fanning J, Mullen SP, McAuley E. Increasing physical activity with mobile devices: a meta-analysis. J Med Internet Res 2012;14(6):e161.

[88] Bort-Roig J, Gilson ND, Puig-Ribera A, Contreras RS, Trost SG. Measuring and influencing physical activity with smartphone technology: a systematic review. Sports Med 2014;44(5):671–86.

[89] Van Camp CM, Hayes LB. Assessing and increasing physical activity. J Appl Behav Anal 2012;45(4):871–5.

[90] Cohn AM, Hunter-Reel D, Hagman BT, Mitchell J. Promoting behavior change from alcohol use through mobile technology: the future of ecological momentary assessment. Alcohol Clin Exp Res 2011;35(12):2209–15.

[91] Weaver ER, Horyniak DR, Jenkinson R, Dietze P, Lim MS. "Let's get Wasted!" and other apps: characteristics, acceptability, and use of alcohol-related smartphone applications. JMIR Mhealth Uhealth 2013;1(1):e9.

[92] Bewick BM, Trusler K, Barkham M, Hill AJ, Cahill J, Mulhern B. The effectiveness of web-based interventions designed to decrease alcohol consumption—a systematic review. Prev Med 2008;47(1):17–26.

[93] Armstrong AW, Watson AJ, Makredes M, Frangos JE, Kimball AB, Kvedar JC. Text-message reminders to improve sunscreen

II. SUPPORT ACROSS THE CONTINUUM

use: a randomized, controlled trial using electronic monitoring. Arch Dermatol 2009;145(11):1230–6.

[94] Brewer AC, Endly DC, Henley J, Amir M, Sampson BP, Moreau JF, et al. Mobile applications in dermatology. JAMA Dermatol 2013;149(11):1300–4.

[95] Buller DB, Berwick M, Lantz K, Buller MK, Shane J, Kane I, et al. Smartphone mobile application delivering personalized, real-time sun protection advice: a randomized clinical trial. JAMA Dermatol 2015;151(5):497–504.

[96] Webb TL, Joseph J, Yardley L, Michie S. Using the internet to promote health behavior change: a systematic review and meta-analysis of the impact of theoretical basis, use of behavior change techniques, and mode of delivery on efficacy. J Med Internet Res 2010;12(1):e4.

[97] Collins L, Baker T, Mermelstein R, Piper M, Jorenby D, Smith S, et al. The Multiphase Optimization Strategy for engineering effective tobacco use interventions. Ann Behav Med 2011;41(2):208–26.

[98] Nilsen W, Kumar S, Shar A, Varoquiers C, Wiley T, Riley WT, et al. Advancing the science of mHealth. J Health Commun 2012;17(Suppl. 1):5–10.

[99] Kumar S, Nilsen WJ, Abernethy A, Atienza A, Patrick K, Pavel M, et al. Mobile health technology evaluation: the mHealth evidence workshop. Am J Prev Med 2013;45(2):228–36.

[100] Mohammadzadeh N, Safdari R, Rahimi A. Cancer care management through a mobile phone health approach: key considerations. Asian Pac J Cancer Prev 2013;14(9):4961–4.

CHAPTER

7

Early Detection in the Age of Information Technology

Ekland Abdiwahab MPH[1], Stephen H. Taplin MD, MPH[1], Gloria Coronado PhD[2], Heather Dacus DO, MPH[3], Melissa Leypoldt RN[4] and Celette Skinner PhD[5]

[1]Healthcare Delivery Research Program, Division of Cancer Control and Population Science, National Cancer Institute, Rockville, MD, United States [2]Kaiser Permanente Center for Health Research, Portland, OR, United States [3]New York State Department of Health, Albany, NY, United States [4]Division of Public Health, Nebraska Department of Health and Human Services, Lincoln, NE, United States [5]Department of Clinical Sciences, UT Southwestern Medical Center, Dallas, TX, United States

OUTLINE

7.1 Introduction	124
7.2 Epidemiology	124
7.2.1 Breast Cancer	124
7.2.2 Cervical Cancer	125
7.2.3 Colorectal Cancer	125
7.2.4 Lung Cancer	125
7.3 Early Detection	125
7.3.1 Screening	126
7.3.2 Breast Cancer Screening	126
7.3.3 Cervical Cancer Screening	127
7.3.4 Colorectal Screening	127
7.3.5 Lung Cancer Screening	128
7.3.6 High-Risk Individuals	128
7.4 The Process of Care	128
7.4.1 Screening Is a Process Not a Test	128
7.4.2 Organized Versus Opportunistic Screening Programs	129
7.5 The Challenge of Early Detection	129
7.5.1 Failure to Screen	131

7.5.2 Failure to Detect	131
7.5.3 Failure During the Follow-Up	131
7.6 Communication Challenges	132
7.6.1 Use of IT in Early Detection	134
7.7 Evidence-Based Solutions	134
7.7.1 Oregon Community Health Information Network	134
7.7.2 New York State Department of Health	136
7.7.3 Parkland Health and Hospital System	137
7.7.4 Nebraska Department of Health and Human Services	138
7.8 Challenges With Using IT	139
7.9 Overcoming Disparities	139
7.10 Looking to the Future	139
List of Acronyms and Abbreviations	140
Acknowledgments	140
References	140

B. Hesse, D. Ahern & E. Beckjord: Oncology Informatics.
DOI: http://dx.doi.org/10.1016/B978-0-12-802115-6.00007-0

7.1 INTRODUCTION

Cancer remains the second leading cause of mortality in the United States accounting for more than 575,000 deaths annually; approximately 23% of all-cause mortality [1]. Cancer not only affects the individuals diagnosed, but also their families, communities, and society as a whole. Medical costs associated with cancer care have increased substantially; costs were estimated at $124.6 billion in 2010 alone and are projected to reach $173 billion by 2020 [2]. In addition, lost productivity due to cancer-related premature death is estimated to be $147.6 billion annually by 2020 [3]. Cancer is increasingly becoming a global epidemic and low-resourced countries are being disproportionately impacted. According to the latest estimates from the International Agency for Research on Cancer (IARC), there were approximately 14.1 million new cases of cancer and 8.2 million deaths globally in 2012 alone [4]. Though there have been advancements in prevention, early detection, and treatment, 80% of cancer mortality will occur in developing countries by 2020 where many of these advances are not currently available [5,6].

There are four clear opportunities where early detection can impact cancer diagnoses: screening for breast, cervical, and colorectal cancers among average-risk people, and screening for lung cancer among high-risk individuals [7–10]. While many think that the increased survival associated with screening is the justification for doing it, that is not the case. The challenge with screening is that it introduces lead time bias; lead time is the period of additional time someone is aware of their cancer diagnosis. For example, if there are two individuals and one of them has their cancer detected by screening at age 55 while the other had it diagnosed at age 59 but both die of cancer at age 60, screening did not confer a survival advantage. The only difference here is that the first person lived with their cancer for 5 years while the second lived with it for 1 year. Because of lead time, the benefit of screening is only certain when two groups of people are randomly assigned to receive or not receive the screening test. When fewer people die of cancer in the screened group then this is evidence that the screening test is efficacious. Such studies have been carried out for breast, colorectal, and lung cancer. As for cervical cancer, screening has been shown to be effective because population-level screenings offered by several Nordic countries demonstrated reductions in cervical cancer mortality during the years screenings were offered. When screening was removed, because of a lack of clarity about the reason for the mortality reduction, mortality rates rose again. With the reinstation of screenings mortality rates dropped once more. The reduced mortality in trials and large population studies are the reason screening is recommended for these four cancer types [8,9,11]. Despite evidence for the efficacy of screening in experimental trials for these cancers, challenges remain for implementation in clinical practice.

This chapter considers the epidemiology of the four cancers (breast, cervical, colorectal, and lung) recommended for screening by the United States Preventive Services Task Force (USPSTF), the complexity of early detection, and how information technology (IT) can support and simplify the work associated with it. Simplification is important because within each type of screening there are multiple activities that require coordination among providers, patients, family, and the people within institutions whose behavior can facilitate or inhibit early detection and diagnosis. We use the definition of health information technology (HIT) as "the application of information processing involving both computer hardware and software that deals with the storage, retrieval, sharing, and use of health care information, data, and knowledge for communication and decision making" [12]. While HIT offers many conceptually appealing solutions to the challenge of coordinating care, it is in many cases easier to conceive of electronic solutions than implement them. Our primary purpose is to articulate the work and associated activities of early detection, summarize what we know about how IT can support that work, imagine future uses, and identify some early signs of success that encourage pursuing the gap between conception and implementation of IT that will improve care.

7.2 EPIDEMIOLOGY

7.2.1 Breast Cancer

Breast cancer is the second leading cause of cancer-related morbidity and mortality for women in the United States. In 2014 alone there were an estimated 232,670 new cases of breast cancer and roughly 40,000 deaths [13]. In the United States, a woman has a 12.8% chance of developing breast cancer in her lifetime [14]. Age-adjusted breast cancer incidence rates have remained stable from 2001 through 2010 in every racial and ethnic group except for African American women who have shown a significant increase [15]. Although mortality rates have steadily declined, African American women continue to have the highest mortality rates of any racial/ethnic group [13]. Breast cancers can be classified according to two hormone-receptors and a human epidermal growth factor receptor (HER2) [16]. A large proportion of breast cancers in the United States are estrogen receptor (ER) positive. ER positive tumors tend to also be progesterone receptor (PR) positive. Tumors that are estrogen and progesterone positive can be treated with hormone therapies that block the body's ability to either produce these hormones or interfere with the activities of the hormones. Cancers that are ER or PR negative lack these hormone receptors and are therefore not treated with hormone therapy. Women whose tumors lack one or both of these receptors (ER+/PR−, ER−/PR+, or ER−/PR−) experience higher rates of mortality than those that are ER+/PR+ [17]. Approximately 25–30% of breast cancers are found to be HER2 positive. HER2 positive tumors are more aggressive and less likely to respond to therapies than hormone-stimulated breast cancer. The development of therapies that target this receptor in the past 20 years have helped to drastically improve survival rates [18]. Triple negative breast cancer is categorized as being negative for the estrogen, progesterone, and HER2 receptors (ER−/PR−/Her2/neu−). Triple negative breast cancer is a much more aggressive subtype and incidence and mortality rates for this subtype tend to be disproportionately high in African American and Sub-Saharan African women [19,20].

Globally, breast cancer is the most prevalent cancer among women. In 2012, there were 1.7 million new cases of breast cancer and roughly 522,000 deaths. Although breast cancer accounts for 25% of all new cancer cases in women globally, incidence and mortality rates vary across countries [4]. The highest rates of breast cancer can be found in Western Europe and North America, though mortality rates are highest in Melanesia and Western Africa [4].

7.2.2 Cervical Cancer

Due to major advancements in prevention and early detection, cervical cancer is no longer a leading cause of cancer morbidity or mortality among women in the United States [15]. Cervical cancer occurs because of the presence of the human papilloma virus. Vaccination against human papilloma virus is capable of preventing the occurrence of cervical cancer. In 2014, there were an estimated 12,360 new US cases of cervical cancer and approximately 4020 deaths [13]. Between 1975 and 2011 the overall cervical cancer incidence and mortality rates decreased by 54% and 60%, respectively [14]. Although African American women have seen the largest drop in cervical cancer incidence rates between 1973 and 2007, they continue to have the highest mortality rates [21,22]. Hispanic women have the highest incidence rates, and women who live in the South have both the highest incidence and mortality [22]. Globally, cervical cancer is the fourth most common cancer in women. In 2012, there were an estimated 528,000 new cases and 266,000 deaths. Less developed countries suffer the greatest burden of cervical cancer incidence and mortality. Roughly 85% of all new cases and 87% of deaths occur in less developed regions. Cervical cancer accounts for 12% of all cancers in less developed regions [4].

7.2.3 Colorectal Cancer

In the United States, colorectal cancer is the third most prevalent cancer and the third leading cause of cancer mortality in men and women [13]. An estimated 136,830 Americans were diagnosed with colorectal cancer in 2014 and approximately 50,310 died [13]. Colorectal cancer rates have declined for both sexes, however, incident and mortality differences persist [15]. Although Hispanic men, Hispanic women, and Asian/Pacific Islander women are more likely to be diagnosed with colorectal cancer than any other racial/ethnic group, African Americans of both sexes are more likely to die from the disease [14,15]. Worldwide, colorectal cancer is the third most prevalent cancer in men and the second most prevalent cancer in women. In 2012, roughly 1.4 million individuals were diagnosed with colorectal cancer and 694,000 died. There is gender and geographic variability in colorectal cancer incidence and mortality globally. The incidence, mortality, and 5-year prevalence are higher for males than females. Although the incidence of colorectal cancer is higher in more developed countries, less developed regions suffer from higher mortality rates [4].

7.2.4 Lung Cancer

In the United States, lung cancer is the second most prevalent cancer among both men and women, and it remains the leading cause of cancer death [13]. There were an estimated 224,210 new cases and 159,260 deaths from lung cancer in 2014 [13]. As a result of public health measures aimed at reducing smoking rates, lung cancer incidence and mortality rates have been steadily declining the last two decades [14]. Although rates continue to decline, there are gender and geographic disparities in incidence and mortality. Minority populations continue to experience an increased burden of lung cancer. African American males in particular have the highest incidence and mortality rates of any other group [15]. In addition, individuals living in the rural South are more likely to be diagnosed with lung cancer than those living in other US geographic areas [23]. Globally, lung cancer remains the leading cause of cancer morbidity and mortality. Roughly 1.8 million new cases were diagnosed in 2012, accounting for 12.9% of all new cancer diagnosis. Mortality from lung cancer accounts for 20% of all cancer deaths; this translates to 1.6 million deaths in 2012 alone. Both incidence and mortality rates of lung cancer are highest among men in developed nations [4].

7.3 EARLY DETECTION

The task of cancer early detection encompasses at least two types of medical care: (1) screening for cancer precursors or early forms of cancer that when treated change the natural history of the disease and reduce mortality, and (2) responding to symptoms and signs of early cancer to reduce the morbidity and potentially the mortality of cancer.

7.3.1 Screening

While screening is intuitively appealing, the challenge of proving that it confers a mortality benefit has occupied researchers, policy makers, and health care organizations for decades. Screening is considered beneficial if it results in the extension of life that otherwise would not have been observed in the absence of screening. This means that screening detects cancer in the pre-clinical stage and treatment is more effective in cancers that are screen-detected as opposed to cancers found in the absence of screening. Screening should result in the reduction of mortality, and in the case of colorectal and cervical cancers, the identification and subsequent removal of precancerous lesions or polyps have been shown to reduce the incidence of colorectal and cervical cancers [24,25].

When implementing population-based screening programs, the potential benefits of screening described above must be assessed against the potential harms of screening. These harms include false positive readings that result in increased stress and anxiety, complications associated with diagnostic investigation, and toxicity associated with cancer therapies. Additionally, many are now concerned about overdiagnosis of cancers when screening finds a precancerous or cancerous condition that would otherwise not have affected the individual during his or her lifetime. There are also harms associated with false negative readings which may include a false sense of being disease free and potential advancements in disease progression without appropriate treatment [8,9]. Screenings that are shown to be efficacious in experimental settings (ie, randomized controlled trials) may not be effective in the real world due to the unpredictable nature of the context in which screening is implemented. Multiple requirements must be fulfilled in order to fully realize the value proposition of screening; ideally, screening should be: inexpensive; conducted if the disease has a recognizable presymptomatic phase; result in cancer detection that affords more effective treatment than waiting for more advanced disease; acceptable to those being screened; and conducted when there are adequate resources for diagnosis and treatment [26].

Population-based estimates of screen-detected versus symptom-detected cancers are difficult to find, but one study of breast cancer in New Hampshire suggested that 54% (123/228) within their state-based registry were found by screening exams and another in New Mexico suggested it was 58% over a 5-year period [27,28]. In the United Kingdom where an active nationwide colorectal

cancer screening program was fully implemented using fecal immunochemical tests (FITs), 67.6% were screen-detected over a 3-year period from 2007 to 2010 [29]. Evaluation of invasive and micro-invasive cervical cancers diagnosed during a 12-year implementation period of a cervical cancer screening program in two districts of the United Kingdom (Southampton and South West Hampshire) showed that 33% were screen detected among screening eligible women [30]. These numbers are from regions with organized programs and yet many cancers continue to be detected through means other than screening. Finding cancers through both symptomatic detection and screening are therefore both important methods of reducing the impact of this disease. In this subsequent section we summarize the evidence for screening, US and global guidelines for screening, and current screening rates.

7.3.2 Breast Cancer Screening

Mammography, low-dose X-ray images of the breast, is used both as a screening and diagnostic tool. The use in screening has been riddled with controversy and some of that controversy is actually good news [31]. Part of the challenge is that the trials were conducted when treatment was not as effective as it is today. Whether the benefits of screening shown in trials that were implemented many years ago are comparable to screenings conducted today can never be fully resolved. Despite the controversy, and debates about the details of trials, most agree that randomized trials have demonstrated benefits of screening for breast cancer [32]. Furthermore, subsequent observational studies in countries with large programs have also shown a benefit. A 30-year follow-up study by Tabar and colleagues showed a 27–31% reduction in breast cancer mortality for women who received screening mammography [33]. In addition, after evaluating screening strategies using six model estimates, Mandelblatt and colleagues found strategies that employed biennial screenings were the most efficient (used the least resources while reducing mortality) [34]. The effectiveness of screen-film mammography in detecting tumors has been shown to be comparable to digital mammography except digital mammography has been shown to be more accurate in women under the age of 50, those who have dense breast tissue, and women who are premenopausal or perimenopausal [35].

Based on findings from a meta-analysis of randomized-controlled mammography trials, the USPSTF recommends biennial screening mammography for women 50–74 years of age. Women who are younger than 50 are advised to consult their physician to determine individual benefits or harms of getting a mammogram. The USPSTF notes there is insufficient evidence that women 75 years or older would benefit or be harmed by mammography. The USPSTF recommends against clinical breast exams and instruction in breast self-exams because no benefit has been shown for either [7]. The World Health Organization (WHO) makes recommendations for mammograms based on two criteria: age and setting. The WHO recommends that women 50–69 years of age who live in well-resourced settings receive biennial screenings. The WHO recommends that countries with strong health systems but with areas of limited resource settings create population-based mammography screening programs only if the health care system can withstand a population-based design and shared decision making strategies can be implemented. However, the WHO advises that clinical breast examinations which are low-cost may be implemented if ongoing studies provide evidence for their efficacy. The WHO advises against creating a population-based screening program for women 40–49 and 70–75 [36].

In addition to mammography, magnetic resonance imaging (MRI) is used for breast cancer screening in a subset of the population. MRI uses electron magnets to create fields that change the alignment of the protons within the hydrogen atoms in the water and fat of tissue. As the proton changes the direction of its alignment it releases energy [37]. Fat, fibrous tissue, normal cells, and cancer release the proton energy differentially and the differences are analyzed to create an image. MRI is recommended by some for women who have a 20–25% lifetime risk for breast cancer [38]. This recommendation is not based on results from randomized controlled trials, but rather from the performance characteristics of MRI in women for whom standard digital mammography has not performed well.

In the United States, between 2000 and 2010, the number of women who received annual screening mammograms remained stable; however, variability across demographic characteristics persisted. Approximately 72.4% of women who were eligible based on age were screened in 2010. Screening rates were lowest among Asian women (64.1%), the uninsured (38.2%), individuals without usual source of care (36.2%), those in the United States less than 10 years (46.6%), and individuals with less than a high school certificate (58.3%) [39].

7.3.3 Cervical Cancer Screening

Large time series analyses within the population of Nordic countries have built a convincing case for the benefits of screening for cervical cancer [40,41]. Pap testing, the process of collecting and analyzing cells scraped from the cervix, and human papillomavirus (HPV) testing, the examination of the cervical cells for the HPV, have been demonstrated to be effective screening tools [8,25,42]. Although there is controversy associated with the effectiveness of visual inspection with acetic acid

(VIA; the application of acetic acid to the cervix and observing a color change to indicate abnormality) as compared to Pap, there is evidence to show that it is an inexpensive and effective screening tool in low-resourced settings where diagnosis and treatment are assured [43].

The USPSTF recommends a Pap smear every 3 years for women 21–65, or a combination of Pap smear and HPV testing every 5 years for women 30–65. The USPSTF advises against cervical cancer screening in the following groups: women 21 years or younger, women older than 65 who have had a history of screening and who are not at high risk for cervical cancer, and women who have had a hysterectomy and do not have a history of cervical cancer. The USPSTF does not consider screening effective if HPV testing is implemented alone or in combination with Pap smear in women younger than 30 years of age [8]. The WHO recommends that women 30 years and older get screened every 3–5 years; women who are 30–49 years are given screening priority. The WHO makes cervical cancer screening recommendations based on the context of the screening program and the resources available. In low-resourced regions where a screening program is in place and resources are available for subsequent tests, HPV testing and VIA are recommended, either in combination or alone. If a screening program is not in place, VIA alone is recommended. For programs that are able to provide colposcopy and cytology, cytology, or HPV testing followed by colposcopy is recommended [44]. Although a small dip in cervical cancer screening rates was observed between 2000 and 2010, approximately 83% of eligible American women (21–65 years old) reported getting the recommended Pap screening within 3 years according to the 2010 National Health Interview Survey (NHIS). Consistent with variability among demographic groups observed in mammography screening, Pap rates were lowest among Asian women (75.4%), uninsured women (63.8%), and women without usual source of care (64.9%) [39].

7.3.4 Colorectal Screening

Randomized controlled trials have demonstrated a benefit of colorectal cancer screening [45–47]. Flexible sigmoidoscopy, colonoscopy, and fecal occult blood testing (FOBT) have been shown to be effective tools at detecting both precancerous and cancerous polyps [48]. The USPSTF recommends colorectal screening with high sensitivity FOBT annually, sigmoidoscopy every 5 years with FOBT every 3 years, or screening with colonoscopy every 10 years for individuals aged 50–75. The USPSTF does not recommend routine screening for individuals aged 76–85 but it does recommend shared decision making in this age group, and it does not recommend screening for individuals older than 85 years of age [10]. Colorectal cancer screening varies globally. Many high- and middle-income countries have established guidelines for population-based screenings, whereas challenges still remain in low-income regions. The European Union currently only recommends FOBT for men and women aged 50–74, with screening intervals no more than 2 years apart; sigmoidoscopy no less than every 10 years and no more than 20 years only if performed in an organized program [49]. In the United States, colorectal screening rates significantly increased between 2000 and 2010. In 2010, 58.6% of adults reported having received one of the recommended colorectal screening tests. There was significant demographic variability in screening; Whites (59.8%), non-Hispanics (59.9%), individuals who are US born (60.5%), college graduates (67.3%), individuals with usual source of care (62.4%), and adults 67–74 years of age were more likely to be up to date [39].

7.3.5 Lung Cancer Screening

Lung cancer screening has only recently been approved as an effective method of screening in high-risk populations [9]. Early randomized controlled trials showed no mortality benefit of lung cancer screening using X-ray and sputum cytology [50]. However, more recent studies using low-dose computed tomography (CT) have shown it to be an effective method of identifying lung cancer at an early stage [51,52] and superior to radiography in reducing mortality [53]. The USPSTF recommends annual lung screening with low-dose CT for individuals 55–80 years of age who have a 30 pack-year smoking history and who currently smoke or have quit smoking within the past 15 years. Screening should be suspended for individuals who have not smoked for at least 15 years [9]. Although low-dose CT is currently in use in many low-, middle-, and high-income countries, there are currently no lung cancer screening recommendations by the WHO. This is based on the WHO's interpretation that for the global population, where resource use is also an important consideration, there is insufficient evidence that the benefits of using low-dose CT for lung cancer screening outweigh the harms [54]. Lung cancer screening rates are unavailable as the test was recently approved for population-level screening in the United States, but rates are expected to increase as the test is recommended to those at highest risk and the screening is now covered by insurance.

7.3.6 High-Risk Individuals

High-risk individuals; those who carry a genetic mutation (eg, *BRCA*, lynch syndrome); cancer survivors; individuals with HIV/AIDS or those who are immunosuppressed; or individuals who are at particular risk due to behavioral or environmental factors (eg, exposure to certain chemicals and radiation) need to consult with a physician to determine appropriate screening initiation and intervals [25,55–59].

7.4 THE PROCESS OF CARE

In order to better address challenges associated with screening, it is helpful to think of it as a process with multiple interacting players and pieces rather than simply a test. In this section we elaborate on the process of cancer screening and the ways that IT may be used to address failures in this process.

7.4.1 Screening Is a Process Not a Test

Screening entails a complex set of interactions within the multilevel context of care [60]. That context includes (1) the national policy and guidelines; (2) the community culture and expectations; (3) the organizational structure and culture where the screening is occurring; and (4) the individual patient culture, knowledge, and expectations [61]. The screening process includes multiple steps: offering screening, performing screening, and managing the follow-up after the screening test is performed. The latter must assure that those with abnormalities are evaluated and those with negative results are reassured while remaining appropriately vigilant for symptoms that should be evaluated. Interactions between patients and providers may vary within each step of testing, evaluation, and follow-up. All of these interactions may be further complicated by organizational and/or practice characteristics and system-level policies (Fig. 7.1).

Patient-Provider Interactions: An individual patient's desire to participate in the decision-making process during screening varies and can be influenced by individual characteristics such as age, education, and health knowledge [62]. Patient engagement is often affected by time constraints and providers are often faced with competing priorities such as managing chronic illnesses like hypertension, or cardiovascular disease. This may result in screening initiation either being delayed or never being initiated. It may also mean that patients are not able to make an informed choice.

Provider and Organizational Interactions: Characteristics of an organization including (1) culture, (2) organizational policies, including incentives, and (3) clinical information system may facilitate or inhibit a provider's screening patterns [63]. A study by Zapka et al. of 761 primary care providers in three different health organizations found that providers' perceptions of their organizations' policies and culture surrounding screening influenced their efforts to screen [64]. Although, there is some recent evidence for the effectiveness of incentive programs specifically in Pap screening, there has been insufficient evidence for their overall effectiveness [65,66].

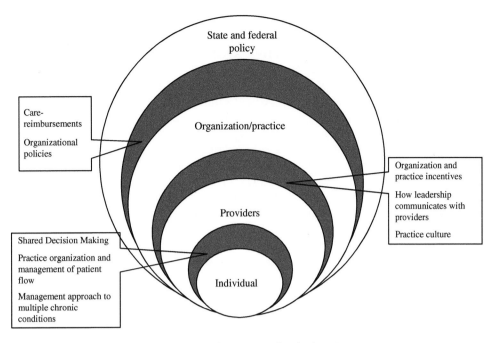

FIGURE 7.1 Multiple levels of interaction that occur during the process of early detection.

Organizational and State/Federal Policies: The ability of an individual to be screened may also be influenced by the interactions between organizations and larger sectors of influence such as federal or state policy. An analysis of Medicaid data from 46 states and the District of Columbia by Halpern and colleagues found that although there were mixed associations between increasing Medicaid reimbursements for screening tests and screening rates, there was a positive association between increasing Medicaid reimbursements for office visits and screening rates. Increasing reimbursements for office visits increased the odds of screening for breast, cervical, and colorectal cancers by 2–9% [67]. In addition, organizational policies that reduce the number of times that patients need to move between providers, that promote organized communication with patients, and that generally support continuity of care facilitate screening in practice [63].

7.4.2 Organized Versus Opportunistic Screening Programs

Because of the complexity of the screening process, there is a spectrum of implementation strategies from organized programs to opportunistic screening. Many high- and middle-income countries including the Netherlands, United Kingdom, Canada, Republic of Korea, and Argentina have organized screening programs. Organized programs are defined as those that actively invite eligible individuals from a target population usually based on age and geographical area. There

is usually a centralized management structure with responsibility for implementation of the steps of the screening process, and evaluation of its overall quality. They use systematic recall to provide follow-up care to individuals who are found to have an abnormal screening. They consistently provide quality assurance, and link their database with other systems, such as cancer registries and death registration systems, to monitor the effectiveness of their programs. The main goal of organized screening is to increase screening participation, and assure that test performance and treatment are achieving the expected outcomes. Services are usually provided for free and programs work to assure that participants all receive the same quality of care. On the contrary, many high-income countries such as the United States, France, Germany, and Japan have opportunistic screening programs. Screenings are provided on a patient request basis or are recommended by providers during routine care. Comparably organized screening programs have been shown to be more accurate and more cost-effective than unorganized programs [68,69].

7.5 THE CHALLENGE OF EARLY DETECTION

There are many ways in which a patient may enter the cancer detection process, and many factors that affect that entry and the progression to diagnosis. To evaluate these factors we use a multilevel ecological framework that examines how the individual, provider, and environment each influence early detection and cancer screening service utilization [70]. The problem of early detection, whether by screening or symptomatic presentation, is that it requires coordination across multiple steps of care and involves multiple providers [71]. An individual who needs to be screened must first have the opportunity to discuss their test options and preferences with their provider and then they must be provided the tests they choose. Ensuring that patients access appropriate tests could prove to be challenging under certain circumstances. For example, screening for cervical cancer may be initiated and completed in a primary care physician's office but mammography requires referral to a radiologist. Once an individual is screened they must be notified of any abnormalities, referred for additional evaluation when it is indicated, and then referred to the appropriate provider to initiate therapy if a cancer is detected. Across these multiple steps in care there are many opportunities for confusion among individuals seeking care and those that provide care thus leading to breakdowns in the screening process. Failure at any

point of the process limits the impact of early detection to reduce morbidity and mortality in persons with disease (Fig. 7.2). Organized screening programs are an attempt to prevent failures in the process by establishing an infrastructure to assure the steps occur. However, in the setting of heterogeneous models of care delivery, like the United States, a centrally organized national program is impossible. The closest the United States has come to an organized program is the National Breast and Cervical Early Detection Program, and even in this program delivery is organized through state centers [72]. Another common model of organized programs within the United States is managed care. Managed care organizations are able to centralize screening and outreach efforts, and monitor quality of care [73]. However, even under such a system, breakdowns still occur [74,75]. For example, in a population of women enrolled in a managed care plan for at least 3 years, more than half of the late-stage breast and invasive cervical cancers occurred among women who had not been screened (52% of late stage breast and 56% of invasive cervical cancers). Of those that initially screened negative, 39.5% and 32%

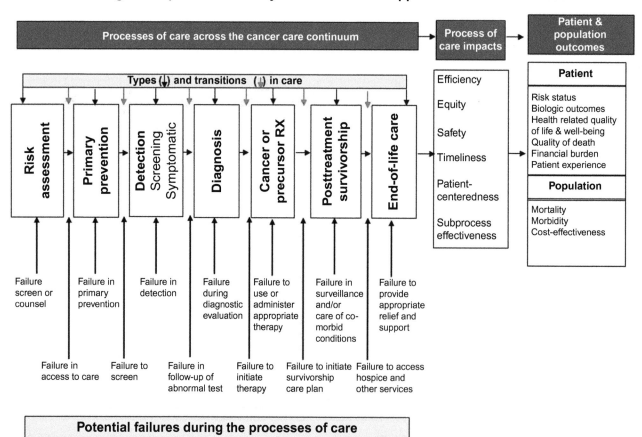

Linking the steps of care in early cancer detection: opportunities for informatics

FIGURE 7.2   Potential points of failure during screening and early detection. *Source: Adapted from [91] and [123].*

were later to be found to have late stage breast and invasive cervical cancers, respectively. In addition, between 8.8% and 13% screened positive but waited more than a year to get a diagnostic mammogram [73,75]. The questions then become, what contributes to these failures and can the causes be addressed by HIT?

7.5.1 Failure to Screen

To assess whether or not IT can remedy the problem, we must first look at the patient-level, provider-level, and system-level factors that lead to screening failures. The breakdowns associated with late-stage cancers can occur during the initiation of screening, during detection, or during follow-up of abnormal screening results. Several patient-level factors can impact whether they decide to participate in cancer screening. Some of these factors may be amenable to interventions including an individual's confidence in the test to detect an abnormality, how important they perceive screening to be in the absence of clinical symptoms, fear that an abnormality may be found, lack of knowledge of the test, and concerns over discomfort of the test [76,77]. Health care provider behavior may have screening promoting or inhibiting effects. Behaviors such as communication about family history and encouraging screening have been shown to be predictors of screening uptake [78]. Several studies have also shown that system-level factors are important to increasing screening [79]. One such factor is the electronic health record (EHR) system with provider reminders/provider prompts. This has been shown to encourage providers to offer screening during the course of care (inreach), and can impact their ability to send letters to patients' homes to remind them when they are due for screening (outreach). Both inreach and outreach reminders have been demonstrated to increase screening rates [80]. For the initiation of screening, HIT that educates and informs patients during decision making may be helpful. If patients are knowledgeable about the recommended screening and their risks for cancer, then they are better positioned to make an informed decision. Similarly, decision support tools that promote providers' knowledge and interaction with patients about the screening choices that exist could also be helpful. Finally, HIT may be useful to organizations by helping them aggregate the data of the patient population they serve in order to assess screening rates and to help cue them to screen patients through automated inreach or outreach reminders.

7.5.2 Failure to Detect

Assuming that screening occurs, there are still challenges associated with how the screening tests are performed [31,54]. There are several performance measures of the screening tests that must be considered and which have been associated with overdiagnosis and missed cases. A test's ability to identify cancer when it is present (sensitivity) and be negative when cancer is absent (specificity) has implications for false positive and false negative rates. The higher the sensitivity of a test, the fewer cancers are missed. Often a test can be made to be very sensitive. If radiologists called every screening mammogram abnormal they would find most cancers. But that is clearly not a successful strategy because many people without cancer would be referred for further evaluation and biopsy. Under these circumstances the test would have a low specificity. There is almost always a tradeoff between sensitivity and specificity so it is important to monitor each.

This tradeoff in sensitivity and specificity is driven by the fundamental characteristics of the test as well as the human factors associated with performing and interpreting it. There may be differences in how cells are collected and preserved at the time of Pap test or, how the technicians position a woman during a mammogram. Both affect the quality of the test. There may also be differences in the providers' ability to correctly interpret a test. Cytologists must review thousands of cells submitted in PAP tests and recognize those that are abnormal. Radiologists must recognize the 4–6 cancers in every thousand set of mammograms. Furthermore, that recognition is affected by patient characteristics like the density of the breast tissue, and the time since previous mammogram, which in turn affects the size of any tumor present [81,82]. There has been substantial hope that software installed in digital mammography machines, computer-assisted detection (CAD), would address the challenge of optimizing sensitivity and specificity, but the hope has not been realized. Sensitivity and specificity have not improved despite these efforts, though reimbursement for the service continues [83,84]. While the challenge is clear in mammography, variability in detection also exists for interpreting fecal immunochemical testing for evidence of blood in stool, performance of colonoscopy to identify polyps and cancers, or finding abnormal cells in a Pap smear [85–87]. CAD has been proposed for both Pap and colonoscopy interpretation but remains experimental [88,89].

7.5.3 Failure During the Follow-Up

Even if an abnormality is found during the screening process there may be failures that occur during the follow-up of abnormal test and during the diagnostic evaluation. These failures may be associated with individual-level factors including being low-income, perceptions of discrimination, the ability of the patient to understand and interpret the test results, and access to facilities that provide screening and evaluation services [90]. Failures may also be due to provider-level factors such as whether they perform the diagnostic evaluation correctly, and whether the results of the evaluation are communicated to the patient [90,91]. Communication, whether it be between the patient and provider, within an organization, or between organizations, appears to be a continuing thread in the failures observed in early detection and may be a point of intervention [92]. This is further explored in the chapter by Hesse, "Communication Science: Connecting Systems for Health." Here again, HIT offers an opportunity to improve the process by helping to ensure that providers are informed of which patients had an abnormal test result, which patients received a follow-up evaluation, and which patients need referral for cancer treatment. One challenge, however, is that the information that a primary care physician needs to assess the status of a patient in the screening process depends upon data that may be in multiple provider systems. For example, if a patient has an abnormal mammogram, the result is found in the radiology system. Easy transfer of that data to the referring physician depends upon having interoperable information systems. Interoperability of HIT is therefore fundamental to bridging the steps of the screening process that cross institutions and provider groups.

7.6 COMMUNICATION CHALLENGES

Challenges remain in linking all of the players and processes involved in early detection [63]. Much of the screening process depends on shared knowledge and interdependent activities that need to be executed with minimal confusion and anxiety for patients. HIT continues to hold promise for assisting in the process, but to fully achieve this promise more must be done to resolve institutional and human challenges [93]. For example, there is the fundamental human challenge of communication triangulation that must be addressed when managing the steps of screening or diagnosis (Fig. 7.3). Generally, a patient has at least two providers involved in screening, and almost always involved in the diagnosis of cancer. Once a screening test is ordered or an abnormality is found, the information must be shared in a manner that is easily understood by the patient and providers involved in executing the next step in care. If the patient is responsible for acting as liaison between their primary care physician and the provider responsible for the next step in the care process, there is potential for confusion. Similarly, if the providers communicate with each other and not the patient, there is also room for confusion. Care is more

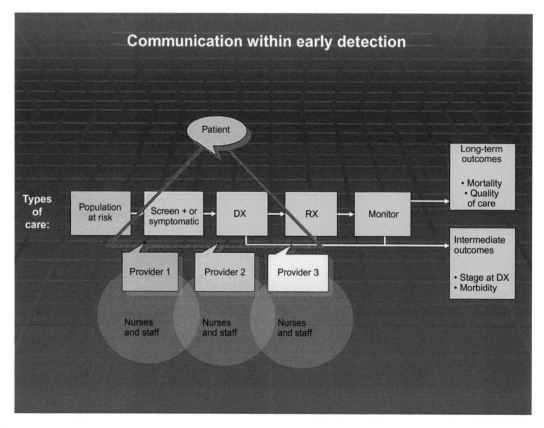

FIGURE 7.3 Communication between patients and providers during early detection.

supportive of the patient if there is joint understanding of the issues [94]. If individuals managing the work of early detection do not recognize their interdependence, they do not manage it well. Team researchers studying teamwork have recognized this for some time, and that recognition is now dawning in medical care [94,95]. As might be expected, some of the necessary work to understand the human factors involved in shared work is occurring outside of the technical world of HIT. The field of relational coordination, defined as a "mutually reinforcing process of communicating and relating for the purpose of task integration" is growing and providing evidence that the ways in which people interact greatly affects the quality and outcomes of their work [96]. The Agency for Healthcare Research and Quality (AHRQ) has developed a training program for teams in hospitals and has demonstrated reductions in medication errors when providers are trained to work in teams [97]. Metrics of relational coordination now exist to evaluate teamwork within and across organizations [96]. To further our knowledge in the field of relational coordination, we need to begin exploring how technology can support these human interactions.

A key strategy to support human interaction is minimizing information overload [93]. It is not sufficient to just remind physicians of their daily tasks; there is now strong evidence that information overload contributes to mistakes in health care settings [93]. HIT can be used to help track where individuals are positioned in the screening process (eg, due for screening, considering options, scheduling the screening test, due for follow-up) and identify the tasks the physician must complete. Ideally, HIT would only provide the most pertinent information and reminders at the appropriate times in the process while distributing the work among the team thereby reducing workload [93]. For example, if the providers within a practice discussed screening and came to a consensus on a practice-level policy regarding how they will implement screenings, the information system could help them accomplish this. Once a practice agrees on how they want to manage abnormal screening tests, the practice could clarify responsibilities of each team member. The team members could then jointly manage the steps in the screening process for multiple individuals under their care. The patient needs to be informed as to whether or not they are responsible for making the appointment to see the next provider in the process; if HIT could automatically generate appointments it would help alleviate patient responsibility and reduce failures in initiating follow-up. A key goal of HIT must be to sort information and reduce burden on practicing clinicians so they can concentrate on supporting their patients and their patients' families who are attending to abnormalities and/or treatments.

There is great deal of concern that HIT is not achieving this end and may in fact be contributing to workload. Primary care providers on average spend an extra hour in clinic after their scheduled work hours to complete medical records; few are satisfied with reminders for cancer screening (38% for breast, 37% for colorectal, and 31% for cervical); and most (54%) continue to use free text to document patient history [98]. One way to help address these provider challenges with using HIT is to have HIT developers spend time in clinical settings in order to help them understand the work that is being carried out before they begin to conceptualize and develop these tools [93]. When new tools are developed they need iterative, longitudinal testing to ensure that they facilitate work that is needed prospectively rather than retrospectively. Identifying potential barriers in the clinical setting may not be intuitive for HIT developers and others involved in the engineering of HIT, therefore it is imperative that physicians and other members of their team become more actively involved in the development of these tools.

Early detection is not an independent process but rather a process that it is nested within the overall delivery of care. Screening may take place as part of, or in conjunction with, preventive care services such as physical activity and diet counseling, or during the treatment of morbid conditions like hypertension or cardiovascular disease. While reminders can increase compliance with guidelines and reduce errors in recommending unnecessary testing or failing to recommend necessary testing, there is also evidence they are ignored 49–96% of the time [99]. Although HIT may offer solutions to help physicians prioritize tasks, simply alerting physicians that a patient is due for screening based on criteria such as age may create problems. Physicians may learn to ignore the reminders in the face of competing tasks. To rectify this issue, providers need to get input from patients to determine shared priorities, and then use HIT to help them realize those priorities.

Information systems could be used to document and remind both the physician and patient of their roles and responsibilities based on the priorities they set together. For example, in the short term, controlling hypertension is more important than providing information about screening; therefore reminders for patients to receive a checkup for hypertension could be sent prior to a reminder to obtain cancer screening. In addition to reinforcing shared established priorities for care, HIT could also reinforce guidelines. Providers need simple methods to establish and renew their guidelines to reflect the latest science and up-to-date options for an individual. When controversies regarding screening guidelines arise it should be easy to document the source of the controversy for physician reference without interrupting the course of care.

7.6.1 Use of IT in Early Detection

Screening is clearly a complicated process. Despite the push for HIT as a tool to improve the quality of health care delivery and to enable meaningful use of data at the patient and population levels [100], IT use in early detection has been quite limited and variable. The most common use of IT has been to gather data about the screening process. Using IT in this manner allows for the identification of factors that impact screening at the population-level that may not be readily apparent at the individual or organizational level. The Breast Cancer Surveillance Consortium (BCSC) has a 20-year history of using data collected in the course of screening mammography to evaluate how mammography works in clinical practice [101]. The BCSC has produced more than 400 articles that demonstrate the variation in performance, as well as improvement in mammography over time, and has become a major source of data for policy makers (www.breastscreening.cancer.gov consulted March 28, 2015). The BCSC is a good example of the potential for data collected in the course of clinical care to help generate insights that can improve clinical practice. Similarly, Population-based Research Optimizing Screening through Personalized Regimens (PROSPR) is a set of research organizations and health care providers that are collaborating and building several networks to capture data relevant to the screening process for breast, colorectal, and cervical cancers across the United States (www.Healthcaredelivery.cancer.gov/PROSPR, consulted March 28, 2015). There have also been comprehensive programs that have helped to: (1) identify who is due for screening among the thousands eligible; (2) mail reminders when an individual is due for screening; and (3) track those with abnormalities to be sure they are evaluated and treated [73]. However, these are the exceptions to the norm. Automated reminders that notify the physician in the course of a visit are more commonly used [80]. But these systems do not allow physicians to identify patients who did not receive follow-up care after an abnormal result. In 2007, about 16% of primary care physicians reported use of reminders for mammography, 16% for PAP tests, and 21% for colorectal cancer screening during the course of care [80]. More providers received a report regarding their screening level (30% mammography, 31% Pap testing, 12% colorectal cancer screening) but few receive information about failures in follow-up testing [80,90]. To fully support the entire screening process information systems must help identify the people who are due for screening and track them through the entire process [102].

Below are examples of how IT has been used to not only better understand failures in early detection but to address failures in the process. Cowburn and colleagues used electronic health record (EHR) data from Oregon and California community health centers to understand the association between cervical cancer screening and insurance status [103]. Others have used IT to assess quality measures of cancer screening within organizations. Friedberg and colleagues assessed structural factors at primary care practices and found that the use of EHRs were associated with higher performance outcomes including increased screening for breast and cervical cancers [104].

Green et al. found that participants who were tracked via EHR-linked mailings were two times more likely to be current on their colorectal cancer screening. The effects were more pronounced in participants who were contacted by an individual and guided through the steps in the screening process in addition to being tracked via EHR [105]. Interventions have also shown that IT can be used to help providers comply with screening guidelines [106,107].

The examples above have provided hints of the potential of IT to improve screening. The advent of funding for IT implementation in primary care has opened the door to more comprehensive approaches that may build on these examples. In 2009, the Health Information Technology for Economic and Clinical Health (HITECH) Act provided incentives for the adoption of EHRs. By December 2014, nearly 71% of primary care physicians had adopted some type of EHR (www.healthit.gov consulted March 28, 2015). The next section reveals four examples of exciting approaches to using IT to improve cancer screening in clinical practice.

7.7 EVIDENCE-BASED SOLUTIONS

7.7.1 Oregon Community Health Information Network

The Oregon Community Health Information Network (OCHIN) was constructed to support the implementation of EHRs in Federally Qualified Health Centers (FQHCs) and community clinics. They have central servers that support the use of a single commercial system (Epic) in more than 70 clinics that spread from California to Massachusetts. In this example, a research team is building and testing an intervention on the foundation of the Epic system supported by OCHIN.

The Strategies and Opportunities to Stop Colorectal Cancer (STOP CRC) study is a pragmatic trial to assess the effectiveness of EHR clinical decision support tools to improve rates of colorectal cancer screening in FQHCs. The STOP CRC intervention uses EHR-embedded reports to identify patients due for colorectal screening and mails them fecal FIT kits. The base program has three main steps: (1) mail an introductory and educational letter to patients meeting the correct criteria;

(2) mail FIT kits to patients due for screening; and (3) mail a reminder letter to anyone who has not returned a kit.

The primary analysis follows a cluster-randomized design that involves 26 clinics affiliated with 8 FQHCs, all of which use Epic© [108]. The project adapts the tools in All scripts© [109] and tests their implementation in four additional clinics affiliated with a single health center. Investigators sought to design user-friendly, adaptable, and scalable tools. The pragmatic study was based on a pilot showing a 38 percentage point increase in colorectal cancer screening when reminders were mailed directly to patients associated with one health center [110].

The investigators worked with OCHIN to build EHR tools that could perform key functions: (1) using real-time EHR data, *identify* patients due for colorectal cancer screening; (2) *enable clinic workflow* to support the mailing of reminders to patients (eg, lab ordering and address correction); and (3) *track* patients due for subsequent intervention steps or *follow-up* care of patients with abnormal test results [111].

While performing these functions, the software also supports new work processes. For example, it supports removing patients with invalid contact information or who are ineligible for screening, and allowing for lab orders to be placed outside of the typical workflow of in-clinic visits. The tools rely on direct electronic interface with the laboratory that processes the fecal tests, thus allowing for real-time updates to the registry.

In addition to customizing software that could do the above functions, this team also worked with the intervention clinics to develop the human activities that would use the IT functionality to augment, rather than replace, their care. Examples of the human functions were:

1. Clinic staff running reports that list all patients due for colorectal cancer screening based on specific criteria (eg, age and time since previous screening). The EHR identifies eligible patients at different time points (ie, when initially overdue, when a reminder is due weeks later).
2. Clinic staff reading reports and removing patients from the mailings when they contained invalid addresses or when flagged by clinicians as ineligible (Fig. 7.4).

The STOP CRC team used a participatory process to develop the software and engaged clinical staff to enhance the usability and acceptance of the tools. They gathered information in three ways: (1) One-on-one meetings with EHR site specialists to gather information on the current use of the EHR for documenting colorectal screening events; (2) 1- to 2-hour biweekly meetings with EHR tool developers, clinic staff (operations directors and EHR site specialists), and research staff, and three 4-hour work sessions to define the tool specifications; (3) monthly meetings with EHR site specialists and clinicians from each site to identify and prioritize needed refinements after the tools were implemented.

The program adds reporting and workflow capabilities to an existing EHR that tracks receipt of preventive care services (eg, Health Maintenance in Epic). Providers can therefore identify patients who are poor candidates for colorectal cancer screening and postpone Health Maintenance alerts; this removes ineligible patients

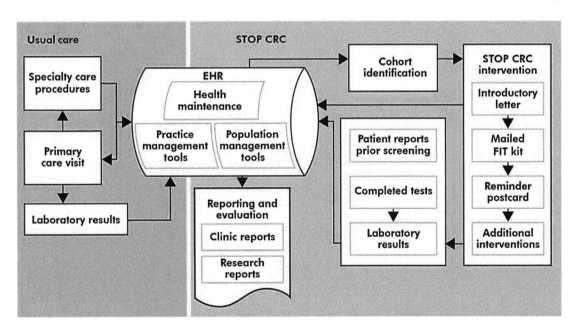

FIGURE 7.4 Schematic of OCHIN workflow.

from the list of those who need to get reminders for screening. Investigators identified additional functionality that would improve the program's efficiency, such as batch ordering FIT tests for a large group of patients at one time. They also modified the tools to be able to remind patients regardless of how they received their FIT, whether through the mail or during a clinic visit.

The team encountered several challenges that deserve mention. First, the inconsistent capture of historical colonoscopy limited their ability to identify patients due for screening. Primary care EHRs that link to claims data can confirm receipt of a colorectal procedure but provide no information on clinical findings. Clinically relevant information can often be found in scanned reports, rather than in discrete fields. Technological solutions are still needed to facilitate the transfer of clinically relevant data from specialty care to primary care.

In addition, programs delivered in safety net clinics face unique challenges identifying patient status. For example, the date of the most recent clinic visit is often used as proxy to determine whether a patient is established at a given clinic. STOP CRC faced additional challenges when ongoing changes in patients' insurance status and income levels complicated billing for tests performed outside of clinical encounters. To address this challenge, investigators limited eligibility to patients who had a clinic visit within the previous year. Ongoing quality assurance is imperative to ensure that programming scripts and algorithms function as intended.

Clinical decision support tools enable a direct-mail intervention to improve rates of colorectal cancer screening. The tools also provide opportunities for clinical teams to track and monitor their progress. Delivering colorectal cancer screening outside of the clinical encounter is thought to save time and reach a broader population as compared to delivering it during an in-person visit. Also, the ordering of a lab test for a group of patients identified as eligible deserves further exploration across EHR platforms. Refinements to the tools may be needed to deliver the right level of intervention; for example, patients who have been screened in the past are more likely to complete future screening, whereas those who have not may need further prompting. Well-designed decision support tools can enhance the sustainability of an intervention over the long run. Sustainability can be enhanced if the tools are amenable to being easily adapted to local contexts, for example, leveraging existing patient portals. Finally, engaging staff in tool development may aid in further refinement and adherence to the program.

7.7.2 New York State Department of Health

In the next example, the New York State Department of Health (NYSDOH) has designed an innovative model to increase screening across New York State (NYS) FQHCs

by linking FQHC data into a platform that FQHCs can use to compare screening across the state and within their practice; this database acts as a clinical information system, commonly referred to as a cancer screening registry, for connected FQHCs within the state.

With funding from the Centers for Disease Control and Prevention (CDC), the NYSDOH, in collaboration with the Community Health Care Association of New York State (CHCANYS), the state's Primary Care Association, and IPRO-Improving Healthcare for the Common Good, the Quality Improvement Organization for NYS, is implementing a 5-year demonstration project to evaluate the use of HIT and quality measurement to increase breast, cervical, and colorectal cancer screening rates among participating FQHCs. The project focuses on the development and use of a cancer screening registry within the CHCANYS Center for Primary Care Informatics (CPCI), a data warehouse and analytics and reporting solution that extracts information nightly from FQHC EHRs, calculates performance measures using uniform specifications, and features a dashboard with expanded functionality where FQHC staff can compare performance internally and to other connected FQHCs. The data warehouse also provides clinical workflow tools such as patient visit planning and referral management reports. Key project goals are to interface at least 75% of NYS's FQHCs to the CPCI, work through all of the project's phases with at least 36 FQHCs and their practice sites, and increase cancer screening rates across FQHCs by a minimum relative increase of 5–10% over baseline by June 2017.

As of January 2015, 35 FQHCs and their affiliated sites representing every region of the state, and 7 EHR products, are interfaced with the CPCI. Three cohorts are enrolled for targeted interventions. The first cohort of 12 FQHCs completed all initial phases of the project by December 2014. The first cohort represents 62 practice sites and a nearly 400,000 patient population eligible for cancer screening. Based on a baseline formal assessment in 2013, this cohort is high functioning in terms of HIT and Patient Centered Medical Home (PCMH)-recognition status; 56% had reached National Committee for Quality Assurance Level 3 PCMH status (an additional 23% reported working on achieving Level 3 status) and 75% have at least a half time equivalent person dedicated to meaningful use adoption. For baseline data validation, reviewers compared CPCI registry data with data available within EHRs. Of the total random sample of nearly 5700 EHR records reviewed in comparison to CPCI registry data, the rate of agreement between the two sources ranged from 78.5% to 83.2%, with the CPCI reporting screening rates that were 3–18% lower than manual review of the EHR.

Three categories of data quality errors leading to the inability to calculate accurate metrics were identified and became a focus of data quality improvement efforts: *erroneous inclusion/exclusions* (eg, inclusion of dental clinics in the count of practice sites); *inappropriate use of codes/data mapping* (eg, urine occult blood counting as a FOBT), and *inconsistent workflow processes* (eg, entering results in free text fields). Key findings of a precollaborative workflow survey completed by FQHC staff include the existence of cancer screening policies/protocols in each FQHC but variability in, or lack of, clear and consistent cancer screening recommendations, follow-up management protocols, and data documentation guidance. Common improvements by cohort 1 during the collaborative were:

1. Establishing policies and procedures to record data in EHR structured fields
2. Developing a center-wide comprehensive cancer screening policy
3. Offering fecal screening tests as an option for colorectal cancer screening
4. Utilizing additional CPCI functionality to establish workflows for patient visit planning and implementing use of brief previsit team huddles.

Over the course of the 12-month learning collaborative, aggregate screening rates, as reported by the Center for Primary Care Informatics (CPCI) across the first 12 FQHCs involved in this effort, increased respectively for breast, cervical, and colon cancer from 38.8 to 42.6%, 48.4 to 52.4%, and 28.0 to 43.5%. These absolute changes represent relative increases of 9.7, 8.3, and 55.4 percentage points. These improvements are likely the result of a combination of mapping fixes to the CPCI made based on data validation findings as well as data capture and clinical quality improvements implemented during the 12-month learning collaborative. Additional analyses are seeking to determine improvements that are attributable to the mapping fixes versus the learning collaborative quality improvement work that was instituted.

Challenges arising thus far include competing priorities at the FQHCs and maintaining workflow and data quality improvements long-term. These challenges are exacerbated by staff turnover, limited staff time, and EHR-related obstacles such as needing to continuously identify and correct mapping errors that arise as a result of EHR product or metric specification/payment code updates.

Preliminary data from an ongoing evaluation demonstrate the promise that the establishment of a planned approach to cancer screening across FQHCs can be supported by an EHR-based registry with additional focus on data quality as well as quality improvement coaching to improve clinical workflow. Initial results are consistent with previous studies [112,113]. Acknowledging that practice transformation requires more than a time-limited quality improvement intervention [113], future directions for this project include training and technical assistance to FQHCs in the use of CPCI/registry-based referral management and patient visit planning report tools, as well as development and training in the use of data self-validation tools. Sustainability of project outcomes will be dependent on a number of factors, including the provision of additional quality improvement coaching via the current project, other resources where possible, and assisting FQHCs to normalize new ways of working that were shown during the collaborative to improve outcomes and were deemed of value by clinical care teams and FQHC leadership.

7.7.3 Parkland Health and Hospital System

In this third example, the Parkland-UT Southwestern PROSPR Center, funded by the National Cancer Institute, has done a great deal of work around user-centered EHR design in order to follow a cohort of more than 70,000 primary care patients eligible for colorectal cancer screening.

In this urban, safety-net system, investigators developed and implemented the Parkland-UT Southwestern Colonoscopy Reporting System (CoRS), an EHR-based system that uses the *NoteWriter* feature in Epic (EHR, Epicare, Madison, WI) to match colonoscopic findings with guideline-consistent surveillance recommendations. This allows for the generation of tailored colonoscopy results and recommendation letters for both patients and referring physicians. CoRS was developed with input from a varied group of stakeholders including gastroenterology (GI) faculty, fellows, and laboratory staff; institutional leadership; primary-care providers; IT staff; and English- and Spanish-speaking patients.

Using features built into the system, colonoscopists are able to answer questions about the clinical encounters and pathology findings to determine appropriate follow up. Pathology results can be accessed through the Epic *In Basket* feature. Examples of questions include (1) the reason for the colonoscopy (screening, surveillance, or diagnostic); (2) whether the cecum was successfully intubated; (3) quality of the bowel prep; (4) family history of colorectal cancer; (5) number of polyps; and (6) the "worst" finding on the pathology report. The system then generates guideline-based follow-up [114,115]. To facilitate easy and accurate data collection, a "toggle bar" allows simultaneous access to the endoscopy and pathology reports while clinicians answer questions.

Once completed, CoRS generates a progress note documenting colonoscopy findings and surveillance recommendations in the EHR. This information is then available to all specialty providers as well as the referring physician and colonoscopist. In addition, tailoring algorithms in the Epic *NoteWriter* function generate a plain-language English and Spanish letter for both the referring provider and patient that contains the findings and recommendations for repeat screening or surveillance based on national guidelines [114,115]. When there is flexibility, users choose from several guideline-based intervals. For example, because current US Multi-Society Task Force on Colorectal Cancer guidelines recommend repeat colonoscopy any time within 3 years for 10 or more adenomatous polyps, users have an option of repeat colonoscopy in 3–6 months, 1, 2, or 3 years (but not 5 or 10 years). Patient letters are printed by administrative staff and sent via US mail and providers' versions of the letter are routed to their electronic in-boxes.

Colonoscopists quickly adopted CoRS. CoRS "went live" in December 2013 and in June 2014 investigators assessed its usability by surveying the 18 colonoscopists in the safety-net's GI practice (100% response) [116]. More than three-quarters agreed or strongly agreed that CoRS is easy to use (83%), provides guideline-based follow-up recommendations (89%), improves quality of Spanish-language letters (94%), and is something they would recommend for adoption at other institutions (78%). More than half agreed that the system led to improvement in the colorectal cancer screening practice (56%) and made their work easier (61%), with most of those who did not agree being neutral. Utilization was 84% during the first 6 months and increased to nearly 99% over the next 6 months. Most cases in which colonoscopists did not use it were within the first 60 days of implementation. Based on feedback from users, investigators worked to make slight amendments to CoRS during the first few months.

The Parkland-UT Southwestern CoRS is a novel EHR-based tool that is well-accepted by clinicians and provides guideline-based recommendations and standardized results communications to patients and providers. Continued stakeholder engagement of GI faculty and fellows during development and the early implementation period, along with live technical assistance, were crucial to improving acceptance and adoption for CoRS. Because of the overwhelmingly positive response, the University of Texas Southwestern is considering expanding CoRS for use with standard colonoscopies, rather than only those with polyps, and to implement it in the University practice, not just the safety-net system in which it was created.

7.7.4 Nebraska Department of Health and Human Services

In this final example, the Nebraska Department of Health and Human Services Women's and Men's Health Program has recently leveraged financial resources and talents from three CDC grants to support a new model of change within the state's health care system to increase breast, cervical, and colorectal cancers screenings rates. Data from 2013 for Nebraska's FQHCs show that screening rates vary widely between each facility, but are generally lower than comparable statewide estimates. Colorectal cancer screening rates at the FQHCs ranged from 5% to 42% compared to the state rate of 65%; cervical cancer screening rates ranged from 36% to 71% compared to the state rate of 77%; and breast cancer screening rates at the FQHCs ranged from 19% to 46% compared to state rate of 73%. This new model (referred to as the Community Health Hub (CHH) model) focuses on the state's FQHCs with some input from local health departments; all seven of Nebraska's FQHCs are participating.

Teams at each FQHC utilize three documents: (1) the *Clinic-Based Environmental Scan*; (2) the *Clinic-Community Resource Scan*; and (3) the *Evidence-Based Strategies*. These documents will help the teams capture information from their EHRs in order to establish baseline screening rates, describe the demographics of the clinic's client population, and set goals for improvements in screening rates and patient outcomes. These three documents were designed to work together to guide the process of change within each FQHC.

The *Environmental Scan* is an assessment of how each clinic environment supports screening utilization, follow-up, and referral as appropriate for abnormal findings. To complete the document, each FQHC must utilize its EHR, review clinic policies and standing orders around preventive screenings, review patient pathways to care within the clinic, and review education provided to patients concerning preventive screenings and their results. The *Clinic-Community Resource Scan* is designed for the FQHCs to perform a needs assessment of the resources and supports for healthy behaviors provided at the community level, including linkages between the community and the FQHC through existing referral mechanisms. This provides each FQHC with the opportunity to enumerate and evaluate existing resources and supports within the community and suggests possibilities for building new partnerships within the community. The *Evidence-Based Strategies* document provides the specific framework for systems change within each FQHC. Based on the summaries of the *Clinic-Based Environmental Scan* and the *Clinic-Community Resource Scan* documents, each FQHC identifies screening priorities and goals for the next phase of the project.

Utilizing the EHR is essential for implementing the strategies chosen—identifying clinic patients eligible for screening; documenting recalls, reminders, follow-up, and referrals for specialized care; documenting sources of referral to the clinic through community linkages; and quality improvement and evaluation.

Since the initiation of the project, two FQHCs are now in their second year of the CHH project. These two facilities have shown one-year gains from baseline across all three cancer screening tests. Cervical cancer screening rates increased an average of 13%, while the improvements in colorectal cancer screening rates were less impressive, averaging just 5%. Improvements in breast cancer screening rates showed the most variability, with an increase of 7% at one facility and 28% at the other.

Despite some initial successes, several challenges have caused delays in initiation of the process and in meeting deadlines for the required deliverables. Challenges have included staff turnover and shortages, and the availability of resources across the clinic sites. For example, three of the FQHCs serve large urban areas and these facilities have the largest staff and capacity to devote to the CHH project. The other four FQHCs serve rural populations and have a smaller number of staff, thereby making it difficult for them to split time between clinic duties and the CHH project.

Throughout the implementation process, the FQHCs have raised the issue of initiative fatigue. One potential solution may be the hiring of personnel to assist FQHCs on-site. Assistance could include providing expertise in areas such as data analysis, policy development, training, and quality improvement. For those FQHCs that are unable to fully utilize their EHR, technical assistance including instruction on the full range of features available within their EHR to monitor trends in screening within their clinic, and to evaluate the effect of the evidence-based strategies they introduce into their practice.

The interventions described above are great examples of ways that organizations are currently using IT to address the myriad of challenges in early detection. Using IT, OCHIN has developed an approach to help clinicians identify patients who have failed to screen. By engaging stakeholders, UT Southwestern is simplifying the process of follow-up and notifications for both physicians and patients. The Nebraska Department of Health and Human Services is using IT for process improvement and surveillance purposes. Finally, the NYSDOH is using IT to essentially create a cancer screening registry for the whole state. These are all great examples of how organizations at the local or state level can identify their own unique challenges associated with early detection and can address those challenges through IT.

7.8 CHALLENGES WITH USING IT

Although the examples above demonstrate ways that HIT is currently being used to reduce failures within the system, there are many challenges associated with the use of HIT. HIT may be used to improve follow-up of abnormal cancer screening, but if errors within the technology exist it may be rendered useless. Singh et al. conducted a mixed methods study to determine whether workflow-related or technical factors were associated with the lack of physician follow-up of 40% of positive FOBTs. They identified a technical error in the configuration of the EHR used by the facility in their study. After

correcting this technical problem, the lack of follow-up decreased nearly sixfold (29.9–5.4%) [117].

For example, EHR as a standalone may not impact quality of care; the context in which care is taking place needs to be evaluated. A study by Kern et al. assessed the effects of EHRs within PCMHs and found that the quality of care provided by physicians in PCMH groups was 6% higher than in the EHR group alone [118]. This suggests that other factors, such as organizational policies and practices in conjunction with EHR, may have synergistic effects on the quality of care. Although HIT in some ways was intended to improve physician workload, in many instances the use of EHR has been deemed burdensome. A study by Makam et al. found that 51% of providers surveyed in 11 internal medicine and family practices in Texas found the reminders generated by EHRs to be unreliable and inaccurate [98]. The issue of technology inhibiting workflow has also been raised. Although a sample of medical care providers considered a web-based decision aid for colorectal cancer as promising, there was concern about how to integrate this type of technology into the daily workflow [119]. Unexpected outcomes of using EHRs have also been observed in medical settings; this includes facilitating medical errors [120], unintentionally diverting resources from average-risk patients to high-risk or symptomatic patients [121], and despite attempts to improve racial/ethnic disparities, there is some evidence that the use of EHR alone may not reduce cancer screening disparities between White and non-White patients [122].

7.9 OVERCOMING DISPARITIES

While IT offers hope for addressing health disparities, there are limitations to what it can do. As noted in the examples above, OCHIN and Nebraska are working with FQHCs to address screening failures. Although the Affordable Care Act has increased access to screening exams for low-income populations, many low-income populations who do not have citizenship will be unable to access these services. Other ways that IT may not help to reduce disparities include organizational or personal resistance to the use of IT, and social and behavioral factors that create barriers to screening in general.

7.10 LOOKING TO THE FUTURE

There are large gaps between the potential and the realization of IT in practice. Some of those gaps are amenable to insights gained through research on how people work, what people want, and how shared knowledge is achieved. We need clinicians and health services researchers to identify what work needs to be done to address failures in the care process and to envision innovative ways that IT can help to address these failures. We also need a better understanding of the limitations of IT. Human-to-human communication (whether between two or more providers or between patients and providers) is paramount to ensuring that patients get quality care; therefore, it is important that we identify when communication is necessary across the trajectory of care, and move toward optimizing these interactions (using IT when strategic and/or appropriate) instead of assuming or expecting that IT will do this for us. Consideration of what is needed in the future benefits from a multilevel perspective: individuals, teams, and organizations. We need more information about how individuals access and use information efficiently in the course of care. This work needs to also examine how that access supports rather than hinders the relationships between provider and patients. How IT supports or hinders teamwork also needs closer examination so that shared work becomes easier. How organizations create physical structures that support the use of IT and link their IT to other organizations involved in care all need examination. Finally, we need more information about how IT can routinely aggregate the experience of patients in a care process and provide meaningful analysis and reporting so that the providers and organization continually improve care.

The use and benefits of IT in early detection is still in its infancy. A total of 71% of primary care providers now have EHR and that means we can begin to identify new problems and solutions. The next 20 years need to be devoted to reducing information burden, linking patients to the information they want, and to connecting all the providers involved in care to a common narrative about that care. Realizing the potential of IT will depend upon the active articulation of health care needs by the groups of people involved, active listening by the people developing the tools, and the recognition where IT can help and where humans need to use their unique abilities unencumbered by technology. We have only just begun.

LIST OF ACRONYMS AND ABBREVIATIONS

AHRQ Agency for Healthcare Research and Quality
BCSC Breast Cancer Surveillance Consortium
CAD Computer-assisted detection
CDC Centers for Disease Control and Prevention
CHCANYS Community Health Care Association of New York State
CHH Community Health Hub
CoRS Colonoscopy Reporting System
CPCI Center for Primary Care Informatics
CT Computed tomography
EHR Electronic health record
FQHC Federally Qualified Health Center
ER Estrogen positive

FIT Fecal immunochemical test
FOBT Fecal occult blood testing
FQHC Federally Qualified Health Center
GI Gastroenterology
HER2 Human epidermal growth factor receptor 2
HIT Health information technology
HITECH Health Information Technology for Economic and Clinical Health
HPV Human papillomavirus
IARC International Agency for Research on Cancer
IT Information technology
MRI Magnetic resonance imaging
NHIS National Health Interview Survey
NYS New York State
NYSDOH New York State Department of Health
OCHIN Oregon Community Health Information Network
PCMH Patient Centered Medical Home
PR Progesterone positive
PROSPR Population-based Research Optimizing Screening through Personalized Regimens
STOP CRC Strategies and Opportunities to Stop Colorectal Cancer
USPSTF United States Preventive Services Task Force
VIA Visual inspection with acetic acid
WHO World Health Organization

Acknowledgments

The authors would like to acknowledge the following individuals and organizations for their contribution to the projects featured in this chapter.

OCHIN: Beverly B Green, MD, MPH; Jen Coury, MA; Amanda F. Petrik, MS.

Parkland: Katharine McCallister; Wendy Bishop, MS; Joanne M. Sanders, MS; Samir Gupta, MD; Ethan A. Halm, MD; Amit G. Singal, MD; Shaun Wright, BS.

New York State Department of Health: Ian Brissette, PhD; Erin Shortt, MPH; Gina O'Sullivan, MPH; Lisa Perry, MPP, MBA; Kathy Alexis, MPH, CHES; Diane Ferran, MD, MPH; Shoshanna Levine, MPH, CPH; Alan Silver, MD, MPH; Veronica Pryor, RN, BSN, MPA; Ti-Kuang Lee, Sc.M.; Thomas Huang, BS, MS.

Nebraska Department of Health and Human Services:
Bryan Rettig, MS; Charles Drew Health Center; Community Action Partnership of Western Nebraska Health Center; Good Neighbor Community Health Center; Heartland Health Center; Midtown Health Center; OneWorld Community Health Centers, Inc.; People's Health Center.

Disclaimer: The opinions expressed here are those of the authors and cannot be construed to reflect the views of NCI or the Federal Government.

References

[1] Hoyert DL, Xu J. Deaths: preliminary data for 2011. Natl Vital Stat Rep 2012;61(6):1–51.
[2] Mariotto AB, Yabroff KR, Shao Y, Feuer EJ, Brown ML. Projections of the cost of cancer care in the United States: 2010–2020. J Natl Cancer Inst 2011;103(2):117–28.
[3] Bradley CJ, Yabroff KR, Dahman B, Feuer EJ, Mariotto A, Brown ML. Productivity costs of cancer mortality in the United States: 2000–2020. J Natl Cancer Inst 2008;100(24):1763–70.
[4] Ferlay J, Soerjomataram I, Dikshit R, et al. Cancer incidence and mortality worldwide: sources, methods and major patterns in GLOBOCAN 2012. Int J Cancer 2015;136(5):E359–86.

[5] Rastogi T, Hildesheim A, Sinha R. Opportunities for cancer epidemiology in developing countries. Nat Rev Cancer 2004;4(11):909–17.

[6] Kanavos P. The rising burden of cancer in the developing world. Ann Oncol 2006;17(Suppl. 8):viii15–viii23.

[7] Nelson HD, Tyne K, Naik A, Bougatsos C, Chan BK, Humphrey L. Screening for breast cancer: an update for the U.S. Preventive Services Task Force. Ann Intern Med 2009;151(10):727–42.

[8] Moyer VA. Screening for cervical cancer: U.S. Preventive Services Task Force recommendation statement. Ann Intern Med 2012;156(12):880–91. W312.

[9] Moyer VA. Screening for lung cancer: U.S. Preventive Services Task Force recommendation statement. Ann Intern Med 2014;160(5): 330–8.

[10] Whitlock EP. Screening for colorectal cancer: a targeted, updated systematic review for the U.S. Preventive Services Task Force. Ann Intern Med 2008;149(9):638–58.

[11] Nelson HD, Tyne K, Naik A, Bougatsos C, Chan BK, Humphrey L. Screening for breast cancer: an update for the U.S. Preventive Services Task Force. Ann Intern Med 2009;151(10):727–42.

[12] HRSA. What is health IT? <http://www.hrsa.gov/healthit/toolbox/oralhealthittoolbox/introduction/whatishealthit.html/> [accessed 30.07.15].

[13] Siegel R, Ma J, Zou Z, Jemal A. Cancer statistics, 2014. CA Cancer J Clin 2014;64(1):9–29.

[14] Howlader N, Noone A, Krapcho M, et al. SEER cancer statistics review, 1975–2008, vol. 19. Bethesda, MD: National Cancer Institute; 2011.

[15] Edwards BK, Noone AM, Mariotto AB, et al. Annual report to the nation on the status of cancer, 1975–2010, featuring prevalence of comorbidity and impact on survival among persons with lung, colorectal, breast, or prostate cancer. Cancer 2014;120(9): 1290–314.

[16] Sorlie T, Perou CM, Tibshirani R, et al. Gene expression patterns of breast carcinomas distinguish tumor subclasses with clinical implications. Proc Natl Acad Sci U S A 2001;98(19):10869–74.

[17] Dunnwald LK, Rossing MA, Li CI. Hormone receptor status, tumor characteristics, and prognosis: a prospective cohort of breast cancer patients. Breast Cancer Res 2007;9(1):R6.

[18] Hudis CA. Trastuzumab—mechanism of action and use in clinical practice. N Engl J Med 2007;357(1):39–51.

[19] Tao L, Gomez SL, Keegan TH, Kurian AW, Clarke CA. Breast cancer mortality in African-American and non-Hispanic white women by molecular subtype and stage at diagnosis: a population-based study. Cancer Epidemiol Biomarkers Prev 2015;24(7): 1039–45.

[20] Ly M, Antoine M, Dembele AK, et al. High incidence of triple-negative tumors in sub-Saharan Africa: a prospective study of breast cancer characteristics and risk factors in Malian women seen in a Bamako university hospital. Oncology 2012;83(5):257–63.

[21] Adegoke O, Kulasingam S, Virnig B. Cervical cancer trends in the United States: a 35-year population-based analysis. J Womens Health 2012;21(10):1031–7.

[22] Benard VB, Thomas CC, King J, Massetti GM, Doria-Rose VP, Saraiya M. Vital signs: cervical cancer incidence, mortality, and screening-United States, 2007–2012. MMWR Morb Mortal Wkly Rep 2014;63(44):1004–9.

[23] Underwood JM, Townsend JS, Tai E, et al. Racial and regional disparities in lung cancer incidence. Cancer 2012;118(7):1910–8.

[24] Winawer SJ, Zauber AG, Ho MN, et al. Prevention of colorectal cancer by colonoscopic polypectomy. The national polyp study workgroup. N Engl J Med 1993;329(27):1977–81.

[25] Schiffman M, Castle PE, Jeronimo J, Rodriguez AC, Wacholder S. Human papillomavirus and cervical cancer. Lancet 2007;370(9590):890–907.

[26] Wilson JMG, Jungner G, Principles and practice of screening for disease. Geneva: Public Health Papers (34). World Health Organization; 1968. p. 9–17.

[27] Poplack SP, Tosteson AN, Grove MR, Wells WA, Carney PA. Mammography in 53,803 women from the New Hampshire Mammography Network. Radiology 2000;217(3):832–40.

[28] Hill DA, Nibbe A, Royce ME, et al. Method of detection and breast cancer survival disparities in Hispanic women. Cancer Epidemiol Biomarkers Prev 2010;19(10):2453–60.

[29] Gill MD, Bramble MG, Hull MA, et al. Screen-detected colorectal cancers are associated with an improved outcome compared with stage-matched interval cancers. Br J Cancer 2014;111(11):2076–81.

[30] Herbert A, Anshu Gregory M, Gupta SS, Singh N. Invasive cervical cancer audit: a relative increase in interval cancers while coverage increased and incidence declined. BJOG Int J Obstet Gynaecol 2009;116(6):845–53.

[31] Gotzsche PC, Jorgensen KJ. Screening for breast cancer with mammography. Cochrane Database Syst Rev 2013;6:CD001877.

[32] Tabar L, Vitak B, Chen HH, et al. The Swedish two-county trial twenty years later. Updated mortality results and new insights from long-term follow-up. Radiol Clin North Am 2000;38(4):625–51.

[33] Tabar L, Vitak B, Chen TH, et al. Swedish two-county trial: impact of mammographic screening on breast cancer mortality during 3 decades. Radiology 2011;260(3):658–63.

[34] Mandelblatt JS, Cronin KA, Bailey S, et al. Effects of mammography screening under different screening schedules: model estimates of potential benefits and harms. Ann Intern Med 2009;151(10):738–47.

[35] Pisano ED, Gatsonis C, Hendrick E, et al. Diagnostic performance of digital versus film mammography for breast-cancer screening. N Engl J Med 2005;353(17):1773–83.

[36] Bramley D, Murad HM, Sepulveda C, Heneghan C, Gartlehner G, Norris S. WHO position paper on mammography screening. Geneva: World Health Organization; 2014.

[37] Edelman RR, Warach S. Magnetic resonance imaging (2). N Engl J Med 1993;328(11):785–91.

[38] Saslow D, Boetes C, Burke W, et al. American cancer society guidelines for breast screening with MRI as an adjunct to mammography. CA Cancer J Clin 2007;57(2):75–89.

[39] Center for Disease Control and Prevention Cancer screening—United States, 2010. MMWR Morb Mortal Wkly Rep 2012;61(3): 41–5.

[40] Day NE. Effect of cervical cancer screening in Scandinavia. Obstet Gynecol 1984;63(5):714–8.

[41] Bigaard J, Hariri J, Lynge E. Cervical cancer screening in Denmark. Eur J Cancer 2000;36(17):2198–204.

[42] Ronco G, Dillner J, Elfström KM, et al. Efficacy of HPV-based screening for prevention of invasive cervical cancer: follow-up of four European randomised controlled trials. Lancet 2014;383(9916):524–32.

[43] Sankaranarayanan R, Esmy PO, Rajkumar R, et al. Effect of visual screening on cervical cancer incidence and mortality in Tamil Nadu, India: a cluster-randomised trial. Lancet 2007;370(9585):398–406.

[44] Broutet N, WHO Guideline Development Group, WHO Methods Group, and WHO External Review Group. WHO guidelines for screening and treatment of precancerous lesions for cervical cancer prevention. Geneva: World Health Organization; 2013.

[45] Mandel JS, Bond JH, Church TR, et al. Reducing mortality from colorectal cancer by screening for fecal occult blood. Minnesota Colon Cancer Control Study. N Engl J Med 1993;328(19): 1365–71.

[46] Hardcastle JD, Chamberlain JO, Robinson MHE, et al. Randomised controlled trial of faecal-occult-blood screening for colorectal cancer. Lancet 1996;348(9040):1472–7.

[47] Kronborg O, Fenger C, Olsen J, Jørgensen OD, Søndergaard O. Randomised study of screening for colorectal cancer with faecal-occult-blood test. Lancet 1996;348(9040):1467–71.

[48] Zauber AG, Lansdorp-Vogelaar I, Knudsen AB, Wilschut J, van Ballegooijen M, Kuntz KM. Evaluating test strategies for colorectal cancer screening: a decision analysis for the U.S. preventive services task force. Ann Intern Med 2008;149(9):659–69.

[49] The Blue Sheet. Chevy Chase MD: F - D- C Reports, Inc., 1996.

[50] Marcus PM, Bergstralh EJ, Fagerstrom RM, et al. Lung cancer mortality in the Mayo Lung Project: impact of extended follow-up. J Natl Cancer Inst 2000;92(16):1308–16.

[51] Henschke CI, McCauley DI, Yankelevitz DF, et al. Early Lung Cancer Action Project: overall design and findings from baseline screening. Lancet 1999;354(9173):99–105.

[52] Humphrey LL, Deffebach M, Pappas M, et al. Screening for lung cancer with low-dose computed tomography: a systematic review to update the US Preventive Services Task Force recommendation. Ann Intern Med 2013;159(6):411–20.

[53] Aberle DR, Adams AM, Berg CD, et al. Reduced lung-cancer mortality with low-dose computed tomographic screening. N Engl J Med 2011;365(5):395–409.

[54] Bach PB, Mirkin JN, Oliver TK, et al. Benefits and harms of CT screening for lung cancer: a systematic review. JAMA 2012;307(22): 2418–29.

[55] Easton DF. How many more breast cancer predisposition genes are there? Breast Cancer Res 1999;1(1):14–17.

[56] Campeau PM, Foulkes WD, Tischkowitz MD. Hereditary breast cancer: new genetic developments, new therapeutic avenues. Hum Genet 2008;124(1):31–42.

[57] Johns LE, Houlston RS. A systematic review and meta-analysis of familial colorectal cancer risk. Am J Gastroenterol 2001;96(10):2992–3003.

[58] Grulich AE, van Leeuwen MT, Falster MO, Vajdic CM. Incidence of cancers in people with HIV/AIDS compared with immunosuppressed transplant recipients: a meta-analysis. Lancet 2007;370(9581):59–67.

[59] Engels EA, Biggar RJ, Hall HI, et al. Cancer risk in people infected with human immunodeficiency virus in the United States. Int J Cancer 2008;123(1):187–94.

[60] Taplin SH, Dash S, Zeller P, Zapka J. Screening. New York, NY: Springer; 2006.

[61] Taplin SH, Clauser S, Rodgers AB, Breslau E, Rayson D. Interfaces across the cancer continuum offer opportunities to improve the process of care. J Natl Cancer Inst Monogr 2010;2010(40):104–10.

[62] Hanoch Y, M-ST Rolison JJ, Omer Z, Ozanne E. Shared decision making in patients at risk of cancer: the role of domain and numeracy. Health Expect 2014;18:2799–810.

[63] Anhang Price R, Zapka J, Edwards H, Taplin SH. Organizational factors and the cancer screening process. J Natl Cancer Inst Monogr 2010;2010(40):38–57.

[64] Zapka JG, Puleo E, Taplin S, et al. Breast and cervical cancer screening: clinicians' views on health plan guidelines and implementation efforts. J Natl Cancer Inst Monogr 2005;2005(35):46–54.

[65] Sabatino SA, Lawrence B, Elder R, et al. Effectiveness of interventions to increase screening for breast, cervical, and colorectal cancers: nine updated systematic reviews for the guide to community preventive services. Am J Prev Med 2012;43(1):97–118.

[66] Kaczorowski J, Hearps SJ, Lohfeld L, et al. Effect of provider and patient reminders, deployment of nurse practitioners, and financial incentives on cervical and breast cancer screening rates. Can Fam Physician 2013;59(6):e282–9.

[67] Halpern MT, Romaire MA, Haber SG, Tangka FK, Sabatino SA, Howard DH. Impact of state-specific Medicaid reimbursement and eligibility policies on receipt of cancer screening. Cancer 2014;120(19):3016–24.

[68] Sankaranarayanan R. Screening for cancer in low- and middle-income countries. Ann Glob Health 2014;80(5):412–7.

[69] Miles A, Cockburn J, Smith RA, Wardle J. A perspective from countries using organized screening programs. Cancer 2004;101(5 Suppl):1201–13.

[70] Phillips KA, Morrison KR, Andersen R, Aday LA. Understanding the context of healthcare utilization: assessing environmental and provider-related variables in the behavioral model of utilization. Health Serv Res 1998;33(3 Pt 1):571–96.

[71] Zapka J, Taplin SH, Ganz P, Grunfeld E, Sterba K. Multilevel factors affecting quality: examples from the cancer care continuum. J Natl Cancer Inst Monogr 2012;2012(44):11–19.

[72] Lee NC, Wong FL, Jamison PM, et al. Implementation of the national breast and cervical cancer early detection program: the beginning. Cancer 2014;120(Suppl. 16):2540–8.

[73] Taplin SH, Ichikawa L, Buist DS, Seger D, White E. Evaluating organized breast cancer screening implementation: the prevention of late-stage disease? Cancer Epidemiol Biomarkers Prev 2004;13(2):225–34.

[74] Taplin SH, Ichikawa L, Yood MU, et al. Reason for late-stage breast cancer: absence of screening or detection, or breakdown in follow-up? J Natl Cancer Inst 2004;96(20):1518–27.

[75] Leyden WA, Manos MM, Geiger AM, et al. Cervical cancer in women with comprehensive health care access: attributable factors in the screening process. J Natl Cancer Inst 2005;97(9):675–83.

[76] van Dam L, Korfage IJ, Kuipers EJ, et al. What influences the decision to participate in colorectal cancer screening with faecal occult blood testing and sigmoidoscopy? Eur J Cancer Prev 2013;49(10):2321–30.

[77] Taplin SH, Montano DE. Attitudes, age, and participation in mammographic screening: a prospective analysis. J Am Board Fam Pract 1993;6(1):13–23.

[78] Courtney RJ, Paul CL, Sanson-Fisher RW, et al. Individual- and provider-level factors associated with colorectal cancer screening in accordance with guideline recommendation: a community-level perspective across varying levels of risk. BMC Public Health 2013;13:248.

[79] Stone EG, Morton SC, Hulscher ME, et al. Interventions that increase use of adult immunization and cancer screening services: a meta-analysis. Ann Intern Med 2002;136(9):641–51.

[80] Yabroff KR, Zapka J, Klabunde CN, et al. Systems strategies to support cancer screening in U.S. primary care practice. Cancer Epidemiol Biomarkers Prev 2011;20(12):2471–9.

[81] Carney PA, Miglioretti DL, Yankaskas BC, et al. Individual and combined effects of age, breast density, and hormone replacement therapy use on the accuracy of screening mammography. Ann Intern Med 2003;138(3):168–75.

[82] Yankaskas BC, Taplin SH, Ichikawa L, et al. Association between mammography timing and measures of screening performance in the United States. Radiology 2005;234(2):363–73.

[83] Fenton JJ, Taplin SH, Carney PA, et al. Influence of computer-aided detection on performance of screening mammography. N Engl J Med 2007;356(14):1399–409.

[84] Fenton JJ, Xing G, Elmore JG, et al. Short-term outcomes of screening mammography using computer-aided detection: a population-based study of medicare enrollees. Ann Intern Med 2013;158(8):580–7.

[85] Young GP, Symonds EL, Allison JE, et al. Advances in fecal occult blood tests: the fit revolution. Dig Dis Sci 2015;60(3):609–22.

[86] Robertson DJ, Kaminski MF, Bretthauer M. Effectiveness, training and quality assurance of colonoscopy screening for colorectal cancer. Gut 2015;64(6):982–90.

[87] Zhao L, Wentzensen N, Zhang RR, et al. Factors associated with reduced accuracy in Papanicolaou tests for patients with invasive cervical cancer. Cancer Cytopathol 2014;122(9):694–701.

[88] Summers RM, Yao J, Pickhardt PJ, et al. Computed tomographic virtual colonoscopy computer-aided polyp detection in a screening population. Gastroenterology 2005;129(6):1832–44.

[89] Bengtsson E, Malm P. Screening for cervical cancer using automated analysis of PAP-smears. Comput Math Methods Med 2014;2014:842037.

[90] Zapka J, Taplin SH, Price RA, Cranos C, Yabroff R. Factors in quality care—the case of follow-up to abnormal cancer screening tests—problems in the steps and interfaces of care. J Natl Cancer Inst Monogr 2010;2010(40):58–71.

[91] Zapka JG, Taplin SH, Solberg LI, Manos MM. A framework for improving the quality of cancer care: the case of breast and cervical cancer screening. Cancer Epidemiol Biomarkers Prev 2003;12(1):4–13.

[92] Zapka JG, Puleo E, Taplin SH, et al. Processes of care in cervical and breast cancer screening and follow-up—the importance of communication. Prev Med 2004;39(1):81–90.

[93] Karsh B-T. Clinical practice improvement and redesign: how change in workflow can be supported by clinical decision support. Rockville, MD: AHRQ; 2009. 43 pages Publication No. 09-0054-EF.

[94] Taplin SH, Weaver S, Chollette V, et al. Teams and teamwork during a cancer diagnosis: interdependency within and between teams. J Oncol Pract 2015;11(3):231–8.

[95] Taplin SH, Weaver S, Salas E, et al. Reviewing cancer care team effectiveness. J Oncol Pract 2015;11(3):239–46.

[96] Gittell JH, Beswick J, Goldmann D, Wallack SS. Teamwork methods for accountable care: relational coordination and TeamSTEPPS(R). Health Care Manage Rev 2015;40(2):116–25.

[97] King HB, Battles J, Baker DP, et al. TeamSTEPPS: team strategies and tools to enhance performance and patient safety. In: Henriksen K, Battles JB, Keyes MA, Grady ML, editors. Advances in patient safety: new directions and alternative approaches (Vol 3: Performance and Tools). Rockville (MD): Agency for Healthcare Research and Quality; 2008.

[98] Makam AN, Lanham HJ, Batchelor K, et al. Use and satisfaction with key functions of a common commercial electronic health record: a survey of primary care providers. BMC Med Inform Decis Mak 2013;13:86.

[99] MQSA (Mammography Quality Standards Act) final rule released. American College of Radiology. Radiol Manage 1998;20(4):51–5.

[100] (PCAST) PCoAoSaT. Report to the president realizing the full potential of health information technology to improve healthcare for Americans: the path forward; 2010.

[101] Ballard-Barbash R, Taplin SH, Yankaskas BC, et al. Breast Cancer Surveillance Consortium: a national mammography screening and outcomes database. AJR Am J Roentgenol 1997;169(4):1001–8.

[102] Taplin SH, Rollason D, Camp A, diDonato K, Maggenheimer E. Imagining an electronic medical record for turning cancer screening knowledge into practice. Am J Prev Med 2010;38(1):89–97.

[103] Cowburn S, Carlson MJ, Lapidus JA, DeVoe JE. The association between insurance status and cervical cancer screening in community health centers: exploring the potential of electronic health records for population-level surveillance, 2008–2010. Prev Chronic Dis 2013;10:E173.

[104] Friedberg MW, Coltin KL, Safran DG, Dresser M, Zaslavsky AM, Schneider EC. Associations between structural capabilities of primary care practices and performance on selected quality measures. Ann Intern Med 2009;151(7):456–63.

[105] Green BB, Wang CY, Anderson ML, et al. An automated intervention with stepped increases in support to increase uptake of colorectal cancer screening: a randomized trial. Ann Intern Med 2013;158(5 Pt 1):301–11.

[106] Broach V, Day L, Barenberg B, Huang S, Kenton K, White P. Use of electronic health record-based tools to improve appropriate use of the human papillomavirus test in adult women. J Low Genit Tract Dis 2014;18(1):26–30.

[107] White P, Kenton K. Use of electronic medical record-based tools to improve compliance with cervical cancer screening guidelines: effect of an educational intervention on physicians' practice patterns. J Low Genit Tract Dis 2013;17(2):175–81.

[108] Epic, inventor. Verona, WI United States. 2014.

[109] Scripts A, Inventor. Chicago, IL United States. 2014.

[110] Coronado GD, Vollmer WM, Petrik A, et al. Strategies and opportunities to STOP colon cancer in priority populations: pragmatic pilot study design and outcomes. BMC Cancer 2014;14:55.

[111] Coronado GD, Burdick T, Petrik A, Kapka T, Retecki S, Green B. Using an automated data-driven, EHR-embedded program for mailing fit kits: lessons from the STOP CRC pilot study. J Gen Pract 2014;2.

[112] Taplin SH, Haggstrom D, Jacobs T, et al. Implementing colorectal cancer screening in community health centers: addressing cancer health disparities through a regional cancer collaborative. Med Care 2008;46(9 Suppl. 1):S74–83.

[113] Shaw EK, Ohman-Strickland PA, Piasecki A, et al. Effects of facilitated team meetings and learning collaboratives on colorectal cancer screening rates in primary care practices: a cluster randomized trial. Ann Fam Med 2013;11(3):220–8. S1-8.

[114] Winawer SJ, Zauber AG, Fletcher RH, et al. Guidelines for colonoscopy surveillance after polypectomy: a consensus update by the US Multi-Society Task Force on Colorectal Cancer and the American Cancer Society. CA Cancer J Clin 2006;56(3):143–59. quiz 84–5.

[115] Lieberman DA, Rex DK, Winawer SJ, et al. Guidelines for colonoscopy surveillance after screening and polypectomy: a consensus update by the US Multi-Society Task Force on Colorectal Cancer. Gastroenterology 2012;143(3):844–57.

[116] Skinner CS, Gupta S, Halm E, et al. Development of the Parkland-UT Southwestern Colonoscopy Reporting System (CoRS) for evidence-based colon cancer surveillance recommendations. JAMIA 2015.

[117] Singh H, Wilson L, Petersen LA, et al. Improving follow-up of abnormal cancer screens using electronic health records: trust but verify test result communication. BMC Med Inform Decis Mak 2009;9:49.

[118] Kern LM, Edwards A, Kaushal R. The patient-centered medical home, electronic health records, and quality of care. Ann Intern Med 2014;160(11):741–9.

[119] Jimbo M, Shultz CG, Nease DE, Fetters MD, Power D, Ruffin IV MT. Perceived barriers and facilitators of using a Web-based interactive decision aid for colorectal cancer screening in community practice settings: findings from focus groups with primary care clinicians and medical office staff. J Med Internet Res 2013;15(12):e286.

[120] Koppel R, Metlay JP, Cohen A, et al. Role of computerized physician order entry systems in facilitating medication errors. JAMA 2005;293(10):1197–203.

[121] Bian J, Bennett CL, Fisher DA, Ribeiro M, Lipscomb J. Unintended consequences of health information technology: evidence from veterans affairs colorectal cancer oncology watch intervention. J Clin Oncol 2012;30(32):3947–52.

[122] Mishuris RG, Linder JA. Racial differences in cancer screening with electronic health records and electronic preventive care reminders. J Am Med Inform Assoc 2014;21(e2):e264–9.

[123] Taplin SH, Rodgers AB. Toward improving the quality of cancer care: addressing the interfaces of primary and oncology-related subspecialty care. J Natl Cancer Inst Monogr 2010;(40):3–10.

8

Informatics Support Across the Cancer Continuum: Treatment

Bradford Hirsch MD, MBA and *Amy P. Abernethy MD, PhD*

Flatiron Health, New York, NY, United States

O U T L I N E

8.1 Overview   145
  8.1.1 Evidentiary Uncertainty   146
  8.1.2 Limitations of Guidelines   147
  8.1.3 Balancing Survival and Quality of Life 147
  8.1.4 Market Evolution   148

8.2 Data Aggregation   148
  8.2.1 Providers and Networks   148
  8.2.2 Tumor Registries   148
  8.2.3 Secondary Data Sources   149
  8.2.4 Translating Data Into Action   149

8.3 Data Optimization   149
  8.3.1 Addressing the Gap in Codified,
     Standardized Data   149
  8.3.2 NLP and ML   150
  8.3.3 Use Case   151

8.4 Patient Insights to Optimize Care   151
  8.4.1 Patient-Reported Outcomes   151

8.4.2 Sensors   152
8.4.3 Use Case   152

8.5 Genomics in the Care Continuum   153
  8.5.1 Use Case   153

8.6 The Tooling Required   153
  8.6.1 Analytic Approaches   153
  8.6.2 Data Visualization and Accessibility 154
  8.6.3 Clinical Decision Support as a Tool for
     Clinicians   154
  8.6.4 Training the Workforce   154

8.7 Novel Organizational Approaches   155

8.8 Summary   155

List of Acronyms and Abbreviations   155

References   156

8.1 OVERVIEW

Oncology is at a turning point in the treatment of disease. We are transitioning from a time in which few treatments are available for a given cancer type to one with numerous options. For instance, there have been six new treatments approved for the treatment of kidney cancer between 2005 and 2012 [1], and all but one of these are recommended as a first line treatment option in the kidney cancer treatment guidelines published by the National Comprehensive Cancer Network (NCCN) [2]. Most of these new agents were only compared against placebo in their pivotal clinical trials, so their comparative effectiveness is unknown. And, the impact of treatment in later lines of therapy is also unknown, despite the fact that kidney cancer patients are receiving up to eight lines of therapy

B. Hesse, D. Ahern & E. Beckjord: Oncology Informatics.
DOI: http://dx.doi.org/10.1016/B978-0-12-802115-6.00008-2

[3]. At the end of the day, the answer to a core question in oncology is largely unknown for many common cancer types: What is the appropriate sequence of therapies, and what is their impact on disease and patient outcomes?

To date, clinicians have relied on randomized controlled trials (RCTs) to generate the majority of the data supporting approaches to a given patient; however, there are a number of dramatic limitations to this approach. First, RCTs sacrifice external validity for the sake of internal validity, meaning that they tightly control the patient population and settings to make certain that the results of the study are reflective of those achieved by the included population. However, the patient population is not necessarily representative of those seen in community practices, where 85% of care is delivered, due to strict inclusion/exclusion criteria [4–6] and the fact that as few as 2% of patients take part [7,8]. Second, as an increasing number of drugs are approved, there is inadequate comparative effectiveness research (CER) showing which agent is better for a specific patient. The largest driver of the paucity of data is the cost and time required to perform an RCT for every question that comes up in practice. As agents make it to market, it would take years to run large, head-to-head trials comparing them directly to others that may be available for the same indication. By the time the results would be available, the treatment options would have evolved, likely limiting the relevance of the results. This is not an efficient approach. And, third, the patient's experience is not adequately captured today [9,10]. While RCTs report on the adverse events and other patient-centric outcomes that occur among enrolled patients, it is very difficult to personalize the results to a given patient.

While questions remain about the utility of real-world data and informatics to guide therapies, the time has arrived for a fundamental change in how clinicians approach treatment in oncology. The breadth and depth of data being generated from care has risen dramatically. Health policy is helping to drive this change, including the passage of the Health Information Technology for Economic and Clinical Health (HITECH) Act in 2009, part of the American Recovery and Reinvestment Act, and the Affordable Care Act in 2010. The penetration of electronic health records (EHRs) in oncology clinics has increased and the headwinds are pushing the field yet further thanks to initiatives such as Meaningful Use [11] and changes from fee for service (FFS) models to value-based reimbursement. All of these factors lead to the increasingly ubiquitous availability of clinical data, which can be matched with claims, genomic, and other data sets to allow for the generation of meaningful insights in how best to care for a patient across multiple decision points such as treatment selection and avoidance of hospitalization.

The first key to improving and personalizing treatment is to leverage this real-world data to better understand the care being delivered across the entire population of people affected by cancer and identify opportunities for optimization. With millions of patients treated every day in the United States, capturing and analyzing data on even a small proportion would allow for the generation of meaningful insights into how to improve care. For example, how many lines of therapy are appropriate in breast cancer before the toxicity outweighs the benefit? Among bladder cancer patients for which there are numerous second line agents included in the guidelines, but none that are shown to impart substantial benefit, can we identify subsets of patients who are more likely to respond to one agent versus another? With a large enough sample size, and continued optimization of the validity of the insights being generated, new findings could be prospectively validated over time as part of a process that can unfold much more quickly and inexpensively than a traditional RCT.

8.1.1 Evidentiary Uncertainty

There has been an exponential increase in the volume of published oncology literature, much of which focuses on very nuanced aspects of treatment. It is hard for a practicing clinician to keep up with, and make sense of, this rapidly accruing and often contradictory information, resulting in an information paradox in health care. As an example, recent studies on the use of docetaxel chemotherapy early in the treatment of prostate cancer have yielded conflicting results. The "Chemohormonal Therapy versus Androgen Ablation Randomized Trial for Extensive Disease in Prostate Cancer" (CHAARTED) was presented during the plenary session at the American Society of Clinical Oncology (ASCO) Annual Meeting in 2014 [12]. The results showed that treating select prostate cancer patients with chemotherapy early in their disease course extended overall survival from 32.2 months in the control arm to 49.2 months in the experimental arm ($p = 0.0013$). A similar trial in Europe showed a difference in overall survival of only 54.2 months in the control arm versus 58.9 months in the experimental arm (hazard ratio 1.01, confidence interval 0.75–1.36) [13]. Despite enrolling 1175 patients in the two trials and relying on experts who know the data intimately to interpret the results, there is still disagreement as to how to apply them to clinical practice [14,15]. Some experts recommend waiting for the results of the "Systemic Therapy in Advancing or Metastatic Prostate Cancer: Evaluation of Drug Efficacy" (STAMPEDE) trial [16], the results of which are not yet published, before changing the standard of care. Many similar examples exist where, despite the completion of large RCTs, nuanced differences in inclusion/exclusion criteria, variations in trial design and analysis, and conflicting results leave questions unanswered. Practicing clinicians are left drowning in data but still unclear how to proceed with respect to a specific patient.

One way of dealing with this complexity is to move toward increased specialization within community practices wherein clinicians focus on the treatment of only a few subtypes of cancer. This approach has been standard practice in academic settings but it is now being seen in the community as well. However, specialization alone will not address the problem, as the contradictory issues of large data volume but weak clinical guidance exist even within very specific manifestations of cancer. If we do not generate the data to understand the nuances of care and the informatics-based support systems with which to integrate it into practice, no matter how specialized medical oncologists become, they will still struggle to provide optimal care. Furthermore, the nature of referral patterns do not lend themselves to specialization at the physician level in the community.

8.1.2 Limitations of Guidelines

Cancer care guidelines were developed as a tool to provide roadmaps for managing complex treatment decisions. Care guidelines help to overcome evidentiary uncertainty by convening expert panels to provide consensus recommendations for the treatment of specific cancer types. However, the guidelines oversimplify recommendations, remain relatively nonspecific due to their inclusive nature, and are slow to evolve. For example, the last time that ASCO updated its guideline on the use of growth hormones in supportive care was in 2006 [17]. The NCCN is more timely in its approach, releasing yearly updates on nearly all of their guidelines [18]; however, a great deal changes even within a year. New RCTs and observational studies are published. New agents are approved. It would be nearly impossible for the NCCN to convene its committees to update their recommendations every time a new study is published.

Because recommendations are consensus driven, experts must be called together to reach agreement on each step in the guideline. As a result, patients may be treated based on information that could be outdated by months or even years. Furthermore, many of the nuances of care decisions can be lost in guidelines that only include broad recommendations based on factors such as stage of disease, performance status, and genomic signature, stopping well short of aspects such as comorbidities or personal patient preference. If clinicians are truly relying on these sources to guide the care they deliver, a new, or at least reimagined, solution is needed.

8.1.3 Balancing Survival and Quality of Life

Treatment choices in oncology are meant to balance the desire to maximize overall survival with the need to ensure tolerability and maintenance of quality of life (QOL). Currently, the data needed to inform these decisions are missing in oncology. While RCTs focus on the risks and benefits at the population level, even with "definitive" evidence of benefit, it can be exceedingly difficult to apply the results of a collection of clinical trials to a patient sitting in front of a clinician.

An example can be drawn from the treatment of advanced pancreatic cancer. The available options to control the disease have limited benefit. Per the NCCN guidelines, there are four options that are considered "category one recommendations" for patients with good performance status, meaning those for which the option has the strongest supporting evidence: single agent gemcitabine, gemcitabine+ erlotinib, gemcitabine+ paclitaxel, or FOLFIRINOX (5FU+ oxaliplatin+ irinotecan) [19]. The final two options are identified as the "preferred" choices.

The advantage of FOLFIRINOX over single agent gemcitabine was demonstrated in a trial of 342 patients with chemotherapy naïve, metastatic pancreatic cancer who were randomized to one of the two treatments [20]. The FOLFIRINOX arm resulted in an objective response rate of 32% versus 9% with single agent gemcitabine and an overall survival of 11.1 versus 6.8 months. However, toxicity was much higher in the FOLFIRINOX arm including grade 3 or 4 neutropenia (46% vs 21%), febrile neutropenia (5.4% vs 1.2%), vomiting (15% vs 8%,), diarrhea (13% vs 2%), and peripheral neuropathy (9% vs 0%), to name a few. There were also limitations to the trial that may lead to an underestimation of the differential toxicity, particularly that it included a younger, healthier population than that seen in the community.

Now consider an elderly woman weighing her treatment options in conjunction with her doctor. Is a median extension of survival of 4.3 months worth the risk of the treatment-related morbidity? Will the potential survival benefit be shorter for this patient since she is elderly? Will she suffer from a higher rate of toxic effects? Will toxicity limit fundamental components of her QOL, such as her ability to get around, make meals for herself, or visit her grandchildren? No one knows. How can her doctor confidently conduct that conversation, particularly in the absence of adequate supporting evidence or a clear mechanism with which to personalize the recommendations?

Yet, the expectation that clinicians will provide personalized cancer treatment recommendations is expanding. There is strong conviction that oncologists should be matching drugs to biomarkers that predict response and tolerability, and that the patient's specific characteristics should be matched to those agents with the optimal balance of benefits and toxicity. In other words, there is the expectation of multivariable tailoring of treatment decisions, incorporating a multitude of details including patient, disease, financial, social, and health delivery related factors. However, evidence-based decision-making based upon a traditional RCT paradigm can only partially solve this need. We must devise systems to support such approaches.

8.1.4 Market Evolution

These concerns about evidentiary uncertainty, lack of timely guidelines, and limited integration of QOL data are not new; however, changes in reimbursement and payer expectations are providing incentives to address them in real-world practice. Prior to the integration of EHRs into the clinic and the wide availability of secondary data sources, there was very little transparency as to the care being delivered. This is changing with the consolidation of clinical data among a core group of provider networks (eg, Flatiron Health, US Oncology) and health systems (eg, Partners Healthcare, Carolinas Health Care System).

To date, clinicians have been paid in a FFS model in which an increase in care (ie, scans ordered, treatments delivered) leads to an increase in revenue, providing conflicting incentives for providers. In February 2015, US Department of Health and Human Services Secretary Sylvia Burwell announced a plan to increase the percentage of value-based payments to 30% by 2016 and 50% by 2018 [21]. The Centers for Medicare and Medicaid Services (CMS) also proposed that, of the remaining FFS contracts, 85% must include quality and efficiency metrics by 2016. Soon thereafter, CMS introduced the Oncology Care Model, which they will begin piloting in conjunction with other payers in 2016. The stated goal is to "align financial incentives to improve care coordination, appropriateness of care, and access to care for beneficiaries undergoing chemotherapy" [22]. To do so, they are providing a per-beneficiary-per-month payment for the duration of a given episode of care to pay for supportive services and coordination. They are also providing a performance-based payment in which providers will share in savings that are generated after predefined threshold and quality metrics are met, which will be based on historical trends. Private payers have already been experimenting in the space, however the involvement of CMS is likely to make the trend far more defined [23].

Payer-driven approaches to care coordination and optimization will continue to be diverse (ie, pathway-driven treatment choices, oncology medical home models, bundled payments); however, all have fundamental alignment in that they will require real-time decisions about patient treatment from across the portfolio of available choices, the characteristics of a given patient, and the underlying value of a given approach. Without the use of data and technology to support their implementation, it will undoubtedly be a failed experiment.

8.2 DATA AGGREGATION

Despite widespread agreement that informatics holds great promise in optimizing the treatments being delivered in oncology, there is a lack of clarity as to the specific solutions and approaches. EHRs are evolving to support better documentation, data capture, and the provision of treatment decision support; however, this is only one aspect of the greater issue. The key questions are (1) how to aggregate the data across fragmented providers and systems; (2) how to access critical data elements hidden in unstructured documents; (3) what approaches are available to improve the data being captured; and (4) what tools are available to then make data useful? In support of the first question, there are a few key players of note including provider networks, tumor registries, and secondary data sets; exemplar strengths and weaknesses are discussed next. We address the other questions subsequently.

8.2.1 Providers and Networks

There is an effort within oncology to aggregate data on the patients receiving care in the community. There are numerous groups involved, including hospitals, health systems, and community-based networks. A handful stand out in the present landscape due to the breadth of the market they touch, including Flatiron Health and US Oncology. The two organizations capture nearly half of all patients treated in the community setting across the United States.

Flatiron Health and US Oncology each offer proprietary EHRs (OncoEMR and iKnowMed, respectively) to member practices and are therefore able to both define data quality and ensure aggregation at scale for the community practices with which they have agreements. While they are unique in scale, they provide examples of the opportunities available to both understand and drive treatment in oncology. Their relationship with sites moves beyond the EHR alone, including services such as practice management support, clinical decision support, and laboratory services. These efforts further expand the breadth of available data, providing the opportunity to extract and normalize data from a variety of data sources (eg, EHRs, claims, practice management systems) in order to populate data warehouses.

8.2.2 Tumor Registries

The most widely known examples of cancer data aggregation across disparate sites are tumor registries. The registry system was formalized in 1992 as part of the Cancer Registries Amendment Act. Administered by the Centers for Disease Control and Prevention (CDC), the resulting National Program of Cancer Registries

(NPCR) is meant to "help us understand [cancer] better and use our resources to the best effect in prevention and treatment" [24]. Prior to the introduction of the legislation, there were 10 states with no registries. Registries now cover 96% of the US population [25]. Medical facilities, largely consisting of hospitals, employ *cancer registrars* whose job it is to review the records of cancer patients and transfer that information into a local data capture system. The registrars then submit data both to the NPCR and the National Cancer Institute's (NCI's) Surveillance, Epidemiology, and End Results (SEER) Program.

8.2.3 Secondary Data Sources

There are numerous other data sources that are complementary to those captured in the direct provision of care. ASCO is introducing the Cancer Learning Intelligence Network for Quality (CancerLinQ) [26], a movement in partnership with SAP to assemble data from practices across the country, with the intention of feeding the data back for performance and quality benchmarking, among other metrics (see Chapter 1: Creating a Learning Health Care System in Oncology). NCI's SEER program has been aggregating cancer data since 1973 from population-based cancer registries to "provide data on cancer statistics in an effort to reduce the burden of cancer among the US population" [27]. SEER data is often matched with Medicare claims data to make it yet more robust, in that treatment and outcome data can be linked to disease characteristics. There are also more targeted data sets of importance such as the clinical trial data aggregated by the CEO Roundtable on Cancer as part of the Project Data Sphere Initiative [28]. These examples are just the tip of the iceberg, and more like them will exist over time.

8.2.4 Translating Data Into Action

Each of the data sources has its strengths and limitations. For example, despite the best intentions with the tumor registries, there are significant restraints to their use at scale due to issues such as the delay in data availability, limited scope of the data due to the reliance on completely manual abstraction of selected elements, and lack of national interoperability of the local systems. Despite such issues, there is great promise in the ability to aggregate data.

8.3 DATA OPTIMIZATION

Without improving data quality and making it accessible and actionable, the promise will not be realized. Along these lines, there are a few key needs to drive success including improvements in the capture of standardized,

codified data and the use of informatics-enabled tools such as natural language processing (NLP) and machine learning (ML) to drive accessibility and utility.

8.3.1 Addressing the Gap in Codified, Standardized Data

What are the deficiencies in our current process of data collection and aggregation? EHRs remain digital versions of paper charts, largely consisting of free text clinical notes that are difficult to parse. While there are codified elements, they are often limited and have not been carefully designed to meet the needs of varied stakeholders. Key data elements are buried in the free text of documents such as clinical notes, radiology reports and pathology reports. To further complicate the situation, many "reports" are really just pictures— digital images—representing medical documentation faxed between clinicians and scanned into the chart. Data are not structured in an electronic format and therefore cannot be easily aggregated or analyzed. This is a by-product of how medicine is practiced and documented (predominantly in narrative form), and the lack of incentives for EHRs to improve data capture facilities (and, when they do, it makes the doctor less efficient, producing backlash).

Meanwhile, harnessing data to improve treatment decision-making requires a spectrum of codified, consistently defined elements. Examples of important cancer-related variables that need to be consistently captured, but often are not, include stage of disease, comorbid illnesses, biomarker results, oral therapies received, response to therapy, symptom profiles, and QOL. A number of efforts have been taken to drive consensus around the key variables to collect, in what care settings, and use of consistent definitions; however, uptake of these recommendations outside of the clinical research setting remains limited. In a discussion of *Data Standards, Data Quality and Interoperability* by the American Health Information Management Association (AHIMA), data standards are described as "documented agreements on representations, formats, and definitions of common data. Data standards provide a method to codify in valid, meaningful, comprehensive, and actionable ways, information captured in the course of doing business" [29]. Consistent collection of a group of core data elements with related data standards, beyond just the capture of vital signs and lab results, would represent a powerful step forward.

There are a number of standard development organizations (SDOs) that have made strides in this area but that has not translated into widespread uptake at the data element level in routine practice. For instance, Health Level Seven (HL7) was first developed in 1987 to drive a framework around the retrieval and sharing of health information. This has been critical for clinical data to be exchanged across systems. Many others have been developed for specific areas of importance, such as the Digital Imaging and Communications in Medicine (DICOM) for imaging and National Council for Prescription Drug Programs (NCPDP) for pharmacy data. Within the HL7 framework, the Consolidated Clinical Document Architecture (C-CDA) also marks a step forward, which is largely a library of different templates that can be transferred between organizations, including such documents as a Continuity of Care Document (CCD), Diagnostic Imaging Report (DIR), and Progress Note. However, the fields within these elements are left open to definition.

These standards allow the transfer of data, but stop short of defining the elements themselves. The Systemized Nomenclature of Medicine—Clinical Terms (SNOMED-CT), and others like it, help to provide a framework for the relationship between concepts and their hierarchical structure, but also do not ensure consistent definitions of individual elements. There are examples of the next step; however, they are limited. The Clinical Data Interchange Standards Consortium (CDISC) works to ensure data standards and interoperability in medical research, based on the acknowledgment that the "data content, structure, and quality of the data models are of paramount importance" [30]. They have gained traction in the research community but this too has not been integrated within EHRs in practice. Whether a group such as CDISC is able to drive standardization, and whether there is a business case for wider adoption, remains a point of discussion.

Regardless of the mechanism by which it is achieved, the key is to advance the availability of codified data. While other techniques will be discussed subsequently to augment it, the upfront capture facilitates accuracy and completeness. Organizations (eg, hospitals, health systems, and provider networks) are in a unique position to advance this cause, as are EHR providers. By convening stakeholders, identifying those elements that are key to success, and then defining the workflow for their capture, one can maximize their completeness and utility. Leveraging standards that are being advanced by SDOs is a logical starting place, as compared to attempting to reinvent the wheel repeatedly.

8.3.2 NLP and ML

Even with consensus on elements of interest, and definitions thereof, a number of roadblocks remain. It is not possible to ask clinicians to enter every variable due to the inefficiencies it would introduce into clinical care. Of those that are too time-consuming, complex, or peripheral, some may reside in unstructured fields (ie, free text), scanned reports, and secondary data

sources. Examples of different potential issues abound: (1) Pathologic reviews are often performed outside of a given clinical practice and the resulting reports are returned to clinicians via fax. They are then scanned into the record, but not included as codified or searchable elements. The most important elements of the results may also be summarized in the free text of a clinician's note, but these too are inaccessible for analysis. (2) Oral chemotherapies are often prescribed for patients using written scripts and filled outside of the treating clinician's office. Because data are not routinely transferred between the varied stakeholders in the market, clinicians are unlikely to have access to the resulting prescribing data held by payers, making it very difficult to utilize these data to guide care. This is in comparison to infused agents, which are well captured because they are directly administered within the clinic setting. (3) Symptoms are not included in codified elements, but instead are buried in the free text of a clinician's note, if they are captured at all. The decision to include a given adverse event, and the severity attributed to it, is reflective of the clinician's interpretation of the patient's status during a hurried interview, as opposed to the direct report from the patient.

NLP and ML are potential tools that can help make data that is presently unstructured accessible. NLP was defined in the *Journal of Oncology Practice* in 2011 as "a sub discipline of computer science that is dedicated to the analysis of unstructured natural language text and speech. Although true understanding of natural languages by computers is an elusive goal, there have been great advances recently in the application of automated methods to extract structured information from unstructured text" [31]. There have been numerous examples of the application of this technology to clinical practice with results that have been improving over the past few years.

Attempts to extract medical problem lists from narrative text using NLP have been occurring for well over a decade [32]. The difficulties in using NLP remain daunting, having to deal with issues such as how to handle abbreviations and the development of phenotypic algorithms [33,34]. Success in building models becomes critical in the attempt to leverage data to better understand the care being delivered.

On the other hand, using ML offers a distinct, but complementary functionality. It leverages computing power to iteratively improve on the quality of an algorithm or approach, without being explicitly programmed to do so. An oft quoted definition was supplied by Tom Mitchell, "A computer program is said to learn from experience with respect to some class of tasks and performance measures, if its performance at tasks, as measured by the performance measure, improves with experience" [35].

A prime example of the use of ML in cancer treatment can be seen from a 2002 article in *Nature Medicine* in which ML was used to develop a prediction model for outcomes related to diffuse large B-cell lymphoma [36]. In the study, researchers analyzed 6817 genes from patients treated with cyclophosphamide, adriamycin, vincristine, and prednisone (CHOP) chemotherapy to see if a signature could be identified that indicated potentially curable disease. The result was an algorithm that categorized patients into groups with very different overall survival, using the ML to iteratively hone the model. Since its publication, the article has been referenced more than 2000 times.

8.3.3 Use Case

In oncology, the potential use cases abound where codified data, NLP, and ML could be leveraged to improve the treatment of patients. A basic use case applies to attempts to understand the ideal treatment of advanced kidney cancer. As referenced earlier, many new treatments are being approved, with limited CER available with which to inform clinicians of the ideal treatments to use in a given setting.

Ensuring accurate capture of basic demographics, disease characteristics, pathologic markers, and outcomes are critically important. For instance, the definition and capture of "disease progression" does not presently occur in many systems, yet it is important. Surrogates can be used, if captured, such as discontinuation of a treatment, however the data is not always collected and, when it is, it doesn't include information about the reason for the switch (eg, progression, toxicity, cost). This element is critically important to provide a data set with utility.

Despite the best efforts of stakeholders to increase the capture of key elements, there will always be those that are not captured and are buried in unstructured text fields such as the symptoms a patient is experiencing and nuances of radiology findings. The incremental value of these data points is high so developing NLP to aggregate it, if guided by stakeholders who can identify the key needs, will provide substantial benefit. By aggregating data with this depth and breadth at scale, key insights can be generated that far outstrip the capabilities possible with claims data alone.

As the data sets grow to truly represent "big data," defined by the three V's of velocity (or speed of data generation), variety (or forms of data being generated), and volume (or scale of data), ML will become increasingly useful to make sense of it. As shown in the lymphoma example, as the complexity of genomics alone grows, it becomes helpful to have tools to parse and learn from the data in a way that explicit programming makes difficult. By applying ML to the identified data elements, both from codified data and those derived from NLP, the opportunity to drive entirely new insights into the treatment of kidney cancer emerges.

8.4 PATIENT INSIGHTS TO OPTIMIZE CARE

Regardless of the strength of codified elements, NLP, and ML, the voice of the patient is not captured within the record. Research shows that the interpretation of a patient's status by a clinician is often biased, usually toward underreporting [37]. Clinicians have limited time with a patient and see them only episodically, so their view cannot fully encompass and represent the patient experience.

As an example, a clinician may see a patient immediately prior to each cycle of chemotherapy, which is often the time at which the patient feels his or her best, as opposed to the point at which the chemotherapy is at its maximum effect. Patients often do not want to burden a clinician or are not as worried since they are out of the acute phase, further limiting the exchange of key data points, such as reports of symptoms or side effects. Finally, clinicians often choose to document certain patient characteristics more fully, such as those areas where they have interventions that are likely to provide benefit. The result is that the data do not exist within the record to drive insights, regardless of the complexity of the approach used.

Advances in technology and its penetration in society allow for new mechanisms to directly integrate the patient voice. *Patient-generated data* is commonly used to describe this area. The PRO Task Force of the Patient-Centered Outcomes Research Institute (PCORI) recently defined *patient generated data* (see Chapter 16: "Crowdsourcing Advancements in Health Care Research: Applications for Cancer Treatment Discoveries") to include "health history, symptoms, biometric data, treatment history, lifestyle choices, and other information— created, recorded, gathered, or inferred by or from patients or their designees (ie, care partners or those who assist them) to help address a health concern" [38]. As described, the breadth and depth of this data can be daunting, including everything from vital signs ascertained at home via biometric sensors to simple responses to questionnaires. Patient-reported outcomes (PROs) and sensors represent low-hanging fruit in oncology that can be leveraged to understand the patient experience and guide care.

8.4.1 Patient-Reported Outcomes

PROs refer to the collection of data directly from patients using validated measurement instruments, largely consisting of surveys. The term "PRO" was introduced for regulatory purposes by the US Food and Drug Administration (FDA) [39]; however, it is a bit confusing, because PROs do not consist purely of outcomes metrics. They can include everything from descriptive to explanatory to prognostic data points, asking questions ranging from frequency of diarrhea to work status [40–42]. The tools themselves span the gamut from highly curated and psychometrically validated tools to those that are introduced based on their face validity (eg, "Do you have nausea?").

8.4.2 Sensors

Sensors are increasingly worn in the community today, meant largely to help facilitate health and wellness-related goals. Many commercial devices are available, such as those made by FitBit and Misfit. Various goals have been put forward as to the number of steps that a person should take in a day, often ranging from 5000 to 10,000. With the introduction of the Apple Watch and the HealthKit, these areas have gained yet more traction. In a *Forbes* article, the use of these devices was referred to as "wellutainment" due to the limited scientific validity of the metrics and the cut-points being used [43]. The devices largely meet wellness and entertainment goals, as opposed to rigorous medical needs. Interestingly, the fitness device makers themselves point to engagement as the goal, as opposed to accuracy [44]. Recent studies out of the University of Pennsylvania and the American Council on Exercise have also shown the variability among commercial fitness trackers [45].

However, there is an increasing integration of sensors into the clinic. Hospital systems and technology companies are enabling ways to use the data to drive care. For instance, Duke University, Stanford University, Mayo Clinic, and Cleveland Clinic were all early pilot sites for Apple's HealthKit, assessing the use of patient-generated data to understand the clinical experience and drive care decisions [46]. Companies such as Validic are further enabling the data to be standardized and normalized across devices, before being supplied to insurers and large wellness programs.

In oncology, there are a number of validated metrics which are measured using sensor technologies and have been shown to be meaningful. For example, several trials have shown a relationship between moderate to vigorous physical activity (MVPA), sedentary time (SED), and QOL. A recent study of 199 breast cancer survivors demonstrated that the amount of MVPA and SED that patients experience is significantly related to their levels of pain ($p = 0.02$), fatigue ($p = 0.01$), and dysphoria ($p = 0.03$) [47]. Another study of 177 breast cancer survivors found that patients spend an average of 78% of their time sedentary and that MVPA worsens over the 12 months after therapy [48]. A study of 181 colorectal cancer survivors found a significant difference in health-related quality of life (HRQOL) between the highest and lowest quartiles of MVPA ($p = 0.014$) [49]. Furthermore, it was found that participants who achieved 150 minutes

of MVPA per week had 18% higher HRQOL than those who reported no MVPA [50] and that fatigue mediates the association between MVPA and HRQOL [51].

Even more nascent, yet equally important, is the analysis of sleep among oncology patients. The rate of sleep disturbance experienced by cancer patients is said to range from 25% to 59% [52–54]. In one study, 51% of women being treated for breast cancer reported sleep difficulties, with 19% meeting the criteria for insomnia syndrome [55]. This in turn was associated with impaired function, lower HRQOL and increased health care use. A randomized trial among breast cancer patients further showed that treating insomnia led to lower levels of depression/anxiety and greater global HRQOL [56]. Insomnia is said to occur when sleep is disturbed more than three times per week with an impact on sleep efficiency (ratio of sleep time to time spent in bed falls).

8.4.3 Use Case

The use of patient-generated data, including PROs and sensors, may seem abstract, but is tangible today. Let's take an example of Barry, a patient recently diagnosed with pancreatic cancer. He is 84 years old and has advanced disease, but has an excellent functional status when seen, spending little of the day in bed, has maintained his weight, and states that he wants to be "as aggressive as possible." He is started on FOLFIRINOX, an aggressive chemotherapy regimen consisting of three agents. In usual care, he is seen a few weeks later when he is next due for his second cycle of chemotherapy. While he struggled mightily after receiving the first treatment, he feels better by the time of the follow-up visit, does not want to burden his clinician, and does not want to "give up" by being taken off therapy so he minimizes his difficulties when speaking with the clinician. If his PRO and sensor data—gathered continuously between clinical encounters—is available for review, the clinician will see the reality. He went from being quite active before starting treatment to nearly purely sedentary. He had poor sleep efficiency and no MVPA. He also rated his nausea at 10/10 after treatment and his QOL, shown in aggregate scores of individual PRO questions, had a dramatic decline. At the very least, this data would lead to discussions about dose reductions, but it may lead to a reevaluation about whether FOLFIRINOX is the right approach to his care.

The utility of the data is threefold: (1) it can be used to capture deep, rich data on the patient experience in the course of real-world clinical practice in a cost-effective manner; (2) the data can be used to differentiate agents used within routine care; and (3) it provides guidance for future research that will allow for personalization of care through better targeting of agents to specific patient populations and that will allow for the development of interventions to improve QOL, outcomes, and adherence.

8.5 GENOMICS IN THE CARE CONTINUUM

Genomics represent another area of great promise, with limited success to date. When the human genome was decoded in 2003, there was great promise as to its use to guide care and maximize outcomes. At the 10-year anniversary of the completion of the first sequence, many opined about how expectations had not been met despite a decade of focus [57]. In oncology specifically, strides have been made, although as was discussed more broadly, a lot can still be done.

A number of genomic signatures are consistently used in oncology in the treatment of patients. Examples include *EGFR* and *BRAF* mutations in lung cancer and melanoma patients, respectively. In both cases, treatments have been developed that are shown to be particularly effective in patients with these mutations, allowing for the targeting of drugs to those in which they are likely to be particularly effective, as opposed to the use of conventional chemotherapy in all comers, independent of the likelihood of impact. Unfortunately, there are limited examples of the successful development of companion diagnostics to guide therapies.

To continue to advance the paradigm, genomic data must be captured in new ways and the annotation of biospecimens must be robust. Genomic data is available for a limited number of patients and largely captured in unstructured fields. Test results are often faxed to a clinic, the report may be scanned into the chart and the relevant results may be dictated into the clinical note. In this situation, nowhere is this data directly input into codified fields. The result is that it is difficult to drive discovery as genomic results cannot be matched to response to agents or patient outcomes at scale.

While little progress has been made in capturing the data, the amount of data being generated is growing exponentially. Companies like Foundation Health and Claris make testing available to patients for a wide variety of mutations that might drive their disease. Many genomic tests do not have specific drug targets today, but new drugs are likely to be discovered over time that will enable increasingly personalized treatment. Since the genomics tests are run outside of the clinical systems in which care is delivered, an opportunity is missed if that information is not directly tied back to the clinical data and biospecimens of a given patient. As the cost of whole genome sequencing falls and new technologies gain steam, the need will become yet more pressing.

8.5.1 Use Case

Barry, our 84-year-old patient with advanced pancreatic cancer, has his tissue sent for whole genome sequencing to see if any target might be apparent to guide therapy in later lines of treatment. Unfortunately, none are identified so he proceeds with chemotherapy. The results of his tests are scanned into the chart, but since no target is identified, they do not make it into his clinical note or any codified fields.

Two months later, a new agent is identified for which Barry is an excellent candidate. In a setting in which his clinical and genomic data were matched, a clinician could search across his or her pancreatic cancer patient population for any matches that might exist, but this was not available and therefore Barry did not receive the agent. Furthermore, the company producing the drug was looking for patients known to have the mutation so they could perform further testing on available biospecimens. Unfortunately, the ability did not exist to make the connection to the tissue, further delaying discovery.

8.6 THE TOOLING REQUIRED

8.6.1 Analytic Approaches

Another key is the robustness of data analytics. While data warehouses once had significant limitations, the evolution of technology allows them to be quite robust, integrating numerous source systems into a centralized repository providing the opportunity to ask broad questions of the data. Aggregation alone cannot overcome the limitations of the data without tools such as improved codified capture and NLP, but being able to generate insights about the strengths and limitations of the data is a critical first step in improving its quality.

The analysis of the data is a key step toward making it "useful." For instance, one would imagine that a "line of therapy" would be easily defined for a given patient as the regimen that they received at a given point in time and that treatment sequencing would be very straightforward, reported as the sequential provision of therapies. In reality, the definition of a line of therapy can be quite complex. For instance, does treatment with a given agent, followed by a 6-month break, and then resumption of the same agent signify a new line of therapy or continuation of the same? How is maintenance therapy captured? In a multidrug regimen, how is the discontinuation or exchange of one of the agents handled? While these are not insurmountable issues, they require agreement as to the approach and clear definitions prior to moving forward. They also require a complete picture from the applicable data sources in order to avoid errors, including data on infusional agents, oral agents, lab results, scan results, and the input of clinicians.

It is the output of analytics such as this that become critically important to guide care. Physician dashboards are examples of a way in which analytics can be used to optimize treatment. After information about lines of therapy is generated, it can be used to understand overall treatment patterns, outcomes by treatment pattern, reimbursement variations, guideline compliance, and the quality of care. When fed back to physicians, this can be a powerful driver of decisions and outcomes.

8.6.2 Data Visualization and Accessibility

Another key learning is the importance of visualization and user experience in any interface that is developed to support clinical decisions. In many health care applications, functionality is prioritized over design, leading to data being presented in nonintuitive interfaces and in a manner inconsistent with the workflow related to it. Crucial to the success of this work is the ability to translate it to a mechanism that clinicians and others can integrate into workflow and understand in real time. There is ongoing work about what is most easily digested by clinicians and most useful (see Chapter 11: "Data Visualization Tools for Investigating Health Services Utilization Among Cancer Patients" and Chapter 15: "Extended Vision for Oncology: A Perceptual Science Perspective on Data Visualization and Medical Imaging").

8.6.3 Clinical Decision Support as a Tool for Clinicians

A daunting array of data points has been discussed—structured data, unstructured data, literature, guidelines, patient-generated data, genomics—each of which play a critical role in the treatment of a given patient. The reality is that a clinician cannot be expected to efficiently integrate all of these data points at any given time. Personalized, evidence-based care delivery therefore necessitates the use of decision support tools in order to optimize care. At their most basic, these tools help to provide structured support for a given decision.

US Oncology uses its "Clear Value Plus" (CVP) program to support treatment selection [58]. Through a partnership with the NCCN, committees within the US Oncology Network review key NCCN Guidelines and develop business rules based on key disease criteria to guide the choice of treatments for patients within the Network. In areas where there are multiple potential treatment choices, other aspects of decisions such as estimations of value are integrated into the decision process to result in portfolio of treatments that are "on pathway." A web-based interface is used to capture a few key clinical elements (eg, diagnosis, stage, line of therapy) from the EHR. For those elements that are missing, the clinicians are asked to supply them.

CVP represents a step forward in optimizing treatment, but more is possible. To truly personalize care, other aspects of a patient's case should be integrated such as functional status as generated by sensor data,

patient characteristics as generated by PROs, differences in patient copays using insurer/claims data, and genomic signatures that predict response to a given therapy. The integration of many of these elements remains a few years from reality, but the roadmap to the new paradigm is being developed now.

Additional steps have been taken by groups such as IBM with its Watson Health initiative. The Watson Health team uses cognitive computing, described as an attempt to "provide machine-aided serendipity by wading through massive collections of diverse information to find patterns and then apply those patterns to respond to the needs of the moment" [59] to guide treatment selection. IBM explains that they "bring together clinical, research, and social data from a diverse range of health sources, creating a secure, cloud-based data sharing hub, powered by the most advanced cognitive and analytic technologies" [60]. As opposed to the more controlled approaches such as that outlined by US Oncology, this methodology attempts to leverage the power of computing to drive understanding. The Watson Health team has partnered with institutions like Memorial Sloan Kettering Cancer Center [61] and MD Anderson Cancer Center [62] over the last few years, and to date, remain in the discovery phase of this endeavor.

As these pilots evolve, payers can leverage tools to assess utilization and the value of care being delivered, supporting oncology medical home models, bundled payments, and accountable care organizations. Further efforts will be made in areas such as adverse event management and supportive care guidance [63]. At the end of the day, clinical decision support is critical for all aspects of personalization in cancer care.

8.6.4 Training the Workforce

A final key element in the drive to leverage informatics for clinicians is that they need to be prepared to generate and use the tools. Many argue that comfort with informatics is a generational issue that will solve itself as new doctors join the workforce. This is partially true but to wait for the workforce to turn over would preclude the use of the tools for a few more decades. Further, the more tech savvy generation of clinicians does not necessarily understand the complexity of data models and evidence generation that underlies these tools. One of the goals mentioned in the prior section is to make the interfaces as intuitive as possible, but it is still critical that those using it know the relative strength of the underlying data, what they can do to optimize it, and how to ask questions of the data.

To begin to close this gap, certification programs are being established to train clinicians. One such program is the Learning Health System Training Program (LHSTP) at the Duke University School of Medicine.

All trainees participate in classes on data generation, analysis, and visualization. Those with a greater interest apply to a more in-depth program, which includes a case study wherein each participant chooses an informatics topic of interest. They then spend months understanding how to design and execute informatics-related projects. Another example is Duke's Masters in Clinical Informatics program, which trains clinicians, alongside data scientists and executives, about the nuances of informatics. The goal of all of these endeavors is to bring stakeholders together to develop a common language and understanding.

8.7 NOVEL ORGANIZATIONAL APPROACHES

Beyond traditional stakeholders such as health systems, tumor registries, and provider networks, a number of new organizations have been developed that attempt to leverage informatics and the established infrastructure to drive our understanding of care and to develop novel approaches to the generation of new knowledge with which to guide treatment. Examples include the National Institutes of Health (NIH) Collaboratory, FDA Sentinel Initiative, and PCORNet.

The NIH Collaboratory has as a mission statement the desire to "strengthen the national capacity to implement cost-effective large-scale research studies that engage healthcare delivery organizations as research partners" [64]. As an extension of this focus, a core need is to aggregate the data that is collected, and presently siloed, across integrated university health systems, such as Duke, Harvard, and Johns Hopkins, to enable pragmatic clinical trials. An example project is entitled *Strategies and Opportunities to Stop Colorectal Cancer*, which the Kaiser Foundation Research Institute leads [65]. More than 200 federally qualified health centers are banding together to test a culturally tailored colorectal screening program by leveraging systems of care.

Taking a different tack, the FDA Sentinel Initiative is leveraging relationships with data partners and health systems to perform drug safety monitoring. Established in May 2008, the FDA uses the initiative to investigate signals of adverse events that might be of concern for agents that are on the market. Queries are sent to participating institutions about a given agent and the occurrence of the events of concern. The execution of the queries is not yet automated due to governance, privacy, and other considerations; however, responses can quickly be returned and aggregated for near real-time insights into the experience of patients on various agents. An example publication was able to assess guideline adherence to glucose screening prior to treatment initiation across a national cohort of patients [66].

Finally, PCORNet takes yet another different approach, focusing on the generation of patient-centered outcomes in the research that it funds. The goal of PCORNet is to "improve the nation's capacity to conduct CER efficiently by creating a large, highly representative network for conducting clinical outcomes research" [67]. Interestingly, the network is made of a mixture of Clinical Data Research Networks, representing large institutions, and Patient Powered Research Networks, representing patient groups that propose creative ways to capture and aggregate data [68].

8.8 SUMMARY

The opportunity to improve and personalize care in oncology by leveraging informatics is dramatic. To drive improvement, there needs to be an optimization of the quality of the data through processes such as improved codification and standardization and the use of NLP and ML. There also needs to be a focus on generating and integrating secondary data such as patient-generated data. Finally, we must develop the tools to feed the data back to the point of care through analytics, visualizations, and decision support tools. The ideal result would be an entirely new body of evidence being used to optimize the outcomes of vulnerable cancer patients.

LIST OF ACRONYMS AND ABBREVIATIONS

5FU Fluorouracil
AHIMA American Health Information Management Association
ASCO American Society of Clinical Oncology
CancerLinQ Cancer Learning Intelligence Network for Quality
CCD Continuity of Care Document
C-CDA Consolidated Clinical Document Architecture
CDC Centers for Disease Control and Prevention
CDISC Clinical Data Interchange Standards Consortium
CER Comparative effectiveness research
CHAARTED Chemohormonal Therapy versus Androgen Ablation Randomized Trial for Extensive Disease in Prostate Cancer
CHOP Cyclophosphamide, adriamycin, vincristine, and prednisone
CMS Centers for Medicare and Medicaid Services
CVP Clear Value Plus
DICOM Digital Imaging and Communications in Medicine
DIR Diagnostic Imaging Report
EHR Electronic health record
FDA Food and Drug Administration
FFS Fee for service
HITECH Health Information Technology for Economic and Clinical Health
HL7 Health Level Seven
HRQOL Health-related quality of life
LHSTP Learning Health System Training Program
ML Machine learning
MVPA Moderate to vigorous physical activity
NCCN National Comprehensive Cancer Network
NCI National Cancer Institute

NCPDP National Council for Prescription Drug Programs
NIH National Institutes of Health
NLP Natural language processing
NPCR National Program of Cancer Registries
PCORI Patient-Centered Outcomes Research Institute
PCORNet Patient-Centered Outcomes Research Network
PRO Patient-reported outcome
QOL Quality of life
RCT Randomized controlled trial
SDO Standard development organization
SED Sedentary time
SEER Surveillance, Epidemiology, and End Results
SNOMED-CT Systemized Nomenclature of Medicine—Clinical Terms
STAMPEDE Systemic Therapy in Advancing or Metastatic Prostate Cancer: Evaluation of Drug Efficacy

References

[1] Centerwatch. Approved drugs by therapeutic area [Internet]; 2015 [cited June 22, 2015]. Available from: <http://www.centerwatch.com/drug-information/fda-approvals/drug-areas.aspx?AreaID=12>.

[2] National Comprehensive Cancer Network. NCCN clinical practice guidelines in oncology (NCCN Guidelines): Kidney cancer. Ft. Washington, PA; 2014.

[3] Harrison MR, George DJ, Walker MS, Chen C, Korytowsky B, Kirkendall DT, et al. "Real world" treatment of metastatic renal cell carcinoma in a joint community-academic cohort: progression-free survival over three lines of therapy. Clin Genitourin Cancer 2013;11(4):441–50.

[4] Zulman DM, Sussman JB, Chen X, Cigolle CT, Blaum CS, Hayward RA. Examining the evidence: a systematic review of the inclusion and analysis of older adults in randomized controlled trials. J Gen Intern Med 2011;26(7):783–90.

[5] Elting LS, Cooksley C, Bekele BN, Frumovitz M, Avritscher EB, Sun C, et al. Generalizability of cancer clinical trial results: prognostic differences between participants and nonparticipants. Cancer 2006;106(11):2452–8.

[6] Sorbye H, Pfeiffer P, Cavalli-Bjorkman N, Qvortrup C, Holsen MH, Wentzel-Larsen T, et al. Clinical trial enrollment, patient characteristics, and survival differences in prospectively registered metastatic colorectal cancer patients. Cancer 2009;115(20):4679–87.

[7] Murthy VH, Krumholz HM, Gross CP. Participation in cancer clinical trials: race-, sex-, and age-based disparities. JAMA 2004;291(22):2720–6.

[8] Sateren WB, Trimble EL, Abrams J, Brawley O, Breen N, Ford L, et al. How sociodemographics, presence of oncology specialists, and hospital cancer programs affect accrual to cancer treatment trials. J Clin Oncol 2002;20(8):2109–17.

[9] Hirsch BR, Abernethy AP. Incorporating the patient's voice in the continuum of care. J Natl Compr Cancer Netw 2013;11(1):116–8.

[10] Howie L, Hirsch B, Locklear T, Abernethy AP. Assessing the value of patient-generated data to comparative effectiveness research. Health Aff 2014;33(7):1220–8.

[11] Blumenthal D, Tavenner M. The "meaningful use" regulation for electronic health records. N Engl J Med 2010;363(6):501–4.

[12] Sweeney C, Chen Y-H, Carducci MA, et al. Impact on overall survival with chemohormonal therapy versus hormonal therapy for hormone-sensitive newly metastatic prostate cancer: an ECOG-led phase III randomized trial. J Clin Oncol 2014;35:5s.

[13] Gravis G, Fizazi K, Joly F, Oudard S, Priou F, Esterni B, et al. Androgen-deprivation therapy alone or with docetaxel in non-castrate metastatic prostate cancer (GETUG-AFU 15): a randomised, open-label, phase 3 trial. Lancet Oncol 2013;14(2):149–58.

[14] Armstrong AJ. In hormone-naive metastatic prostate cancer, should all patients now receive docetaxel? No, not yet. Oncology 2014;28(10) 881, 883.

[15] Suzman DL, Antonarakis ES. In hormone-naive metastatic prostate cancer, should all patients now receive docetaxel? Yes; we must beware of drawing conclusions from a subset analysis. Oncology 2014;28(10) 880, 882.

[16] Clinicaltrials.gov. STAMPEDE: Systemic Therapy in Advancing or Metastatic Prostate Cancer: Evaluation of drug efficacy: a multi-stage multi-arm randomised controlled trial [Internet]; 2015 [cited June 22, 2015].

[17] Smith TJ, Khatcheressian J, Lyman GH, Ozer H, Armitage JO, Balducci L, et al. 2006 update of recommendations for the use of white blood cell growth factors: an evidence-based clinical practice guideline. J Clin Oncol 2006;24(19):3187–205.

[18] National Comprehensive Cancer Network. NCCN Clinical Practice Guidelines in Oncology (NCCN Guidelines): Myeloid growth factors. Ft. Washington, PA; 2014.

[19] National Comprehensive Cancer Network. NCCN Clinical Practice Guidelines in Oncology (NCCN Guidelines): Pancreatic cancer. Ft. Washington, PA; 2014.

[20] Conroy T, Desseigne F, Ychou M, Bouche O, Guimbaud R, Becouarn Y, et al. FOLFIRINOX versus gemcitabine for metastatic pancreatic cancer. N Engl J Med 2011;364(19):1817–25.

[21] Keckley P. HHS doubles down on the shift from volume to value. H&HN Daily; February 2, 2015.

[22] Center for Medicare and Medicaid Services. Oncology Care Model request for applications [Internet]; 2015 [cited June 22, 2015]. Available from: <http://innovation.cms.gov/Files/x/ocmrfa.pdf>.

[23] Newcomer LN, Gould B, Page RD, Donelan SA, Perkins M. Changing physician incentives for affordable, quality cancer care: results of an episode payment model. J Oncol Pract 2014;10(5):322–6.

[24] Center for Disease Control and Prevention. Cancer Registries Ammendment Act [Internet]; 2012 [cited June 22, 2015]. Available from: <http://www.cdc.gov/cancer/npcr/amendmentact.htm>.

[25] Centers for Disease Prevention and Control. National Program of Cancer Registries [Internet]; 2013 [cited June 22, 2015]. Available from: <http://www.cdc.gov/cancer/npcr/about.htm>.

[26] American Society of Clinical Oncology. CancerLinQ [Internet]; 2015 [cited June 22, 2015]. Available from: <http://cancerlinq.org/>.

[27] National Cancer Institute. Surveillance, Epidemiology, and End Results Program [Internet]; 2015 [cited June 22, 2015]. Available from: <http://seer.cancer.gov/about/>.

[28] CEO Roundtable on Cancer. Project Data Sphere [Internet]; 2015 [cited June 22, 2015]. Available from: <https://http://www.projectdatasphere.org/projectdatasphere/html/home.html>.

[29] American Health Information Management Association. Data standards, data quality, and interoperability [Internet]; 2013 [cited June 22, 2015]. Available from: <http://library.ahima.org/xpedio/groups/public/documents/ahima/bok1_050482.hcsp?dDocName=bok1_050482>.

[30] Clinical Data Interchange Standards Consortium. CDISC vision and mission [Internet]; 2015 [cited June 22, 2015]. Available from: <http://www.cdisc.org/CDISC-Vision-and-Mission>.

[31] Warner JL, Anick P, Hong P, Xue N. Natural language processing and the oncologic history: is there a match? J Oncol Pract 2011;7(4):e15–9.

[32] Meystre SM, Haug PJ. Comparing natural language processing tools to extract medical problems from narrative text. AMIA Annu Symp Proc 2005:525–9.

[33] Younghui W, et al. A comparative study of current clinical natural language processing systems on handling abbreviations in discharge summaries. AMIA Annu Symp Proc 2012;2012:997–1003.

[34] Liao KP, Cai T, Savova GK, Murphy SN, Karlson EW, Ananthakrishnan AN, et al. Development of phenotype algorithms using electronic medical records and incorporating natural language processing. BMJ 2015;350:h1885.

[35] Mitchell T. Machine learning. New York City: McGraw Hill; 1997.

[36] Shipp MA, Ross KN, Tamayo P, Weng AP, Kutok JL, Aguiar RC, et al. Diffuse large B-cell lymphoma outcome prediction by gene-expression profiling and supervised machine learning. Nat Med 2002;8(1):68–74.

[37] Basch E, Bennett A, Pietanza MC. Use of patient-reported outcomes to improve the predictive accuracy of clinician-reported adverse events. J Natl Cancer Inst 2011;103(24):1808–10.

[38] Shapiro MF, Johnston D, Wald J, Mon D. Patient-generated health data [Internet]; 2012 [cited June 22, 2015]. Available from: <http://www.rti.org/pubs/patientgeneratedhealthdata.pdf>.

[39] Food and Drug Administration. Guidance for industry: patient reported outcomes measures: use in medical product development to support labeling claims; December 2009.

[40] Cella D, Webster K. Linking outcomes management to quality-of-life measurement. Oncology 1997;11(11A):232–5.

[41] Coates A, Porzsolt F, Osoba D. Quality of life in oncology practice: prognostic value of EORTC QLQ-C30 scores in patients with advanced malignancy. Eur J Cancer 1997;33(7):1025–30.

[42] Dancey J, Zee B, Osoba D, Whitehead M, Lu F, Kaizer L, et al. Quality of life scores: an independent prognostic variable in a general population of cancer patients receiving chemotherapy. The National Cancer Institute of Canada Clinical Trials Group. Qual Life Res 1997;6(2):151–8.

[43] Shaywitz D. Pressed to demonstrate utility, digital health struggles—just like traditional medicine. Forbes 2014;January 7.

[44] Comstock J. Fitness device makers say engagement, not accuracy, is most important. MobiHealth News 2015;February 18.

[45] Case MA, Burwick HA, Volpp KG, Patel MS. Accuracy of smartphone applications and wearable devices for tracking physical activity data. JAMA 2015;313(6):625–6.

[46] Pema G. Standford and Duke hospitals working with Apple for pilots. Healthcare Informatics 2014;September 14.

[47] Sabiston CM, Brunet J, Vallance JK, Meterissian S. Prospective examination of objectively assessed physical activity and sedentary time after breast cancer treatment: sitting on the crest of the teachable moment. Cancer Epidemiol Biomarkers Prev 2014;23(7):1324–30.

[48] Trinh L. Physical and psychological health among breast cancer survivors: interactions with sedentary behaviour and physical activity. Presented at CPHA in 2014.

[49] Vallance JK, Boyle T, Courneya KS, Lynch BM. Associations of objectively assessed physical activity and sedentary time with health-related quality of life among colon cancer survivors. Cancer 2014;120(18):2919–26.

[50] Lynch BM, Cerin E, Owen N, Hawkes AL, Aitken JF. Prospective relationships of physical activity with quality of life among colorectal cancer survivors. J Clin Oncol 2008;26(27):4480–7.

[51] Buffart LM, Thong MS, Schep G, Chinapaw MJ, Brug J, van de Poll-Franse LV. Self-reported physical activity: its correlates and relationship with health-related quality of life in a large cohort of colorectal cancer survivors. PLoS One 2012;7(5):e36164.

[52] Davidson JR, MacLean AW, Brundage MD, Schulze K. Sleep disturbance in cancer patients. Soc Sci Med 2002;54(9):1309–21.

[53] Savard J, Villa J, Ivers H, Simard S, Morin CM. Prevalence, natural course, and risk factors of insomnia comorbid with cancer over a 2-month period. J Clin Oncol 2009;27(31):5233–9.

[54] Palesh OG, Roscoe JA, Mustian KM, Roth T, Savard J, Ancoli-Israel S, et al. Prevalence, demographics, and psychological associations of sleep disruption in patients with cancer: University of Rochester Cancer Center-Community Clinical Oncology Program. J Clin Oncol 2010;28(2):292–8.

[55] Savard J, Simard S, Blanchet J, Ivers H, Morin CM. Prevalence, clinical characteristics, and risk factors for insomnia in the context of breast cancer. Sleep 2001;24(5):583–90.

[56] Savard J, Simard S, Ivers H, Morin CM. Randomized study on the efficacy of cognitive-behavioral therapy for insomnia secondary to breast cancer, Part II: Immunologic effects. J Clin Oncol 2005;23(25):6097–106.

[57] Varmus H. Ten years on—the human genome and medicine. N Engl J Med 2010;362(21):2028–9.

[58] McKesson Speciality Health. Clear Value Plus [Internet]; 2014 [cited June 22, 2015]. Available from: <http://sites.mckesson.com/mscs/documents/products/Value_Pathways_and_Clear_Value_Plus_Sell_Sheet.pdf>.

[59] Wikipedia. Cognitive computing [Internet]; 2015 [cited June 22, 2015]. Available from: <https://en.wikipedia.org/wiki/Cognitive_computing>.

[60] International Business Machine Corporation. Watson Health [Internet]; 2015 [cited June 22, 2015]. Available from: <http://www.ibm.com/smarterplanet/us/en/ibmwatson/health/>.

[61] Kris MG. How Memorial Sloan-Kettering is training Watson to personalize cancer care. Atlantic 2013;April 8.

[62] Upbin B. IBM's Watson now tackles clinical trials at MD Anderson Cancer Center. Forbes 2013;October 18.

[63] Hoverman JR, Klein I, Harrison DW, Hayes JE, Garey JS, Harrell R, et al. Opening the black box: the impact of an oncology management program consisting of level I pathways and an outbound nurse call system. J Oncol Pract 2014;10(1):63–7.

[64] National Institute of Health. Health care systems research collaboratory [Internet]; 2015 [cited June 22, 2015]. Available from: <https://http://www.nihcollaboratory.org/about-us/Pages/default.aspx>.

[65] National Institute of Health. UH3 project: Strategies and opportunities to stop colorectal cancer in priority populations [Internet]; 2015 [cited June 22, 2015]. Available from: <https://http://www.nihcollaboratory.org/demonstration-projects/Pages/STOPCRC.aspx>.

[66] Food and Drug Administration. Adherence to guidelines for glucose assessment in starting second generation antipsychotics [Internet]; 2014 [cited June 22, 2015]. Available from: <http://www.mini-sentinel.org/communications/mini-sentinel_publications/details.aspx?ID=268>.

[67] Patient Centered Outcomes Research Institute. PCORnet [Internet]; 2015 [cited June 22, 2015]. Available from: <http://www.pcornet.org/about-pcornet/>.

9

Survivorship

Ellen Beckjord PhD MPH[1], G.J. van Londen MD, MS[2] and
Ruth Rechis PhD[3]

[1]Population Health Program Design and Engagement Optimization, UPMC Health Plan, Pittsburgh,
PA, United States [2]Division of Hematology-Oncology, Department of Medicine,
University of Pittsburgh, Pittsburgh, PA, United States [3]Programs & Strategy,
LIVESTRONG Foundation, Austin, TX, United States

OUTLINE

9.1 Cancer Survivorship	**159**
9.1.1 Definitions	160
9.1.2 Population Data on Survivorship	160
9.1.3 Recommendations for Survivorship	161
9.1.4 Overview of the Chapter	161
9.2 Challenges in Survivorship	**162**
9.2.1 Physical, Emotional, and Practical Sequelae and Late Effects	162
9.2.2 Adopting and Maintaining Positive Health Behaviors	163
9.2.3 Information Seeking and Processing	163
9.2.4 Care Coordination and Defining a Model of Survivorship Care	164
9.2.5 Survivorship Care Plans and Survivorship Care Planning	165
9.3 Opportunities for Informatics-Based Solutions	**167**
9.3.1 Internet and Informatics Use Among Cancer Survivors	167
9.3.2 Informatics-Enabled Survivorship Care Plans and Care Planning	169
9.3.3 Data Liquidity and Interoperability	171
9.3.4 mHealth and Context-Aware, Real-Time Intervention	171
9.3.5 Rapid Learning Systems in Survivorship Care	172
9.3.6 Measure Standardization	173
9.4 Envisioning a Future State	**174**
9.4.1 Leveraging "Long Data" in Survivorship	174
9.4.2 Example Informatics-Based Solutions to Achieve Essential Elements of Care	174
9.5 Conclusions	**176**
List of Acronyms and Abbreviations	**176**
References	**176**

When I finished my last cycle of chemotherapy, in April 2014, friends and family congratulated me on being "done." What they couldn't know was that in some ways the hardest part of my cancer experience began once the cancer was gone. **Suleika Jaouad, Lost in Transition After Cancer, New York Times, March 2015**

9.1 CANCER SURVIVORSHIP

Individuals with a personal history of cancer—referred to herein as "cancer survivors" or "survivors"—number more than 14 million Americans. Over the course of their lifetime, one in two men and one in three women will

B. Hesse, D. Ahern & E. Beckjord: Oncology Informatics.
DOI: http://dx.doi.org/10.1016/B978-0-12-802115-6.00009-4

be diagnosed with cancer [1]. In 1971, when President Nixon declared a "war on cancer," average 5-year survival rates for cancer were only at 51% [2]. Today, the landscape is significantly different: for adults diagnosed with cancer between 2003 and 2009, 5-year survival rates are nearly 70% [1]. Survival statistics are even more favorable for children diagnosed with cancer, as nearly 80% survive for 5 years or longer [3]. For some types of cancer, conditional survival statistics show that after a certain period of time, the history of a cancer diagnosis no longer negatively impacts life expectancy. For most cancers, the likelihood of survival increases with each year the individual survives, and for early stage breast and colorectal cancers, after surviving for between 3 and 15 years, there is no evidence that the diagnosis of cancer contributes to excess mortality in this group compared to cancer-free peers [4].

9.1.1 Definitions

However, this "booming" population of cancer survivors [5] is still relatively new within the cancer community. The term "survivorship" first appeared in the literature in 1984, when "survivorship" was specifically identified as a topic of importance in nursing research [6]. At the founding meeting of the National Coalition of Cancer Survivorship (NCCS) in 1986, the term "cancer survivor" was defined emphatically and broadly. The NCCS declared "an individual is considered a cancer survivor from the time of diagnosis through the balance of his or her life" [7]. This definition, which has been widely adopted, including by the National Cancer Institute (NCI), also includes other individuals directly affected by the diagnosis, such as family, friends, and caregivers [7]. Here we will use the term "cancer survivor" or "survivor" to refer to the individual diagnosed with cancer, and will mostly focus on the time in survivorship that occurs after primary treatment ends; however, other chapters in this book will specifically address survivorship during treatment (Chapter 8, "Informatics Support Across the Cancer Continuum: Treatment") and the impact of cancer on family, friends, and caregivers (Chapter 10, "Advanced Cancer: Palliative, End of Life, and Bereavement Care").

9.1.2 Population Data on Survivorship

Fig. 9.1 shows the rapid growth in the number of cancer survivors alive in the United States over the last 40 years, with projections for even more accelerated growth in the decades to come. This growth, which is largely due to advances in early detection and treatment (please see Chapters 7, "Early Detection in the Age of Information Technology"; and 8, "Informatics Support Across the Cancer Continuum: Treatment" in this book

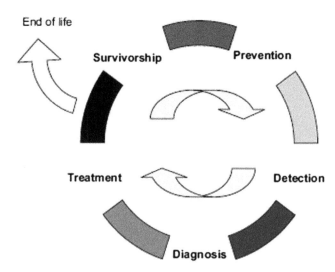

FIGURE 9.1 The cancer control continuum (revisited). *Source: Rowland JH, Bellizzi KM. Cancer survivors and survivorship research: a reflection on today's successes and tomorrow's challenges. Hematol Oncol Clin North Am 2008;22(2):181–200.*

for in-depth coverage of these topics), in many ways represents an enormous public health success.

But the rapid growth of cancer survivors over a relatively short period of time has two important implications. First, it has fundamentally challenged the notion of the "cancer continuum," which, until very recently, was commonly depicted in a linear fashion beginning with primary prevention, following to secondary prevention, then treatment, survivorship, and end-of-life (segments that are paralleled by the chapters in this section of this book). But near the end of the first decade of the new millennium, the structure of this continuum was called into question in two ways. McCabe argued that if there had previously been any question about the appropriateness of including "survivorship" as a distinct portion of the cancer continuum, given the size of this population, there could be no question about it now, saying "we have before us a unique opportunity to assure the inclusion of survivorship ... as a formal [part] of the health care continuum" (p. 2; [8]. And Rowland and Bellizzi called for "revisiting" the cancer continuum, suggesting that rather than depicting the continuum in a linear fashion, that it be represented cyclically (Fig. 9.2). This would be more accurate, they argued, as such large numbers of cancer survivors are surviving for such substantial lengths of time that they actually cycle back into the beginning of the continuum, where primary prevention, screening, and, if necessary, treatment for recurrence or a new primary cancer diagnosis become important [2]. These earlier phases of the cancer control continuum are perhaps even more important for this group, as survivors are at increased risk for another cancer diagnosis, given their diagnosis and treatment histories [9].

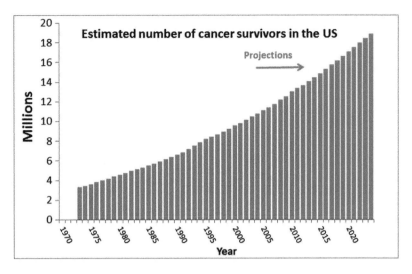

FIGURE 9.2 The number of cancer survivors alive in the United States. *Source: National Cancer Institute's Office of Cancer Survivorship (http://cancercontrol.cancer.gov/ocs/statistics/statistics.html) which cites DeSantis C, Chunchieh L, Mariotto AB, et al. Cancer Treatment and Survivorship Statistics, 2014. CA: A Cancer J Clin 2014. In press.*

A second result of the rapid growth of cancer survivors has been how research and practice have responded to this population, including informatics-related research and practice. When Nixon's "war on cancer" commenced, research devoted to cancer survivors was scarce, and was almost exclusively focused on issues related to describing quality of life (QOL), primarily during treatment. This was not unreasonable, as nearly half of all individuals diagnosed with cancer could not be expected to survive for any substantial length of time, and so research was heavily geared toward understanding how to preserve as much of a survivor's QOL for the remainder of their lives. But as survival has increased, research and practice have evolved. Starting in the 1990s, survivorship research began to address interventions to *improve* QOL and health outcomes for cancer survivors, both during and after treatment [10].

9.1.3 Recommendations for Survivorship

In 2005, the Institute of Medicine (IOM) released a landmark report titled "From Cancer Patient to Cancer Survivor: Lost in Transition" that made a series of recommendations for research and practice devoted specifically to the period of survivorship that occurs after treatment ends [11]. As shown in Table 9.1, the IOM's recommendations for survivorship research and practice cover a broad amount of territory, commensurate with the wide array of issues and needs that exist within this population. In general, in the nearly 30 years since the NCCS proposed a definition of "cancer survivor," the research on this population has not caught up to the new definition of the cancer control continuum, and there is a need for more research devoted to primary

and secondary prevention among cancer survivors, as well as a need for continued investigations into interventions that are intended to improve survivor health-related quality of life (HRQOL; [12]).

All of this, we will see, has implications for informatics in the context of cancer survivorship. Cancer survivors, like most Americans, are heavily engaged in the use of informatics, and even more so in some cases, such as use of the Internet to look for cancer information [13]. By 2020, when the population of cancer survivors approaches 18 million (see Fig. 9.1), more than half (63%) of cancer survivors will be aged 65 years and older. This cohort, then, would have been 48 years old in 2003, when, according to the NCI's Health Information National Trends Survey (HINTS), roughly 58% of Americans were online, and they would have been 58 in 2013, when HINTS suggested that Internet penetration reached nearly 80% [14]. As such, the largest age demographic within the growing population of cancer survivors were likely still part of the workforce when the Internet came of age in the United States, and were likely exposed to the Internet in the context of their employment. As such, this suggests that survivors, on the whole, are well-positioned to benefit from use of informatics applications.

9.1.4 Overview of the Chapter

Research and practice devoted to survivorship stands to benefit from informatics in a number of ways as well. The next section of this chapter will provide an overview of the most common challenges encountered by cancer survivors and the most significant challenges facing survivorship research and practice. The following section

TABLE 9.1 Ten Recommendations from the IOM "Lost in Transition" Report

1. Health care providers, advocates, and other stakeholders should raise awareness of the needs of cancer survivors, establish cancer survivorship as a distinct phase of cancer care, and act to ensure the delivery of appropriate survivorship care.
2. Patients completing primary cancer treatment should be provided with a comprehensive care summary and follow-up plan written by the health care provider(s) who provided cancer treatment.
3. Systematically developed evidence-based clinical practice guidelines, assessment tools, and screening instruments should be developed to manage late effects of cancer and its treatment.
4. Quality of survivorship care measures should be developed through public/private partnerships and quality assurance programs implemented by health systems to monitor and improve the care that all survivors receive.
5. The Centers for Medicare & Medicaid Services, National Cancer Institute (NCI), Agency for Healthcare Research and Quality, the US Department of Veterans Affairs, and other quality organizations should support demonstration programs to test models of coordinated, interdisciplinary survivorship care in diverse communities and across systems of care.
6. Congress should support the Centers for Disease Control and Prevention, the States, and other collaborating institutions in developing comprehensive cancer control plans that include survivorship care. Community-based services and plans generated by public health agencies or public health practitioners are the key to establishing successful disease prevention activities of relevance to cancer survivors.
7. NCI, professional associations, and voluntary organizations should expand and coordinate efforts to provide educational opportunities to health care providers to equip them to address the health care and quality of life issues facing cancer survivors.
8. Employers, legal advocates, health care providers, sponsors of support services, and government agencies should act to eliminate discrimination and minimize adverse effects of cancer on employment, while supporting cancer survivors with short- and long-term limitations in ability to work.
9. Federal and state policy makers should act to ensure that all cancer survivors have access to adequate and affordable health insurance; insurers and payers of health care should recognize survivorship care as an essential part of cancer care and design benefits, payment policies, and reimbursement mechanisms to facilitate coverage for evidence-based aspects of care.
10. The NCI and funding agencies as well as private health insurers should increase their support for survivorship research and expand mechanisms for its conduct. New research initiatives focused on cancer patient follow-up are urgently needed to guide effective survivorship care.

will review informatics-based solutions to these challenges. Finally, we will end with future visioning for how informatics can be broadly used to support survivors and survivorship research and practice.

9.2 CHALLENGES IN SURVIVORSHIP

Though the hope after a cancer diagnosis is always for survivorship, survivorship often comes at a high cost

[15]. For many survivors, the sequelae of treatment and resulting late effects—physical, emotional, or practical consequences of cancer or its treatment that can occur years after treatment ends—create a health experience that is akin to living with a chronic disease [16,17]. However, like other chronic disease models, this is really the only common denominator among individuals who are cancer survivors. What late effects are experienced, for how long, and to what degree of severity are highly variable and a function of the cancer diagnosis, its treatment, and person-level biomedical and sociodemographic factors [16]. In this way, all that informatics has to offer health care is brought to bear in survivorship, as the individualized health experiences of survivors and the resulting need for highly coordinated care both lead to challenges that informatics is uniquely positioned to address.

9.2.1 Physical, Emotional, and Practical Sequelae and Late Effects

Although the physical and emotional late effects of cancer and its treatment vary across survivors, the most common physical late effects include cardiovascular; pulmonary; gastrointestinal; rheumatologic; endocrine; renal; sensory/neurologic [18]; neurological; lymphatic; genitourinary; and second malignancies [19]. Given that the majority of cancer survivors are age 65 or older, some have called for a specific conceptual model of elderly survivorship that would address, in addition to the issues previously listed, frailty, nutritional needs, and premorbid cognitive disruption [20].

In addition to physical clinical late effects, other behavioral and psychosocial significant recovery issues commonly encountered during survivorship include fatigue; emotional distress; concerns about body image; sexual health issues; infertility; fears of recurrence; post-traumatic stress disorder (PTSD); and family/caregiver stress [21]. Estimates of how many survivors experience these recovery issues and to what extent vary in the literature. In two surveys of adult cancer survivors within 5 years of diagnosis conducted by the LIVESTRONG Foundation in 2006 and 2010 ($n = 2910$), almost 90% of respondents reported to be dealing with at least one physical concern (eg, fatigue); 90% reported to be dealing with at least one emotional concern (eg, emotional distress); and 45% reported to be dealing with at least one practical concern related to their cancer diagnosis (eg, financial issues) [22]. With respect to the degree to which these concerns interrupt daily life, there is some consistency across the literature in identifying a "significant minority" of survivors (20–30%) whose physical, emotional, or practical concerns cause clinically significant levels of disruption [23].

9.2.1.1 Fear of Recurrence

Perhaps the most common concern among cancer survivors is fear of recurrence of cancer. While this is understandable and manageable for most survivors who encounter fears of recurrence primarily around dates of follow-up tests and screenings, it represents an important target for surveillance and treatment as fear of recurrence is closely associated with broader issues of anxiety and depression [24]. A common clustering of recovery issues seen in survivors is the challenging "trifecta" of pain, depression, and fatigue [25–27]. Unfortunately, the evidence suggests that recovery issues in survivorship tend to be enduring, rather than transitory [26,28,29], and a number of studies have shown that younger survivors experience more recovery issues than older survivors [28].

9.2.1.2 Long-Term Health Status

Additionally, these recovery issues lead to generally poorer health status among cancer survivors than age-matched cancer-free peers. Compared to individuals without a personal history of cancer, cancer survivors have higher rates of problems with pain, emotional distress, insomnia, and a generally higher burden of comorbid conditions [30]. They are also more likely to have a mental health diagnosis and utilize more outpatient mental and physical health treatment [31]. For survivors of childhood cancer specifically, as adults, these survivors have twice the number of health conditions compared to their cancer-free siblings [32], and 40% experience moderate to severe late-effects in adulthood [33].

9.2.1.3 Existential Issues

While there is evidence that many cancer survivors experience posttraumatic growth as part of their cancer experience (eg, [34]), for many there are also existential, identity-related challenges. These challenges are often a function of a desire on the part of the survivor to return to "normal" after cancer, and an expectation on the part of the people in their lives that they will do so. Much like the spirit of the quote that begins this chapter, many survivors are distressed to realize that the myriad of challenges commonly encountered in survivorship make it difficult to feel like a return to "normal" is possible, and make it very challenging to celebrate that cancer is "over" [17]. This can lead to feelings of guilt on the part of the survivor, who may struggle with trying to balance seeking care for late effects and enduring concerns while also experiencing gratitude for being alive, especially while others they may have encountered during their cancer journey succumbed to their illness [35]. Survivors may also experience frustration and confusion over their need for continued intervention to resolve survivorship challenges at a time when they no longer think of themselves as a current cancer patient [36].

9.2.2 Adopting and Maintaining Positive Health Behaviors

Another assumption that is often not accurate is that cancer survivors will use their cancer experience as motivation to improve health behaviors, particularly after treatment ends. Indeed, adopting and maintaining better health behaviors is as or more important for cancer survivors as compared to individuals without a cancer history, as obesity, sedentary lifestyle, poor nutrition, and smoking are all associated with increased risk for recurrence and mortality [37], and meeting healthy behavior guidelines are key to lowering the risk of adverse late effects [38]. But available data do not suggest that survivors differ from cancer-free normative peers when it comes to rates of tobacco use, fruit and vegetable consumption, physical activity, or body mass index (BMI). In a study of more than 36,000 cancer survivors, the American Cancer Society (ACS) found that less than 20% of cancer survivors were meeting current fruit and vegetable consumption recommendations and less than 50% were meeting current physical activity recommendations. And these percentages were worse than success rates of the general population. While most survivors were not using tobacco, the ACS found that fewer than 5% of survivors in the study were simultaneously meeting recommendations for all three recommendations (fruit and vegetable consumption; physical activity; smoking). At the same time, the ACS found that participation in health behaviors—physical activity specifically—was associated with better HRQOL among survivors ([39]; for an in-depth discussion of using informatics to affect behavior in the context of cancer, please see Chapter 12, "Oncology Informatics: Behavioral and Psychological Sciences" in this book).

9.2.3 Information Seeking and Processing

Given the broad range of challenges faced by cancer survivors and confusing, sometimes conflicting, recommendations about what they should do to achieve and maintain optimal health and wellness during survivorship, it is not surprising that this population has a significant number of information needs. In a population-based study of 1040 adult posttreatment survivors of colorectal or bladder cancers or non-Hodgkin lymphoma or leukemia, more than 50% of survivors reported to needing more information about tests and treatments they should receive during survivorship; health promotion and what health behavior recommendations to adopt; side effects and symptoms they could expect to encounter and what to do about them; and interpersonal and emotional challenges [40].

Survivors seek cancer-related information at a higher rate than the general population (more than 60% of cancer survivors have looked for cancer information compared to less than 30% of Americans with no cancer history) and high levels of cancer information seeking are maintained even after more than a decade since time since diagnosis [13]. When survivors have significant information needs, it can threaten their sense of self-efficacy in survivorship. This is particularly concerning, as self-efficacy appears to serve a protective effect for survivors in preventing clinically significant levels of emotional distress in survivors [41]. Though self-efficacy varies considerably among survivors, unfortunately, it tends to be lowest among survivors who are experiencing challenges such as fatigue, pain, and depression [42]. As such, promoting self-efficacy among survivors, including through empowering their information search and processing experiences, is a high priority.

9.2.4 Care Coordination and Defining a Model of Survivorship Care

Promoting self-efficacy among cancer survivors can also occur through the provision of coordinated, patient-centered cancer care. Using the IOM's definition of patient-centered care as a foundation [43], patient-centered cancer care has been recently defined by LIVESTRONG as cancer care that considers the survivor as a whole person, beyond their disease, from the time of diagnosis through the balance of their life; is respectful of the survivor's preferences, needs, and values related to the involvement of their family and friends in their care; empowers the survivor to participate in their care in a way that is consistent with their preferences, needs, and values; and requires that multiple levels of the cancer care delivery are designed to accommodate the needs of survivors and caregivers, acknowledging that the care delivery system must support providers to function effectively [44].

9.2.4.1 Care Coordination

However, given the relatively new status of this large and fast-growing population, models of survivorship care, patient-centered or otherwise, have not caught up to demand. One of the biggest challenges in providing high-quality, patient-centered care to cancer survivors is the degree to which survivorship care requires a high level of care coordination. Meyers and colleagues define care coordination as having two core functions: the transfer of information and establishing accountability among members of a care team [45]. Care coordination is central to other newer models of health care, such as Patient-Centered Medical Homes and Accountable Care Organizations, and the task of achieving high-quality care coordination is equally challenging in these models as it is in survivorship care. In all instances, given

the degree to which information exchange and ease of identifying accountability are fundamental to care coordination, informatics is a necessary, though often not sufficient, solution to helping care coordination occur.

Given the impending boom of cancer survivors (many of whom will be older and thus suffer from multiple comorbidities) and the relative shortage of providers, the care for cancer survivors will become more strained and will need to be restrategized. One possible solution for this relative discrepancy includes the leveraging into the cancer care paradigm of a more prominent role for primary care providers (PCPs), who often already provide essential care for cancer survivors [7]. Another health care provider with whom coordination is often necessary—though too often underutilized—is the palliative care provider [46] (please see Chapter 10, "Advanced Cancer: Palliative, End of Life, and Bereavement Care" in this book for an in-depth discussion of palliative care in cancer survivorship). A third category of health care providers instrumental in survivorship, though like palliative care providers are often underutilized, are providers who can deliver psychosocial care [47,48]. The provision of psychosocial care in cancer survivorship was highlighted both in 2008 by the IOM report "Cancer Care for the Whole Patient: Meeting Psychosocial Health Needs" [49] and the 2012 American College of Surgeons standard requiring systematic distress screening for cancer survivors by 2015 [50]. Unfortunately, at the current time, there is limited to no adequate reimbursement for most cancer survivorship-related clinical services, including the necessary coordination of care; the onsite availability of crucial clinical services (eg, nutrition, physical therapy, navigators); as well as the e-mail and phone-mediated provision of supportive care (which becomes more prominent in the posttreatment-phase since survivors are less frequently seen in a health care provider's office).

9.2.4.2 Communication Is Key

In addition to lack of reimbursement as a challenge to delivery of survivorship care, communication challenges exist as well. Both during and after treatment, health care for the cancer survivor almost inevitably will involve multiple specialists creating, from the start, some significant communication challenges [51,52]. These challenges are not only reserved for communication between providers in the context of care coordination; challenges also exist in provider communication with survivors. Patient-centered cancer communication is a multidimensional charge for the health care provider caring for a cancer survivor. In addition to keeping the survivor on-track with follow-up surveillance to detect recurrence or new disease, the provider must also deal with survivors' uncertainties about recurrence; respond to their dynamic emotional states; promote adherence to recommended follow-up tests and treatments; and promote understanding of an oftentimes complex and evolving health care regimen [53].

While there is broad agreement that care coordination and communication are key to the provision of patient-centered cancer and survivorship care, there is currently no standardized approach to delivering survivorship care [54]. Relatedly, and more concerning, is that many cancer survivors are not receiving care for physical, emotional, and practical concerns in the posttreatment period. Though the majority of survivors report to be dealing with at least one physical and/or emotional concern in the posttreatment period, in a 2010 survey by the LIVESTRONG Foundation, only 67% of survivors said they received any care for their posttreatment physical concerns, and only 41% of survivors said they received any care for their posttreatment emotional concerns [22]. When survivors who did not receive posttreatment care were asked why they had not received care, most (55%) said they had "learned to live with" their posttreatment physical, emotional, and practical concerns [55]. As Dr Michael Feuerstein, Founder and Editor-in-Chief of the *Journal of Cancer Survivorship* described when recounting his own cancer journey put it: "*I had many consultations with no single provider coordinating care. Coordination was left to me ... my overall care was fragmented, which is illustrative of how the health care system currently responds to the needs of cancer survivors*" (p. 114; [56]). Clearly there is an enormous opportunity to do better.

9.2.5 Survivorship Care Plans and Survivorship Care Planning

Survivorship has come to be understood as a highly transitional time when, like other transitions in health care, the risk of "falling through the cracks"—whether it be information falling through the cracks or cancer survivors' concerns—is high [57]. Few expect that an exclusively oncologist- or PCP-led model of survivorship care will emerge as a solution to doing a better job of meeting the needs of cancer survivors [58]. As such, if care coordination will be an unavoidable challenge in survivorship care, solving the challenge of care coordination in survivorship care requires a reliable operationalization of the processes for information exchange and establishment of accountability that are integral to care coordination. In the 2005 "Lost in Transition" IOM report, the survivorship care plan (SCP), which includes a treatment summary (TS), was first proposed as this operationalization. The IOM report recommended that the SCP include multiple components addressing treatment history and follow-up care recommendations (Box 9.1).

Over the past decade, in the wake of the 2005 IOM report, two things have happened. First, SCPs became,

---

BOX 9.1

RECOMMENDED COMPONENTS OF SCPS

- Cancer type, treatments received, and their potential consequences
- Specific information about the timing and content of recommended cancer follow-up
- Recommendations regarding preventive practices and how to maintain health and well-being
- Information on legal protections regarding employment and access to health insurance
- The availability of psychosocial services in the community

Adapted from Hewitt M, Greenfield S, Stovall E, editors. From cancer patient to cancer survivor: lost in transition. Washington (DC): National Acadamies Press; 2005.

---

in a way, a beacon of hope for solving the challenges in providing better care to cancer survivors and were identified as the most promising solution to the care coordination challenges in survivorship care [59]. There were multiple calls for specific "transition visits" at the end of primary treatment in which the SCP would be delivered to the cancer survivor, thus demarcating the end of primary treatment and the beginning of survivorship care. The survivor, then, armed with the SCP, would no longer get "lost" in the transition [60].

9.2.5.1 Challenges to the Delivery of SCPs

As a result, research began to detail the results of the provision of SCPs to cancer survivors. This has led to the second event of significance in the wake of the IOM report: it has become clear that SCPs alone fall short of overcoming the challenges in survivorship care, and that informatics will be key to solving those challenges and realizing the full potential of both SCPs and survivorship care *planning*. In perhaps the most in-depth process investigation of the provision of SCPs, Dr Carrie Stricker and her colleagues studied the degree to which SCPs provided by LIVESTRONG Survivorship Centers of Excellence (Centers) adhered to the recommendations of the IOM regarding what SCPs should contain, and also how long it took to prepare and deliver the SCP to a survivor. The LIVESTRONG Centers involved multiple academic medical centers that partnered with community settings of cancer care [61]. These partnerships were funded by the LIVESTRONG Foundation, in part, to investigate different models of survivorship care and interventions such as the provision of SCPs. The Survivorship Centers of Excellence were all NCI-designated comprehensive cancer centers and were some of the most prestigious academic settings in the United States. In short, if any settings of cancer care were to be able to achieve a "slam dunk" when it came to the provision of SCPs, it would be the LIVESTRONG Centers.

Stricker and her colleagues [62] found that, despite the enormous amount of work the Centers were putting into SCPs, they were not reliably creating SCPs that included the elements recommended by the IOM (Box 9.1) and that the process of creating and delivering the SCP was not scalable or sustainable. Only 2 of 13 Centers were delivering SCPs that were in at least 75% concordance with the IOM recommendations. The average level of concordance was only 59%, ranging from 38% to 83%. Over one-third of sites reported that it took more than 1 hour to prepare the SCP, and 30% said it was more than an additional hour to review the SCP with the survivor. Stricker and her colleagues concluded, "if a network of centers with dedicated funding and documented institutional support for survivorship care does not achieve high concordance with IOM recommendations, can widespread concordance with these recommendations be expected?" (p. 366). However, of significant note is that Stricker's study focused on activity in the LIVESTRONG Centers during 2009, during which few sites could leverage an electronic health record (EHR) to create, deliver, or disseminate the SCP. As will be discussed in more detail in the next section of this chapter, the lack of an informatics-based foundation for the SCP was likely a major barrier for the Centers to achieving concordance with the IOM recommendations and to creating and delivering SCPs in a more reasonable amount of time.

Research has also documented shortfalls with respect to the degree to which SCPs are achieving better care coordination. In 2009, the NCI launched the Survey of Physician Attitudes Regarding the Care of Cancer Survivors (SPARCCS) study. SPARCCS involved surveys of 1100 oncologists and 1100 PCPs, with survey questions addressing perceived roles, knowledge, and care practices regarding posttreatment cancer survivors (SPARCCS). One component of these surveys addressed the provision of SCPs on the part of oncologists and the receipt of SCPs on the part of PCPs. In an analysis led by Dr Laura Forsythe, results were encouraging in that PCP receipt of SCPs was associated with better oncologist-PCP communication; better PCP perceptions of care coordination; and greater confidence among PCPs regarding their level of survivorship care knowledge [63]. Unfortunately, the conditions that led to these positive outcomes—oncologist provision of SCPs and PCP receipt of SCPs—were far from the norm. Oncologists reported to "always" or "almost always" provide a SCP to a PCP only 20% of the time, and PCPs reported to "always"

or "almost always" receive SCPs only 13% of the time. The Stricker and Forsythe studies have three things in common. Both were focused on results collected in 2009; both found results that indicated significant problems with the process of creating and delivering SCPs (in the Stricker study, to survivors; in the Forsythe study, to PCPs); and both pointed to early evidence that informatics is instrumental to achieving better results. In their analysis of the SPARCCS study, Forsythe and colleagues found that oncologists were significantly more likely to provide SCPs to PCPs when they used an EHR [63].

Finally, in 2011, Dr Eva Grunfeld and her colleagues published the first randomized trial designed to gage the impact of SCPs on survivorship health outcomes in the *Journal of Clinical Oncology* [64]. These results were presented to the cancer community at the American Society of Clinical Oncology meeting in 2011, and were rather controversial. Grunfeld and colleagues focused their study on 408 early-stage breast cancer survivors who were at least 3 months posttreatment. All participants' care was transferred to their PCP upon conclusion of primary cancer treatment, and all underwent a transition visit with their oncology practice. Between 2007 and 2009, women randomized to the intervention group also received a SCP, which was delivered during a 30-minute nurse-led visit. Additionally, the SCP was provided to the participant's PCP. For 2 years the study tracked a number of outcomes, including cancer-specific distress; general emotional distress; HRQOL; patient satisfaction; and survivor-perceived continuity and coordination of care.

The only difference observed between the survivors who received a SCP and those who did not was that slightly more survivors who received a SCP could identify their PCP as being responsible for their follow-up care. There were no differences observed on any of the other outcomes, and a secondary analysis of the study data showed that the provision of the SCP to the intervention group added $67 to the cost of care and did not result in a significant gain in quality-adjusted life years [65].

9.2.5.2 The Intersection of Survivorship Care Planning and Informatics

Needless to say, between the Stricker, Forsythe, and Grunfeld studies, the initial years of the new millennium were not kind to SCPs. The earlier hopes that SCPs would be a viable solution to survivorships most pressing challenges—supporting surveillance and treatment for late effects; promoting health behaviors; alleviating survivors' information needs; and facilitating care coordination—were all but dashed, and the goal of figuring out how to deliver high-quality, patient-centered survivorship care seemed farther away than ever.

Enter informatics. In a very coincidental, but rather elegant way, informatics and survivorship have come of age together, both gaining traction and visibility with particular speed and emphasis over the last 30 years. Today, it seems that the most promising way forward for survivorship care is a marriage of the two: informatics-enabled survivorship care planning. In 2013, in her seminal commentary in the *Journal of Clinical Oncology*, "Can't See the Forest for the Care Plan: A Call to Revisit the Context of Care Planning," Dr Carly Parry and colleagues noted that, to date, research was suggesting that SCPs were falling short of the potential they were assigned in the early 2000s [66]. But this, they argued, should not be taken as an indication of whether SCPs can or should be routinely provided to cancer survivors so much as an indicator of too narrow a focus on SCPs as a document. Parry argued that there should be less focus on SCPs in isolation and more on the process SCPs are designed to support: survivorship care *planning*. Parry noted that SCPs alone could not be expected to significantly change outcomes for cancer survivors; as she notes, "we cannot expect a document to do the work of a process" (p. 2651, [66]). In response, Parry proposed a conceptual framework for survivorship care planning, and called for continued research on SCPs to incorporate this framework into their research in an effort to support the standardization of processes and measures to more efficiently build the relatively nascent evidence base in survivorship care.

Of greatest interest here is the degree to which informatics looms large in the conceptual framework as a foundational component of survivorship care planning. In Parry's framework, technology is positioned as a foundation to models and processes of survivorship care. In the next section, we will discuss ways informatics could be used—and, to a lesser extent, is already being used—to support innovative solutions to survivorship's most pressing challenges, and how this work, in the context of survivorship care planning, will ultimately offer the best evidence on the impact of survivorship care planning on survivors' HRQOL and health outcomes and lead to the most innovative and impactful uses of informatics to support survivorship care.

9.3 OPPORTUNITIES FOR INFORMATICS-BASED SOLUTIONS

The enormous potential for informatics-based solutions to improve survivorship and survivorship care is a function of two realities. First, cancer survivors are an online population, and are using the Internet at higher rates than the general population for their health. Second, informatics-based solutions are best positioned to be dynamic and personalized in ways that match the highly individualized nature of an individual's journey through cancer survivorship [67].

9.3.1 Internet and Informatics Use Among Cancer Survivors

Cancer survivors look to informatics to manage their health in the posttreatment period, and use the Internet to complement and supplement the care they receive from health care providers. Even more than a decade after diagnosis, more than half of cancer survivors report to have recently looked for cancer information, and between 30% and 50% of them use the Internet as their information source [13]. The Internet plays an even greater role in the information management of longer-term cancer survivors. In general, survivors prefer to use their health care provider as their source of cancer information, but survivors within 1 year of diagnosis are more likely to turn to a health care provider first as compared to survivors 2–10 years postdiagnosis who rely more heavily on the Internet. This is likely because survivors closer to time of diagnosis are still heavily engaged with the medical system and accessing their health care providers through regular clinical encounters [13]. Regular access to health care providers plummets in the posttreatment period, but the presence of cancer in the survivor's life often remains high due to late effects and posttreatment concerns (Fig. 9.3). At this point, the Internet and informatics-based tools are positioned to fill the gap that opens between the presence of the medical system in the survivor's life and the lingering presence of cancer.

Use of informatics in health care has grown rapidly over the past decade and survivors have kept pace. Between 2003 and 2008, there was significant growth in the number of cancer survivors who were online (from 49% to nearly 60%), and during that time, survivors outpaced the general population with respect to the degree to which they used the Internet for health-related purposes [68]. Interestingly, while less education, older age, and non-White race/ethnicity were still barriers to Internet access among cancer survivors, these promoters of the "digital divide" were not barriers to use of the Internet for health among survivors [68].

Indeed, results of an online survey conducted by the LIVESTRONG Foundation in 2010 and harmonized with a dual-frame, nationally representative sample of adults collected through HINTS support the idea that cancer survivors see great potential in informatics for improving their care. The LIVESTRONG survey yielded a sample of 8411 respondents, including 2343 posttreatment cancer survivors, and 5337 with no history of cancer. Comparisons revealed a strong predilection to value health information technology within the cancer-relevant groups, especially among those living with cancer as a chronic disease. In comparison, only about half of the general population, represented in the HINTS data,

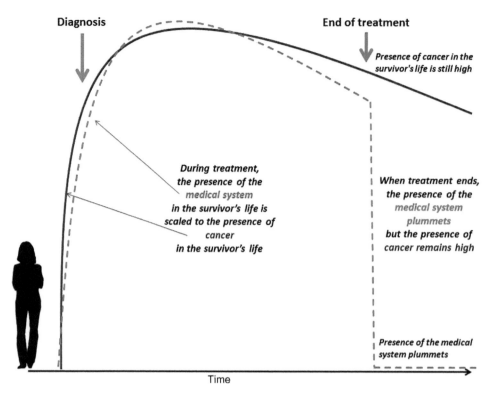

FIGURE 9.3   Relative presence of the medical system and "cancer" before and after treatment ends. *Source: Ellen Beckjord, PhD, MPH.*

showed a similar degree of enthusiasm. When asked about specific functions for EHRs, respondents valued privacy and security above all, followed by improving care coordination and data sharing between providers [69]. One of the most clear ideas shared was that informatics could improve care and save time. As one individual noted, "*I am tired of filling out forms each time I go to another doctor. I think the doctor would have faster access to the patients' information. Too often it is buried in tons of tests, previous visits... the average doctor today doesn't have the time to sift through all that paper. Things get overlooked. The electronic form could be organized and in an easy-to-read format for the doctor and the patient. Each doctor could see what the other specialist had suggested or prescribed*" [70].

9.3.1.1 Internet Cancer Support Groups

However, one of the first and most well-studied examples of using informatics in cancer survivorship existed outside of the medical systems: Internet cancer support groups (ICSGs). ICSGs have a number of advantageous features, including making it possible for survivors to connect to one another despite geography. This can be particularly useful for survivors diagnosed with rarer cancers who may not have a peer within their health care system or geographical area to connect to who is coping with the same disease. A second advantage to ICSGs is that they allow survivors to give and receive support from anywhere, usually from home, which can

be more convenient than traveling to a facility to attend a support group. This convenience is especially appealing when survivors are in active treatment and may not be feeling well, or when they are recovering from treatments such as surgery. Despite the prevalence of ICSGs, they are not utilized as frequently as the Internet generally by cancer survivors [68]. Dr Eun-Ok Im proposed a conceptual model of the factors that influence ICSG use, and through a review of the literature, found support for the model [71]. Dr Im found that sociodemographic factors; cultural factors; Internet use; and level of health care, psychosocial, or information needs were associated with ICSG use. Specifically, Im found that White survivors were most likely to use ICSGs, as were survivors with higher levels of depression; women; survivors of higher socioeconomic status; and survivors with higher levels of psychosocial needs.

Few empirical studies of ICSGs have utilized designs that allow for investigations of the impact of ICSG participation on survivor health outcomes. Those that have reveal mixed results; while participants generally report positive experiences with ICSGs, there is no substantial evidence at this time that ICSGs significantly improve mood, adjustment to cancer, or self-rated health [72]. One exception is studies of the Cancer Health Enhancement Support System (CHESS), developed by Dr David Gustafson and colleagues at the University of Wisconsin [73]. CHESS is not an ICSG, but does provide an online forum for the receipt and delivery of social support among cancer survivors. Studies of CHESS have suggested that it positively impacts social support, participation in health care, and health information competence (for an in-depth review of CHESS, please see Chapter 10, "Advanced Cancer: Palliative, End of Life, and Bereavement Care" in this book).

9.3.1.2 Consumer-Facing Applications

In his broad, and now dated, review of consumer health informatics applications commissioned by the Agency for Healthcare Research and Quality (AHRQ), Dr Christopher Gibbons went beyond ICSGs and into the realm of consumer-facing informatics applications [74]. Dr Gibbons found that informatics-based applications for health covered a wide variety of conditions, including cancer, but also health promotion (eg, physical activity, smoking cessation); chronic disease management; and mental health. Generally, Gibbons concluded, these applications show considerable promise for improving health and wellness, but he also asserted that the real role of consumer health informatics is to improve the efficacy of health care interventions delivered by people. Striking this balance, and designing informatics applications that are useable both by the target patient population *and* the providers who care for members of the population is critical [75]. For example, in a study of CHESS with more than 400 breast cancer survivors, women randomized to use CHESS or randomized to have a human mentor to help them navigate their cancer experience had better information competence and emotional processing outcomes compared to a control group. However, women randomized to a fourth group that received both CHESS and the human mentor did better than either group that got the single intervention alone [76].

Informatics-based interventions for cancer survivors of all kinds are still relatively new, and the evidence base to reliably estimate their impact does not yet exist. However, preliminary reviews support the notion that informatics-based interventions positively impact survivors' HRQOL [77]. But direct intervention is really only the tip of the iceberg. The potential of informatics to benefit survivors by being used as a foundation to create positive, proactive decisional architectures around relevant "points-of-choice"—or times when survivors are making decisions about behavior, health care, or other health-relevant events—is much greater [78].

9.3.2 Informatics-Enabled Survivorship Care Plans and Care Planning

To this end, informatics-enabled SCPs and survivorship care planning hold incredible promise to significantly improve the survivorship landscape. Informatics is uniquely suited to address two significant barriers to allowing SCPs to reach their full potential. First, survivorship is a highly individualized experience. The challenges that any one individual encounters during survivorship are a function of their type of cancer, the treatments they received, any preexisting comorbid conditions they may have had, and their premorbid and current socioeconomic statuses and sociocultural environment. In short, one size will never fit all when it comes to SCPs, so using informatics to make it easy to personalize care plans is absolutely necessary. Second, and related, is that survivorship is a dynamic and heterogeneous journey [17,51]. What a survivor needs from their SCP or from the care planning process at one stage of their survivorship journey may be very different from what they need at the next. In this way, unless the SCP that serves as the informational foundation of good survivorship care planning is an evolving, dynamic, "living and breathing" set of recommendations, it will not reach optimal usefulness over time [56,79].

9.3.2.1 EHR-Enabled SCPs

SCPs that use EHRs as a foundation are much better positioned to be agile and nimble in this way. EHR-enabled SCPs are better positioned to stay current with the survivor's needs, so long as the assumption that their current needs are accurately documented in the EHR. However, there are two major challenges to this assumption: first, the evidence suggests that relatively few survivors receive care for their posttreatment physical, emotional, and practical concerns. Data from the LIVESTRONG Surveys of People Affected by Cancer found that among survivors with posttreatment physical concerns, only 67% received care for their concerns; among survivors with posttreatment emotional concerns, only 47% received care; and among survivors with practical concerns, only 37% received care [22]. If few survivors are receiving care for their posttreatment concerns, then the process of using the EHR as a reliable foundation for a current take on their needs—which would involve assessment and documentation during a clinical encounter—is not viable. The second and related challenge to EHR-enabled SCPs has to do with the general challenges of delivering survivorship care. A serious barrier to moving toward standardized models of survivorship care planning and care delivery is that most of the activities involved, including the creation and delivery of SCPs (EHR-enabled or otherwise), are not reimbursable care events, thus discouraging providers from engaging in these activities over and above their already strained schedules [80].

Despite these barriers, EHR-enabled SCPs are uniquely positioned to overcome them. A high priority for increasing the frequency with which SCPs are created, delivered to a survivor, and delivered to other providers in the survivor's health care ecosystem to support care coordination is to make the process of creating the SCP more efficient and work-flow aligned. Here, informatics and the EHR are instrumental. Not only can use of the EHR as a foundation for SCPs and survivorship care planning more broadly help the content of SCPs and care planning evolve and remain current with the survivor's dynamic needs, but an informatics foundation can also significantly increase the efficiency with which SCPs are created [81]. Using the EHR as a foundation, much of the information in an SCP related to the details of the cancer diagnosis, treatment received, and follow-up recommendations can be automatically populated into the EHR, saving time and effort on the part of the provider and clinic staff. This model was used in one of the only published demonstrations of SCP delivery that actually showed a financial return on the investment of the SCP creation and delivery process. Rosales and colleagues detailed their SCP model with descriptions of how the EHR was used to populate key components of the SCP, leading to the creation and delivery of the SCP occurring in less than 1 hour. In addition, they discussed ways of billing for the SCP process and found that after accounting for the time it took to create and deliver the EHR-enabled SCP, that there was an average 6% return on the investment after receiving reimbursement [82].

This likely reflects the future direction of SCP creation and survivorship care planning more generally—using the EHR and other informatics-based systems to largely automate the process of creating the SCP; to keep it current and evolving in tandem with survivor needs; and to share it for the purposes of care coordination with other providers involved in the posttreatment care of the cancer survivor, most notably, their PCP. Achieving this future state will be a significant step forward in overcoming current challenges related to providers creating SCPs that adhere to the IOM's recommendations as far as what content the SCP should include [62], and to providers sharing and reliably receiving SCPs within the survivor's health care ecosystem [63]. Two studies that specifically focus on EHR-generated SCPs have been done at the University of Wisconsin. In [83], Tevaarwerk and colleagues examined the provision of an EHR-generated SCP to 38 breast cancer survivors who were between 4 months and more than 4 years postdiagnosis. Using the elements of SCPs outlined by the IOM as the standard, they found that only a minority of elements could be automatically populated in the EHR-generated SCP. However, the electronic infrastructure that supported the SCP allowed for relatively easy manual entry of information, resulting in the median time for SCP creation to be 3 minutes (range 2–12 minutes). The EHR-generated SCP was made available to survivors online; 95% found it to be easily accessible and survivors spent, on average, about 12 minutes reading their SCP.

The second study from this group [84] examined PCP (n=72) reactions to SCPs that were not only generated by the EHR but were delivered to the PCP via the EHR. PCPs responded overwhelmingly favorably to the SCPs, both with respect to content (88% found the information useful and 82% said it supported clinical decision making) and with respect to receiving the SCP via the EHR. In fact, 89% of PCPs said that receiving an SCP via an EHR would be critical to their actually using it in care for cancer survivors.

Additionally, in 2013, the LIVESTRONG Foundation, the ACS, Baptist Memorial Cancer Center, the Abramson Cancer Center of the University of Pennsylvania, and OncoLink (powered by Penn Medicine) launched a 2-year project to prepopulate an SCP with relevant data elements from the National Cancer Database cancer registry and EHRs. Using this automated tool, the study is evaluating the feasibility of implementing this plan with clinicians; patients; and survivors of prostate, colorectal, and breast cancer across multiple sites. Results from this research are forthcoming.

9.3.2.2 Internet-Enabled SCPs

To date, however, more common than EHR-enabled SCPs are Internet-based SCPs, which have advantages in terms of giving more survivors access to SCPs and to making the creation of them more efficient. But Internet-based SCP creation does not achieve the goal of using the SCP as a dynamic and evolving document upon which to anchor high-quality, coordinated survivorship care planning, as the creation of the document occurs outside the context of an informatics-enabled health care system. Nonetheless, there are some important successes worth noting in what has been learned from observations of Internet-enabled SCPs. In one of the earliest examples of an Internet-based SCP, a system called OncoLife was made available to cancer survivors between 2007 and 2008 [85]. More than 3300 individuals accessed the OncoLife tool; 63% of these individuals were survivors and 25% were health care providers. OncoLife users could input cancer and treatment history data into OncoLife, and calling upon best practice-based recommendations, OncoLife would create an individualized SCP. Though significant challenges to this model include the reliance on the user to populate key elements of the SCP (rather than an automated, and likely more reliable, population by the EHR) and the lack of EHR integration to evolve or update the SCP, it is important to note that only 12% of survivors who made use of OncoLife reported to have previously received survivorship information of any kind. In this way, the OncoLife Internet-based SCP filled an important gap for these users.

9.3.3 Data Liquidity and Interoperability

Scaling the creation and provision of SCPs through EHRs will rely heavily upon data sharing and data liquidity, or more generally, interoperability (for an in-depth review of these issues, please see Chapter 3, "Cancer Clinical Research: Enhancing Data Liquidity and Data Altruism" in this book). Interoperability has proven to be a stubborn and significant rate-limiting step in health informatics, in the context of survivorship and more broadly. While the past several years have seen enormous growth in the degree to which the Internet and other informatics-based tools are being used to document, measure, and track health outcomes, the promise of this growth has largely yet to be realized because of challenges in interoperability. Lack of interoperability limits the use of informatics in survivorship care planning in two fundamental ways. First, without the data liquidity required to pull clinical data from informatics-enabled medical systems into care planning tools such as SCPs, adoption of SCPs will remain low [86]. Second, informatics-based SCPs cannot be shared across settings of care if the settings do not use interoperable informatics systems. Unfortunately, this is not an uncommon scenario. Highlighting the importance of interoperability, the US Department of Health and Human Service's Office of the National Coordinator for Health Information Technology (the ONC) has identified interoperability as a critical goal for 2015.

9.3.3.1 Privacy and Security

But the barriers to interoperability and the resulting data-sharing that interoperability can enable have not just been technical in nature. Some have been socio-cultural, though the significance of those barriers has evolved rapidly. At the beginning of the millennium, there were robust national conversations around the privacy and security implications of informatics-enabled medicine. Many of these conversations pointed to concerns among patients and health care consumers about the privacy and security of their own health information. But most recently, it seems that while there continues to be broad agreement that privacy and security are critical to the success of informatics-enabled health care, that patients are ready for it and willing to take on any risks informatics might pose, as these risks are less significant than the potential benefits that could be realized when informatics is more broadly and consistently leveraged in medicine [87]. Data from studies of the Veteran's Administration's (VA) health care system (one of the most mature informatics-enabled health care systems in the world) show that the vast majority of veterans (nearly 80%) want others to be able to access their personal health record, including others who are outside of the VA health care system, for the purposes of coordinating

care [88]. Data from the 2013 to 2014 administration of HINTS found that fewer Americans were "very concerned" about the privacy or security of their health information being sent electronically between health care providers (about 19%) as compared to health information being shared via fax (about 25%) [89]. HINTS also showed that 84% of Americans believed their health information was kept in electronic format by their health care providers, and that 75% of Americans were confident in the privacy and security of that information. In a 2010 LIVESTRONG survey targeted to cancer survivors, more than 70% said that health care providers should be able to share information electronically [70].

Practice is slowly catching up to potential. In 2013, Jensen and colleagues reviewed 27 electronic patient-reported outcomes (ePRO) systems used in cancer care [90]. ePRO systems capture patient-reported data electronically, such as on a computer, tablet, or mobile device, and are a critical part of an informatics-enabled cancer care system. ePRO processes in cancer care allow for potential integration of survivor (patient)-reported data with the clinical data in the EHR, and when used together, can create a reliable and evolving picture of the survivor's current needs. Jensen's review found that of the 27 cancer care ePRO systems reviewed, 12 were linked to an EHR and 5 were linked to a patient portal. Clinical integration and actionable reporting structures that make use of ePRO data were noted as continued challenges that have yet to be fully addressed.

9.3.4 mHealth and Context-Aware, Real-Time Intervention

One way that survivor-reported outcomes can be captured outside of clinical encounters is through use of a mobile device. mHealth has been referred to as the "killer app" in the field of informatics because of how ubiquitous mobile devices have become, and how intimately users engage with them, uniquely positioning the mobile device to provide continual assessment of the user's state [91]. The rise of mHealth has spawned work on ecological momentary interventions (EMI), or real-time intervention [92], sometimes informed by ecological momentary assessment (EMA), real-time data collection [93]. In an early and important paper on the topic of mHealth, Dr William Riley described how the advent of mHealth would challenge the very foundation of many theories in behavioral medicine. These theories, Riley and his colleagues argued, were organized around relatively static conceptualizations of experience and behavior. In contrast, mHealth allows for a richer assessment and appreciation of the dynamic nature of human experience and behavior, thus enabling a whole new cadre of context-aware and nimble interventions for promoting health and wellness [94]; for a full discussion of innovative methods in oncology informatics, please see Chapter 18, "A New Era of Clinical Research Methods in a Data-Rich Environment" in this book.

Given the dynamic and evolving nature of survivorship, mHealth applications are particularly well suited for use among cancer survivors. Much like EHRs can be used to provide a dynamic foundation for SCPs and survivorship care planning by updating information about the survivor's status at the point of care, mHealth offers a vehicle for even more fine-grained assessment and intervention [92]. Currently, there are no completed and published studies of how EMA-informed EMI can be used to promote health and wellness during survivorship. However, this will not likely be the case for long, and it is easy to imagine many excellent mHealth use cases for addressing some key survivorship challenges. For example, while there is currently no evidence that a diagnosis of cancer on its own promotes significant changes in health behavior, there is reason to believe that if health behavior change interventions were well-timed during survivorship that perhaps interventions and resulting behavior change would be more successful [95]. If a survivor used an mHealth application to track their symptoms over time, and EMI was made available in ways that matched intervention to current symptoms, survivors may be more likely to adopt behavior changes that would have a direct impact on their HRQOL.

9.3.4.1 OncoKompass

An example of a system that is aiming to achieve context-aware, real-time intervention for cancer survivorship is OncoKompass [96]. The OncoKompass application, which has been funded by the Netherlands Cancer Society and Alpe d'HuZes Foundation, has the potential to enhance not only the efficiency of ePRO collection but also the provision of supportive care. The goals of OncoKompass are to support the growing number of cancer survivors and their HRQOL; their functional status; and the more efficient use of health care as well as support providers who may not have the time, resources, or expertise to engage in ongoing symptom management. OncoKompass allows survivors to assess independently their own HRQOL (physical, psychological, social, and existential domains) and lifestyle habits, whenever they want to, in a serial manner, in the comfort of their home. The results are processed in real-time and the survivor receives an immediate summary of their well-being scores and advice concerning supportive care and lifestyle (supported by evidence-based knowledge and decision support algorithms). Based on the individual's well-being profile and survivors' preferences, users can be directed toward guided self-care approaches or referrals to professional care providers.

This application has been created by a team in the Netherlands through a rigorous development process that consists of three phases to optimize uptake by users and providers: design of the program (driven by stakeholders' input), feasibility testing, and evaluation of outcomes. The needs assessments that served as the foundational information for creation of the OncoKompass system probed patients, providers, as well as a random sample from the general Dutch population about their needs and preferences with respect to eHealth and tiered supportive care [97]. The results of feasibility and outcome testing are to be published soon, and have led to the impending release of the next version of "OncoKompas 2.0." Through further testing upon launch of the application, the developers hope to learn more about determinants of successful triage and supportive care provision and thereby continue to refine their system to further optimize outcomes. They also will perform further research on the reach, cost-effectiveness, adoption, implementation, and maintenance of the application.

9.3.5 Rapid Learning Systems in Survivorship Care

An inevitable result of making broader use of informatics in survivorship care is more data being available for use in cancer care. This is whether it be via use of the EHR as a foundation for more dynamic SCPs and care planning; use of ePRO systems to capture more survivor-reported outcomes at the point-of-care; or use of mHealth to capture survivor-generated data outside the clinical context on an episodic or continual basis. Consistent with recommendations from the 2005 "Lost in Transition" IOM report, there are four ways this influx of data can be used to improve survivorship care: (1) the data can be used to create an evidence base for best practices in survivorship care; (2) the data can be used as a source of surveillance across settings of care; (3) the data can indicate when intervention is needed to resolve late effects; and (4) the data can be the communication foundation for improved care coordination [75]. These data uses are consistent with the notion of a "learning system" in cancer care [98].

The 2012 IOM report "Better Care at Lower Cost: The Path to Continuously Learning Health Care in America" identified seven characteristics of a learning health care system [99]: (1) provide real-time access to knowledge; (2) use informatics to capture experiences of care; (3) engage and empower patients; (4) provide incentives for care delivery that are aligned with high-value care; (5) offer full transparency related to the provision of care and the data collected; (6) are supported by a leadership-instilled culture that values continuous learning; and (7) are maintained by supportive system competencies. Learning health care systems are a wonderful example of a vision that is not born out of imagining how technology can be used in the context of cancer care, but of identifying technology as critical to realizing the critical components an imagined future of cancer care.

9.3.5.1 Value Propositions of a Learning System

Informatics is central to learning health care systems because of their reliance on data liquidity and interoperability [98]. In the context of cancer, learning health care systems offer a huge value proposition. First, at the level of medical discovery and care delivery, cancer care is rapidly and continually evolving. As a result, what we know and understand about survivorship and late effects today will likely not be useful knowledge and understanding in a decade, when the treatments received by people newly diagnosed with cancer may be significantly different than the treatments received by people diagnosed just 10 years before [100]. Learning health care systems in cancer are critical to allowing survivorship to stay ahead of the curve on identifying the late effects that accompany future treatments and the most efficient ways for resolving them.

A second value proposition of a learning health care system in cancer is that learning systems would significantly expedite the creation of the evidence base that is so badly needed for identifying and disseminating best practices in survivorship care [101]. Long-term cancer survivors are still such a relatively new population, with even more nascent models of care delivery to support them, that learning systems used to continually capture data at the point of care would be invaluable for standardizing care delivery and refining best practices to provide the most efficient and high-impact care to cancer survivors. Providing evidence-based care in survivorship will require the generation and accumulation of care-based evidence though a learning health care system.

Furthermore, learning health care systems can also incorporate survivor-generated data from outside of the clinical encounter, whether by use of mHealth, EMA, or passively sensed data. In this way, learning health care systems can specifically include the voice of the survivor and include their experiences in the creation of the evidence base that results from the continual capturing and interpreting of data [98]; please see Chapter 8, "Informatics Support Across the Cancer Continuum: Treatment" in this book for a detailed overview of learning health care systems in cancer treatment.

9.3.6 Measure Standardization

A critical practice to fully realize the potential of learning health care systems in survivorship care is the standardization of measures used to capture outcomes [66]. Capturing more data will not necessarily expedite the creation of an evidence base in survivorship care if the data are not able to be harmonized across populations, settings of care, or other factors. Measure standardization is really the third leg of the stool in "rapid, responsive, and relevant research"—the kind of research

that will lead to the efficient construction of an evidence base and reduce the typically lengthy time between a discovery in research and implementation in practice [102]. In addition to an informatics infrastructure that will support the reliable capture of high-volume data and the use of that infrastructure as part of a learning health care system, measure standardization is a necessary component of ensuring that the data that are captured can be aggregated in meaningful ways to support more reliable inferences about the best practices leading to optimal outcomes.

9.3.6.1 The Grid-Enabled Measures Care Planning Initiative

There are challenges to the standardization of clinical data in survivorship care, but perhaps even more challenging is standardizing the capture of outcomes related to survivor-reported measures of psychosocial outcomes or measures of processes of care delivery. For example, a barrier to optimizing the provision of psychosocial care in survivorship is that there is limited comparability across studies of psychosocial interventions for cancer survivors because so many measures are used to capture the most common intervention targets, such as symptoms of depression and HRQOL [103]. Measures of priority outcomes of survivorship care planning are equally widely distributed. To address this, in 2012, NCI conducted a large-scale initiative using technology-mediated social participation and their Grid-Enabled Measures (GEM) platform [104]. The initiative, titled GEM-Care Planning, or GEM-CP, used a segment of the GEM website to capture all existing measures being used in studies of survivorship care planning. This first phase of the initiative, the "populate" phase, invited researchers from all over the world who were conducting or interested in conducting survivorship care planning research to upload metadata about the constructs and measures they thought were best for use in this area (and, if publicly available, the measures themselves). In 6 months, the GEM-CP community (which was constituted of 477 user visits over the course of the initiative) proposed 51 constructs and 124 measures as important to the study of survivorship care planning.

The "rate" phase followed the "populate" phase. Armed with metadata about the proposed constructs and measures, and with the capability within the GEM-CP web-based workspace to offer comments on the proposed constructs and measures, the user community rated each construct and measure. Using this rating system, the community drove consensus toward a more narrow set of constructs and measures for survivorship care planning research. The 51 constructs and 124 measures initially proposed narrowed to 20 constructs and associated measures that were rated an average of four stars (out of a possible five). In this way, the GEM-CP initiative provided guidance to the community of researchers and practitioners devoted to advancing survivorship care planning by pointing to the measures that received the most support for use. Over time, these results have the potential to help standardize measurement in survivorship care planning research, thus speeding up the pace at which research results can build the evidence base in best practices, and can point to gaps where measures still need to be developed to capture critical components of survivorship experiences and care.

9.4 ENVISIONING A FUTURE STATE

At the 2015 meeting of the American Medical Informatics Association, Dr Karen DeSalvo gave a keynote address. She was currently serving as the lead of the ONC. In her remarks, she acknowledged that "big" data were perhaps the most popular data of the day, but encouraged the audience to also consider the notion of "long" data, or data that, independent of volume, would follow individuals and/or populations over time and across settings (see [105] for more details on the ONC's vision for how informatics can be used to support quality in health care).

9.4.1 Leveraging "Long Data" in Survivorship

Long data are the end-game in survivorship. Long data are instrumental to following survivors over the course of their lives, whether it be from pediatric cancer care into adulthood; from adolescent and young adult cancer care into adulthood; or from adult cancer care to geriatric medicine [106]. Long data are also the substrate for better coordination across the multiple specialties that are not the exception but the rule in survivorship care: medical oncology, radiation oncology, surgical oncology, PCPs, and other specialties for comorbid conditions. And long data become central to adequately capturing information that is relevant to heritable forms of cancer. As genomics continues to change the landscape of cancer and more heritable factors are identified as risks for the family members of the individual diagnosed with cancer, long data will be the means by which historical data about family members can be made actionable for the care of family members in the present [107]. And finally, long data are the foundation of a cancer care system that provides relational, rather than transactional, support, or support that is less episodic and more continual across the course of a survivor's life [108].

Without informatics, long data and the existence of a learning health care system to capitalize on them in cancer care are impossible. Currently, in 2015, we are not there yet, but we can begin to envision what this future might look like in survivorship care, and how informatics-enabled, data-driven survivorship care can

achieve the "P4" future of medicine: predictive, preventive, personalized, and participatory [109]. The last "P" in P4, *participatory*, has become even more central in medicine in the wake of the participatory Web, or "Web 2.0" [110,111]. When long data support a learning health care system and that system enables data liquidity—including the flow of data from the system to the survivor and back—survivors will be more empowered than ever to truly be a part of their health care team.

9.4.1.1 Health Equity in Survivorship

It is important to note in looking to a more informatics-enabled survivorship care future that it will always be important to be mindful of disparities in informatics access and use. As the Internet has become nearly ubiquitous in modern American life as well as the use of devices to access it, the "digital divide" has, to some extent, closed. But there will always be the information "haves" and "have nots" [112], and a future that looks to use of informatics to improve survivorship care cannot leave some survivors behind. Informatics has so much to offer to cancer survivors and to the individuals who devote their careers to research and practice in survivorship. For survivors in particular, their HRQOL during survivorship has been conceptualized as a function of the balance between their stressors and the available resources to help them cope with those stressors [113]. As such, we must always pay attention to how survivors can either leverage informatics directly or how informatics can be leveraged on their behalf to equip them with the resources they need on their survivorship journey.

9.4.2 Example Informatics-Based Solutions to Achieve Essential Elements of Care

The LIVESTRONG Foundation has been at the forefront of equipping survivors with the resources that they need, and in 2011, with the goal of making progress in building consensus in the survivorship community around how to best address the needs of posttreatment survivors, the Foundation convened 125 leaders, stakeholders, experts, cancer survivors, and cancer survivor advocates to build consensus on identifying the essential elements of survivorship care delivery [114]. An "element" of survivorship care was defined as a descriptor of some component of health care that is discrete enough to be actionable (ie, provides enough information to communicate how the element might function as part of survivorship care) but not overly prescriptive (ie, does not include specific directions on implementation, since specific needs will vary significantly across survivor populations and survivorship care settings).

Through multiple consensus-building exercises, meeting attendees created a list of 20 essential elements of survivorship care delivery (Table 9.2). These

TABLE 9.2 Essential Elements of Survivorship Care and Informatics-Based Strategies for Implementation

Essential elements of survivorship care	Informatics-based implementation strategy
CONSENSUS ELEMENTS	
Survivorship care plan (SCP), psychosocial care plan, and treatment summary	Informatics-enabled SCPs that evolve with the survivors' changing needs and are accessible online by the survivor and any providers on the survivor's care team.
Screening for new cancers and surveillance for recurrence	Reminder systems through the electronic health record (EHR) and consumer health informatics applications to keep survivors and their providers on track with personalized screening recommendations. Use of mobile applications and wearable devices to track symptoms and prompt screening when necessary.
Care coordination strategy that addresses care coordination with primary care providers (PCPs) and primary oncologists	Use of informatics-enabled, interoperable SCPs that serve as an actionable foundation for communication between oncologists and PCPs.
Health promotion education	Engaging, multimedia content accessible on a variety of platforms on a number of topics addressing health promotion topics relevant to survivorship.
Symptom management and palliative care	Use of mobile application and wearable devices to track symptoms (with resulting data available for import into the EHR) for proactive symptom management in collaboration with the care team, including via telehealth. Use informatics-enabled EHRs to coordinate care at an early stage with palliative care providers to help decrease the probability of symptom escalation.
HIGH-NEED ELEMENTS	
Late-effects education	Engaging, multimedia content accessible on a variety of platforms on a number of topics addressing topics relevant to late effects.
Psychosocial assessment	Screening for distress and other psychosocial outcomes on a regular basis both in-clinic and outside of clinical encounters via web-based and/or mobile assessments.
Comprehensive medical assessment	Comprehensive medical assessments are enabled by interoperability between electronic records maintained across settings of care for the cancer survivor, as well as between the clinical informatics infrastructure and any data that survivors themselves are capturing and tracking using consumer health informatics tools.
Nutrition services, physical activity services, and weight management	Health promotion and positive health behaviors are supported by consumer health informatics systems. Engagement in health promotion and health behavior change is prompted in timely ways through use of informatics-enabled sensing of relevant changes in the survivor's lifestyle or health status.
Transition visit and cancer-specific transition visit	Transition visits can be held virtually with the survivor and representatives from oncology and primary care. The informatics-enabled SCP serves as the evolving foundation for the transition and subsequent follow-up care.
Psychosocial care	Distress screening prompts electronic referral to psychosocial care when necessary. Receipt of care is tracked by interoperable EHR systems across physical and behavioral health.
Rehabilitation for late effects	Referral for rehabilitation is sent through the EHR and the survivors' progress is shared with their PCP and oncologist.
Family and caregiver support	Families and caregivers can, with the survivor's permission, access relevant electronic health information to maintain situational awareness. Online communities are available where family members and caregivers can receive and provide social support.
Patient navigation	Survivors can access navigators telephonically, online, or use virtual navigators to answer their questions about processes of care.
Educational information about survivorship and program offerings	Online education about a variety of topics in survivorship is available in multiple formats (text, video) and accessible on any device.
STRIVE ELEMENTS	
Self-advocacy skills training	Online skills training makes use of peer support with virtual communities of survivors who have completed training made available to new trainees to share experiences and provide support.
Counseling for practical issues	Informatics-enabled SCPs link survivors to available sources of practical support, such as the Patient Advocacy Foundation (www.patientadvocate.org)

(Continued)

TABLE 9.2 (Continued)

Essential elements of survivorship care	Informatics-based implementation strategy
Ongoing quality improvement activities	At the system level of survivorship care, metrics are captured and tracked on the number of survivors who receive informatics-enabled SCPs and who have survivor-generated data captured outside of the clinical encounter integrated into their EHR and SCP.
Referral to specialty care	Referrals occur electronically via the EHR and the informatics-enabled SCP serves as the foundation of data sharing and care coordination for all members of the survivor's care team.
Continuing medical education	Online continuing medical education addresses issues related to the evolving state of the population of cancer survivors alive in the United States; changes in survivorship trajectories based on advances in primary treatment; and ways to use informatics to support survivorship care.

20 elements were organized into tiers, the definitions of which were intended to provide guidance on the way in which medical settings might consider each in their design and delivery of survivorship care. Elements were placed in tiers in the order which most closely reflects their rank order based on the results of the consensus-building exercises. The five Tier 1 "consensus" elements were ranked consistently high in every consensus building exercise. The 10 Tier 2 "high need" elements were not identified as "essential" with the same degree of consensus as those in Tier 1, but multiple analyses of the data from the consensus-building exercises identified these elements as having strong and distinguishing support as essential elements of survivorship care delivery. Finally, the five Tier 3 "strive" elements had less consensus than those in Tiers 1 and 2, but still received substantial support from a significant minority of meeting attendees as worthy of inclusion as "essential."

Based on a vision for the future that projects ways in which informatics will be used in survivorship care, Table 9.2 lists the essential elements of survivorship care with examples of how informatics could be—and in some cases, is already being—used to implement them as part of survivorship care delivery.

9.5 CONCLUSIONS

In every way, the future of survivorship looks bright. Survivors will continue to live longer past their time of diagnosis; models of survivorship care will continue to evolve and become more robust and available; and SCPs and survivorship care planning will move closer to achieving their full potential in helping survivors to live well and healthy. Informatics, at every level from the health care system to the survivor, will be instrumental to achieving this future. For the large population of cancer survivors that will only continue to grow over time, informatics will be key to optimizing their care and health outcomes.

LIST OF ACRONYMS AND ABBREVIATIONS

ACS American Cancer Society
AHRQ Agency for Healthcare Research and Quality
BMI Body mass index
CHESS Cancer Health Enhancement Support System
EHR Electronic health record
EMA Ecological momentary assessment
EMI Ecological momentary interventions
ePRO Electronic patient-reported outcomes
GEM Grid-Enabled Measures
GEM-CP GEM-Care Planning
HINTS Health Information National Trends Survey
HRQOL Health-related quality of life
ICSGs Internet cancer support groups
IOM Institute of Medicine
NCCS National Coalition of Cancer Survivorship
NCI National Cancer Institute
ONC Office of the National Coordinator for Health Information Technology
PCP Primary care provider
PTSD Posttraumatic stress disorder
QOL Quality of life
SCP Survivorship care plan
SPARCCS Survey of Physician Attitudes Regarding the Care of Cancer Survivors
TS Treatment summary
VA Veterans Administration

References

[1] American Cancer Society Cancer facts & figures 2014. Atlanta, GA: American Cancer Society; 2014.
[2] Rowland JH, Bellizzi KM. Cancer survivors and survivorship research: a reflection on today's successes and tomorrow's challenges. Hematol Oncol Clin North Am 2008;22(2):181–200. v.
[3] Howlader NNA, Krapcho M, editors. SEER cancer statistics review, 1975–2011. Bethesda, MD: National Cancer Institute; 2014.
[4] Janssen-Heijnen M, Houterman S, Lemmens V, Brenner H, Steyerberg E, Coebergh J. Prognosis for long-term survivors of cancer. Ann Oncol 2007;18(8):1408–13.
[5] Parry C, Kent EE, Mariotto AB, Alfano CM, Rowland JH. Cancer survivors: a booming population. Cancer Epidemiol Biomarkers Prev 2011;20(10):1996–2005.

[6] Carter B. Cancer survivorship: a topic for nursing research. Oncol Nurs Forum 1984;16:435–7.

[7] Ganz PA. Survivorship: adult cancer survivors. Prim Care 2009;36(4):721–41.

[8] McCabe M. Living well: a goal for all patients. Oncology (Williston Park) 2009;23(4 Suppl Nurse Ed):10.

[9] Ng AK, Travis LB. Second primary cancers: an overview. Hematol Oncol Clin North Am 2008;22(2):271.

[10] Meneses K, Benz R. Quality of life in cancer survivorship: 20 years later. Semin Oncol Nurs 2010;26(1):36–46.

[11] Hewitt M, Greenfield S, Stovall E, editors. From cancer patient to cancer survivor: lost in transition. Washington, DC: National Acadamies Press; 2005.

[12] Harrop JP, Dean JA, Paskett ED. Cancer survivorship research: a review of the literature and summary of current NCI-designated cancer center projects. Cancer Epidemiol Biomarkers Prev 2011;20(10):2042–7.

[13] Hesse BW, Arora NK, Burke Beckjord E, Finney Rutten LJ. Information support for cancer survivors. Cancer 2008;112(11 Suppl):2529–40.

[14] National Cancer Institute. Health Information National Trends Survey Online Codebook; 2013, <http://hints.cancer.gov>.

[15] Campbell M, Mayer D, Abernethy A, Carroll S. Cancer survivorship. N C Med J 2008;69(4):322.

[16] Rowland JH, Aziz N, Tesauro G, Feuer EJ. The changing face of cancer survivorship. Semin Oncol Nurs 2001;17(4):236–40.

[17] Stanton AL, Revenson TA, Tennen H. Health psychology: psychological adjustment to chronic disease. Annu Rev Psychol 2007;58:565–92.

[18] Miller KD, Triano LR. Medical issues in cancer survivors—a review. Cancer J 2008;14(6):375–87.

[19] Stricker CT, Jacobs LA. Physical late effects in adult cancer survivors. Oncology (Williston Park) 2008;22(8 Suppl Nurse Ed):33–41.

[20] Bellury LM, Ellington L, Beck SL, Stein K, Pett M, Clark J. Elderly cancer survivorship: an integrative review and conceptual framework. Eur J Oncol Nurs 2011;15(3):233–42.

[21] Alfano CM, Rowland JH. Recovery issues in cancer survivorship: a new challenge for supportive care. Cancer J 2006;12(5):432–43.

[22] Beckjord EB, Reynolds KA, van Londen GJ, Burns R, Singh R, Arvey SR, et al. Population-level trends in posttreatment cancer survivors' concerns and associated receipt of care: results from the 2006 and 2010 LIVESTRONG surveys. J Psychosoc Oncol 2014;32(2):125–51.

[23] Foster C, Wright D, Hill H, Hopkinson J, Roffe L. Psychosocial implications of living 5 years or more following a cancer diagnosis: a systematic review of the research evidence. Eur J Cancer Care (Engl) 2009;18(3):223–47.

[24] Deimling GT, Bowman KF, Sterns S, Wagner LJ, Kahana B. Cancer-related health worries and psychological distress among older adult, long-term cancer survivors. Psychooncology 2006;15(4):306–20.

[25] Shi Q, Smith TG, Michonski JD, Stein KD, Kaw C, Cleeland CS. Symptom burden in cancer survivors 1 year after diagnosis: a report from the American Cancer Society's Studies of Cancer Survivors. Cancer 2011;117(12):2779–90.

[26] Harrington CB, Hansen JA, Moskowitz M, Todd BL, Feuerstein M. It's not over when it's over: long-term symptoms in cancer survivors—a systematic review. Int J Psychiatry Med 2010;40(2):163–81.

[27] Patrick DL, Ferketich SL, Frame PS, Harris JJ, Hendricks CB, Levin B, et al. National Institutes of Health State-of-the-Science Conference Statement: symptom management in cancer: pain, depression, and fatigue, July 15–17, 2002. J Natl Cancer Inst Monogr 2004;32:9–16.

[28] Brant JM, Beck S, Dudley WN, Cobb P, Pepper G, Miaskowski C. Symptom trajectories in posttreatment cancer survivors. Cancer Nurs 2010.

[29] Bennett JA, Cameron LD, Brown PM, Whitehead LC, Porter D, Ottaway-Parkes T, et al. Time since diagnosis as a predictor of symptoms, depression, cognition, social concerns, perceived benefits, and overall health in cancer survivors. Oncol Nurs Forum 2010;37(3):331–8.

[30] Mao JJ, Armstrong K, Bowman MA, Xie SX, Kadakia R, Farrar JT. Symptom burden among cancer survivors: impact of age and comorbidity. J Am Board Fam Med 2007;20(5):434–43.

[31] Earle CC, Neville BA, Fletcher R. Mental health service utilization among long-term cancer survivors. J Cancer Surviv 2007;1(2):156–60.

[32] Wells RJ. Chronic conditions in adult survivors of childhood cancer. Curr Oncol Rep 2007;9(6):435–6.

[33] Blaauwbroek R, Groenier KH, Kamps WA, Meyboom-de Jong B, Postma A. Late effects in adult survivors of childhood cancer: the need for life-long follow-up. Ann Oncol 2007;18(11):1898–902.

[34] Stanton AL, Bower JE, Low CA. Posttraumatic growth after cancer Calhoun LG, Tedeschi RG, editors. Handbook of posttraumatic growth: research and practice. Mahwah, NJ: Routledge; 2014. p. 138–75. ISBN: 1317778006, 9781317778004.

[35] da Silva G, dos Santos MA. Stressors in breast cancer posttreatment: a qualitative approach. Rev Lat Am Enfermagem 2010;18(4):688–95.

[36] Deimling GT, Bowman KF, Wagner LJ. Cancer survivorship and identity among long-term survivors. Cancer Invest 2007;25(8):758–65.

[37] Ligibel J. Lifestyle factors in cancer survivorship. J Clin Oncol 2012;30(30):3697–704.

[38] Carmack CL, Basen-Engquist K, Gritz ER. Survivors at higher risk for adverse late outcomes due to psychosocial and behavioral risk factors. Cancer Epidemiol Biomarkers Prev 2011;20(10):2068–77.

[39] Blanchard CM, Courneya KS, Stein K. Cancer survivors' adherence to lifestyle behavior recommendations and associations with health-related quality of life: results from the American Cancer Society's SCS-II. J Clin Oncol 2008;26(13):2198–204.

[40] Beckjord EB, Arora NK, McLaughlin W, Oakley-Girvan I, Hamilton AS, Hesse BW. Health-related information needs in a large and diverse sample of adult cancer survivors: implications for cancer care. J Cancer Surviv 2008;2(3):179–89.

[41] Philip EJ, Merluzzi TV, Zhang Z, Heitzmann CA. Depression and cancer survivorship: importance of coping self-efficacy in post-treatment survivors. Psychooncology 2013;22(5):987–94.

[42] Foster C, Breckons M, Cotterell P, Barbosa D, Calman L, Corner J, et al. Cancer survivors' self-efficacy to self-manage in the year following primary treatment. J Cancer Surviv 2015;9(1):11–19.

[43] Institute of Medicine Delivering high-quality cancer care: charting a new course for a system in crisis. Washington, DC: The National Academies Press; 2013.

[44] LIVESTRONG Foundation Patient-centered cancer care: opportunities for innovation. Austin, TX: LIVESTRONG Foundation; 2015.

[45] Meyers D, Peikes D, Genevro J, Peterson G, Taylor EF, Lake T, et al. The roles of patient-centered medical homes and accountable care organizations in coordinating patient care. Rockville, MD: Agency for Healthcare Research and Quality; 2010.

[46] Bull JH, Abernethy AP. Expanding use of palliative care in the oncology setting. N C Med J 2014;75(4):274–8.

[47] Jacobsen PB, Wagner LI. A new quality standard: the integration of psychosocial care into routine cancer care. J Clin Oncol 2012;30(11):1154–9.

[48] Jacobsen PB, Holland J, Steensma DP. Caring for the whole patient: the science of psychosocial care. J Clin Oncol 2012;30:1151–3.

[49] Institute of Medicine Cancer care for the whole patient: meeting psychosocial health needs. Washington, DC: National Acadamies; 2008.

[50] American College of Surgeons. Cancer program standards 2012, version 1.1: ensuring patient-centered care; [cited March 2012], <http://www.facs.org/cancer/coc/programstandards2012.html>.

[51] Ganz PA, Casillas J, Hahn EE. Ensuring quality care for cancer survivors: implementing the survivorship care plan. Semin Oncol Nurs 2008;24(3):208–17.

[52] Hesse BW, Beckjord E, Rutten LJ, Fagerlin A, Cameron LD. Cancer communication and informatics research across the cancer continuum. Am Psychol 2015;70(2):198–210.

[53] Epstein RM, Street RL. Patient-centered communication in cancer care: promoting healing and reducing suffering. Bethesda, MD: National Cancer Institute; 2007. NIH Publication No. 07-6225, Contract No.: NIH Publication No. 07-6225.

[54] McCabe MS. Living beyond cancer: survivorship is more than surviving. Nat Clin Pract Urol 2007;4(11):575.

[55] Rechis R, Reynolds KA, Beckjord EB, Nutt S, Burns RM, Schaefer JS. "I Learned to Live With It" is not good enough: challenges reported by post-treatment cancer survivors in the LIVESTRONG surveys. Austin, TX: LIVESTRONG; 2011.

[56] Feuerstein M. The cancer survivorship care plan: health care in the context of cancer. J Oncol Pract 2009;5(3):113–5.

[57] Grunfeld E, Earle CC. The interface between primary and oncology specialty care: treatment through survivorship. J Natl Cancer Inst Monogr 2010;2010(40):25–30.

[58] Howell D, Hack TF, Oliver TK, Chulak T, Mayo S, Aubin M, et al. Models of care for post-treatment follow-up of adult cancer survivors: a systematic review and quality appraisal of the evidence. J Cancer Surviv 2012;6(4):359–71.

[59] McCabe MS, Jacobs L. Survivorship care: models and programs. Semin Oncol Nurs 2008;24(3):202–7.

[60] Seehusen DA, Baird D, Bode D. Primary care of adult survivors of childhood cancer. Am Fam Physician 2010;81(10):1250–5.

[61] Shapiro CL, McCabe MS, Syrjala KL, Friedman D, Jacobs LA, Ganz PA, et al. The LIVESTRONG survivorship center of excellence network. J Cancer Surviv 2009;3(1):4–11.

[62] Stricker CT, Jacobs LA, Risendal B, Jones A, Panzer S, Ganz PA, et al. Survivorship care planning after the Institute of Medicine recommendations: how are we faring? J Cancer Surviv 2011;5(4):358–70.

[63] Forsythe LP, Parry C, Alfano CM, Kent EE, Leach CR, Haggstrom DA, et al. Use of survivorship care plans in the United States: associations with survivorship care. J Natl Cancer Inst 2013;105(20):1579–87.

[64] Grunfeld E, Julian JA, Pond G, Maunsell E, Coyle D, Folkes A, et al. Evaluating survivorship care plans: results of a randomized, clinical trial of patients with breast cancer. J Clin Oncol 2011;29(36):4755–62.

[65] Coyle D, Grunfeld E, Coyle K, Pond G, Julian JA, Levine MN. Cost effectiveness of a survivorship care plan for breast cancer survivors. J Oncol Pract 2014;10(2):e86–92.

[66] Parry C, Kent EE, Forsythe LP, Alfano CM, Rowland JH. Can't see the forest for the care plan: a call to revisit the context of care planning. J Clin Oncol 2013;31(21):2651–3.

[67] Hesse BW. Harnessing the power of an intelligent health environment in cancer control. Stud Health Technol Inform 2005;118:159–76.

[68] Chou WY, Liu B, Post S, Hesse B. Health-related Internet use among cancer survivors: data from the Health Information National Trends Survey, 2003–2008. J Cancer Surviv 2011;5(3):263–70.

[69] Beckjord EB, Rechis R, Nutt S, Shulman L, Hesse BW. What do people affected by cancer think about electronic health information exchange? Results from the 2010 LIVESTRONG Electronic Health Information Exchange Survey and the 2008 Health Information National Trends Survey. J Oncol Pract 2011;7(4):237–41.

[70] Rechis RNS, Beckjord E. The promise of electronic health information exchange: a LIVESTRONG report. Austin, TX: LIVESTRONG; 2011.

[71] Im EO. Online support of patients and survivors of cancer. Semin Oncol Nurs 2011;27(3):229–36.

[72] Hong Y, Pena-Purcell NC, Ory MG. Outcomes of online support and resources for cancer survivors: a systematic literature review. Patient Educ Couns 2012;86(3):288–96.

[73] Gustafson DH, Hawkins R, Boberg E, Pingree S, Serlin RE, Graziano F, et al. Impact of a patient-centered, computer-based health information/support system. Am J Prev Med 1999;16(1):1–9.

[74] Gibbons MC, Wilson RF, Samal L, Lehman CU, Dickersin K, Lehmann HP, et al. Impact of consumer health informatics applications. Evid Rep Technol Assess 2009(188):1–546.

[75] Hesse BW, Suls JM. Informatics-enabled behavioral medicine in oncology. Cancer J 2011;17(4):222–30.

[76] Hawkins RP, Pingree S, Baker T, Roberts LJ, Shaw B, McDowell H, et al. Integrating eHealth with human services for breast cancer patients. Transl Behav Med 2011;1(1):146–54.

[77] Agboola SO, Ju W, Elfiky A, Kvedar JC, Jethwani K. The effect of technology-based interventions on pain, depression, and quality of life in patients with cancer: a systematic review of randomized controlled trials. J Med Internet Res 2015;17(3):e65.

[78] Hesse BW, Ahern DK, Woods SS. Nudging best practice: the HITECH act and behavioral medicine. Transl Behav Med 2011;1(1):175–81.

[79] Silver JK. Strategies to overcome cancer survivorship care barriers. PM R 2011;3(6):503–6.

[80] Earle CC, Ganz PA. Cancer survivorship care: don't let the perfect be the enemy of the good. J Clin Oncol 2012;30(30):3764–8.

[81] Beckjord E. The need for focus on outcomes and the role of informatics. J Oncol Pract 2014;10(2):e93–4.

[82] Rosales AR, Byrne D, Burnham C, Watts L, Clifford K, Zuckerman DS, et al. Comprehensive survivorship care with cost and revenue analysis. J Oncol Pract 2014;10(2):e81–5.

[83] Tevaarwerk AJ, Wisinski KB, Buhr KA, Njiaju UO, Tun M, Donohue S, et al. Leveraging electronic health record systems to create and provide electronic cancer survivorship care plans: a pilot study. J Oncol Pract 2014;10(3):e150–9.

[84] Donohue S, Sesto ME, Hahn DL, Buhr KA, Jacobs EA, Sosman JM, et al. Evaluating primary care providers' views on survivorship care plans generated by an electronic health record system. J Oncol Pract 2015;24:003335.

[85] Hill-Kayser CE, Vachani C, Hampshire MK, Jacobs LA, Metz JM. An internet tool for creation of cancer survivorship care plans for survivors and health care providers: design, implementation, use and user satisfaction. J Med Internet Res 2009;11(3):e39.

[86] Gillespie G. HealthVault: PHRs still growing, but is the industry even ready? Health Data Manag 2010;18(6):70–2.

[87] Hoffman S. Electronic health records and research: privacy versus scientific priorities. Am J Bioeth 2010;10(9):19–20.

[88] Zulman DM, Nazi KM, Turvey CL, Wagner TH, Woods SS, An LC. Patient interest in sharing personal health record information: a web-based survey. Ann Intern Med 2011;155(12):805–10.

[89] Patel V, Beckjord E, Moser RP, Hughes P, Hesse BW. The role of health care experience and consumer information efficacy in shaping privacy and security perceptions of medical records: national consumer survey results. JMIR Med Inform 2015;3(2):e14.

[90] Jensen RE, Snyder CF, Abernethy AP, Basch E, Potosky AL, Roberts AC, et al. Review of electronic patient-reported outcomes systems used in cancer clinical care. J Oncol Pract 2014;10(4):e215–22.

[91] Atienza AA, Patrick K. Mobile health: the killer app for cyber-infrastructure and consumer health. Am J Prev Med 2011;40(5 Suppl. 2):S151–3.

[92] Heron KE, Smyth JM. Ecological momentary interventions: incorporating mobile technology into psychosocial and health behaviour treatments. Br J Health Psychol 2010;15(Pt 1):1–39.

[93] Shiffman S, Stone AA, Hufford MR. Ecological momentary assessment. Annu Rev Clin Psychol 2008;4:1–32.

[94] Riley WT, Rivera DE, Atienza AA, Nilsen W, Allison SM, Mermelstein R. Health behavior models in the age of mobile interventions: are our theories up to the task? Transl Behav Med 2011;1(1):53–71.

[95] Oestreicher P. Cancer survivors' health behaviors present challenges and teachable moments for oncology nurses. ONS Connect 2007;22(5):20–1.

[96] OncoKompass2.0; 2015, <http://www.samenlevenmetkanker.nl/?p=305-Oncokompas2.0>.

[97] Lubberding S, van Uden-Kraan CF, Te Velde EA, Cuijpers P, Leemans CR, Verdonck-de Leeuw IM. Improving access to supportive cancer care through an eHealth application: a qualitative needs assessment among cancer survivors. J Clin Nurs 2015;24(9–10):1367–79.

[98] Abernethy AP, Etheredge LM, Ganz PA, Wallace P, German RR, Neti C, et al. Rapid-learning system for cancer care. J Clin Oncol 2010;28(27):4268–74.

[99] IOM (Institute of Medicine) Best care at lower cost: the path to continuously learning health care in America. Washington, DC: The National Academies Press; 2013.

[100] Rowland JH, Hewitt M, Ganz PA. Cancer survivorship: a new challenge in delivering quality cancer care. J Clin Oncol 2006;24(32):5101–4.

[101] Hudson MM, Landier W, Ganz PA. Impact of survivorship-based research on defining clinical care guidelines. Cancer Epidemiol Biomarkers Prev 2011;20(10):2085–92.

[102] Riley WT, Glasgow RE, Etheredge L, Abernethy AP. Rapid, responsive, relevant (R3) research: a call for a rapid learning health research enterprise. Clin Transl Med 2013;2(1):10.

[103] Jacobsen PB, Jim HSL. Consideration of quality of life in cancer survivorship research. Cancer Epidemiol Biomarkers Prev 2011;20(10):2035–41.

[104] Parry C, Beckjord E, Moser RP, Vieux SN, Padgett LS, Hesse BW. It takes a (virtual) village: crowdsourcing measurement consensus to advance survivorship care planning. Transl Behav Med 2015;5(1):53–9.

[105] Office of the National Coordinator for Health Information Technology. Connecting health and care for the nation: a ten-year vision to achieve an interoperable health IT infrastructure. Retrieved from: <http://healthit.gov/sites/default/files/ONC10yearInteroperabilityConceptPaper.pdf2014>.

[106] Jacobs LA, Palmer SC, Schwartz LA, DeMichele A, Mao JJ, Carver J, et al. Adult cancer survivorship: evolution, research, and planning care. CA Cancer J Clin 2009;59(6):391–410.

[107] Jacobs LA, Giarelli E. A model of survivorship in cancer genetic care. Semin Oncol Nurs 2004;20(3):196–202.

[108] Hesse BW, et al. Outside the box: will information technology be a viable intervention to improve the quality of cancer care? J Natl Cancer Inst Monogr 2010;2010(40):81–9.

[109] Khoury MJ, Gwinn ML, Glasgow RE, Kramer BS. A population approach to precision medicine. Am J Prev Med 2012;42(6):639–45.

[110] Lo B, Parham L. The impact of web 2.0 on the doctor-patient relationship. J Law Med Ethics 2010;38(1):17–26.

[111] Hesse BW, Hansen D, Finholt T, Munson S, Kellogg W, Thomas JC. Social participation in health 2.0. Computer (Long Beach Calif) 2010;43(11):45–52.

[112] Viswanath K, Kreuter MW. Health disparities, communication inequalities, and eHealth. Am J Prev Med 2007;32(5 Suppl.):S131–3.

[113] Andrykowski MA, Lykins E, Floyd A. Psychological health in cancer survivors. Semin Oncol Nurs 2008;24(3):193–201.

[114] Rechis R, Beckjord E, Arvey S, Reynolds KA, Goldrick D. The essential elements of survivorship care: a LIVESTRONG brief report. Austin, TX: LIVESTRONG; 2012.

CHAPTER

10

Advanced Cancer: Palliative, End of Life, and Bereavement Care

Lori L. DuBenske PhD[1], Deborah K. Mayer PhD[2] and David H. Gustafson PhD[3]

[1]Department of Psychiatry, School of Medicine and Public Health, University of Wisconsin–Madison, Madison, WI, United States [2]School of Nursing, University of North Carolina Lineberger Comprehensive Cancer Center, Chapel Hill, NC, United States [3]Center for Health Enhancement Systems Studies, University of Wisconsin–Madison, Madison, WI, United States

OUTLINE

10.1 Introduction	182
10.1.1 Symptom Management	182
10.1.2 Decision Making	183
10.1.3 Caregiving and Bereavement	184
10.2 Opportunities for eHealth to Address Needs in Advanced Cancer Care	184
10.2.1 Opportunity for Symptom Management	186
10.2.2 Opportunity for Decision Making	187
10.2.3 Opportunity for Bereavement	189
10.3 A Case Example: CHESS—The Comprehensive Health Enhancement Support System	190
10.3.1 CHESS and Symptom Management	191
10.3.2 CHESS for Caregiving and Bereavement	192
10.3.3 Lessons From CHESS Development and Implementation	193
10.3.4 Lessons From CHESS Evaluation	196
10.4 Future Directions for Research	197
10.4.1 Research Design	197
10.4.2 Patient Outcomes	197
10.4.3 Decision Making Research	198
10.4.4 Economic Outcomes	199
10.4.5 Family Involvement	199
10.5 Future Directions for Development and Implementation	200
10.6 Conclusion	200
List of Acronyms and Abbreviations	201
Acknowledgments	201
References	201

B. Hesse, D. Ahern & E. Beckjord: Oncology Informatics.
DOI: http://dx.doi.org/10.1016/B978-0-12-802115-6.00010-0

10.1 INTRODUCTION

Today, one in every four deaths in America is due to cancer and in 2016 about 595,690 Americans, or about 1630 people per day, are expected to die of cancer [1]. The diagnosis of advanced cancer often inflicts fear, despair, and hopelessness on patients and loved ones. Advanced stage disease may be diagnosed at the onset, may culminate due to disease progression despite treatment, or manifest from recurrence after a period of remission. While the former is often an abrupt entry into mortality salience and issues of end of life, the later may require an additional psychological shift from prior focus on treatments with intent for cure and extending survival to acceptance of incurable disease with increased palliative care efforts and preparing for end of life. The challenges facing advanced disease include symptom management and the reduction of both physical and psychological suffering, complex decision making regarding treatment and the weighing of quality of life versus chances for life extension, and the inclusion of family members who are central to patient support and care. Throughout advanced disease, critical questions arise: What do patients want at the end of life? Where do they prefer to die? What measures do they want taken to extend life? What personal activities or events do they want to prioritize? The personal process of acceptance and understanding of the transition to end of life is unique for each individual who faces it. Patients deserve personalized care.

Yet, research suggests that patients are not receiving the end-of-life care that they desire. This significant gap between what people say they want and what actually happens has been documented in a number of studies [2,3]. For example, in a large-scale study funded by the Robert Wood Johnson Foundation, most patients with serious illness said they would prefer to die at home; however, the majority (55%) actually died in hospitals [3]. Furthermore, they showed that care was rarely aligned with patients' reported preferences, despite extensive nursing efforts to align their care with their wishes. They concluded that patients often prefer a more conservative pattern of end-of-life care than they receive. Accordingly, the practice patterns of the hospital may override patient's wishes in care delivered at end of life. These findings call for innovative approaches to care that help ensure that patients and their families identify their preferences and values, communicate these clearly with each other and the treatment teams, and assist providers in directing care that aligns with their patients' intentions for care.

Another gap exists between what people would like to share about their end-of-life wishes and what actually occurs with their family members or health care providers [2]. Understanding patient and family preferences and values can guide efforts for symptom management, facilitate decision making, and to the extent care aligns with these preferences and values, ease family bereavement. This chapter aims to identify the opportunities for informatics in addressing the challenges of advanced disease, end of life, and bereavement through discussion of critical care issues, examples of existing eHealth applications, and discussion of future directions.

10.1.1 Symptom Management

Palliation is about physical and psychosocial symptom management and supportive care at any stage of the cancer journey but is especially important as the disease progresses [4]. With advanced cancer, the focus of treatment often shifts to symptom management and palliative care, with the potential extension of life, rather than cure. The most common symptoms with advanced cancer include pain, fatigue, and depression [5]. Pain management is one of the most important aspects of advanced cancer care, and is addressed best through aggressive therapy and rigorous assessment. Despite studies suggesting pain control can be achieved for 80% of cancer patients, pain remains a significant problem for two-thirds of those with advanced stage or metastatic disease [6]. Pain is often underassessed, underreported, and undertreated [7] and is associated with significant impairment in overall quality of life [8]. Patients and families alike report that pain is the most worrisome aspect of cancer and they have a high need for information regarding pain management [8–10]. Although pain is a critical symptom for focus in and of itself, pain also serves as a prototype example with applications for addressing numerous other cancer-related symptoms.

Early treatment of pain leads to better pain control. Rigorous assessment of pain is necessary at all stages of treatment. One study found that nearly one-third of patients who reported mild pain after receiving their initial treatment had pain that progressed to moderate to severe pain by the time of their first follow-up visit, suggesting more frequent monitoring and reporting of pain is necessary to optimize pain control [11]. This may be even more critical for advanced stage disease when time between appointments may be longer and disease is progressing rather than improving.

In addition to physical distress, The Institute of Medicine (IOM) [12] called for greater efforts to decrease psychosocial distress among cancer patients. In 2012, the Commission on Cancer of the American College of Surgeons released new accreditation standards to include the screening of all cancer patients for psychosocial distress [13]. However, these general guidelines leave room for much variance in the timing, frequency, or mechanism of such assessment. Depressed mood is the most common psychological symptom in patients with cancer [14]. Depressive symptoms range in severity from sadness and crying, to clinical syndromes including hopelessness, helplessness, lack of motivation and withdrawal, and even suicidal thinking, and are associated with marked distress and disability. More severe symptoms of depression are associated with more prolonged hospital stays, physical distress, poorer treatment adherence, lower quality of life, increased desire to hasten death, and completed suicide. Furthermore, the suicide rate for cancer patients is over twice the rate of the general population [15]. Oncologists miss many cases of depression [16]. Improvements are needed in identifying depression along with providing treatment. Educating patients of their risk for depression and the availability of help combined with improved targeted assessment may increase use of resources and follow-up in clinic.

Management of pain, fatigue, and depression rely on the patient's subjective report of symptom burden. Thus, interventions addressing communication about such subjective symptoms between patients and the clinical care team are crucial to quality of life. Patient beliefs that "complaining" about pain, being tired, and mood issues are not appropriate topics for clinic discussion or may be embarrassing to report in front of family can compromise information exchange between the patient and clinician, resulting in less-than-ideal care. Furthermore, the patient's symptom distress and progressive disease can also interfere with information exchange, often requiring a family caregiver to provide information to the clinical team on the patient's behalf.

While oncology clinicians could provide needed symptom management and psychological support, barriers include: (1) time constraints within clinic visits that limit the scope of symptoms that are assessed; (2) avoidance of discussions of psychosocial issues, whether from clinician discomfort or concern for time; and (3) clinicians may underestimate the needs of patients/families [6,17,18]. In attempting to overcome these barriers, one study had nurses repeatedly communicate caregivers' and patients' concerns, including pain control, to physicians—yet patient symptoms did not improve [19]. A similar study found improved patient symptoms only for those patients who reported greater symptom severity initially [20]. Prescheduled, clinician-initiated communication may not impact symptom management because it does not occur when patients or family may most need help. A more proactive intervention that ensures timely communication initiated by patients and/or their family outside of scheduled appointments may better overcome these barriers.

While cancer invades the body of an individual, its impact ripples throughout the social network of the individual with cancer. Most cancer care is provided in the outpatient setting, leaving patients and their caregivers responsible for implementing pain management regimens [21]. Patients at all stages of cancer often rely on support from family and friends. Dependence on such support increases as disease progresses: care demands increase with regard to symptom management while simultaneously the patient's physical and mental ability to care for and advocate for oneself may diminish [100]. In meeting such demands while facing the end of life for a loved one, these informal caregivers are at risk for caregiving burden, depression, and anxiety [17,22].

As mentioned previously, pain and other symptom management is a significant concern involving family caregivers in advanced cancer care. Caregivers need symptom management information throughout the cancer care trajectory, including advanced stage disease and end of life [9]. As cancer progresses, effective pain management depends on the caregiver's knowledge, attitudes, and skills in implementing and supervising prescribed regimens, safeguarding the medication supply at home, and the ability to solve complex and ever-changing problems [20,23]. Similar challenges arise with other symptoms and side effects. The caregiver's interaction with the clinician at the clinic visit is the conduit between the caregiver's ability to understand health information and having their needs met [24]. Accordingly, pain information (eg, knowledge of medications) is not enough and may not be mutable within the clinic visit. This is supported by research demonstrating educational interventions have had limited effect on patient pain [25]. But interventions that facilitate caregiver interactions about pain (ie, assessing/reporting pain, discussing concerns) may bridge the gap between pain knowledge and pain management.

10.1.2 Decision Making

There are many decision making points along the cancer journey and include decisions about continuing treatment (or not) in the face of progressive disease and other aspects of care. Talking about and making decisions can be difficult for all involved (including patient, caregiver, and providers), and may or may not occur in a timely manner. Failure to plan for end of life increases the risk of a "bad" death—one that is inconsistent with one's preferences and values and extends unnecessary physical or psychological suffering for the dying individual and/or their loved ones. Yet, decisions regarding end-of-life care are becoming more complex. With increasing cancer treatment options and clinical trials of experimental treatments, patients may receive multiple medical trials for hope of extended life. These treatments often come at some cost, including physical side effects, time and effort to return to the clinic for appointments, or delay in seeking other supportive care such as hospice. Furthermore, patients always face the decision to continue treatment or not, although many patients do not think that is a decision. Other decisions include options for receiving second opinions and choices of where to receive care. All of these decisions occur within the context of the individual's cultural, religious, legal, and ethical considerations [26,27]. Each transition along the cancer journey offers the opportunity to make decisions that are consistent with a patient's values and preferences for care, some with consequences that impact the nature of end-of-life care, for better or for worse.

Family members are frequently involved in end-of-life decisions, either jointly with the patient or as a surrogate for the patient [27]. Advance care planning allows patients to document their plans and preferences to guide surrogate decision making when illness or injury impedes the patient's ability to think or communicate about health decisions. However, fewer than 50% of seriously or terminally ill people have an advance directive filed in their medical record [28]. Furthermore, even with an advance directive, surrogate decision makers may not be able to predict their loved one's wishes amongst the complex physical and psychological symptoms of the disease [29]. The establishment of effective end-of-life care and decision making supports is dependent upon consideration of family system dynamics and the needs of a variety of configurations of potential users.

At varying points patients may face the decision between aggressive, potentially (although low probability) life extending treatment versus forgoing aggressive treatment and focusing solely on supportive care. For some patients with metastatic disease, they may live for years receiving one form of treatment after another. Depending on the type of cancer, it can be difficult to determine when it is best to stop treatment. For example, certain chemotherapy treatments can cause heart damage, and judgments between whether survival would be extended or shortened through additional chemotherapy are difficult. Further, the decision to forgo an offered treatment may be resisted from either one's own or social perceptions of "giving up."

Hospice provides an alternative for end-of-life care. Hospice offers comprehensive interdisciplinary end-of-life care that addresses the physical, psychosocial, and spiritual needs of terminally ill individuals and their families and provides bereavement support to families after an individual's death. Depending on the facility, hospice services may be offered in an inpatient setting, or more often, through outpatient services provided at the patient's home. Hospice was initially established in the United States in the 1970s and has since evolved into an integrated part of US health care [30], with improved symptom management, quality of life, and patient and family satisfaction over standard care. While less than 25% of US deaths are caused by cancer, people with cancer make up 36.9% of hospice admissions [31]. Percentages of cancer patients who receive hospice care at end of life vary across studies and by treatment location, with reports as low as 31% to reportedly as high as 74% by state in 2010 [32]. While hospice may not be preferred or appropriate for everyone, currently many terminally ill cancer patients who may benefit from hospice care do not receive it. Furthermore, admissions to hospice are often too late for patients to fully benefit from the comprehensive services available. Despite being designed for lengthier supportive care, in 2010 the average length of stay in hospice for patients with cancer was 9.1 days [33]. Inordinately short length of stay at hospice can create organizational, clinical, and/or emotional problems for all involved (patient, family, provider, payers) [34].

10.1.3 Caregiving and Bereavement

For family members and loved ones, the trajectory of cancer includes adjustment after their loved one has died. End-of-life caregiving and decision making difficulty can have a lasting impact on the family [35]. Unresolved questions of treatment decision making, decision regret, and questioning the quality of their delivery of care and support puts these informal caregivers at risk for unresolved or complicated grief. Caregivers also experience many of their own physical and psychosocial issues while caring for a loved one with cancer, especially toward the end of life. For bereaved caregivers, poor quality of life and increased psychiatric illness has been associated with their loved one dying in the hospital [36].

Bereaved loved ones commonly review and continue to have questions about the cancer care process. However, when the patient dies, the family is suddenly extracted from the support system of the oncology clinic where they have turned for answers throughout the cancer journey. There is a need for continuity of support for family caregivers across the bridge from active caregiving to grief resolution.

10.2 OPPORTUNITIES FOR EHEALTH TO ADDRESS NEEDS IN ADVANCED CANCER CARE

Dramatic changes in the experience of death have occurred over the past century in America [37]. Previously, death commonly occurred in the home with family present and active in supportive care. The gradual shift toward institutionalization of medical care and hospital deaths removed the family from the dying experience. Today, economic trends toward shorter hospital stays and greater home delivery of care, combined with medical advances that extend length of life with terminal disease, creates a situation of greater home-based care for extended time, as well as returning the dying process to home. However, this is not simply a return to the "old way." End of life has changed in America in several critical ways. The family make-up is smaller, spousal availability is lower due to high divorce rates, and geographic distance minimizes extended family care. Likewise, advances in medicine have significantly extended the length of time of care, as well as complexity of home care regimens. Together there are more competing demands between family caregiving and other life stressors, including the need for caregivers to maintain employment for insurance, and multiple generations of care recipients as adult children balance care for their offspring as well as their dying parents. Economic demands drive home care away from direct supervision of medical providers. At the same time, the complexity of care regimens leaves caregivers feeling less competent and more dependent on communication and guidance from clinicians. In addition, shifts to patient-centered care guide the inclusion of patients

and their families in medical decision making and setting priorities; however, this role may be intimidating to some who feel unprepared or underinformed to take such responsibility when facing the high stakes of cancer care. Accordingly, families today are often unprepared to face the physical, functional, and psychological demands of caring for the dying at home.

Informatics and communication technology can meet some of these modern challenges and may offer proactive solutions to support patients and families throughout the cancer trajectory, even when facing end of life and bereavement. One of the key components in palliative care is communication [27]. eHealth systems can facilitate communication in many critical areas, between patients, providers, family caregivers, social networks, and organizations (see Fig. 10.1). Greater health care need has been associated with greater use of eHealth systems. The degree of disease burden and complexity of cancer care lends itself to higher care needs, as well as needs that extend beyond the scheduled clinic visit. Thus, the oncology setting is a ripe environment for the application of such eHealth systems. Studies have shown that cancer patient use of these systems exceeds that reported in other populations, both by a greater proportion of the population and also greater intensity of use [38]. These technologies can help extend

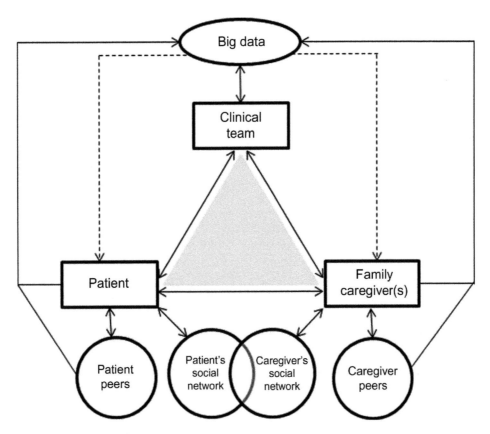

FIGURE 10.1 Channels of communication that offer opportunities for informatics in advanced cancer.

and enhance the care the patient and caregiver receive and may improve the quality of care delivered but are underdeveloped and underutilized in these settings [26]. For an in-depth discussion of communication technology, please see Chapter 13, "Communication Science: Connecting Systems for Health" in this book.

10.2.1 Opportunity for Symptom Management

There is a tremendous opportunity for technology solutions that facilitate communication for improved symptom management both within and beyond the clinical encounter. Technology is increasingly being used within the clinic setting for obtaining electronic self-report measures of patient symptom severity. Tablet devices allow patients to complete questionnaires such as symptom ratings or the distress thermometer, and can instantly translate item responses into scale scores or graphic representation for ease of clinician identification of critical issues for follow-up. Such technology was demonstrated in the Electronic Self-Report Assessment–Cancer (ESRA-C) [39] to assess quality of life issues in the oncology outpatient clinic visit. While in the clinic waiting room, patients completed questionnaires on touch screen notebook computers. Upon completion, the ESRA-C automatically generated a color graphical summary that flagged any issues reported above a set threshold of distress. While these summaries were printed and provided to the clinician immediately before the clinic visit, technology exists that would allow such data to be delivered via the electronic health record (EHR). Use of ESRA-C increased discussion of quality of life issues without extending the length of the clinical encounter. This example demonstrated the potential of informatics to be used as an extension of the face-to-face clinical encounter to increase symptom reporting and facilitate communication regarding symptom management.

Family caregivers of people with cancer specifically desire increased communication with the treatment team. Problems often arise between clinic visits, requiring patients and family caregivers to make decisions of triage, medication adjustments, or decisions regarding need for emergency room visits or waiting symptoms out until the clinic opens. The need for guidance outside of clinic hours and willingness to seek this through eHealth technologies is demonstrated by the finding that one-third of cancer-related eHealth system use occurred outside of oncology clinic hours [38]. While communication technology is often used to gather information, its promise of symptom management lies in yielding the ability to connect with the clinical team between visits for symptom reporting and management. Project ENABLE (Educate, Nurture, Advise Before Life Ends) [40], a telephone-based, nurse-led palliative care intervention that addressed patients' physical and psychosocial needs as

well as the need for care coordination, improved quality of life in patients with advanced cancer. Another intervention, The Assessing Caregivers for Team Intervention through Videophone Encounters (ACTIVE) [41], uses videophone technology; family caregivers of home-hospice patients participated remotely in interdisciplinary team meetings. This study revealed that caregivers readily participated primarily by asking questions related to pain management. These examples yield evidence for the roles of distant rather than in-person interventions.

Beyond direct clinician contact, caregivers seek skills training and advice in delivering practical aspects of home-based care [42]. One-on-one training is costly and has limitations in the timeliness of its delivery. Many needs arise unexpectedly. Likewise, providing the extensive education and training necessary to prepare caregivers for numerous possibilities would be impractical and unnecessarily burdensome to caregivers and medical staff. Technology holds the potential to offer anytime access to tailored instruction and remote advisors. Additional pilot work from the ACTIVE intervention has demonstrated the utility of videophone technology for delivering problem-solving therapy to family caregivers of hospice patients [41]. In addition to such professional resources, opportunities exist for caregivers to benefit from connecting with other caregivers to share information, learning from each other care strategies that are often learned through trial and error in critical moments of home care. The Canadian Virtual Hospice [43] offers online palliative care and end-of-life information, along with personal stories of those who experienced hospice care, but without direct clinician–patient contact.

Building on these information interventions, novel educational interventions may include a library of instructional videos that could offer needed technical guidance in the delivery of care as situations arise. Interactive instruction may offer assessment points and opportunities for tailored feedback to guide subsequent instruction. Furthermore, the system could build in thresholds or system alerts that would trigger contact with a live health professional. Any or all of these services could be driven by predictive analytics. Such systems are capable of monitoring data and using algorithms to predict important events that require intervention, and subsequently either deliver the intervention directly (eg, show an instructional video) or trigger an intervention from an outside source (eg, alert the oncology triage nurse of a particular patient's need). The combination of automated services with the availability of remote nursing consultant or a caregiver case manager could prove powerful. This idea has been implemented in the Comprehensive Health Enhancement Support System (CHESS) module for addiction treatment [44]. CHESS is delivered through a web-enabled mobile device and collects data (eg, sleeplessness and relationships quality) on a weekly basis to assess the patient's relative risk of relapse by weighing risk and protective factors in their lives. This information is processed through a Bayesian statistical model and if the risk of relapse exceeds a predefined level, an alert is sent (according to a plan developed by the patient and providers) to key supporters and to the patient themselves [44].

Even when avenues for clinic contact are available, patients and families may be reluctant to report symptom distress out of fear of being a burden to the clinical team. Clinical staff encouragement to call may be perceived as a gesture of kindness rather than as truly desired or permissive. However, technology can overcome such resistance. Research has demonstrated that people may be more willing to disclose concerns or symptoms online rather than in direct contact [45,46]. In addition, the nature of offering a communication channel that is explicitly for symptom reporting may be more permissive, in a sense justifying contact by the very nature that a mechanism for such contact was developed and administered by the treatment team. Such indirect validation may prove quite powerful to increase reporting, both electronically and within the interpersonal clinic encounter.

Informatics systems may also solicit reporting from an identified family caregiver, offering them access to the treatment team as well as a mechanism to offer their perceptions and concerns independent of the patient. This can be a critical gateway for caregiver support, particularly in situations when patients may put their best foot forward during contact with the clinical team, and then suffer at home. When the team understanding of the patient's situation is discordant from how it is actually experienced at home, support for the caregiver is reduced and caregiver burden is heightened. Box 10.1 provides a quote from a bereaved caregiver reflecting on her experience of struggling to communicate the nature of her husband's suffering from advanced cancer. A direct communication line to the clinical team to share observations in the moment of

patient suffering may offer insight that is difficult to confront directly with the patient at the time of the office visit. Beyond assessing symptom status, informatics systems can track and convey trends in symptom distress over time. This information can improve care decisions over retrospective reports or the single appointment's focus on current distress. For example, trends in a patient's pain level may be evaluated within the context of other symptoms, treatments, or medications to inform changes in medication regimen or other care strategies (eg, adjusting timing of short-acting vs long-acting narcotics around the treatment cycle). Later in this chapter, we illustrate such services through our case example of CHESS for advanced stage cancer.

10.2.2 Opportunity for Decision Making

Cancer patients now have multiple choices in how they approach death [47]. The medical system's shift from a patriarchal to a shared decision-making framework calls for health decisions to result from a collaborative, fully informed decision-making process that includes the patient, family, and health care professionals. However, patients and family members often do not feel competent or empowered to make these complex decisions. Further, some prefer to defer decision making to experts. To help increase comfort in the decision process, shared decision-making skills may be improved by providing structure and guidance in deliberating about decision-related preferences and values [48,49]. Patient and family members often have vast differences in opinion regarding treatment decisions and care, with hospice use among the most common areas of disagreement [50]. Decision conflict can create tension in the patient–family relationship and impair decision making and care planning [51]. There is a need for services that facilitate family communication and improve patients' and family satisfaction with treatment decisions, particularly at end of life [27].

Computer-assisted interventions represent an additional approach to patient education and support that may extend, enhance, or offer advantages over professionally directed interventions in their capacity to provide widespread dissemination and contain costs. A patient's and/or family member's decision is often strongly influenced by personal values, beliefs, and emotions, unlike a clinician's decision that is usually based on symptoms and diagnosis [48,52]. Decision aids allow users to consider their options in light of their own values and weigh preferences based on impact on life factors that are most important for them [53]. This is critical for end-of-life choices where there are poor prognostics, no clear "right" choice, and personal meaning to life is most sacred. For example, for some, the devastating effects of further treatment on their physical functioning,

---

BOX 10.1

I was with my husband on a daily basis and could see the decline in his health, physical abilities, and emotional state, but when I tried to relay this to the [clinical team] it was seemingly ignored. They chose to focus on test, scans, and bloodwork... they only saw him for a very short time and he always wanted to put his best foot forward. When he was at home he would cry in my arms... When I could no longer "rah-rah-rah" I shut down and went through his last few months feeling unsupported.

mobility, and energy may be too much of a burden on quality of life for their remaining time and that is more important than extending life. Whereas for others, the opportunity to be involved in research that may impact others may give their life and their death more meaning and motivate them to continue with experimental treatment at the potential cost of side effects that impact quality of life. Decision aids have the potential to help people assess the potential impact of their options selectively on issues most important to them. Systems that facilitate patient and family understanding of treatment choices, potential risks and benefits, and survival rates and prognostics may facilitate informed decisions to further seek treatment or to end active treatment for focus solely on palliative efforts.

Decision aids have been developed as adjuncts to counseling so patients can learn about the benefits and risks, consider personal values, and participate with their clinician in shared decision making. Studies of decision aids have shown that treatment choices become more reflective of personal values when patients use decision aids to deliberate about personal probabilities and values for each outcome [48]. In addition, cancer-related decision aids have been shown to be acceptable to patients and to increase patient knowledge and decision involvement, realistic expectations of outcomes, and decision satisfaction while they reduce decisional conflict [48,54]. However, while many decision supports exist for early-stage cancer, very few address advanced cancer. And while there are growing numbers of decision aids for end-of-life choices, many are proprietary and privately accessible, with limited research support of their efficacy [28].

Historically, decision aids have treated patients as isolated decision makers, where the patient is the sole user of the decision aid [51]. However, increasing understanding of family involvement in treatment decisions, particularly at end of life, necessitates that we expand models of decision aids to assist family members in the decision process as well. While individual values clarification is an essential step toward informed decision making, understanding the values and preferences of other decision participants is also important [49]. In a prostate cancer decision aid study, patients and partners were shown to have different values for treatment outcomes [55]. This points to the as yet undeveloped potential of decision aids to be used to improve communication through identifying value discordance, in turn facilitating joint decision making when desired or preferred.

Informatics applications show promise in the ability to develop algorithms from large patient data sets to establish reasonable probabilities and pathways for the end-of-life experience, potentially more accurately than clinician prognostics. People with terminal illness commonly question and can even fear the process of dying. They wonder how the disease will progress and what the last phases of life will entail. Often patients may have assumptions of how they will die that can create death anxiety. Systems that can map out the most likely courses of illness and the final dying experience have the potential to mitigate this anxiety. However, with that also comes the risk of presenting anxiety-provoking information to some. Therefore, systems need to address the complexity of this information delivery by balancing it with actions for care directives that offer hope for management of suffering through preparation.

People with cancer face many decisions throughout their journey; some are obvious decisions (Do I take treatment?) and some less obvious (Should I get another opinion?). Patients with advanced cancer are trying to balance the quantity and quality of their lives and the decisions that will foster both. But as the disease progresses, a shift occurs that directs the emphasis on quality of life more than quantity of life. That shift may be explicit or implicit based on the preferences of the patient, their family, and their health care provider. Patients may interpret the information they are given and not realize they are being given choices about their care [56]. And the discussions are more nuanced than asking if patients have advanced directives, are considered "Do Not Resuscitate" (DNR) or if power of attorney (POA) documents are in place.

Similarly, end-of-life planning in the form of POA or advanced directives may be delayed by belief or pressure to "think positive" [29] or superstition or cultural taboo that talking about death may hasten it. Alternatively, emotions evoked from thinking about end of life are difficult for some to face and may lead to avoidance. Patients, their families, and their providers may all have different preferences for information sharing and in making decisions about treatment and care toward the end of life [57]. Much work has gone into educating health care professionals about having difficult conversations but more needs to be done to align patient understanding and preferences with others [58].

Decision making regarding hospice exemplifies several of the communication issues that complicate end-of-life decision making. The decision of whether and when hospice is right for the individual is a dynamic and multidimensional process involving a range of personal, medical, social, financial, and psychological factors. This decision is complicated by several specific factors. As hospice requires patients forgo further life-sustaining treatment (ie, experimental chemotherapy), patients must consider large amounts of complex information about treatment options and services available, often weighing quality versus quantity of life and facing uncertainty [54,59,60]. The circumstances surrounding hospice referral are challenging, as patients are typically referred to hospice near end of life, often within days of death, when symptoms may be severe [59,61]. Hospice referrals are often delayed due to misconceptions by patients, families, or clinical staff [54,101]. While the majority of those enrolled in hospice were first told of hospice by their health care provider [62], many patients are never informed of hospice. Common reasons for postponing or rejecting hospice include perceptions of hospice as medical failure, denial by patient, family, and/or the clinician, poor communication regarding the hospice option, and patient values [47]. Studies show clinicians frequently wait until patients are very ill before initiating discussions regarding preferences for end of life, and many times the patient is unable to participate in the decision-making process [63]. Clinicians often have incomplete understanding of hospice or are uncomfortable with discussing hospice [64]. Often patients and families are frustrated with the lack of end-of-life conversation, but are reluctant to initiate them.

The period following diagnosis of terminal illness is a critical time for making decisions about care. If information about hospice services is provided during this period, chances are greatly increased that hospice care will be considered [65]. eHealth may be able to facilitate hospice education sooner by circumventing the clinician as the sole gateway to such information. Casarett et al. [59] demonstrated that a simple nontech intervention to improve communication about hospice care can increase hospice enrollment and improve quality of care for nursing home residents at end of life. Initiatives to better support patients and families regarding hospice understanding and decision making are needed to help patients and families who desire hospice care to benefit more fully from hospice [66].

One mechanism for preparing people to address and minimize potential suffering at end of life may be through the virtual exposure to situations they may face. This offers opportunities to make decisions based on values that present themselves when one is able to fully consider realistic possibilities. Technologies such as interactive video or virtual reality simulators may be useful for aiding people to vividly and realistically imagine themselves facing the physical and psychological effects of advanced cancer [29]. Decision aids could walk people through potential paths of end of life, offering probable outcomes to treatment options based on algorithms that leverage large patient data sets of end-of-life experiences.

Decision making is a critical issue in end-of-life planning; alternatively, complications can arise in decision implementation despite best intentions and preparation. The successful implementation of advanced directives and POA rely on access to that documentation at critical times of disease progression. Hard copies may be difficult to access if needs arise outside of the clinic setting where they are filed or patients and families may not bring copies when hospitalized.

EHR data bridges this gap some; however, EHRs are still often accessed only within the organization where they are entered and not shared across medical systems or jurisdictions that utilize different EHR servers. Informatics systems offer potential for important documentation to easily transmit across medical centers, increasing likelihood of accessing and implementing advance directives and POA decisions at critical moments of time sensitivity. For example, universal EHRs would offer access to this documentation at any medical facility. Alternatively, wearable documentation, such as an electronic health bracelet, may allow the patient to carry this information with them in a scannable format that emergency medical providers can instantly access.

On the other hand, discussions around end-of-life decision making are virtually always carried out in the abstract. Before the events begin to unravel, it may be easy to say that heroics should be avoided or that DNR orders should be followed. But when the time comes, positions can change dramatically in either direction (to pursue aggressive efforts to sustain life or take steps to facilitate death). It is a complicated process with no right answer. Personal stories of struggles by other families and how they were resolved may help and can be provided through electronic support systems. Inherently, the value of early decision-making activities may not be so much in having a confirmed decision and pat answer to all end-of-life circumstances, but rather to have had the opportunity to have thought through and identified personal values to serve as guidelines when faced with difficult and often unpredictable situations. Then when faced with critical events, decision makers, whether the patient or family, may be more mentally prepared with the knowledge of the potential types of treatment options, their risks, and likelihood of resulting in desired outcomes and more open to discuss them with their health care providers [27]. This mental preparedness, rather than a fixed decision, may facilitate more value-based decision making, even in crises when decisions may be based on gut instinct rather than calculated risk–benefit evaluation. Further, this preparedness may buffer against later decision regret. The potential for informatics to be able to address more complicated education and decision making around end-of-life choices is there, but currently highly underdeveloped and underutilized [28].

10.2.3 Opportunity for Bereavement

As described before, the questioning of medical decisions and the quality of caregiving and support is a risk factor for complicated bereavement. As such, resources that minimize decision regret and caregiver burden can reduce this risk. Accordingly, much can be done during the caregiving experience to buffer later bereavement difficulty. Informatics has strong potential in this area through the facilitation of family–patient–clinician communication and decision making.

Acceptance of hospice service provides a framework for understanding such potential. While patients and family members feel at the time of hospice enrollment that enrollment is not too late, a significant number of family members change their perception after the patient's death, retrospectively feeling that they had in fact enrolled too late [67]. Caregivers of patients with shorter length of stay are less satisfied with hospice care [51,68], and are at greater risk for a major depressive disorder within the first 6–8 months of bereavement [69]. This is alarming in light of median hospice stay for cancer patients being a mere 9.1 days [33]. Alternatively, the opportunity exists for electronic decision aids to facilitate hospice decision making and yield earlier, more timely referral based on hospice education, evaluation of values, and presentation of probabilities of disease trajectory. However, access to and use of available decision aids about end of life are limited [28]. The hope lies in the potential to not only improve the effectiveness of hospice care for the patient during end of life, but also to reduce retrospective regret for delay of services, in turn reducing depression during bereavement.

Informatics also hold the potential to bridge the gap caregivers experience in losing the support of the cancer community after their loved one dies. Electronic communication can create viable channels of continuous support with peers and other supportive services over caregiving and through bereavement. Such peer support can be a crucial and often single line of validation for caregiver and family reactions and emotional experiences that may feel taboo to express publicly, and particularly in the presence of their loved one. Many caregivers report feelings of anger and resentment for the disease, the demands of caregiving, and being left behind after patient death. However, they also feel guilty for having such feelings, at best editing such expressions with statements that "I shouldn't feel that way, at least I don't have cancer," and at worst holding feelings inside which can create greater psychological burden and morbidity. Connecting caregivers to each other for support offers a safe place, free of judgment, with others who are walking the same unimaginable yet inevitable path. These connections offer validation that can help relieve the unnecessary layer of suffering that is created by negative attributions made about the natural feelings of anger and resentment that might emerge. Addressing caregiver emotional burden during caregiving has the indirect benefit of easing bereavement adjustment [70].

Support can also be extended into bereavement by connecting with others who have lost a loved one to cancer, who faced difficult decisions, witnessed similar human suffering, and face similar despair in their grief. Similarly, these connections continue to offer a place for validation of and expressing feelings of loss, and offer reassurance that one's grief is normal and expected. This is critical in our society that shies away from death, is uncomfortable with grief, and focuses on moving forward. People often feel societal pressures to "get over it," have "closure" and move on. Lay opinion that grief should take 12 months, or one should move through the "stages of grief" offers little solace to those facing difficult loss that do not match these notions. Further, social networks without similar grief experience may directly or indirectly convey their discomfort with addressing grief, either withdrawing from the bereaved or indicating they should move on. These social cues can send the message to the bereaved that they are grieving too long or "wrong," again adding an unnecessary layer of judgment and guilt to an already difficult situation. Connection with others who share their experience can allow the opportunity to express and explore their grief openly, without fear of judgment of burdening others, and to lessen self-judgment. While in-person support groups can offer this experience, barriers to attendance include limited availability, access, and an individual's comfort with meeting strangers. Online chat rooms or discussion boards can overcome these barriers through their anytime/anywhere availability, and freedom of expression via online anonymity.

10.3 A CASE EXAMPLE: CHESS— THE COMPREHENSIVE HEALTH ENHANCEMENT SUPPORT SYSTEM

Online interventions that include palliative care and psychosocial support, among other elements, have rarely been studied; even less studied are online interventions aimed at family caregivers [14]. In the mid-1980s, we began developing and testing the effectiveness of an online information, communication, and coaching system called CHESS [71]. CHESS is a website created by clinical, communication, and systems scientists at the University of Wisconsin. Previous CHESS modules have addressed early stage breast and prostate cancer, and other medical conditions. In 2002, we developed two CHESS modules that broadened CHESS applications in two critical directions. First, they specifically targeted advanced stage disease for breast, prostate, and lung cancer. The shift to advanced stage disease necessitated the inclusion of family caregivers, and in turn the decision to focus the module toward a caregiver audience with attention to both end of life and bereavement.

CHESS provided focused and reliable content, arranged for ease of use, with many types of help in one place. CHESS was designed to: (1) provide well-organized cancer, care-giving, and bereavement *information*; (2) serve as a channel for *communication* with and support from peers, experts, clinicians, and the users' social networks; and (3) act as a *coach* by gathering information from users and providing feedback based on algorithms. CHESS services are listed in Table 10.1 and described in more detail in DuBenske et al. [72]. The efficacy of these modules were tested through two randomized control trials, one for lung cancer and the other for both breast and prostate cancers. Initially the trials called for three study groups: Internet control (no access to CHESS), CHESS, and CHESS with the Clinician Report. Due to low study attrition, we removed one study group in each trial. The lung cancer study retained the Internet

in comparison to CHESS with Clinician Report; the breast and prostate cancers study retained CHESS in comparison to CHESS with the Clinician Report. Details of the study procedures, including participants and study design are reported in DuBenske et al. [73] and Chih et al. [74], respectively. Findings from these studies are reviewed below to demonstrate the potential of such comprehensive eHealth systems.

10.3.1 CHESS and Symptom Management

CHESS addressed symptom management in several ways. It provided disease specific didactic information about treatments and side effects. It included brief tips developed by experts as well as allowed users to post their own tips to share from their learned experience. Online discussion boards allowed users to anonymously

TABLE 10.1 CHESS Services

CHESS service	Description
INFORMATION SERVICES	
Frequently asked questions (FAQs)	Brief answers to common and important questions about the physical and psychosocial aspects of cancer and caregiving; organized by topic.
Library articles	Links to relevant full text articles from scientific and popular press, vetted by CHESS staff for merit
Web links	Links to other high-quality relevant web sites.
Cancer news	Provides summaries of recent cancer-related news and research
Personal stories	First-person narratives of patient and caregiver experiences with cancer.
Caregiver tips	Brief tips organized by topics developed by experts or added by CHESS users.
COMMUNICATION SERVICES	
Discussion groups	Limited access bulletin boards for posting messages to other CHESS users; patient, caregiver, and bereavement groups were separated.
Ask and expert	One-on-one confidential question and answer service with a cancer information specialist.
Personal webpage	Personal bulletin board and interactive calendar. CHESS users could give access to their family and friends. Patient and caregiver users could to share updates, messages, and use a menu to request helpful tasks. Family and friends could post messages and sign up to help.
Clinician report	Provided the oncology clinic team with information from the patient and the caregiver, including symptom distress ratings, questions for the clinic visit, and caregiver ratings of perceived competence in providing care. Alerts were sent to the clinic team to read the report when a symptom distress rating exceeded the threshold, and 2 days prior to a scheduled clinic visit.
COACHING/TRAINING SERVICES	
Health status	Prompts weekly completion of symptom and need assessment. Charts updates of the patient's health status for review. This assessment provides information for the Clinician Report.
Decision aids	Guided decision analysis to help learn about options, clarify values, understand decision consequences, and implement decisions. Included a Treatment Decision Aid for patients and caregivers and a Respite Decision Aid designed for caregivers.
Easing distress	Uses cognitive behavioral therapy principles to help identify emotional distress and apply coping techniques.
Healthy relating	Teaches techniques to increase closeness and decrease conflict in interpersonal relationships.
Action plan	Guides users in planning behavior changes by identifying goals, resources, and ways to overcome barriers.

connect with each other to ask questions and share experiences in managing symptoms and care needs. Overall, we found that in the lung cancer study, the CHESS with Clinician Report group had lower symptom distress than the Internet group across follow-up for months 2–8 while having access to CHESS [75].

The Clinician Report service in CHESS was specifically designed as a channel for assessing and reporting symptoms distress to the clinical team. The Clinician Report appeared as a weekly check-in for both patients and caregivers using CHESS, assessing the physical and psychosocial distress of the patient and caregiver. Ten symptoms of patient physical and psychological distress were assessed using a modification of the Edmonton Symptom Assessment Scale (ESAS) [76]: pain, shortness of breath, nausea, appetite, diarrhea, constipation, fatigue, depression, anxiety, and distress. Symptoms were rated on a 0 (minimal distress) to 10 (maximum distress) Likert-type scale. Any time a patient or caregiver reported that the patient had significant distress on any one symptom (as rated as 7 or higher), CHESS immediately sent an email alert to the clinical team. These alerts afforded clinicians the opportunity to address serious problems that may have gone unnoticed or address them sooner [77], possibly improving symptom management in the CHESS group. The Clinician Report may also have enabled clinicians to better address patient and caregiver concerns at clinic visits. In interviews, some clinicians reported that caregivers using CHESS were more engaged during the clinic visit and better able to describe their concerns and the patient's symptoms [77].

Communicating symptom concerns to the clinician plays a critical role in reducing suffering and optimizing patient outcomes. To examine whether symptom distress was reduced after clinician reports were sent, we conducted a pooled analysis of the two trials comparing the CHESS group to the CHESS with Clinician Report group for lung, breast, and prostate cancers. We examined symptom ratings of 7 or higher (the level an alert email is triggered). For those who had alerts sent to the treatment team, their symptoms improved 53.1% of the time, whereas for the CHESS group without alerts, improvement was reported only 26.2% of the time [78]. By sharing caregiver ratings of patient's symptoms (eg, pain) with their clinician via the Clinician Report, symptom distress was significantly reduced compared to patients whose symptoms were tracked but not shared [21]. In another pooled analysis of these two trials, we noted a benefit of the Clinician Report for caregiver outcomes. At both 6 and 12 months of access to the CHESS system, those with the Clinician Report reported lower levels of negative mood (a composite of depression, anxiety and anger) than those caregivers who had access to CHESS without the Clinician Report [74]. Such findings support the notion that communication of symptoms

to the clinical team, particularly outside the context of scheduled clinic visits, can not only improve symptom management, but can also ease caregiver distress in the process.

During the course of the lung cancer study, it became apparent that caregivers from the Internet group were transitioning to bereavement status more frequently than caregivers in the CHESS with Clinician Report group. We conducted an exploratory survival analysis to investigate this issue. While 2-year survival rates did not differ significantly between groups, median survival was 3.8 months longer for the CHESS with Clinician Report group than the Internet group [75]. This is particularly striking for two reasons. First, 3.8 months of extended life is clinically meaningful for a disease with a median survival of only 8 months. Second, the advantage is similar to the 2.7 month improvement in survival documented in Temel et al.'s [79] work on the benefit if there is early palliative care. Like palliative care, CHESS is designed to promote patient and caregiver engagement in healthcare by providing information and encouraging communication. Unlike palliative care, patients and caregivers using CHESS have anytime access to narratives about and communication with peers who share their treatment and decision-making experiences. They also have an extension of communication via the Clinician Report. As such, CHESS demonstrates the promise for eHealth interventions to reduce suffering for advanced stage and terminal cancer patients, and even lengthen survival.

10.3.2 CHESS for Caregiving and Bereavement

Cancer patients depend on family caregivers for physical and emotional support throughout their disease, especially with disease progression and end of life. Supporting a loved one through the journey of cancer and the trials of end of life can be physically and psychologically demanding on caregivers, who in turn then face bereavement in the aftermath of such intense caregiving. CHESS allocated a variety of resources specifically intended to support caregivers in the instrumental and emotional roles of caregiving. The lung cancer study demonstrated that the CHESS system benefited caregivers. In comparison to the Internet group, caregivers with access to CHESS with the Clinician Report had significantly less burden and negative mood, despite having equal levels of disruptiveness [73]. CHESS was likely unable to reduce the amount of practical tasks with which caregivers needed to engage. However, it is likely that the potential reduction in patient's suffering, opportunities for support and validation from other caregivers, and services to increase caregiver competence in addressing the patient's and their own needs may contribute to lowered perception of burden and negative emotional reactions.

The impact of caregiver burden can be extensive, even complicating later bereavement. In most cases, caregiver support ends when the patient dies. CHESS's advanced breast, prostate, and lung cancer websites represent an innovation in offering caregiver support across the continuum from caregiving through bereavement. Specific resources for bereavement included didactic information and tips related to grief and bereavement, and the additional access to a bereaved caregiver discussion group. Furthermore, bereaved caregivers continued to have access to the entirety of CHESS content, allowing a review of information as they may have questions about care received or decisions made. In fact, when bereaved caregivers sought information services on CHESS, 44% of the time it was related to cancer and current caregiving information rather than bereavement information. They also continued to participate in current caregiver discussion groups if they wanted, and with 41% of bereaved caregiver discussion group activity being in the current caregiver group. This offered an opportunity to extend help to others, which may have been a meaningful outlet and positive opportunity from their bereavement.

Not only was CHESS found to lower caregiver burden during active phases of patient care, caregivers with CHESS also saw continued benefit after their loved one died. In our study, mood was measured in caregiving and bereavement surveys with the Profile of Mood States depression, anxiety, and anger subscales. We looked at predictors of caregiver mood at 3 and 5 months after the patient died. For the Internet group, higher levels of depression and anger prior to patient death predicted higher levels in bereavement. Caregivers with access to CHESS had lower levels of depression and anger in bereavement regardless of levels of depression and anger prior to their loved one's death. Accordingly, CHESS demonstrated that informatics systems can play a continued role in supporting caregivers in adjusting to loss and "reentry" after caregiving.

10.3.3 Lessons From CHESS Development and Implementation

The CHESS advanced cancer websites were a departure from previous CHESS expertise in two critical ways: the focus on end of life and the focus on caregivers. This shift in attention illuminated critical challenges for development and implementation.

One concern regarding web-based support for an advanced cancer population is whether this population would use such a system. Earlier CHESS studies that targeted early stage breast cancer had on average 75% accrual rates. Recruitment of advanced cancer populations to similar CHESS intervention studies proved much more challenging. On average, we had 50% accrual, as low as 42% for prostate cancer and up to 56% for lung cancer [80]. The leading reasons people declined study participation included factors related to the clinical trial itself (eg, survey burden, consent form wording, time commitment, lack of interest in the study), the technology (eg, lack of familiarity or interest in computers, already having access to online or other trusted resources, privacy concerns) or personal characteristics (eg, patient doing well so no need, timing is difficult, feeling overwhelmed, poor caregiver health, individual coping styles). Lung cancer patients, more than breast or prostate cancers, patients cited the use of a computer as the reason for refusal. However, for those enrolled in the CHESS arm of the lung cancer study, 75% of caregivers accessed the CHESS website for an average of 15 sessions, and 50% of patients for an average of 24 sessions. Patient use is particularly positive given patient involvement was optional as the study specifically targeted caregiver involvement.

Reasons for CHESS study decline provide insight into barriers to informatics adoption by patients and families. A detailed discussion of these lessons is provided in Buss et al. [80]. Briefly, however, is the issue of when to present such resources and incorporate them into care. Our experience suggests that disease burden can be a barrier. When compounded with issues of unfamiliar technology, and demands of clinical trial participation, target users may be less willing to set aside time to learn something new when they are already overburdened by their cancer situation or at end of life when time is an especially precious commodity. However, separation of triggering factors (eg, trial-, technology-, or person-related) can guide development and implementation initiatives. For example, people who were resistant because of trial-related factors may still be willing adapters to system implementation. Those with personal factors may or may not adapt, but they highlight the importance of recognizing individual differences and identifying effective timing to embed electronic resources within the care framework. If presented too early or too late, the risk is missing the point of need, or alternatively hitting a time of being overwhelmed (essentially too much need), either of which lends to the rejection of what otherwise may have been a valuable resource. Greater understanding of the critical element of timing is essential for successful implementation.

As many people with advanced cancer are older, concerns for older patient's interest or ability to use computers were raised. However, such concerns are reduced by growing evidence that elderly people successfully use computers [81,82]. 2012 Internet and American Life Project findings illustrate that 59% of those age 65 years or older go online; however, this drops off at around age 75. The average age of our lung cancer participants was 62 years. Seventy-five percent of patients tried the CHESS website, demonstrating the potential for greater motivation and uptake of such systems when facing a

---

BOX 10.2

An elderly woman decided to join the CHESS study as the designated caregiver for her husband who had lung cancer. When assessing her access to a computer, she stated she had never used one. She had used a typewriter some many years ago but explained that her husband had a computer set up in the basement. She had severe arthritis and was unable to go down stairs. Her husband had offered many times to bring the computer upstairs, but she had always declined having no interest or need. When she joined the study she remarked optimistically, "I guess now it's time to bring it [the computer] upstairs."

---

health crisis. This is also illustrated in Box 10.2 by the story of one CHESS participant's change in attitude about using the computer. This reiterates findings that cancer patients have the highest rates of eHealth system use compared to other medical populations, potentially because of greater level of need [38]. Our experience with Medicare patients matches these findings and has demonstrated that elderly people will use computers, and while training and technical support is crucial it need not be time-consuming, and that lack of computer experience is not a barrier to use [83].

We decided to focus the intervention for cancer caregivers, but also provide support to patients. In doing so, we had to decide how to deliver information and services for the appropriate perspective of the user (patient or caregiver) and whether access to information should be shared or separated between members of a given patient-caregiver dyad. User login IDs were associated with user characteristics (eg, patient or caregiver status). This allowed us to tailor content to the specific audience. Accordingly, we could use a sensitive voice in conveying caregiver or patient information. In many instances the information was the same regardless of the user. However, in cases when the perspective may be different (eg, issues of self-care, role changes), we pushed user-specific content. Yet, there seemed to be some value in being able to see the other's perspective. So, in instances when messages changed depending on the user, we offered a link to see the content as delivered from the alternative perspective.

Still, decisions about sharing user-provided content, particularly discussion group messages and Health Tracking data, were more complex. Discussion boards allow users to post messages on a board viewable by other users. Should patients and caregivers participate in the same boards? In some cancer circles, patients and caregivers attend joint support groups. In other circles, these are clearly separated, specifically to allow

participants to express feelings or problems that they might not otherwise share openly with their loved ones. Accordingly, based on feedback from patient and caregiver focus groups, we developed separate and specific discussion groups for patients and caregivers, while leaving one board open to all—the spirituality discussion board for conveying religious or spiritual based messages of hope, faith, and the like.

Patients and caregivers were both assessed about patient symptom status for Health Tracking and, if available, the Clinician Report. Based on professional discussion and focus groups, we felt it important again to allow a place of private messaging, where patient and caregiver did not see each other's reports. However, early considerations overlooked the potential problem of how clinicians may address this information within the clinical encounter. A caregiver brought this to our attention when they questioned how the patient may have heard about concerns they indicated during Health Tracking Check-in. Clinicians also reported concern that the shared viewing of patient and caregiver concerns might prevent honest disclosure [77]. Because we had no way to restrict the clinician from divulging information received in the Clinician Report, our response was to relabel the Check-in assessment to indicate clearly that ratings and other information provided could potentially be learned by their partnered user via the oncologist. These examples highlight considerations for future system design to be aware of sensitivities and expectations for privacy, shared information, and use of the information on the end of the clinical team.

One option we considered was the development of patient controls for setting privacy, allowing the patient to decide whether a caregiver can report privately or in shared space, if at all. Given CHESS was an initial test of such a system and many users were unfamiliar with the technology, we opted to simplify system start up by establishing set privacy rules. However, in our current testing of Elder Tree, an online module to enhance quality of life for elderly who are aging in place, we have experimented with private messaging as a means of allowing elders to decide the degree to which their postings are viewed by the mass of system users versus sending to selected users. Private messaging is actively used between elders on the site, as well as a means of elders contacting the research staff. We have also tested the use of anonymous postings, allowing elders to post comments on discussion boards that are signed "anonymous" rather than with their codename. We have needed to restrict this feature because elders often used it as a safe way to aggressively criticize others. For example, one anonymous post in the spirituality/religious discussion stated "I don't think some of you are literate enough to have read the bible!" Now, all anonymous postings are screened by research staff for approval or moderating before they are posted to the website. Additionally, friends and family can communicate through private messaging with the elder but cannot see what the elder posts in the discussion group. Friends and family have access to a separate discussion group for caregivers. The nature of communication channels and access to friends and family is an important consideration when designing such systems and will likely vary in appropriateness depending on the nature of the intervention and scope of data collected and for what intention.

Another challenge we faced was the difficulty of addressing the topic of dying. Dying is not easily discussed in modern culture and at the least can be a sensitive topic for some, whereas even taboo for others. We set out to design a system that would take people through the trajectory of advanced stage disease, including end of life and caregiver bereavement. We wanted to be proactive in having people consider end of life issues and be prepared. However, we also wanted to balance this with hope. We feared the consequences that being too blunt about dying could deter users. We considered models of expanding available information as patients hit milestones that might make information more relevant; however, without evidence-based milestones, we were uncomfortable serving as the gatekeepers for such information. At a minimum risk the information might come too late. Even more daunting, information might come too early and send someone a message that is misconstrued as diagnostic, with the risk of instilling anxiety or other psychological reactions in the absence of personal contact with the opportunity for clarification and support. In-person conversations have the ability to gage the receiver's reaction to information, and provide support or corrective messaging as needed. But online interventions delivered without personal connection are limited and run greater risk. In the end, we took a more conservative approach of offering end-of-life information to all from the start, clearly labeled on the table of contents, but listed last. Paper prototyping of the web page design and content demonstrated this to be acceptable by many. But it also meant sacrificing the opportunity to guide people to end of life content (eg, hospice, financial, and legal considerations) earlier in the disease process.

The newly developed Clinician Report brought the challenge of how to implement CHESS within medical systems, whereas previous modules had been delivered solely to patient users. This study involved multiple cancer centers that utilized a variety of EHR systems and clinic team configurations. One consideration was who within the clinic should receive the email alerts which were triggered by ratings of high symptom distress of an upcoming scheduled clinic visit (patients entered appointment dates as part of Check-in). We were able to tailor the recipient based on clinic desires. Most clinics opted to have the triage nurse receive these notifications. Some oncologists preferred to receive them as well. While some oncologists opted not to receive the alerts, entrusting them exclusively with their staff, no oncologists elected to be the sole receiver of the alert notifications for concerns about delay in addressing concerns. In addition to email alerts, the Clinician Report was an interactive report that provided oncologists with trend data of each symptom, indicators of the types of information the patient and caregiver had been needing in the CHESS system, a listing of their questions for the scheduled clinic visits, along with assessment of the caregiver's competence in addressing the patient's needs. To be most useful, this information needed to be available at the time of the clinical encounter between the oncologist, patient, and caregiver. Given the early stage of development, we were not able to integrate CHESS within the existing EHRs. Therefore, it required clinic staff to login to a separate website to access this. This proved to be a significant barrier to the use of the interactive report. However, the emailed message of the significant symptom distress still yielded the benefits, as discussed previously. In addition, some triage nurses would print the report to attach to the paper chart for the oncologist to see at the time of the clinic visit. From this, clinic teams requested a redesign of the Clinician Report content to fit into a print format for ease of use. While trend data was not available in this format, the willingness to go through the extra steps to log into CHESS and print the Clinician Report demonstrated a perceived value of the information even in static format. Organizational structure is a critical component for dissemination and implementation of systems like CHESS. Understanding of stakeholder needs, including patients, caregivers, a multidisciplinary team of clinicians, and organizations, is imperative. For successful uptake, systems need to be imbedded within existing infrastructure, including the organizations EHR and the clinic workflow.

In summary, eHealth offers the ability to facilitate communication between multiple users via multiple channels within a single system. This very asset drives complexity. The integration of systems and multiple care providers (eg, oncologists, nurses, primary care providers, surgeons) and care organizations (eg, oncology clinics, home health, hospice) compounds this issue. Throughout all stages of development it is critical to solicit the values, needs, and reactions from the key stakeholders, including patients, families, clinicians, and organizations [41]. Furthermore, there is an increasing role for big data in the development of more accurate predictive analytics to help determine effective timing of system delivery, the delivery of content, and potentially even the content itself [84].

10.3.4 Lessons From CHESS Evaluation

Evaluating effectiveness of systems such as CHESS raises a number of complex issues, especially in the context of end of life. One such issue is deciding what we wish to achieve and therefore what to measure. Are we measuring: symptom distress, survival, quality of life, participation in clinical trials, caregiver burden, anxiety, depression, and family engagement?

As with any research study we need to ensure that what we are measuring is consistent with what the system is designed to do. While this is easy to say, our experience as designers, evaluators, and grant reviewers is that there are often big differences between what is being evaluated and what the system was designed to accomplish. Often we use data, collected for other purposes, to test a system whose intended outcomes are different. A classic situation is related to medication adherence. We can try to use self-report but we know that people overstate their adherence. We could use sensors on the medication bottles but we know that we are really measuring whether the bottle has been opened and not whether the medication has been taken. We could measure refill rates but a patient could doctor shop to obtain more than the prescribed amount of medication. Recognition of those facts early on may force us to reexamine what we are trying to do. If we are trying to reduce medication-related admissions, we might decide that all we really care about is overdose of high-risk medications and could then choose to collect physical symptoms of overdose. The relation between goals and measures often requires more intensive thought than might be expected.

As a comprehensive eHealth tool, CHESS was designed to address a variety of needs that may arise across the advanced cancer trajectory. It included a host of means for providing information, decision aids, support, distress management, and symptom management across a variety of formats. While primary research aims were to test CHESS effectiveness at improving quality of life for patients and caregivers, the system could potentially affect many outcomes of interest. Furthermore, the complexity of the system by design meant that users would seek to meet their individual needs through preferred formats, such that user experiences differed. Accordingly, not all users would benefit equally. Furthermore, we did not select users based on psychological distress, but rather wanted a sample that resembled the general advanced cancer audience to which such a system would someday be broadly disseminated. In doing so, not all users had the specific need that the research aims addressed. Some caregivers had low burden and distress. Some patients were relatively symptom free. Having a sample with high baseline functioning on critical outcome measures can dilute the ability to detect the effectiveness for those in need for the population at large. Is a system designed to support patients and caregivers during cancer and end of life effective even for those who are coping well? The answer is a resounding "Absolutely!"—for some. But this is difficult to assess.

More so, distress is a moving target, with cycles of distress corresponding to treatment effects and disease progression. Caregiver roles and burden are equally dynamic. Therefore, not only is the timing of the intervention critical for motivating system use and offering benefits, but so is the timing of outcome assessments. Is a system designed for symptom management effective? Some times more than others, but if you miss the opportune time in the assessment, you miss the opportunity to detect the system's effectiveness. This was most apparent in the CHESS lung cancer study when we aimed to examine bereavement adjustment at months 1, 2, 3, 5, 7, 10, and 13 after the patient died. However, it was common for us to learn of patient deaths when patient surveys were returned. This commonly meant not knowing of the death until 2–3 months after the fact, delaying the implementation of bereavement support services on CHESS and missing assessment of early bereavement reactions. Other assessment considerations required balancing the burden of surveys for already burdened participants. Regular interval assessments allowed us to project the participant burden, however we likely missed opportunities when difficult situations may have arisen or resolved between surveys. Innovations in methodology that allows for assessment that is event-based rather than interval-based may facilitate data gathering at critical points for understanding dynamic patterns of system use and real effects. Critical targets of cancer interventions, such as patient symptoms reduction and quality of life, are constantly in flux. Here, informatics-based assessment and delivery systems have an advantage. Rather than being dependent on a predetermined schedule, these systems can identify individual changes and events to trigger the delivery of personalized assessments or interventions at critical moments.

The Reach Effectiveness Adoption Implementation Maintenance (RE-AIM) framework [85] is appealing in the sense that it helps direct system evaluation toward elements that will be essential in the eventual implementation and dissemination of the technology. Often research focuses almost exclusively on system impact or effectiveness. RE-AIM reminds us of the importance of issues such the extent to which the patients involved are representative of the patients that might be expected to use the system or the extent to which the clinicians who implement the system are representative of that population. It calls us to focus not only on short-term effects but also what it will take to maintain or sustain a system over the long run and to examine not only what was implemented but also how the implementation took place.

10.4 FUTURE DIRECTIONS FOR RESEARCH

A recent review of eHealth interventions [10] specifically for palliative care demonstrated three critical shortcomings in this field of research: (1) there is a dearth of randomized controlled trials; (2) there is a lack of attention to patient-related clinical outcomes; and (3) family caregivers, despite the critical role they play in patient care, are infrequently included in studies. These issues are common in most areas of health services research, but they are particularly important in palliative care.

Patients' involvement in research is compromised because of their illness progression or active dying. Family can serve as surrogates for data collection; however, many face their own priorities and challenges that limit their desire or availability to participate. Nonetheless, there are ways to conduct ethical research that are minimally invasive. Yet, with our own research, and others, accrual is challenging.

10.4.1 Research Design

While randomized trials are very important, the complexity of research with technology and focus on end of life necessitates understanding that alternative designs can be appropriate under certain circumstances. Examples of such designs include time series, nonequivalent control group, stepped wedge, counterbalancing, among others. One needs to keep in mind that eHealth systems development will not wait for evaluations that take several years. As much as we might wish for time to conduct randomized trials, the literature is rife with warnings that in many cases it is not going to be there [86–88]. A paradigm shift is needed. Opportunities for such alternative research designs are explored in Chapter 18, "A New Era of clinical Trial research Methods in a Data-Rich Environment" by Riley et al. in this book.

We also need to recognize and celebrate the differences between science and engineering. Both are important. Science seeks to understand. It seeks highly controlled situations with very careful use of validated measures. Engineering seeks to solve problems. It operates under time constraints that require efficient use of resources and rapid responses to critical questions. "Good enough" is a fundamental principle of engineering while it may be an anathema to scientists. Both perspectives are important. Both have costs and both have benefits. Given the pressures of progress in eHealth, we may be forced to adopt additional principles of engineering. In fact, that is already happening. One example is the use of factorial designs (a staple of engineering for years) that is being adopted in health services research [89]. Additionally, principles of rapid cycle improvement are being adapted for rapid cycle research.

10.4.2 Patient Outcomes

As Capurro [10] articulates, attention to research outcomes for palliative care interventions is also critical. Quality of life research is plentiful in cancer populations. There is growing awareness of the need for focus on both physical and psychological outcomes to measure quality of life. Even with advanced cancer, much can be done to manage physical symptoms and address psychological reactions to minimize depression and anxiety. However, this requires the patient and caregiver reporting their subjective experience to the treatment team, and, in turn, the treatment team responding to these needs. Research continues to examine barriers to such communication and implementation of eHealth solutions. Examples include the previously described CHESS's Clinician Report and ESRA-C [39]. As such, we continue to need to find systems that facilitate effective communication regarding patient and caregiver needs for symptom management. The evidence base for these communication systems needs to not only demonstrate improved communication, but also that the communication is leading to reduced patient and family suffering. Much clinical communication research focuses on patient's satisfaction. However, satisfaction is not necessarily tied to clinically relevant experience, as patients have biases to hold their oncologist in a positive light, even when suffering.

In the advanced cancer continuum, death is inevitable and the quality of death needs to be evaluated as a critical outcome for patient care initiatives. The IOM defines a good death as "one that is free from avoidable death and suffering for patients, families and caregivers in general accordance with the patients' and families' wishes [90], and reasonably consistent with clinical, cultural, and ethical standards." Throughout cancer treatment, many patients fear suffering at the end of life. And for bereaved family members, the period of active dying serves as a lasting memory of their time caregiving. Although the period of active dying is critical, less research attention has focused on the quality of death. Specifically, very little has examined the role of technology in facilitating this process. One challenge for such research is identifying important outcomes for this. The definition of "good" varies by individual, and despite IOM's definition, patients and providers have their own conceptualizations of what a good death means.

Emmanuel and Emmanuel [91] have identified six domains for measuring and modifying a good death. These include: physical symptoms, psychological and cognitive symptoms, economic and caregiving needs, social relationships and support, spiritual and existential beliefs, and hopes and expectations [91]. Informatics holds the promise to directly and indirectly impact any of these areas by facilitating information exchange. We have discussed some opportunities for physical and psychological symptoms management, as well as mapping expectations for end-of-life planning and decision making. These domains serve as a guide for selecting broader outcomes in consideration of a good death.

10.4.3 Decision-Making Research

Many decision theory models are based on principles of disaggregation and logic. They address the following kinds of concerns: What are the factors involved in the decision? What is the relative importance of these factors? What options are available and how well do these options satisfy these factors. Some disease related events are known but others might occur or might not. What are the probabilities that these events will occur? How should rare events be factored into decision making? Beyond the factors related to a perceived single decision, it is important to recognize that decisions are not isolated incidences. They often create new decisions that must be made. Therefore, there is a need to understand decision making as such a sequence and develop the means to optimize those sequences of decisions rather than optimizing one decision at a time. Research has told us that humans are not particularly good at making complex decisions. Concepts such as anchoring and adjustment, as well as conservatism in probability estimation have demonstrated human frailties [92]. But on the other hand there is evidence that humans do not think about or make decisions in a disaggregated way. But humans will decide.

However, when decisions are too complicated or too emotional, people may avoid decision making or find themselves paralyzed by the process. There are often numerous potential trajectories of advanced cancer that are difficult to predict. Furthermore, facing one's own mortality or that of a loved one can trigger anxiety or sorrow. In an effort to manage these difficult emotions, decision making with regard to end of life planning is often avoided. However, such procrastination or indecision can lead to consequences of care that are incongruent with one's values or desires for a good death.

Decision aids have strong potential to facilitate decision making and implementation with regard to complicated decisions of end of life. Yet the clinical uptake of decision aid implementation has been limited. A general need exists in decision aid research to identify the optimal strategies and the appropriate timing for implementing decision aids [93]. A critical issue for patients with terminal diagnosis is consideration of end of life, most notably the decisions of whether to continue with aggressive treatments and whether and when to enter hospice. As discussed earlier, patients often enter hospice at the very end of life during the phase of active dying. While most patients learn of hospice through their clinician, such referrals often come too late to optimize hospice benefits [63]. We know little about patients' willingness to consider hospice prior to receiving this referral and the majority of hospice research has been conducted after hospice referral or enrollment. Critics of the late referrals often site clinician difficulties in prognosing patient life span or accepting their patient is dying, or the belief that the patient is not ready for hospice as key barriers to earlier referral and hospice enrollment [94,95]. However, patients may be willing to consider such alternatives earlier than clinicians assume [96]. The conditions under which cancer patients and families are open to hospice decision support prior to clinician referral have not been empirically evaluated. While Casarett [51] demonstrated improvements in hospice enrollment by implementing a hospice readiness assessment prior to referral and notifying the clinician when hospice seemed appropriate, there is no research that has used similar methods within a clinic setting, or specifically with cancer patients. Further, this assessment was conducted by hand, rather than implementing technology. Understanding when and under what conditions patients and family members are open to education about end-of-life choices and decision support is essential for the successful adoption of end-of-life decision support that informatics can deliver.

Another crucial area of informatics related to shared decision making is the development of decision aids that allow patients and families to integrate their combined beliefs, perspectives, values, and preferences. The decisions of whether or not to continue aggressive treatment or whether to enroll in hospice are often fueled with emotions and rooted in values. It is not uncommon for patients, family, and even clinicians to have discordant preferences in this regard [97]. While decision aids exist that can allow the patient to reflect on the impact of each potential option on their own values and aid in value-concordant decision making, these have not yet blended the decision preferences of other people who may be critical to the decision-making process. Research is needed in the design, operation and impact of decision aids that include multiple decision makers. How can this more complex data be presented to facilitate rather than complicate decision making? What support is needed when decision makers are discordant? What can technology deliver with regard to helping people resolve discordance versus what in-person support infrastructure is required? Furthermore, one barrier patients can experience in terminating aggressive treatment is concern for "letting down" their oncologist. It is critical that decision aids support honest and open conversations between patients and clinicians, and that they empower patients and family members to express their needs even in the face of real or perceived disagreement with clinician recommendations or preferences.

While quality decision aids yield the potential to facilitate complex decisions, limited literature exists regarding the hospice decision-making process [27,47], and particularly the role decision aids may play in improving this process for patients, their families, and health practitioners. Accordingly, development of hospice decision aids and research that establishes an evidence base for their effectiveness is needed. Critical research outcomes should include acceptance of utilizing the decision aid, rates of hospice acceptance, timing of hospice enrollment, patient and family satisfaction with decision making, and assessment of the quality of death [28].

10.4.4 Economic Outcomes

Making the economic case for informatics interventions at end of life is critical to support widespread implementation that will be dependent on organizations to buy in and maintain services. Costs of cancer care can become enormous, especially during the latter part of life. Chemotherapy, for instance, can be very expensive with very little hope of making a difference. Moreover, it can cause enormous, and useless, suffering. No one is at fault here and yet everyone is. Patients often are not ready to give up. They need to make it to the next birthday, graduation, or holiday. Family members often are not ready either. Clinicians hate to lose a fight and therefore can be inclined to keep going, especially when it is so hard to say that it is time to move in a new direction. So the cards are stacked in favor of keeping on when keeping on only leads to pain and suffering and rising costs. We hate to raise this issue, but costs are a critical issue. America cannot afford to cover such costs. No other country can either, but we appear to be alone in being unwilling to come face to face with these issues. eHealth systems have the potential to help our country to come to terms with this issue. For example, registry systems allow us to examine population management issues that may demonstrate the impact of clinical decisions on costs. Simulations can help examine the relative costs of different kind of strategies. Decision models can help us face the values that do or could drive decisions. Much more work is needed to find ways to use eHealth systems to support clinical and patient/family end-of-life decision making in ways that appreciate the full spectrum of issues at hand.

For implementation, finding economic rationale for use of informatics is also critical. The case of cost-effectiveness will drive the medical system and insurers to put forth the cost to develop and implement such systems. However, determining the impact of eHealth systems is complicated in advanced disease when the outcome will eventually be death. Popular belief might suggest that the extension of life with cancer, a disease treated by costly treatments, would necessarily exacerbate costs. Accordingly, interventions that extend life might overtax an already financial threatened health care system. On the contrary, not only has palliative care been shown to increase length of survival for cancer patients, but has done so with less aggressive treatments. More demonstrations of such cost-effectiveness will provide fuel for organization uptake of informatics solutions.

10.4.5 Family Involvement

As discussed, families play a particularly important role in this stage of life and they are affected very extensively as well. Yet cancer care (like health care in general) is missing a very important opportunity, and that is supporting families so that they can play a more effective role in caring for the patient. Research involving family members and or examining family-related clinical outcomes is disproportionately lacking. Cancer patients, especially toward the end of life, are often unable to make decisions, understand clinicians, or to effectively advocate for themselves. Family caregivers can feel like they are alone in their efforts to support the patient. Clinicians may often ignore family members even though they are in a position to know more about the patient than anyone else. With proper training and support the family member can be a very powerful clinician extender. At the same time, family (especially near a patient's end of life) can suffer from burnout, anger, frustration, depression, anxiety, and physical illness. This not only compounds the difficulty of playing an effective caregiver role, but also leads to health care demands that go beyond but are caused by the cancer itself. As we have demonstrated in our lung cancer study, there are numerous ways in which eHealth can support family caregivers and more research is needed on that subject.

CHESS also demonstrated the potential for an eHealth system to have a positive impact on bereavement. However, further research in areas of minimizing the impact on bereavement is needed. It is anticipated that the effective implementation of end of life and hospice decision aids could minimize decision regret, but this needs to be demonstrated through evidenced-based development and implementation of such decision aids. Further, online support services offer the opportunity for caregivers to connect across geographic distance that may allow finding connections to others who share similar circumstances (even for those caregiving for rare diseases). The degree of anonymity may allow for more open sharing of emotional experience that can be difficult for many to express due to concerns for social stigma. In doing so, they can be validated and have potential to be relieved of that unnecessary layer of suffering during their care that can cause guilt and complicated bereavement. Again, the specific mechanisms of such support and these outcomes need to be examined in larger scale studies. Further, such online discussion boards afford the bereaved a platform for offering something back during their bereavement. The ability to channel grief feelings into meaningful work can be helpful in moving forward after loss and making positive meaning of one's experience. The ability to reflect back may also inform big data that can then help others in mapping likely paths of the end-of-life experience, in turn affording others guidance and more informed and potentially more value-directed decisions.

10.5 FUTURE DIRECTIONS FOR DEVELOPMENT AND IMPLEMENTATION

Cancer informatics has the potential to extend life. One concern is that this extension of life with terminal illness might necessarily extend suffering, either with treatment side effects or disease progression. However, initial exploratory evidence suggests otherwise [77,81]. More definitive support of this will build the evidence base for broad-based adoption of such resources to be built into the care continuum as standard practice for meeting end of life needs. Ideally, such systems would be an inherent component of the infrastructure of cancer care from the earliest point of the cancer trajectory, as an essential and ever-present extension of the clinical team. Then their use is not in itself a marker of a transition to death, but rather part of a continuum of support that is comfortable and trusted, and therefore turned to for trusted care delivery to support the hope for a good death in a similar fashion to the support offered when hoping for cure.

Cancer treatment is often a series of highs and lows. Patients have good days and bad days. Similarly patients and families may need different things at different points in time. eHealth systems need to be designed to respond to the rapidly changing aspects of cancer. We need to design eHealth systems that bring in different content or services at different times.

Specifically related to palliative care, we need to begin creating eHealth modules that integrate the concepts of palliative care as soon as cancer is diagnosed, not at the end. For the sake of this book, palliative care and end of life is a separate chapter from treatment and survivorship. However, these are artificial divides for the sake of organizational simplicity. In reality, these are not separable segments but part of a continuum of the cancer experience. Likewise, development and implementation of informatics systems need to embrace this continuum to provide seamless nonfragmented support from initiatives of early detection, diagnosis, and treatment to survivorship, end of life, and family bereavement. Many of the concepts of palliative care apply to any stage of cancer, and eHealth systems may make it possible to advance their use. For instance, goal clarification is a process that can be beneficial at any stage of life. Cancer can be that "whack on the side of the head" that can initiate such thinking. eHealth can help to make it happen.

Yet it is a classic failing of science to say that humans should meet facts and technology where facts and technology are, not the other way around. We call for people to get better at health care literacy, or learn how to live with standards adopted by computer programmers. But why should people coping with impending loss of a spouse or daughter be expected to adapt to anything at this critical point in time? Technology needs to meet people where they are, not the other way around. Voice navigation and interfaces that are stimulus response compatible (for instance) are not unreasonable things to expect from eHealth systems (refer to Chapter 11, "Data Visualization Tools for Investigating Health Services Utilization Among Cancer Patients," by Onukwugha et al. in this book for further discussion). One could reasonably expect that they would be there. Yes, these are hard things to do; so is dying.

10.6 CONCLUSION

Informatics offers much promise for advanced cancer care by addressing gaps in palliative care, end-of-life care, and bereavement. We have highlighted areas for opportunity in symptom management, decision making and implementation, and family bereavement. Most notably such systems need to be implemented in the very foundation of care, addressing needs as early as possible to be familiar and supportive as needs arise across the continuum of cancer and including multiple vital stakeholders, including informal caregivers. In addition, considerations for the implementation of informatics in end-of-life care must remain critically aware of the sensitive nature of this context and the people involved. End of life is a sacred time and deserving of "high touch," not just "hi tech" solutions [98]. In medical encounters, patients have simultaneous needs to "know and understand and to feel known and understood" [99]. The need to know is satisfied with information; the need to feel known is satisfied by empathic behavior. Informatics clearly speaks to the information end, but cannot leave behind the simultaneous need for empathy and compassion. If delivered cold, it will be rejected and its promise unfulfilled. Informatics offers the opportunity to expand communication, allowing an increased sense of being known by offering personal lines of communication to clinical support around the clock and across geographic distance. The ability to connect with patient or caregiver peers who understand what you are going through can reduce the sense of isolation and increase competence. Decision aids that can facilitate difficult and complicated discussions between decision makers are needed to increase interpersonal understanding, resolve decision discord, and likely yield more informed and more value-consistent decisions. Further, decision aids need to embrace more humanistic decision processes, such as those through narrative rather than logistics. By meeting patients' and family members' information and emotional needs simultaneously, technology is not a substitute for human care at end of life, but rather a lifeline that connects the dying, their family, and their clinical teams to increase human connection and facilitate a good death.

LIST OF ACRONYMS AND ABBREVIATIONS

ACTIVE Assessing Caregivers for Team Intervention through Videophone Encounters
CHESS Comprehensive Health Enhancement Support System
DNR Do Not Resuscitate
EHR Electronic health record
ESAS Edmonton Symptom Assessment Scale
ESRA-C Electronic Self Report Assessment–Cancer
IOM Institute of Medicine
POA Power of attorney
RE-AIM Reach Effectiveness Adoption Implementation Maintenance

Acknowledgments

We thank the National Cancer Institute and National Institute of Nursing Research for their funding of CHESS research, and the Agency for Healthcare Research and Quality for their funding of Elder Tree research. We also thank Haile Behre for programming the CHESS and Elder Tree websites, and the large research teams for their support in developing and managing the websites and studies. We offer special appreciation to the participants in the CHESS and Elder Tree research studies for their generous time and willingness to try something new at such a precious period in their lives.

References

[1] American Cancer Society. Cancer facts and figures 2016; 2016.
[2] California Healthcare Foundation. Final Chapter: Californians attitudes and experiences with death and dying; 2012. Retrieved March 27, 2015 from: <http://www.chcf.org/~/media/MEDIA%20LIBRARY%20Files/PDF/F/PDF%20FinalChapterDeathDying.pdf/>.
[3] The Dartmouth Atlas of Healthcare. End of life care. Retrieved March 30, 2015 from: <http://www.dartmouthatlas.org/keyissues/issue.aspx?con=2944/>.
[4] National Cancer Institute. Palliative Care in Cancer. Retrieved March 30, 2015 from: <http://www.cancer.gov/cancertopics/factsheet/Support/palliative-care/>.
[5] National Cancer Institute. Preparing for end of life. Retrieved March 30, 2015 from: <http://www.cancer.gov/cancertopics/coping/end-of-life/>.
[6] Ferrell B. Pain observed: the experience of pain from the family caregiver's perspective. Clin Geriatr Med 2001;17(3):595–609.
[7] Cohen MZ, Easley MK, Ellis C, Hughes B, Ownby K, Rashad BG, et al. Cancer pain management and the JCAHO's pain standards: an institutional challenge. J Pain Symptom Manage 2003;25(6):519–27.
[8] Müller-Nordhorn J, Roll S, Böhmig M, Nocon M, Reich A, Braun C, et al. Health-related quality of life in patients with pancreatic cancer. Digestion 2006;74:118–25.
[9] DuBenske LL, Wen KY, Gustafson DH, Guarnaccia CA, Cleary JF, Dinauer SK, et al. Caregivers' differing needs across key experiences of the advanced cancer disease trajectory. Palliat Support Care 2008;6(3):265–72.
[10] Capurro D, Ganzinger M, Perez-Lu J, Knaup P. Effectiveness of eHealth interventions and information needs in palliative care: a systematic literature review. J Med Internet Res 2014;16(3):e72.
[11] Yennurajalingam S, Kang JH, Hui D, Kang DH, Kim SH, Bruera E. Clinical response to an outpatient palliative care consultation in patients with advanced cancer and cancer pain. J Pain Symptom Manage 2012;44(3):340–50.
[12] Institute of Medicine Committee on psychosocial services to cancer patients/families in a community setting Cancer care for the whole patient: meeting psychosocial health needs. Washington, DC: The National Academies Press; 2008.
[13] American College of Surgeons Commission on Cancer. Cancer program standards 2012: ensuring patient-centered Care: v1.2.1; 2012. Retrieved from: <https://www.facs.org/~/media/files/quality%20programs/cancer/coc/programstandards2012.ashx/>.
[14] Li M, Fitzgerald P, Rodin G. Evidence-based treatment of depression in patients with cancer. J Clin Oncol 2012;30(11):1187–96.
[15] Anguiano L, Mayer DK, Piven ML, Rosenstein D. A literature review of suicide in cancer patients. Cancer Nurs 2012;35(4):E14–26.
[16] Sharpe M, Strong V, Allen K, Rush R, Maguire P, House A, et al. Management of major depression in outpatients attending a cancer centre: a preliminary evaluation of a multicomponent cancer nurse-delivered intervention. Br J Cancer 2004;90(2):310–3.
[17] Given B, Wyatt G, Given C, Sherwood P, Gift A, DeVoss D, et al. Burden and depression among caregivers of patients with cancer at the end of life. Oncol Nurs Forum 2004;31(6):1105–17.
[18] Wool MS, Mor V. A multidimensional model for understanding cancer pain. Cancer Invest 2005;23(8):727–34.
[19] Porter LS, Keefe FJ, Garst J, McBride CM, Baucom D. Self-efficacy for managing pain, symptoms, and function in patients with lung cancer and their informal caregivers: associations with symptoms and distress. Pain 2008;137(2):306–15.
[20] Mehta A, Chan LS, Cohen SR. Flying blind: sources of distress for family cancer patients managing pain at home. J Psychosoc Oncol 2014;32(1):94–111.
[21] Docherty A, Owens A, Asadi-Lari M, Petchey R, Williams J, Carter YH. Knowledge and information needs of informal caregivers in palliative care: a qualitative systematic review. Palliat Med 2008;22(2):153–71.
[22] Palos GR, Mendoza TR, Liao KP, Anderson KO, Garcia-Gonzalez A, Hahn K, et al. Caregiver symptom burden: the risk of caring for an underserved patient with advanced cancer. Cancer 2011;117(5):1070–9.
[23] Schumacher KL, Koresawa S, West C, Hawkins C, Johnson C, Wais E, et al. Putting cancer pain management regimens into practice at home. J Pain Symptom Manage 2002;23(5):369–82.
[24] DuBenske LL, Chih MY, Gustafson DH, Dinauer S, Cleary JF. Caregivers' participation in the oncology clinic visit mediates the relationship between their information competence and their need fulfillment and clinic visit satisfaction. Patient Educ Couns 2010;81S:S94–9.
[25] Oldenmenger WH, Sillevis Smitt PA, van Dooren S, Stoter G, van der Rijt CC. A systematic review on barriers hindering adequate cancer pain management and interventions to reduce them: a critical appraisal. Eur J Cancer 2009;45(8):1370–80.

[26] Corn M, Gustafson DH, Harris LM, Kutner JS, McFerren AE, Shad AT. Survey of consumer informatics for palliation and hospice care. Am J Prev Med 2011;40(5S2):S173–8.

[27] Wallace CL. Family communication and decision making at the end of life: a literature review. Palliat Support Care 2015;13:815–25.

[28] Butler M, Ratner E, McCreedy E, Shippee N, Kane RL. Decision aids for advance care planning: an overview of the state of the science. Ann Intern Med 2014;161(6):408–18.

[29] Ditto PH, Hawkins NA. Advance directives and cancer decision making near the end of life. Health Psychol 2005;24(4 Suppl.):S63–70.

[30] National Hospice and Palliative Care Organization. History of hospice care. Retrieved March 27, 2015 from: <http://www.nhpco.org/history-hospice-care/>.

[31] National Hospice and Palliative Care Organization. 2013. NHPCO's facts and figures: hospice care in America 2013 edition. Retrieved March 27, 2015 from: <http://www.nhpco.org/sites/default/files/public/Statistics_Research/2013_Facts_Figures.pdf/>.

[32] The Dartmouth Atlas of Healthcare. Percent of cancer patients enrolled in hospice, by interval before death. Retrieved March 30, 2015 from: <http://www.dartmouthatlas.org/data/table.aspx?ind=177/>.

[33] Goodman DC, Morden NE, Chang C, Fisher ES, Wennberg JE. September 4, 2013. Trends in cancer care near the end of life a dartmouth atlas of health care brief. Retrieved March 6, 2015 from: <http://www.dartmouthatlas.org/downloads/reports/Cancer_brief_090413.pdf/>.

[34] Miller SC, Kinzbrunner B, Pettit P, Williams JR. How does the timing of hospice referral influence hospice care in the last days of life? J Am Geriatr Soc 2003;51:798–806.

[35] Bernard LL, Guarnaccia CA. Testing two models of caregiver strain and bereavement adjustment: a comparison of husband and daughter caregivers of breast cancer hospice patients. Gerontologist 2003;43(6):808–16.

[36] Wright AA, Keating NL, Balboni TA, Matulonis UA, Block SD, Prigerson HG. Place of death: correlations with quality of life of patients with cancer and predictors of bereaved caregivers' mental health. J Clin Oncol 2010;28:4457–64.

[37] Lynn J. Sick to death and not going to take it anymore!: reforming health care for the last years of life, vol. 10. Berkeley, CA: University of California Press; 2004.

[38] Gerber DE, Laccetti AL, Chen B, Yan J, Cai J, Gates S, et al. Predictors and intensity of online access to electronic medical records among patients with cancer. J Oncol Pract 2014;10(5):e307–12.

[39] Berry DL, Blumenstein BA, Halpenny B, Wolpin S, Fann JR, Austin-Seymour M, et al. Enhancing patient-provider communication with the electronic self-report assessment for cancer: a randomized trial. J Clin Oncol 2011;28(9):1029–35.

[40] Bakitas M, Lyons KD, Hegel MT, Balan S, Brokaw FC, Seville Effects of a palliative care intervention on clinical outcomes in patients with advanced cancer: the Project ENABLE II randomized controlled trial. J Am Med Assoc 2009;302(7):741–9.

[41] Demiris G, Oliver DP, Wittenberg-Lyles E. Technologies to support end-of-life care. Semin Oncol Nurs 2011;27(3):211–7.

[42] Bee PE, Barnes P, Luker KA. A systematic review of informal caregivers' needs in providing home-based end-of-life care to people with cancer. J Clin Nurs 2009;18(10):1379–93.

[43] Chochinov HM, Harlos M, Cory S, Horst G, Nelson F, Hearson B. Canadian virtual hospice. Psychooncology 2015:253–58.

[44] Chih M, Patton T, McTavish F, Isham A, Judkins-Fisher CL, Atwood AK, et al. Predictive modeling of addiction lapses in a mobile health application. J Subst Abuse Treat 2013;46(1):29–35.

[45] Waterton J, Duffy J. A comparison of computer interviewing techniques and traditional methods for the collection of self-report alcohol consumption in a field study. Int Stat Rev 1984;52:173–83.

[46] Locke SE, Kowaloff HB, Hoff RG, Safran C, Popovsky MA, Cotton DJ, et al. Computer based interview for screening blood donors for risk of HIV transmission. J Am Med Assoc 1992;29:1301–5.

[47] Chen H, Haley WE, Robinson BE, Schonwetter RS. Decisions for hospice care in patients with advanced cancer. J Am Geriatr Soc 2003;51(6):789–97.

[48] O'Connor AM, Fiset V, DeGrasse C, Graham ID, Evans W, Stacey D, et al. Decision aids for patients considering options affecting cancer outcomes: evidence of efficacy and policy implications. J NCI Monogr 1999;25:67–80.

[49] Bowman KW. Communication, negotiation, and mediation: dealing with conflict in end of life decisions. J Palliat Care 2000;16 (Suppl.):S17–23.

[50] Zhang AY, Siminoff LA. The role of the family in treatment decision-making by patients with cancer. Oncol Nurs Forum 2003;30(6):1022–8.

[51] Casarett D, Karlawish J, Morales K, Crowley R, Mirsch T, Asch D. Improving the use of hospice services in nursing homes: a randomized controlled trial. J Am Med Assoc 2005;294(2):211–7.

[52] Gauthier DM. Decision-making near end of life. J Hosp Palliat Nurs 2005;7(2):82–90.

[53] Gustafson DH, Hawkins R, Pingree S, McTavish F, Arora NK, Mendenhall J, et al. Effect of computer support on younger women with breast cancer. J Gen Intern Med 2001;16(7):435–45.

[54] Leighl NB, Butow PN, Tattersall MHN. Treatment decision aids in advanced cancer: when the goal is not cure and the answer is not clear. J Clin Oncol 2004;22(9):1759–62.

[55] Volk RJ, Cantor SB, Cass AR, Spann SJ, Weller SC, Krahn MD. Preferences of husbands and wives for outcomes of prostate cancer screening and treatment. J Gen Intern Med 2004;19(4):339–48.

[56] Mack JW, Walling A, Dy S, Antonio ALM, Adams J, Keating NL, et al. Patient beliefs that chemotherapy may be curative and care received at the end of life among patients with metastatic lung and colorectal cancer. Cancer 2015 Online pub Feb 11, 2015.

[57] Shin DW, Cho J, Kim SY, Chung IJ, Kim SS, Yang HK, et al. Discordance among patient preferences, caregiver preferences, and caregiver predictions of patient preferences regarding disclosure of terminal status and end-of-life choices. Psychooncology 2015;24:212–9.

[58] Myers J. Improving the quality of end-of-life discussions. Curr Opin Support Palliat Care 2015;9(1):72–6.

[59] Casarett D, Crowley R, Stevenson C, Xie S, Teno J. Making difficult decisions about hospice enrollment: what do patients and families want to know? J Am Geriatr Soc 2005;53:249–54.

[60] Matsuyama R, Reddy S, Smith TJ. Why do patients choose chemotherapy near the end of life? A review of the perspective of those facing death from cancer. J Clin Oncol 2006;24(21):3490–6.

[61] Duggleby W, Berry P. Transitions and shifting goals of care for palliative patients and their families. Clin J Oncol Nurs 2005;9(4):425–8.

[62] Vig EK, Starks H, Taylor JS, Hopley EK, Fryer-Edwards K, Pearlman RA. How do surrogate decision makers describe hospice? Does it matter? Am J Hosp Palliat Med 2006;23(2):91–9.

[63] Peppercorn JM, Smith TJ, Helft PR, DeBono DJ, Berry SR, Wollins DS, et al. American society of clinical oncology statement: toward individualized care for patients with advanced cancer. J Clin Oncol 2011;29(6):755–60.

[64] Casarett DJ, Crowley RL, Hischman KB. How should clinicians describe hospice to patients and families? J Am Geriatr Soc 2004;52:1923–8.

[65] Gochman DS, Bonham GS. The social structure of the hospice decision. Hosp J 1990;6(1):15–36.

[66] Farnon C, Hofmann M. Factors contributing to late hospice admission and proposals for change. Am J Hosp Palliat Care 1997;14(5):212–8.

[67] Kapo J, Harrold J, Carroll J, Rickerson E, Casarett D. Are we referring patients to hospice too late? Patients and families opinions. J Palliat Med 2005;8(3):521–7.

[68] Stillman MJ, Syrjala KL. Differences in physician access patterns to hospice care. J Pain Symptom Manage 1999;17(3):157–63.

[69] Bradley EH, Prigerson H, Carlson MDA, Cherlin E, Johnson-Hurzeler R, Kasl SV. Depression among surviving caregivers: does the length of hospice enrollment matter? Am J Psychiatry 2004;161(12):2257–62.

[70] Kim Y, Spillers RL, Hall DL. Quality of life of family caregivers 5 years after a relative's cancer diagnosis: follow-up of the national quality of life survey for caregivers. Psychooncology 2012;21(3):273–81.

[71] Gustafson DH, Wise M, McTavish F, Taylor JO, Wolberg W, Stewart J, et al. Development and pilot evaluation of a computer based support system for women with breast cancer. J Psychosoc Oncol 1993;11(4):69–93.

[72] DuBenske LL, Gustafson DH, Shaw BR, Cleary JF. Web-based cancer communication and decision making systems: connecting patients, caregivers and clinicians for improved health outcomes. Med Decis Making 2010;30(6):732–44.

[73] DuBenske LL, Gustafson DH, Namkoong K, Hawkins RP, Brown RL, McTavish F, et al. CHESS's improves cancer caregivers' burden and mood: results of an eHealth RCT. Health Psychol 2014;33(10):1261–72.

[74] Chih MY, DuBenske LL, Hawkins RP, Brown RL, Dinauer SK, Cleary JF, et al. Communicating advanced cancer patients' symptoms via the Internet: a pooled analysis of two randomized trials examining caregiver preparedness, physical burden, and negative mood. Palliat Med 2013;27(6):533–43.

[75] Gustafson DH, DuBenske LL, Namkoong K, Hawkins R, Chih MY, Atwood AK, et al. An ehealth system supporting palliative care for patients with nonsmall cell lung cancer: a randomized trial. Cancer 2013;119(9):1744–51.

[76] Bruera E, Kuehn N, Miller MJ, Selmser P, Macmillan K. The Edmonton Symptom Assessment System (ESAS): a simple method for the assessment of palliative care patients. J Palliat Care 1991;7:6–9.

[77] DuBenske LL, Chih MY, Dinauer S, Gustafson DH, Cleary JF. Development and implementation of a clinician reporting system for advanced stage cancer: initial lessons learned. J Am Med Inform Assoc 2008;15(5):679–86.

[78] DuBenske LL, Gustafson DH, Chih MY, Atwood AK, Hawkins R, Carmack CL, et al. The effect of on online intervention on symptom distress in patients with nonsmall cell lung cancer: a randomized trial [Abstract]. Ann Behav Med 2013;45(Abstract Supplement):s176.

[79] Temel JS, Greer JA, Muzikansky A, Gallagher ER, Admane S, Jackson VA, et al. Early palliative care for patients with metastatic non-small-cell lung cancer. N Engl J Med 2010;363(8):733–42.

[80] Buss MK, DuBenske LL, Dinauer S, Gustafson DH, McTavish F, Cleary JF. Patient/caregiver influences for declining participation in supportive oncology trials. J Support Oncol 2008;6(4):168–74.

[81] Tennant B, Stellefson M, Dodd V, Chaney B, Chaney D, Paige S, et al. eHealth literacy and Web 2.0 health information seeking behaviors among baby boomers and older adults. J Med Internet Res 2015;17(3):e70.

[82] Choi NG, DiNitto DM. Internet use among older adults: association with health needs, psychological capital, and social capital. J Med Internet Res 2013;15(5):e97.

[83] Gustafson DH, McTavish F, Hawkins RP, Pingree S, Arora N, Mendenhall J, et al. Computer support for elderly women with breast cancer. J Am Med Assoc 1998;280(15):1305.

[84] Groves P, Kayyali B, Knott D, Van Kuiken S. The "big data" revolution in healthcare: Accelerating value and innovation. New York, NY: McKinsey Q; 2013.

[85] Glasgow RE, Vogt TM, Boles SM. Evaluating the public health impact of health promotion interventions: the RE-AIM framework. Am J Public Health 1999;89(9):1322–7.

[86] Trochim W, Cappeleri J. Cutoff assignment strategies. Soc Res Methods 1992;13:190–212.

[87] Hackshaw A, Farrant H, Bulley S, Seckl MJ, Ledermann JA. Setting up non-commercial clinical trials takes too long in the UK: findings from a prospective study. J Res Soc Med 2008;101(6):299–304.

[88] American Cancer Society. Clinical trials: what you need to know. Retrieved March 30, 2015 from: <http://www.cancer.org/acs/groups/cid/documents/webcontent/003006-pdf.pdf/>.

[89] Collins LM, Murphy SA, Strecher V. The multiphase optimization strategy (MOST) and the sequential multiple assignment randomized trial (SMART): new methods for more potent eHealth interventions. Am J Prev Med 2007;32(5):S112–8.

[90] Field M, Cassell C. Approaching death: improving care at the end of life. IOM report. Washington, DC: National Academy Press; 1997.

[91] Emanuel EJ, Emanuel LL. The promise of a good death. Lancet 1998;351:21–9.

[92] Kahneman D. Thinking fast and slow. New York, NY: Macmillan; 2013.

[93] Blank T, Graves K, Sepucha K, Llewellyn-Thomas H. Understanding treatment decision-making: contexts, commonalities, complexities and challenges. Ann Behav Med 2006;32(3):211–7.

[94] Teno JM, Casarett D, Spence C, Connor S. It is "too late" or is it? Bereaved family member perceptions of hospice referral when their family member was on hospice for seven days or less. J Pain Symptom Manage 2012;43(4):732–8.

[95] Friedman BT, Harwood MK, Shields M. Barriers and enablers to hospice referrals: an expert overview. J Palliat Med 2002;5(1):73–84.

[96] Matlock DD, Keech TA, McKenzie MB, Bronsert MR, Nowels CT, Kutner JS. Feasibility and acceptability of a decision aid designed for people facing advanced or terminal illness: a pilot randomized trial. Health Expect 2014;17(1):49–59.

[97] Tan A, Manca D. Finding common ground to achieve a "good death": family physicians working with substitute decision-makers of dying patients. A qualitative grounded theory study. BMC Fam Pract 2013;14(1):14.

[98] Hesse BW, Suls JM. Informatics enabled behavioral medicine in oncology. Cancer J 2011;17(4):222–30.

[99] van Vliet LM, Epstein AS. Current state of the art and science of patient-clinician communication in progressive disease: patients' need to know and need to feel known. J Clin Oncol 2014;32(31):3474–8.

[100] Meeker MA, Finnell D, Othman AK. Family caregivers and cancer pain management: a review. J Fam Nurs 2011;17(1):29–60.

[101] Cleary JF, Carbone PP. Palliative medicine in the elderly. Cancer 1997;80(7):1335–47.

SCIENCE OF ONCOLOGY INFORMATICS

11

Data Visualization Tools for Investigating Health Services Utilization Among Cancer Patients

Eberechukwu Onukwugha MS, PhD[1], Catherine Plaisant PhD[2] and Ben Shneiderman PhD[3]

[1]Department of Pharmaceutical Health Services Research, School of Pharmacy, University of Maryland, Baltimore, MD, United States [2]Human-Computer Interaction Lab, UMIACS, University of Maryland, College Park, MD, United States [3]Computer Science Department, Human-Computer Interaction Lab, UMIACS, University of Maryland, College Park, MD, United States

O U T L I N E

11.1 Introduction	208		11.4 Case Studies	219
11.1.1 Background	208		11.4.1 Introduction to EventFlow and CoCo	219
11.1.2 Purpose of This Chapter	208		11.4.2 Application 1: Algorithm Development Using Claims Data	223
11.1.3 Human-Systems Integration	209		11.4.3 Application 2: Patient Comorbidity and Health Services Utilization	224
11.1.4 Chapter Objectives	209			
11.2 Methods and Data Visualization Tools	209		11.5 Conclusion	227
11.2.1 Techniques	209		List of Acronyms and Abbreviations	228
11.2.2 Software Systems	210		References	228
11.2.3 Strengths and Weaknesses of Available Tools	212			
11.3 Applications of Data Visualization in the Cancer Setting	214			
11.3.1 Basic Cancer Science	214			
11.3.2 Population Statistics	214			
11.3.3 Clinical Applications	216			

B. Hesse, D. Ahern & E. Beckjord: Oncology Informatics.
DOI: http://dx.doi.org/10.1016/B978-0-12-802115-6.00011-2

The greatest value of a picture is when it forces us to notice what we never expected to see.—John Tukey, American Mathematician [1].

11.1 INTRODUCTION

11.1.1 Background

One of the promises of an informatics-infused health care system is the ability to extract meaning from large volumes of data for the purposes of improving the quality of care delivery and for generating new knowledge. Schilsky and Miller illustrate this case aptly in Chapter 1: "Creating a Learning Health Care System in Oncology" as they described a vision for how to leverage informatics data from oncology practices into focused feedback for quality improvement. Likewise, Penberthy, Winn, and Scott presented a vision in Chapter 14: "Cancer Surveillance Informatics" for how electronic health record (EHR) data could be used to complement electronic pathology reports and other types of cancer registry data to offer a more complete view of cancer incidence and progression in the general population.

Unlocking the knowledge embedded within these massively distributed data streams in cancer; however, will require continual progress within the interdisciplinary scientific area of data visualization. Specialists in oncology informatics can benefit from advances in data visualization to make decision making more efficient, to improve systemic outcomes within hospitals and their communities, to engage patients more effectively in their own care, and to facilitate exploration of patterns and trends for hypothesis generation in research. Fortunately, advances in our understanding of how the human perceptual system works (see Chapter 15: "Extended Vision for Oncology: A Perceptual Science Perspective on Data Visualization and Medical Imaging" Horowitz and Rensink), combined with advances in our understanding of how to construct more efficient computer interfaces to support those processes, will put informaticists in good stead as we prepare for active participation in the "learning oncology system" [2].

11.1.2 Purpose of This Chapter

This chapter investigates the possibilities for generating insight and evidence from the strategic application of data visualization tools. While the era of "big data" promises more information for practitioners, patients, researchers, and policy makers, there is limited guidance for analysts about how to leverage the availability of such data. A few key questions must be addressed in order to turn the data into evidence: "How well do we extract insights from the information that is currently available?" "Are we prepared to gain insight directly from the information that is available in massive data sets?" "How well do we leverage longitudinal information that is available?" For big data resources to be more than larger haystacks in which to find precious needles, stakeholders will have to aim higher than increasing computing power and producing faster, nimbler machines. We will have to develop tools for visualizing information; generating insight; and creating actionable, on-demand knowledge for clinical decision making.

The White House press release (March 29, 2012) on the national Big Data Initiative identified two challenges, one of which we address directly in this chapter: (1) develop algorithms for processing massive, but imperfect data and (2) create effective human–computer interaction tools for visual reasoning. These well-crafted challenges position data visualization solidly on the national agenda. Three roles of data visualization address the White House challenges and clarify human participation:

1. Cleaning the often error-laden data. Consider the case in which statistical analyses of 6300 emergency room admission records had failed to account for the eight patients who were entered into the EHR system as being 999 years old. Information specialists will recognize this as a code for "age unknown," but the programs that calculated ages of admitted and discharged patients accepted this as a normal value, thereby distorting the results. A simple bar chart of the ages would have led any viewer to gasp with surprise. This example illustrates a proof of concept and there are an unlimited number of errors that may be missed by algorithms but spotted by experts, such as the patient who was admitted to the emergency room 14 times but discharged only twice. A quick glance at an appropriate visual display enables analysts to confirm the expected and detect the unexpected, especially errors.

2. Supporting exploration and discovery. Analysts typically begin with questions about their data, leading them to choose a particular visualization, such as line charts, size and color-coded scattergrams, maps, networks, and more sophisticated strategies. These analysts may immediately spot surprises or errors, but typically they split a data set to see men or women in separate displays, then group by age or race, and may be focus on patients diagnosed at a later stage of cancer. Insights can lead to bold decisions regarding cancer-directed treatment receipt, treatment initiation, treatment continuation, and management of comorbid conditions.

3. Presenting results. In many cases, the results will be of interest to national leaders, health industry decision makers, and news media viewers. The more

critical challenge with big data is to distill millions of health care data into a few cogent visualizations to guide proximal decision makers including clinicians, patients, and the patients' caregivers.

11.1.3 Human-Systems Integration

The perspectives and work presented in this chapter are guided by a collaborative working relationship between the University of Maryland School of Pharmacy's Department of Pharmaceutical Health Services Research and the Human Computer Interaction Laboratory (HCIL). Work in the HCIL, in turn, represents an interdisciplinary approach to system development based on contributions from the College of Computer, Mathematical, and Natural Sciences and the College of Information Studies at University of Maryland, College Park. The purpose of this overall collaborative relationship is to bring a "human-systems integration" approach to the practice of informatics-supported medicine [3,4]. That is, the purpose is to design systems—in the case of this chapter, data visualization tools—that use computing power to augment and enhance the highly trained expertise of cancer epidemiologists, oncology care teams, health services researchers, and biomedical scientists. It builds on one of the core principles of the National Research Council's (NRC) 2009 report on "Computational Technology for Effective Health Care," which was to design systems that provide improved cognitive support to care teams, administrators, patients, and their caregivers for the purpose of enhancing outcomes. Within the context of this chapter, the human-system integration approach facilitates the development of tools designed for parsing data to generate insight and actionable knowledge, particularly when paired with well-articulated, clinically motivated questions. As data availability grows, it becomes more important to develop methods and approaches for connecting humans with these data sources and systems.

The current Health Information Technology (HIT) systems are ill-suited to establish and maintain these connections and continuously inform patient and provider decision making. As noted by Dimitropoulos [5], health care systems should be data-driven, patient-centered, and continuously improving. For health care systems to effectively inform, influence, and interact with patients, it will require integrating systems that are not currently or widely blended such as hospital, outpatient, pharmacy, and dental systems. As research highlights the importance of holistic cancer care, the role of psychosocial cancer care, a link between comorbidity (chronic disease) and cancer outcomes, as well as a link between dental health and chronic disease, we can no longer afford to deliver cancer care using fragmented care systems. Throughout this section, we emphasize

the importance of leveraging big data and making full use of the longitudinal information available in these data to develop actionable evidence based on human interactions with these data based on review, analysis, synthesis, and discussion.

11.1.4 Chapter Objectives

This chapter section has three objectives: (1) to review the data visualization tools that are currently available and their use in oncology; (2) to discuss implications for research, practice, and decision making in the field of oncology; and (3) to illustrate the possibilities for generating insight and actionable evidence using targeted case studies. The case studies investigated here illustrate the possibilities for research and clinical decision making in situations where the interoperability problem is solved.

11.2 METHODS AND DATA VISUALIZATION TOOLS

There are several different techniques and tools that may be applied to visualizing various types of data sets. This section reviews available techniques and discusses their strengths, weaknesses, and applications to cancer research and practice. The case studies in Section 11.4 focus on the use of two different prototypes of control panels [6] as visualization tools for generating insights from observational data sets including information about individuals diagnosed with cancer.

11.2.1 Techniques

One of the most common techniques for visualizing statistical data within the cancer epidemiological context is the use of Geographic Information Systems (GIS) to portray the distribution of a measured variable on top of an identifiable map, and one of the most common uses of GIS is to create choropleth maps. Brewer [7] described choropleth mapping as a way to visualize data relating to regional geographical locations and divisions, such as state lines and zip codes. Choropleth maps provide policy makers and health officials with a situational awareness of the disease processes that may be at play within their jurisdictions. In some cases, a high incidence of certain types of cancer among a group of people within an identifiable geographical area may signal a public health emergency, known as a "cancer cluster," and might therefore require immediate environmental investigation. In other cases, a high incidence of late-stage disease within certain areas may imply that vulnerable populations are falling outside of the reach of recommended public health primary and secondary prevention measures. Choropleth mapping can also give cancer control planners insight into how certain policies, such as cigarette taxes or indoor smoking prohibitions, may be associated with decreases in preventable disease, such as decreases in lung and bronchus cancers.

Symbols, colors, proportional symbols, icons, and text boxes are all commonly used elements within choropleth mapping. Basic cartographic symbols, such as solid lines depicting geopolitical boundaries or icons depicting identifiable landmarks, can provide a sense of consistency for analysts and an anchor for interpreting the underlying data patterns. Patterns or colors within the geographic units portray levels of the mapped data, which may represent an epidemiologic variable such as prevalence or mortality, or it may portray some type of demographic characteristic. Colors may be utilized to represent data and hierarchy based on hues or lightness [7], or they may also be used to stress extremes in data, drawing attention away from more average results colored in white [8]. For example, darker hues generally suggest a higher frequency, percentage, or magnitude of the underlying variable in a choropleth map. Looking at the mortality maps presented at the National Cancer Institute's (NCI) Surveillance, Epidemiology, and End Results (SEER) website, readers can see how darker hues depict higher incidences of cancer-related mortality across cancer sites. When considering color choices, however, investigators must keep the medium of their visualization in mind as the color's appearance and impact may vary between print, Internet, or presentations [8].

An alternative to using colors or patterns within a choropleth map is to use proportional symbols. Proportional symbols are usually geometric shapes, such as circles or triangles, which vary in size according to the magnitude of the underlying variable. Symbols of a larger size generally depict a greater underlying quantity than symbols of a smaller proportion. Proportional symbols may also be used outside of the context of GIS display to juxtapose magnitudes in more of a categorical sense. Fig. 11.1 illustrates how the National Cancer Institute (NCI) uses icons and animation to represent individualized colorectal cancer risk estimates. Appropriately crafted legends and text boxes are often needed to complete the reader's interpretation of the visual representation and to facilitate general sense-making when working with interactive graphs. Because a user's gaze generally orients to the center of a graphic, it is often useful to place icons and text boxes in a central location [9].

For some purposes, choropleth maps and other data visualization tools may need to portray values from more than one variable. To represent multiple variables, Brewer suggested using one or a combination of the following techniques: overlaying symbols, overlaying patterns, creating series, or combining variables [7]. Colors, bands, and customizable icons are often used

to represent categorical data, while numerical data are often shown with line plots, point plots, and bar charts. Other visualization techniques may also be applied to data to allow investigators to see trends more clearly, such as pan and zoom; animation; filtering; brushing; and linking of different views of the same data, matrices [10], and rate smoothing [11].

Another technique that is commonly used in data visualization is data stream clustering; that is, using a clustering algorithm to reduce the dimensionality or noise associated with high frequency data streams. Chauhan et al. [12] explained how data clustering may be applied to identify and explore data patterns. Hierarchical algorithms are often employed, with either an agglomerative (ie, bottom-up, starting with data points and building clusters) or divisive (ie, top down, beginning with one overarching cluster and then dividing) approach, and clusters may either be density-based or grid-based. Density-based clustering techniques, such as Density Based Spatial Clustering of Applications with Noise (DBSCAN), Ordering Points to Identify the Clustering Structure (OPTICS), and Clustering Based on Density Distribution Function (DENCLUE), form clusters from density distributions directly on databases. On the other hand, grid-based techniques, such as Sting, Wave Cluster, and Clique, cluster statistical data on a uniform grid. Data classing, or use of class breaks, is another common method used for developing choropleth or GIS maps [7]. Data are typically grouped by quantiles, standard deviation, size, equal intervals, or natural breaks [8].

There are several other techniques that may be utilized for data visualization. Vellido et al. [13] touched upon the use of directed graphs, which allow for the visualization of covariates and their relationships, and hierarchical visualizations, which provide detailed information about relationships between and for different hierarchical levels. Map projections are utilized to represent a given geographical area, taking into account the spherical curve of the earth [7]. Neural networks, such as Self-Organizing Map (SOM), may be used for nonlinear projects to "project high dimensional, time-varying information in 2D maps that correlate with diagnostic features" [13], while proximity networks form links between molecular information, pathways, and graphs. Community Health Map allows researchers to easily explore and visualize state and county health patterns [14]. GIS maps are important data visualization tools, as they allow participants' behaviors or characteristics to be linked with particular geographic factors [15].

11.2.2 Software Systems

Incorporating various combinations of the techniques above, many systems have been developed to visualize data. The Hierarchical Clustering Explorer (HCE) has

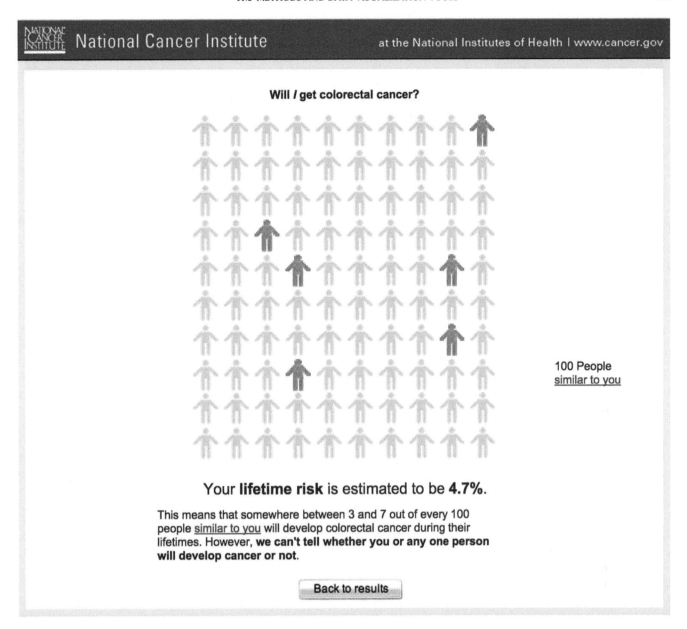

FIGURE 11.1 Using visualization to inform the public. This graphic utilizes icons and animation to present individualized colorectal cancer risk estimates calculated based on the answers to a series of questions collected through a web questionnaire (http://www.cancer.gov/colorectalcancerrisk/), This visualization appear after users review the results and click on a button labeled "Does this mean I will get colorectal cancer?" The position of the darker icons is changed every two seconds to represent randomness [62].

a rank-by-feature framework that allows researchers to choose ranking criteria and visualize results in one-dimensional (histograms) or two-dimensional (scatter plots) projections [16]. A software system called Caregiver is a tool that assists with therapy-related decisions through visualizations of general patient overview, patient cohorts, and individual patients [10]. InfoZoom is a system that ensures displays of data sets will always fit on the selected screen in the form of compressed tables [10,17]. VisPap incorporates both medical images and laboratory data into its scatter plots and parallel coordinate plots, and the Cube uses EHRs to interactively identify and analyze of patterns with two-dimensional parallel planes in a three-dimensional cube display [10,17].

Many systems have been developed to generate and/or base analyses on temporal abstractions. Moskovitch and Shahar [18] described the KarmaLegoSification (KLS) framework that allows for the analyses of multivariate time-series through temporal abstraction, time intervals mining, and pattern classifications. The

Medical Information Visualization Assistant (MIVA) provides a visualization of the numerical value progression of point plots over a period of time [10]. Interactive Parallel Bar Charts (IPBC) is an interactive system that simultaneously analyzes time-series and its associated values from multiple patients as well as sessions [10,17]. Lifelines is a system that illustrates historical data and events from EHRS and allows for aggregation of sets of events [10]. Lifelines2 allows researchers to specify queries with event operators and align records by events [10,19]. The Similan system can also align records, but uses a similarity measure to take into account "addition, removal transposition of events and temporal differences" [10]. Building upon these point-event data projects, EventFlow allows researchers and clinicians to interactively visualize and analyze patterns of medication use from health systems' EHRs [19].

Another type of system is KNAVE II, which utilizes knowledge-based temporal abstraction and allows researchers to interactively visualize and explore temporal abstractions and patterns for single or small sets of electronic health data [10,17]. Building upon KNAVE II, Klimov et al. [17] developed the VISualization of Time-Oriented RecordS (VISITORS) system used for the visualization of multiple patient records. It is able to search and aggregate numerical and categorical data from both raw and abstracted data.

Several proposed systems are currently being developed. Goovaerts [20] described a geostatistical simulation that uses Poisson kriging, p-field simulation, and local clustering to generate risk maps that are more realistic than those formed using solely smoothing methods. West et al. [21] developed two additional prototypes to explore and analyze large data sets through visualization: (1) the radial-coordinates visualization tool incorporates many techniques including colors, lines spreading, parallel and radial coordinates, histograms, and scatter plots, to allow investigators to visualize clusters, data distributions, and individual data sets and (2) the force-directed network visualization tool uses proportional symbols, links, and nodes to explore queries made from particular elements of EHRs.

Harford et al. [22] described a "cancer atlas" system derived from India's Internet-based registry that brings many of the techniques discussed at the beginning of this section into use within a global cancer control context. The system, referred to as GBD *Compare*, allows international users to make comparisons between countries on the global disease burden. As illustrated in Fig. 11.2, the system allows international users to select filtering options on the left side of the screen for two coordinated visualizations. The treemap at the top of the screen represents a type of hierarchical clustering technique while the map at the bottom represents a choropleth mapping technique based on countries as geographical units. The treemap

clusters based on all causes of death, with the size of the rectangle corresponding to the number of deaths and the color hue signifying change over time. Darker hues signify a worsening changing for the cause while lighter hues suggest an improving condition. The overarching color palette for the treemap breaks causes into chronic conditions (blue), infectious disease (brown), and injury (green). The color spectrum used for the choropleth map at the bottom of the screen ranges from dark blue to dark red, with blue signifying low numbers of death and red signifying high numbers.

11.2.3 Strengths and Weaknesses of Available Tools

11.2.3.1 Strengths of Available Tools

The methods described above have varying advantages. Similar to how different hues allow observers to easily distinguish variance, map series allow users to recognize patterns more easily through contrasts between maps. Overlay allows observers to readily identify unreliable data in a particular region, while map projections provide appropriate views of the geographic distributions of diseases [7]. The rate smoothing technique Kafadar [11] described not only mitigates problems that come with utilizing multiple sources, but it also allows investigators to temporarily overlook certain patient characteristics to better visualize patterns. When considering the advantages of density-based clustering, DBSCAN does not require significant information to identify inputs, and OPTICS is able to automatically determine the necessary number of clusters from data sets. On the other hand, grid-based clustering allows for fast processing time [12].

Furthermore, temporal abstractions overcome challenges such as varied frequencies, gaps in data, and working with both time points and intervals [18]. EventFlow allows for easy-to-use interactive visualization, event overlapping, and pattern identification [19]. InfoZoom enables researchers to identify hidden knowledge, and the Lifelines system provides ease of use and access, along with the ability to zoom in and out [10]. The VISITORS system has several strengths. First, it captures data for multiple patients and allows for time and value analysis of clinical data. VISITORS also allows researchers to quickly and accurately answer clinical questions utilizing these temporal abstractions and clinical information [17].

One of the strengths of the radial visualization system prototype designed by West et al. [21] is its ability to utilize numerous techniques to clearly organize data and clusters without muddling the visualization. It is also able to display many different data distributions through multiple axes.

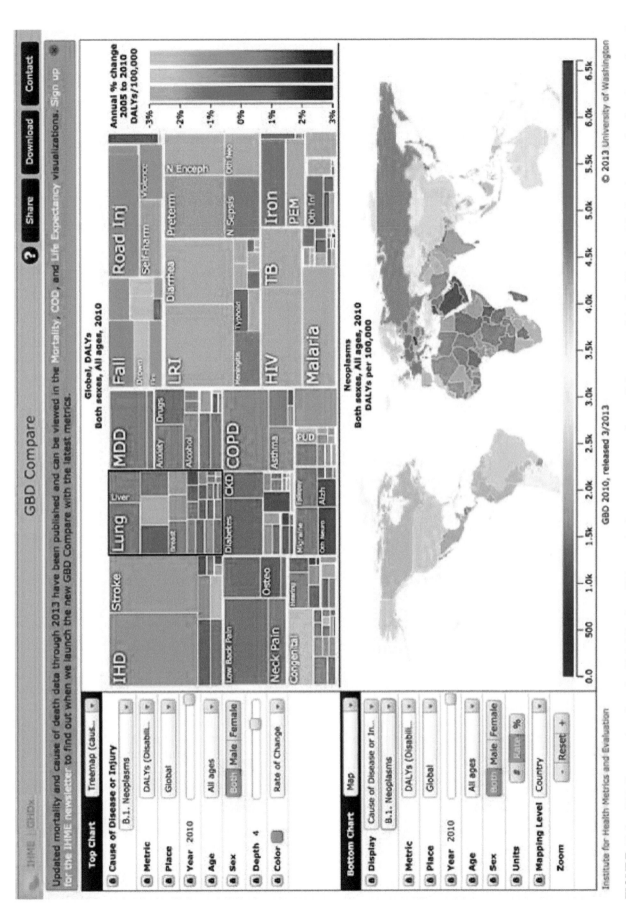

FIGURE 11.2 GBD Compare, based on the Global Burden of Disease. At the top, a treemap shows all the causes of deaths. The size of the box is proportional to the number of deaths, and the color indicates the change over time (light for improving, dark for worsening). Neoplasms are selected, and the map below shows where the disease is most prevalent (http://viz.healthmetricsandevaluation.org/gbd-compare/).

11.2.3.2 *Weaknesses of Available Tools*

It is also important to recognize the weaknesses that visualization methods may have. Utilizing colors becomes a disadvantage when considering individuals with color blindness or color distinguishing deficiencies. Brewer [7] also explained that maps, in general, have several weaknesses such as misleading titles, technological difficulties with sharing maps, and skewed judgment of densities on map projections. Bhowmick et al. [23] found that cancer researchers often face limited data, difficulty in merging data, time-consuming steps, and overly complex software when employing GIS or other spatial analysis software.

Additionally, West et al. [21] explained that different patterns and interpretations may be concluded from alternate views of the same forced-directed network visualization. Likewise, James et al. [8] pointed out that analyses and spatial outcomes may vary greatly, depending on the different techniques investigators may choose to adopt. For example, there are several approaches to establishing cut points; applying Jenks algorithm [24] would cluster data based on their natural breaks, while standard deviations would result in clusters that may be more sparsely dispersed. Clustering techniques have several other disadvantages. It may not take into account the uncertainty associated with predicted risk [20], and different approaches to organizing clusters may result in varied interpretations [13]. Density-based clustering systems are flawed as well. For example, DBSCAN may not be entirely sensitive to all inputs, making it difficult to recognize clusters that are closely related. On the other hand, grid-based clustering is not ideal for irregularly distributed data, as it may not be able to fully capture the cluster quality or time [12].

There are drawbacks to other systems as well. The Caregiver system does not follow patients' development over time [10]. Users need a degree of statistical knowledge to easily and successfully use the HCE system [16]. Vellido et al. [13] discerned that a disadvantage with the Growing Hierarchical Self-Organizing Map (GHSOM) is that investigators would not be able to visualize information from each hierarchal level at the same time. Other techniques, such as directed graphs and proximity networks, have not been well developed. Similarly, several visualization tools are still just developing prototypes [21] or theoretical systems [13,23].

Of the remaining systems previously discussed, Klimov et al. [17] noted that KNAVE II is not an ideal system for large data sets. Because the TimeFinder system is based on time-oriented data, it is not able to focus on a specific set of subjects. Contrarily, Spotfire, SimVis, and Lifelines lack the ability to incorporate or produce high level abstractions such as those focused on time [25]. Lifelines2 and Similan are based on point events rather than time intervals; do not distinguish between data from tests, diagnoses, or treatments; and are not able to display individual record details [10].

11.3 APPLICATIONS OF DATA VISUALIZATION IN THE CANCER SETTING

11.3.1 Basic Cancer Science

Visualization has long been used to complement algorithmic analysis in the basic sciences underlying cancer research. This has been especially true in areas such as genomics in which the amount of raw data to explore for hypothesis generation is simply too large and cumbersome to portray through individual vectors of raw values. The expansive genomic data space lends itself to an exploration of relationships through data visualization. Fig. 11.3, for example, depicts a visualization of whole-genome rearrangements using the *Circos* software package for visualizing data relationships in a circular layout. Circos was developed to give scientists the ability to explore relationships between objects, such as chromosomes and other genomic elements, their size, and orientation in relationship to each other [26]. In Fig. 11.3, the outer ring of the circular graph depicts chromosomes arranged in sequential order from end to end, while the inner ring displays copy-number data in green and interchromosomal translocations in purple for two different tumors. The Circos data visualization package can produce charts with high "data to ink" ratios [28], making the format a highly efficient mechanism to explore relationships in a big data context.

11.3.2 Population Statistics

Aside from using advanced techniques for research purposes, another compelling reason to create data visualization tools is to make the complex incidence and prevalence statistics associated with the national surveillance of cancer trends accessible to journalists, policy makers, and the public [9]. For example, the American Cancer Society (ACS) collaborates with the CDC and NCI to publish an annual compilation of "Cancer Facts and Figures" [29] as a report card on the nation's collective progress against cancer. The report breaks out data from the cancer registries and other surveillance mechanisms to enumerate trends over time, to explore prevalence and mortality as broken out by sociodemographic groupings, and to make distinctions in progress between variants of the disease. These visualizations have employed some of the standard variants of charts and graphs already familiar to most audiences—such as the elements associated with line charts, bar graphs, and

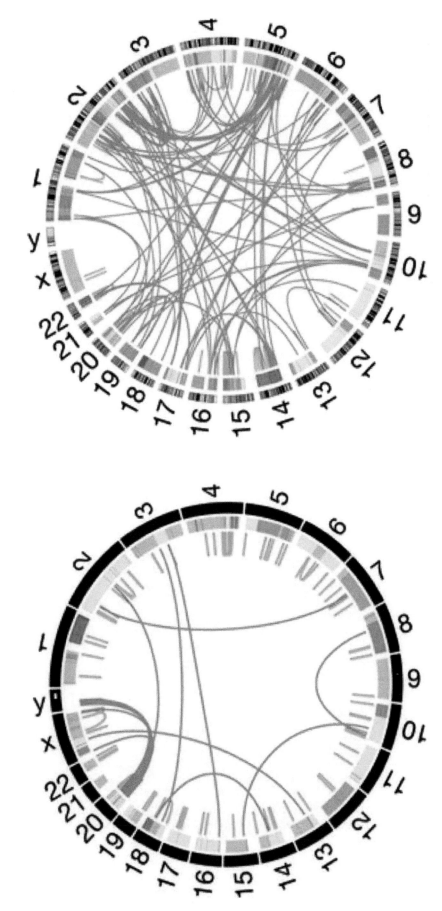

FIGURE 11.3 Visualization of whole-genome rearrangement. Two different tumors are being compared using Circos plots [26] of whole-genome sequence data, showing gene duplications and chromosome rearrangements. The outer ring depicts chromosomes arranged end to end. The inner ring displays copy-number data in green and interchromosomal translocations in purple. *Source: Imielinski M, Berger AH, Hammerman PS, Hernandez B, Pugh TJ, Hodis E, et al. Mapping the hallmarks of lung adenocarcinoma with massively parallel sequencing. Cell 2012;150(6):1107–20 [27].*

pie charts—but more recently have employed new innovations such as the graphical depiction of quantities and numerical trends.

A more recent innovation in communicating to the public, made feasible by diffusion of dynamic HyperText Markup Language (HTML)/web technologies, is the use of publicly facing informatics tools to present interactive data displays for local customization and exploration. Fig. 11.4 presents an image of the US Cancer Statistics Interactive Atlas website hosted by the CDC. This data visualization tool allows analysts to interact with the control box on the left to filter data based on cancer event (eg, incident rate, death rate); cancer site (eg, lung and bronchus, colon and rectum); gender; race/ethnicity; year; and classifying statistic (eg, quintiles). Results are portrayed on a choropleth map at the top center of the screen. A choropleth map uses shading or patterning to fill in geographic areas on a map (eg, states or counties) according to levels of an analytic variable. In this case, the absence of coloring within states indicates an absence of reportable data. Lighter shading indicates a lower value on the outcome variable, while darker shades indicate higher values. Clicking on a state will indicate the ranking of its values within the context of all states' values portrayed graphically within the box at the bottom of the page. The precise numeric values with accompanying confidence intervals are listed in a table on the right, while a player bar in the upper right allows the user to explore trends over time.

More generally, GIS systems are used in the cancer setting to examine data quality [23] and to investigate the association of cancer with socioeconomic, genetic, or environmental factors [7], as they may play a role in the development of cancer. For example, Finney Rutten et al. [30] explored the use of isopleth maps to investigate the distribution of cultural norms and behaviors related to smoking cessation using nationally available data from NCI's Health Information National Trends Survey (HINTS) [31]. Unlike choropleth maps, which display data by filling in geographic units, such as states or counties, with the same shade of color or patterning, isopleth maps portray gradual patterns of change across predefined borders. Weather maps and topographic maps are good examples of isopleth mapping techniques. The isopleth maps for the behaviorally oriented HINTS data illustrated for cancer control planners how beliefs and their concomitant actions can cluster in geographic communities. These maps illustrated how beliefs in the scientific linkage between smoking and cancer were weakest along the Appalachian ridge, which when juxtaposed against the SEER choropleth maps for cancer incidence and mortality corresponded to high cancer mortality rates from lung and bronchus cancer.

Similarly, Chauhan et al. [12] describe the use of DBSCAN, OPTICS, and DENCLUE to visualize cancer clusters using data from two large databases: GLOBOCAN from the International Agency for Research on Cancer and SEER from NCI. SimVis interactively classifies and clusters data from clinical trials and examinations, and visualizations such as caMATCH have been used to identify potential clinical trial patients [14,15]. Spurred by examples such as these, the White House initiated a government-wide effort to make health data from all of the national surveillance programs available to data scientists for the development of usable, transparent interfaces for community planning. On July 10, 2014, the US Department of Health and Human Services included open access to large-scale, health-related databases as an integral part of its Open Government Plan. Examples of open-access data sets, and the data visualization tools being created to access them, can be found at HealthData.gov.

To understand how these new data visualization tools are being utilized in the cancer space, Bhowmick et al. [23] interviewed cancer researchers to identify what aspects of spatial analysis they often employ or consider most useful and suggest features useful for cancer data visualization. The authors observed that cancer control researchers proceed methodically through three phases: (1) a preanalytic phase in exploring and repairing attributes of a given data set; (2) a conceptually exploratory stage, in which scientists explore the nature of preliminary associations; and (3) an analytic phase, in which population estimates are generated, spurious associations are appropriately controlled statistically, and specific conclusions are drawn. What is produced in the analysis phase is then readied for publication. From their interviews, the authors noted that tables and maps are used both in the early exploratory phases of cancer research as well as in the later publication process.

11.3.3 Clinical Applications

As EHR systems become more powerful and greater attention is given to optimizing the use of data for predictive, preemptive, personalized, and participative care [32], then the use of data visualizations within the EHR interface will become more important for allowing analysts to quickly assimilate large amounts of data for clinical purposes. Fig. 11.5 shows a sample screen of a urology EHR system, summarizing the record of a patient with prostate cancer, and using a design similar to early research on Lifelines [33]. In this example, the attending clinical team is given the ability to view the rise and fall of prostate-specific antigen (PSA) levels before and after treatment. The approach typifies an area of human-system integration research aimed at using informatics tools to create better visualizations of temporal patterns

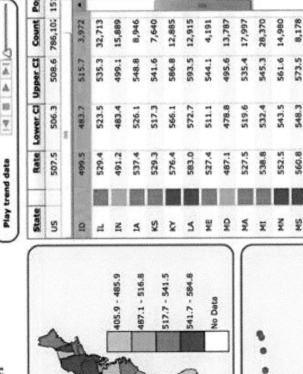
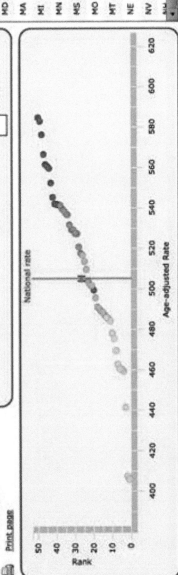
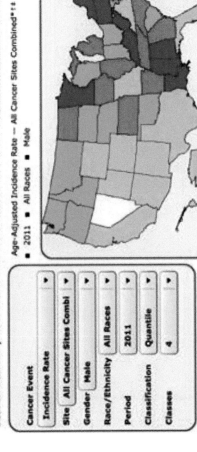
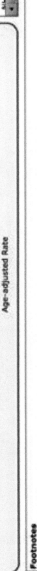
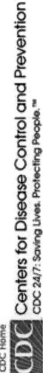

FIGURE 11.4 US Cancer Statistics Interactive Atlas of the CDC (http://nccd.cdc.gov/DCPC_INCA/).

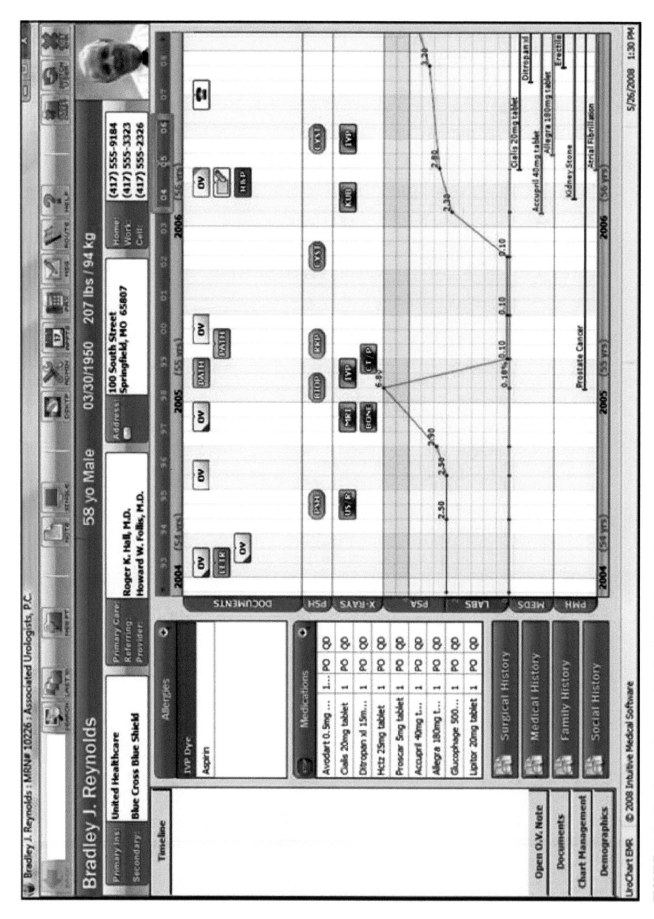

FIGURE 11.5 Visualization of a patient EHR for clinical urology care from IntrinsiQ.

to track the course of treatment over time [34,35], and to reduce discontinuities in care from missed prescriptions [19] or laboratory results [36]. Visualization techniques can also be used at the individual patient level to improve the effectiveness and efficiency of medication reconciliation tasks [37].

When large collections of cancer patient records are available, looking for temporal patterns of treatment, side effects, or outcomes become possible, and visualization can reveal possible linkage to population attributes such as age or gender (Fig. 11.6). Systems such as EventFlow (see case study of Section 11.4) or VISITORS [17] may be used to quickly answer clinical questions. The program VisCareTrails has been to analyze cancer case studies using EHR data. The Cube extracts data from EHR, and VisPap utilizes medical images and laboratory data to interactively visualize patterns [10]. Simpao et al. [39] demonstrated how a visual analytics dashboard in a pediatric hospital's EHR system can be used to optimize drug–drug interaction alerts.

Looking at systems that are currently in place to extract cancer data from EHR and pathology reports, Forman et al. [15] discussed E-path, caBIG's Cancer Text Information Extraction System (caTIES), and MediClass. Information from these databases, in conjunction with data visualization tools described in Section 11.1 may then be used to explore and analyze cancer trends.

Several approaches may not have been applied in the cancer setting yet, but have been effectively used to visualize data in other similarly complex situations. Augmented Interactive Starfield Display uses point plots to display blood glucose readings, while the Web-based interactive visualization system uses data from home monitoring systems to display lung transplant patients' data. Used in intensive care settings, Midgaard "integrates the display of numerical data with graphical representations of medical treatment plans" [10].

Moving forward, visualization systems and programs continue to be developed and incorporated into the cancer setting.

11.4 CASE STUDIES

Case studies provide an ideal framework for illustrating the insights that are possible with these tools. Via targeted case studies, we investigate the utility of two tools, EventFlow and Cohort Comparison (CoCo) that are ideal for investigating longitudinal event sequences. The case studies illustrate the purposeful integration of data visualization and observational data to address questions that are relevant for clinical practice. Using linked cancer registry and health care claims data, we investigate the timing of treatment initiation and health services utilization following the diagnosis of late-stage cancer.

11.4.1 Introduction to EventFlow and CoCo

EventFlow (Fig. 11.7) allows analysts to understand the temporal features and prevalence of the patterns found in a cohort of patients. Fig. 11.7 illustrates dummy data representing 29 men diagnosed with cancer. We use a small sample for clarity of presentation. On the right the timeline shows details of individual records. Triangles represent events. The records have been aligned by the cancer diagnosis date (green event). Users would need to scroll to see all 29 records. In the center, the overview aggregates groups of records with the same sequence of events into horizontal (gray) block stripes that include colored vertical bars representing each event. Within each horizontal block stripe, the height of the vertical bar is determined by the number of patients in the group and the horizontal gap between events is proportional to the average time between events. Reading from the left we can see that all records start with a cancer diagnosis. We can then see the different sequences of treatment with luteinizing hormone-releasing hormone (LHRH) (purple) and radiation therapy (brown). The most common first treatment is the LHRH. The second most common is radiation therapy and we can see that it occurs earlier on average than LHRH as the distance from green to brown is shorter than the distance from green to purple.

The two views (overview and timeline) are coordinated so that when users select records in one view they are highlighted in the other view. The timeline shows the sequencing and timing of therapy for individual patients. EventFlow also includes two separate search interfaces including an advanced graphical user interface that makes it possible for analysts to specify complex temporal queries including temporal constraints and the absence of events [40] (eg, men who did not receive LHRH within 6 months of diagnosis), or search and replace [25]. The combination of those techniques [41] allows analysts to sharpen the focus of an analysis on records exhibiting particular event sequences of interest, for example, considering skeletal complications, analysts could investigate the occurrence of pathological fracture followed by bone surgery then palliative radiation to the bone (RtB).

The second tool, CoCo (see Fig. 11.8), facilitates the identification of salient differences between the temporal patterns found in two separate cohorts of men diagnosed with prostate cancer and identified from the SEER registry data linked with Medicare claims data. In Fig. 11.8, we compare a cohort of 474 stage IV M0 prostate cancer records to a cohort of 2470 stage IV

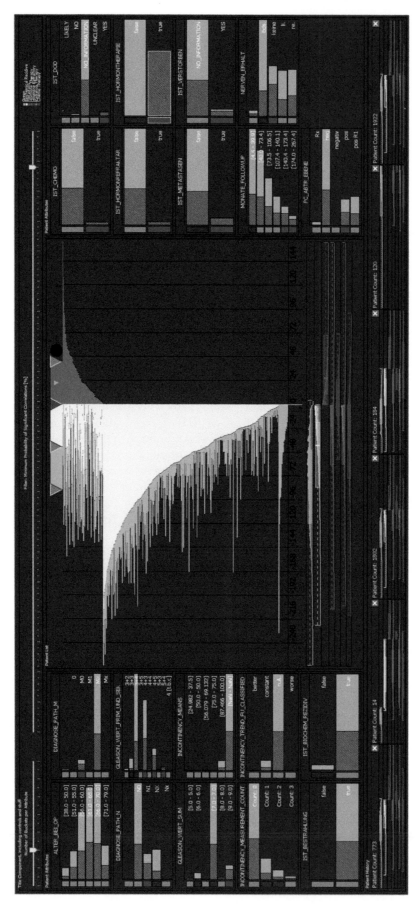

FIGURE 11.6 A visualization of prostate cancer patient records. At the center, the overview of three main stages of the disease are color coded green, yellow, and red. On the side, the distributions of static patient attributes are shown allowing for the selection of subsets of the population and providing insight into differences between groups [38].

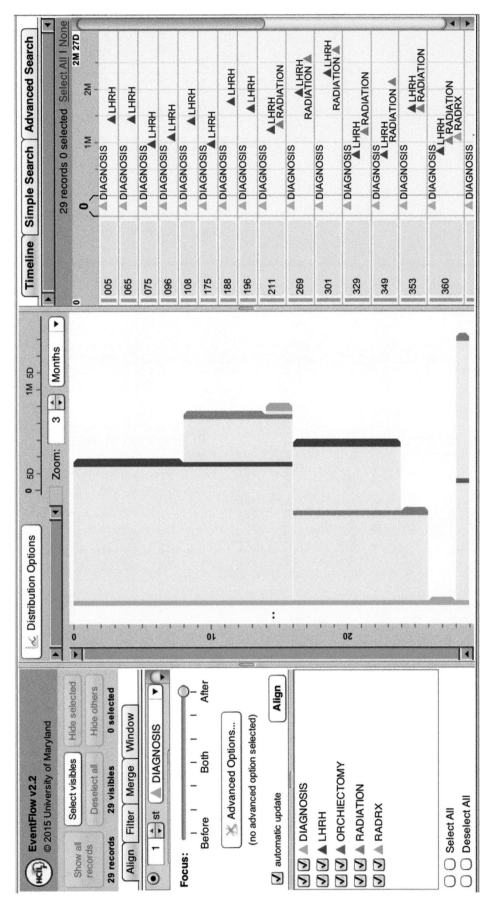

FIGURE 11.7 Illustration of temporal patterns in health care claims data using EventFlow.

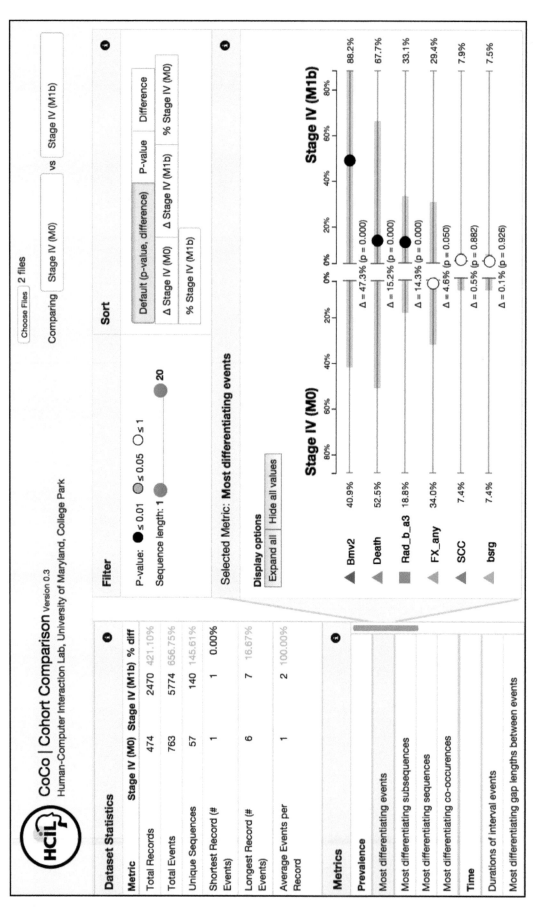

FIGURE 11.8 A screenshot of an early prototype of CoCo, comparing two prostate cancer cohorts: AJCC stage M0 and AJCC stage M1b.

M1b (bone metastatic) prostate cancer records in the 3 months following diagnosis. In pilot work, we proposed an initial taxonomy of metrics (such as differences in the prevalence of events, sequences or subsequences of consecutive events, co-occurrence of events, duration of gaps between events, event attributes—to be refined during the study) [42]. For each metric, CoCo computes a series of statistical tests and presents the results using an interactive user interface. This is a novel approach that combines both statistical methods and a visual representation of the results and encourages rapid hypothesis generation. Users are provided with a set of metrics they can choose from (bottom left), and then review the results of the visualization in the bottom right. Based on our early user tests we find that analysts can usefully incorporate insights from CoCo and EventFlow [43].

11.4.2 Application 1: Algorithm Development Using Claims Data

This case study illustrates an approach that combines the billing information found in claims data with key longitudinal information regarding the timing of health services utilization to isolate probable RtB. Clinical providers and researchers need reliable measures in order to identify treatment receipt and its consequences. Claims data are used to identify treatment and associated consequences in large populations. However, claims-based algorithms used to infer conditions and treatments are error-prone, unless validated, and better algorithms are needed. Research on the development of claims-based algorithms relies on the ability to unlock the rich but incomplete data found in the temporal sequences of events that are available in claims data. However, research on algorithm development has been limited by the lack of a clearly defined approach for unlocking the rich data in temporal patterns and sequences that are available in claims data. These patterns can be first order (eg, interval between events) or second order (eg, patterns of intervals over time for *each* patient and *across* patients) in nature. The first-order events are easily summarized and analyzed using standard statistical methods while the second-order events, as we found out when using standard statistical analysis software, cannot be summarized using standard statistical tools. Another challenge is selecting from competing alternatives to identify the temporal components that are most useful in the algorithms.

Studies using claims data have documented increased mortality and costs associated with bone metastasis (BM) and BM-related complications [44–48]. However, their utility is limited by the fact that the claims algorithms are not validated, are differential [49] (eg, misclassification of metastasis using claims data varies with patient characteristics that also associate with survival), inaccurate [50–52], and can lead to biased conclusions regarding survival [49]. Cooper et al. [53] examined the use of Medicare claims data for identifying the stage of prostate cancer, and found that billing codes had a 78.2% and 72.8% positive predictive value (PPV) for regional and distant prostate cancer, respectively, when compared to medical records. Hassett et al. [50] studied billing codes as indicators for recurrence of prostate cancer after definitive local therapy and reported a maximum PPV of 31%. Results are not unique to prostate cancer. Chawla et al. [49] reported that claims data had a PPV of 65.8% for identifying a diagnosis of distant breast cancer compared to SEER registry data.

Previous studies have identified patients with BM based on the presence of a diagnosis of "secondary malignant neoplasm of bone and bone marrow" [International Classification of Diseases, Ninth Revision, Clinical Modification (ICD-9-CM) 198.5] in claims data. These claims-based algorithms differ in their use of the ICD-9-CM codes. Several studies have defined BM patients as persons with two or more claims encounters including 198.5 anytime on or after the date of the first claim with a diagnosis of cancer [47,48,54]. Other studies have defined BM patients as persons with at least one inpatient claim with the 198.5 code, at least one outpatient claim with the 198.5 code paired with a code for procedures used to diagnose/treat BM, or at least one outpatient physician evaluation and management claim with the 198.5 code [45,46]. Our published results [55] indicate that the approach to measuring BM can impact validity.

Reliable identification of BM is critical for identification of the appropriate clinical subpopulation to study BM complications including RtB. Billing codes available in claims data do not provide information regarding the anatomic site that was treated with radiation therapy. In the absence of these codes, researchers use the BM ICD-9 diagnosis code to identify a BM diagnosis based on claims and then define RtB based on radiation claims occurring after the BM claim [45–47]. The validity of this approach depends on the validity of using BM ICD-9 diagnosis codes to identify a BM diagnosis, a practice which is likely to be unreliable given prior results [50–52] regarding the low sensitivity and PPV of claims-based algorithms to identifying metastasis. In our work, we have found that the duration of radiation therapy can be useful for distinguishing between RtB and radiation to other sites for cancer treatment. As part of the Choosing Wisely campaign, the American Society for Radiation Oncology discouraged routine use of extended fractionation schemes (>10 fractions) for palliation of BM [56], since single fractionation schemes are more convenient for patients and provide comparable pain relief for uncomplicated BM, further indicating the potential utility of duration of radiation therapy for identifying RtB. We investigate the length of therapy and the presence of BM coding on the radiation claim using EventFlow and CoCo.

In Fig. 11.8, the selected metric is the most differentiating event and we could use this information to identify components of an algorithm for identifying RtB separately from radiation to the prostate gland. For example, we see that "Bmv2" (blue rectangle) representing a BM diagnosis code on the health care claim, is found in 40.9% of the M0 records, and 88.2% of the M1b (bone metastatic) records, with a difference of 47%. We also see a difference in the next two most differentiating events: Death and "Rad_b_a3." The former variable, *Death*, represents all-cause mortality while the latter variable, *Rad_b_a3*, represents health care claims for short-course (ie, less than 4 weeks) radiation therapy. We expect that all-cause death and short-course radiation therapy (likely RtB) will be more common in the incident M1b compared to the M0 group within 3 months following diagnosis of prostate cancer. Via this case study using EventFlow output, we illustrate that the presence of a BM code on the radiation claim and the length of radiation therapy may be important for identifying RtB (separately from radiation to the prostate gland) using health care claims data.

11.4.3 Application 2: Patient Comorbidity and Health Services Utilization

Among men diagnosed with prostate cancer, it is commonly stated that they are more likely to die from underlying comorbid conditions (eg, heart failure) than they are to die from the prostate cancer. Much of the research on comorbidity has been conducted among men diagnosed with low or intermediate risk disease [57–60]. Compared to men diagnosed with nonmetastatic cancer, men diagnosed with metastatic prostate cancer are more likely to die from the prostate cancer. It is important that these men receive cancer-directed therapy as soon as possible following diagnosis of late-stage disease. In this application, we investigate whether patient comorbidity status impacts the timing of receipt of cancer-directed therapy and use of other health services including hospital, skilled nursing facility (SNF), and hospice services. We focus on a particularly vulnerable group of cases: men diagnosed with incident bone metastatic disease as identified by the American Joint Committee on Cancer (AJCC) staging information available from the SEER registry. Categories that represented too few patients (ie, $N < 11$) were suppressed in the EventFlow graphic, per the requirements of the SEER-Medicare Data Use Agreement. Specifically, we suppressed the category of Charlson Comorbidity Index (CCI) = 0 in Fig. 11.9 and suppressed the indicator for a hospice admission in Fig. 11.10.

The time to receipt of cancer-directed treatment is plotted in Fig. 11.9 for four groups of men, defined based on their CCI score at the time of diagnosis with bone metastatic disease. The data represented in Fig. 11.9 are based on a stratified random sample of 200 men diagnosed with stage IV M1b (incident BM) prostate cancer between 2005 and 2009 and with at least 1 year of follow-up information following prostate cancer diagnosis. Fifty men were randomly selected from each of the CCI subgroups. We grouped patients based on information in the Medicare claims data from the 12 months prior to the diagnosis of incident M1b prostate cancer. Patients were categorized into groups: missing, 0, 1, and ≥ 2. Of note, the CCI score was categorized as "missing" when no claims were observed during the time 12 months prior to cancer diagnosis.

Given that the patients in this data set were diagnosed with incident M1b prostate cancer, the group with missing CCI score is of particular interest because there were no observed claims for receipt of health services for 12 months prior to the diagnosis of M1b disease and for use in calculating the CCI score. In our prior work [61], we found that these patients are less likely to visit an urologist for a follow-up visit following diagnosis. We found that patients with CCI score coded as "missing" should be studied as a separate group as opposed to combining the "missing" group with the group with CCI score = 0. Our results here are consistent in that we find that the proportion of men who receive treatment is lowest (60%) among the group with CCI coded as "missing," suggesting that the absence of engagement with the health care system prior to diagnosis persists following diagnosis, despite the diagnosis of severe disease (ie, M1b prostate cancer). By comparison, the proportion of men who received treatment was 68% among men with CCI score greater than or equal 2, 76% in the men with CCI score = 1 and greater than 76% in the men with CCI score = 0.

The EventFlow graphic in Fig. 11.9 plots time to receipt of any of the following: orchiectomy, radical prostatectomy, radiation therapy, LHRH agonist, anti-androgen, chemotherapy, and radiopharmaceutical. Fig. 11.9 provides information that is immediately useful for understanding treatment receipt in this sample of men diagnosed with incident M1b prostate cancer. Reading along the y-axis, the height of the light gray panels is informative (or, alternatively, the height of the negative space) for providing information on the proportion of men (not) receiving treatment in a given subgroup. Within each stratum, the height of the *light gray* panel provides information on the proportion receiving cancer-directed treatment, which can then be compared across strata. The height of the white (ie, negative) space provides information on the proportion who did not receive cancer-directed treatment within the timeframe of the follow-up. From Fig. 11.9, we can see that the height of the gray panel is largest among those with CCI score = 0, that is, the healthiest subgroup. The height

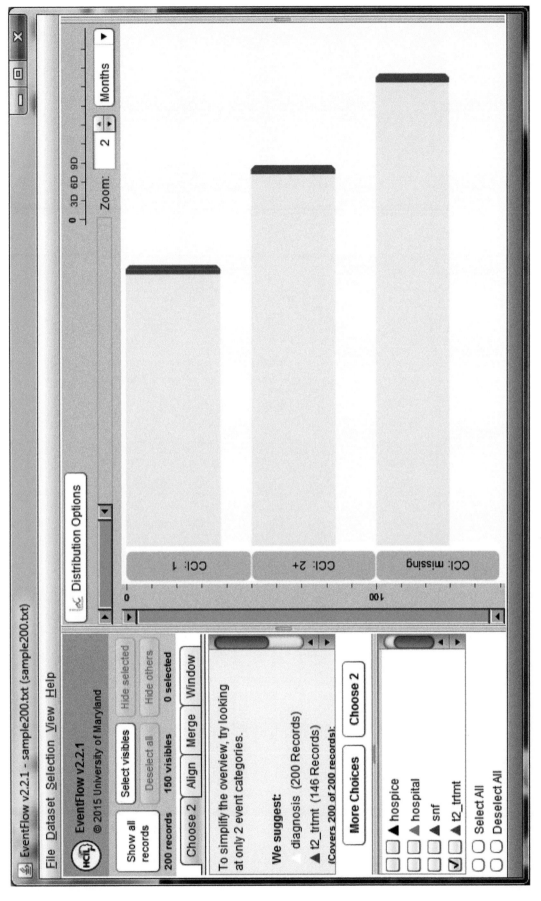

FIGURE 11.9 Time from prostate cancer diagnosis to first treatment in the year following cancer diagnosis, stratified by prediagnosis CCI score (1, ≥ 2, or missing) (CCI= zero was suppressed due to a small sample size, per the Data Use Agreement).

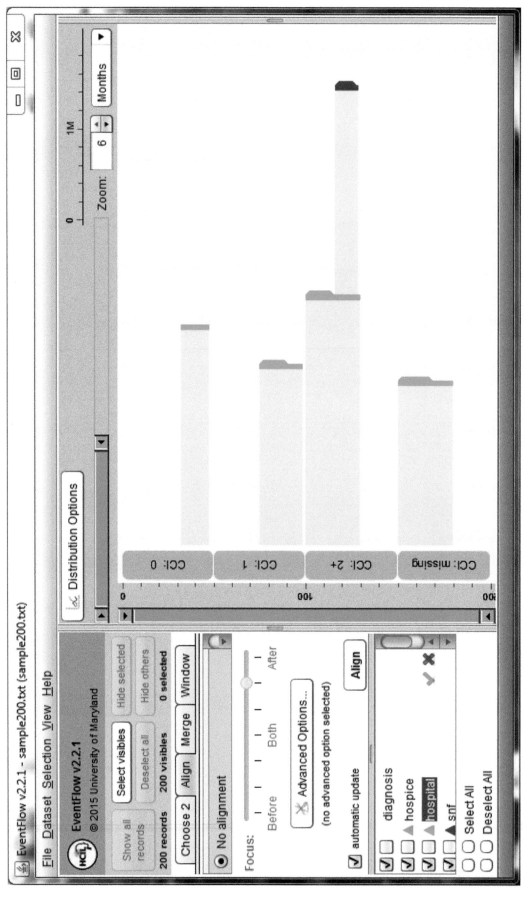

FIGURE 11.10 Time from prostate cancer diagnosis to first hospitalization (green) or SNF stay (blue), stratified by prediagnosis CCI score (0, 1, ≥ 2, or missing) (The indicator for a hospice admission was suppressed due to the small sample size, per the Data Use Agreement).

of the gray panel is smallest among those with CCI = "missing" (those with no health claims for calculating the CCI score during the 12 months prior to their cancer diagnosis). EventFlow also provides information regarding the timing of treatment receipt, via the length of the light gray panel. Comparing across the CCI strata, we see that the time to treatment initiation is shortest among those with CCI score = 0 and longest among those with CCI score = "missing."

The ordering of the light gray and white space is also informative since EventFlow plots the most common events first. Thus, within a given stratum, if treatment receipt is more common than no treatment, the light gray panel will be ordered first (reading top to bottom along the y-axis), followed by the white space. If "no treatment" is more common, the negative space will appear first. In Fig. 11.9, we immediately see that the light gray panel (representing treatment receipt) occurs first among the individuals with few or no comorbidities (CCI = 1 or CCI = 0), indicating that the probability of treatment receipt is higher among the healthier subgroups.

Together, the results from Fig. 11.9 regarding the probability of treatment receipt and timing of treatment initiation suggest that:

1. The group of men with CCI = 2+ are the most vulnerable group among those with nonmissing CCI scores. Compared to individuals with CCI = 0, they are less likely to receive treatment and more likely to receive it in a delayed fashion. The results indicate that comorbidity impacts disease management among those with late-stage prostate cancer, in this case, in terms of their likelihood of receiving critical cancer-directed therapies.
2. The group of men with CCI= missing is also a vulnerable group, and may be *more vulnerable than the group with the highest comorbidity burden*. They are least likely to receive treatment and, when they do receive treatment, exhibit the longest delay in initiating treatment.

Fig. 11.10 provides information regarding time from prostate cancer diagnosis to first hospitalization or SNF stay, stratified by prediagnosis CCI score (0, 1, ≥ 2, or missing). The figure is based on 200 men diagnosed with stage IV M1b (incident BM) prostate cancer between 2005 and 2009 and with at least 1 year of follow-up information following prostate cancer diagnosis. Fifty men were selected from each of the CCI subgroups. The events of interest included time to: all-cause hospitalization and SNF admission. The absence of a shaded light gray area (ie, negative space) indicates that none of the events of interest were observed during the 1 year follow-up period postdiagnosis of incident bone metastatic prostate cancer.

The figure reflecting the proportion and timing of hospitalizations and SNF admissions (Fig. 11.10) indicates that:

1. Hospitalizations (green) are more common than SNF admissions (blue) in the year postdiagnosis in this stratified random sample of 200 men.
2. SNF admissions are most likely in the group with CCI score = 2+.
3. Hospitalizations are more common in the group with CCI = missing and CCI = 2+. The group of patients with a hospitalization is ordered first, followed by the group of patients with no hospitalization events.
4. Hospitalizations are less common in the group with CCI = 0 and CCI = 1. The group of patients with no hospitalization events appears first, followed by the group with hospitalization events.

Note that we have not examined characteristics of the hospitalizations. These characteristics (urgent vs routine admission, length of stay, disease severity index at admission, clinical diagnosis at admission) can be incorporated in Eventflow as attributes in order to provide additional information regarding the hospitalization. As illustrated in these targeted case studies, visualization provides an efficient and intuitive approach to conduct exploratory data analysis of timing and sequencing of events. When supported by a population-based sample of men, these insights from EventFlow can be used to develop formal testable hypotheses (eg, a higher comorbidity index score is associated with a lower probability of treatment receipt) and determine what variables to investigate (eg, an indicator for treatment receipt, time to treatment receipt). The information provided regarding event sequences for patient groups can assist with refining measures, answering questions, and formulating hypotheses for the investigation of cancer-related clinical outcomes.

11.5 CONCLUSION

The easier production of high-quality static graphics, animated weather maps, video presentations, and interactive websites has lowered the barriers to entry into the data visualization product market. However, we are just at the early stages of broadening visual literacy and training a new generation of researchers and decision makers. If data visualization tools that integrate powerful statistical techniques are made commonly available, the benefits could be as potent as the use of graphical user interfaces.

LIST OF ACRONYMS AND ABBREVIATIONS

ACS American Cancer Society
AJCC American Joint Committee on Cancer
BM Bone metastasis
CCI Charlson Comorbidity Index
CDC Centers for Disease Control and Prevention
EHR Electronic health record
GIS Geographic Information Systems
HCIL Human Computer Interaction Laboratory
HINTS Health Information National Trends Survey
HIT Health Information Technology
HTML HyperText Markup Language
ICD-9-CM International Classification of Diseases, Ninth Revision, Clinical Modification
LHRH Luteinizing hormone-releasing hormone
NCI National Cancer Institute
NRC National Research Council
PCAST President's Council of Advisors on Science and Technology
PPV Positive predictive value
PSA Prostate-specific antigen
RtB Radiation to the bone
SEER Surveillance, Epidemiology, and End Results system
SNF Skilled nursing facility

References

[1] Tukey JW. Exploratory data analysis. Reading, MA: Addison-Wesley; 1977.

[2] American Society of Clinical Oncology Accelerating progress against cancer: ASCO's blueprint for transforming clinical and translational cancer research. Alexandria, VA: American Society of Clinical Oncology; 2011.

[3] Hesse BW, Shneiderman B. eHealth research from the user's perspective. Am J Prev Med 2007;32(5 Suppl.):S97–S103.

[4] Shneiderman B, Plaisant C. Designing the user interface: strategies for effective human–computer interaction, 5th ed. Boston, MA: Addison-Wesley; 2010.

[5] Dimitropoulos L. Health IT research priorities to support the health care delivery system of the future. Prepared for the Agency for Healthcare Research and Quality under Contract No290200900023-I. 2014; AHRQ Publication No. 14-0072-EF.

[6] Heer J, Shneiderman B. Interactive dynamics for visual analytics. Commun ACM 2012;55(4):45–54.

[7] Brewer CA. Basic mapping principles for visualizing cancer data using Geographic Information Systems (GIS). Am J Prev Med 2006;30(2 Suppl.):S25–36.

[8] James WL, Cossman RE, Cossman JS, Campbell C, Blanchard T. A brief visual primer for the mapping of mortality trend data. Int J Health Geogr 2004;3(1):7.

[9] Nelson DE, Hesse BW, Croyle RT. Making data talk: communicating health data to the public, policy, and the press. New York: Oxford; 2009.

[10] Rind A, Wang TD, Aigner W, Miksch S, Wongsuphasawat K, Plaisant C, et al. Interactive information visualization to explore and query electronic health records. Found Trends Hum Comput Interact 2013;5(3):207–98.

[11] Kafadar K. Geographic trends in prostate cancer mortality: an application of spatial smoothers and the need for adjustment. Ann Epidemiol 1997;7(1):35–45. [Research Support, U.S. Gov't, Non-P.H.S.].

[12] Chauhan R, Kaur H, Alam MA. Data clustering method for discovering clusters in spatial cancer databases. Int J Comput Appl 2010;10:24–8. (0975–8887) Volume.

[13] Vellido A, Martin JD, Rossi F, Lisboa PJ. Seeing is believing: the importance of visualization in real-world machine learning applications. In: 19th European symposium on artificial neural networks, computational intelligence, and machine learning; 2011.

[14] Shneiderman B, Plaisant C, Hesse BW. Improving health and healthcare with interactive visualization methods. IEEE Comput Spec Issue Chall Inf Vis 2013;46(5):58–66.

[15] Forman MR, Greene SM, Avis NE, Taplin SH, Courtney P, Schad PA, et al. Bioinformatics: tools to accelerate population science and disease control research. Am J Prev Med 2010;38(6): 646–51.

[16] Seo J, Shneiderman B. Knowledge discovery in high-dimensional data: case studies and a user survey for the rank-by-feature framework. IEEE Trans Vis Comput Graph 2006;12(3):311–22.

[17] Klimov D, Shahar Y, Taieb-Maimon M. Intelligent visualization and exploration of time-oriented data of multiple patients. Artif Intell Med 2010;49(1):11–31.

[18] Moskovitch R, Shahar Y. Classification of multivariate time series via temporal abstraction and time intervals mining. Knowl Inf Syst 2014;42:1–40. Accepted: 4 September 2014.

[19] Monroe M, Meyer TE, Plaisant C, Lan R, Wongusphasawat K, Coster TS, et al. Visualizing patterns of drug prescriptions with EventFlow: A pilot study of asthma medications in the Military Health System. HCIL tech report; 2013.

[20] Goovaerts P. Geostatistical analysis of disease data: visualization and propagation of spatial uncertainty in cancer mortality risk using Poisson kriging and p-field simulation. Int J Health Geogr 2006;5:7.

[21] West V, Borland D, Hammond WE. Visualization of EHR and health related data for information discovery. In: Workshop on visual analytics in healthcare; 2013.

[22] Harford JB, Edwards BK, Nandakumar A, Ndom P, Capocaccia R, Coleman MP, et al. Cancer control-planning and monitoring population-based systems. Tumori 2009;95(5):568–78.

[23] Bhowmick T, Griffin AL, MacEachren AM, Kluhsman BC, Lengerich EJ. Understanding the process of cancer data exploration and analysis. Health Place 2008;14(3):576–607.

[24] Jenks GF. The data model concept in statistical mapping. London: George Philip; 1967.

[25] Monroe M, Lan R, Morales J, Shneiderman B, Plaisant C, Millstein J. The challenges of specifying intervals and absences in temporal queries: a graphical language approach Proceedings of the ACM CHI 2013. New York: ACM; 2013, 2349–58.

[26] Krzywinski M, Schein J, Birol I, Connors J, Gascoyne R, Horsman D, et al. Circos: an information aesthetic for comparative genomics. Genome Res 2009;19(9):1639–45.

[27] Imielinski M, Berger AH, Hammerman PS, Hernandez B, Pugh TJ, Hodis E, et al. Mapping the hallmarks of lung adenocarcinoma with massively parallel sequencing. Cell 2012;150(6):1107–20.

[28] Tufte ER. The visual display of quantitative information, 2nd ed. Cheshire, CT: Graphics Press; 2001.

[29] American Cancer Society Cancer facts & figures 2015. Atlanta, GA: American Cancer Society; 2015.

[30] Finney Rutten LJ, Augustson EM, Moser RP, Beckjord EB, Hesse BW. Smoking knowledge and behavior in the United States: sociodemographic, smoking status, and geographic patterns. Nicotine Tob Res 2008;10(10):1559–70.

[31] Nelson DE, Kreps GL, Hesse BW, Croyle RT, Willis G, Arora NK, et al. The Health Information National Trends Survey (HINTS): development, design, and dissemination. J Health Commun 2004;9(5):443–60. discussion 81–84.

[32] Shaikh AR, Butte AJ, Schully SD, Dalton WS, Khoury MJ, Hesse BW. Collaborative biomedicine in the age of big data: the case of cancer. J Med Internet Res 2014;16(4):e101.

[33] Plaisant C, Mushlin R, Snyder A, Li J, Heller D, Shneiderman B. LifeLines: using visualization to enhance navigation and analysis of patient records. In: American Medical Informatics Association 1998 annual fall symposium; 1998.

[34] Plaisant C, Mushlin R, Snyder A, Li J, Heller D, Shneiderman B. LifeLines: using visualization to enhance navigation and analysis of patient records. Proc AMIA Symp 1998:76–80.

[35] Plaisant C, Lam S, Shneiderman B, Smith MS, Roseman D, Marchand G, et al. Searching electronic health records for temporal patterns in patient histories: a case study with microsoft amalga. AMIA Annu Symp Proc 2008:601–5.

[36] Tarkan S, Plaisant C, Shneiderman B, Hettinger AZ. Reducing missed laboratory results: defining temporal responsibility, generating user interfaces for test process tracking, and retrospective analyses to identify problems. AMIA Annu Symp Proc 2011;2011:1382–91.

[37] Plaisant C, Wu J, Hettinger AZ, Powsner S, Shneiderman B. Novel user interface design for medication reconciliation: an evaluation of Twinlist. J Am Med Inform Assoc 2015;22(2):340–9.

[38] Bernard J, Sessler D, May T, Schlomm T, Pehrke D, Kohlhammer J. A visual-interactive system for prostate cancer cohort analysis. IEEE Comput Graph Appl 2015;35(3):44–55.

[39] Simpao AF, Ahumada LM, Desai BR, Bonafide CP, Galvez JA, Rehman MA, et al. Optimization of drug–drug interaction alert rules in a pediatric hospital's electronic health record system using a visual analytics dashboard. J Am Med Inform Assoc 2015;22(2):361–9.

[40] Monroe M, Lan R, Lee H, Plaisant C, Shneiderman B. Temporal event sequence simplification. IEEE Trans Vis Comput Graph 2013;19(12):2227–36.

[41] Shneiderman B, Plaisant C. Sharpening analytic focus to cope with big data volume and variety: ten strategies for data focusing with temporal event sequences, visualization viewpoint. IEEE Comput Graph Appl 2015;35(3):10–14.

[42] Malik S, Du F, Monroe M, Onukwugha E, Plaisant C, Shneiderman B. Comparing cohorts of event sequences with balanced integration of analytics and statistics Proceedings of the ACM 20th international conference on intelligent user interfaces. New York: ACM Press; 2015.38.49

[43] Malik S, Du F, Monroe M, Onukwugha E, Plaisant C, Shneiderman B. An evaluation of visual analytics approaches to comparing cohorts of event sequences. In: EHRVis workshop on visualizing electronic health record data, Paris, France; 2014.

[44] Norgaard M, Jensen AO, Jacobsen JB, Cetin K, Fryzek JP, Sorensen HT. Skeletal related events, bone metastasis and survival of prostate cancer: a population based cohort study in Denmark (1999 to 2007). J Urol 2010;184(1):162–7.

[45] Sathiakumar N, Delzell E, Morrisey MA, Falkson C, Yong M, Chia V, et al. Mortality following bone metastasis and skeletal-related events among men with prostate cancer: a population-based analysis of US Medicare beneficiaries, 1999–2006. Prostate Cancer Prostatic Dis 2011;14(2):177–83.

[46] Sathiakumar N, Delzell E, Morrisey MA, Falkson C, Yong M, Chia V, et al. Mortality following bone metastasis and skeletal-related events among women with breast cancer: a population-based analysis of U.S. Medicare beneficiaries, 1999–2006. Breast Cancer Res Treat 2012;131(1):231–8.

[47] Lage MJ, Barber BL, Harrison DJ, Jun S. The cost of treating skeletal-related events in patients with prostate cancer. Am J Manag Care 2008;14(5):317–22.

[48] Delea T, McKiernan J, Brandman J, Edelsberg J, Sung J, Raut M, et al. Retrospective study of the effect of skeletal complications on total medical care costs in patients with bone metastases of breast cancer seen in typical clinical practice. J Support Oncol 2006;4(7):341–7.

[49] Chawla N, Yabroff KR, Mariotto A, McNeel TS, Schrag D, Warren JL. Limited validity of diagnosis codes in Medicare claims for identifying cancer metastases and inferring stage. Ann Epidemiol 2014;24(9):666–72, 72 e1–2.

[50] Hassett MJ, Ritzwoller DP, Taback N, Carroll N, Cronin AM, Ting GV, et al. Validating billing/encounter codes as indicators of lung, colorectal, breast, and prostate cancer recurrence using 2 large contemporary cohorts. Med Care 2014;52(10):e65–73.

[51] Nordstrom BL, Whyte JL, Stolar M, Mercaldi C, Kallich JD. Identification of metastatic cancer in claims data. Pharmacoepidemiol Drug Saf 2012;21(Suppl. 2):21–8.

[52] Thomas SK, Brooks SE, Mullins CD, Baquet CR, Merchant S. Use of ICD-9 coding as a proxy for stage of disease in lung cancer. Pharmacoepidemiol Drug Saf 2002;11(8):709–13.

[53] Cooper GS, Yuan Z, Stange KC, Dennis LK, Amini SB, Rimm AA. The sensitivity of Medicare claims data for case ascertainment of six common cancers. Med Care 1999;37(5):436–44.

[54] Delea TE, McKiernan J, Brandman J, Edelsberg J, Sung J, Raut M, et al. Impact of skeletal complications on total medical care costs among patients with bone metastases of lung cancer. J Thorac Oncol 2006;1(6):571–6.

[55] Onukwugha E, Yong C, Hussain A, Seal B, Mullins CD. Concordance between administrative claims and registry data for identifying metastasis to the bone: an exploratory analysis in prostate cancer. BMC Med Res Methodol 2014;14:1.

[56] Hahn C, Kavanagh B, Bhatnagar A, Jacobson G, Lutz S, Patton C, et al. Choosing Wisely: the American Society for Radiation Oncology's Top 5 list. Pract Radiat Oncol 2014;4(6):349–55.

[57] Albertsen PC, Moore DF, Shih W, Lin Y, Li H, Lu-Yao GL. Impact of comorbidity on survival among men with localized prostate cancer. J Clin Oncol 2011;29(10):1335–41.

[58] Stattin P. Mortality in older men with low-risk prostate cancer and high comorbidity. J Clin Oncol [Letter] 2015;33(9):1086–7.

[59] Daskivich TJ, Chamie K, Kwan L, Labo J, Dash A, Greenfield S, et al. Comorbidity and competing risks for mortality in men with prostate cancer. Cancer 2011;117(20):4642–50.

[60] Daskivich TJ, Fan KH, Koyama T, Albertsen PC, Goodman M, Hamilton AS, et al. Effect of age, tumor risk, and comorbidity on competing risks for survival in a U.S. population-based cohort of men with prostate cancer. Ann Intern Med 2013;158(10):709–17.

[61] Onukwugha E, Osteen P, Jayasekera J, Mullins CD, Mair CA, Hussain A. Racial disparities in urologist visits among elderly men with prostate cancer: a cohort analysis of patient-related and county of residence-related factors. Cancer 2014;120(21):3385–92.

[62] Han P, Klein W, Killam B, Lehman T, Massett H, Freeman A. Representing randomness in the communication of individualized cancer risk estimates: effects on cancer risk perceptions, worry, and subjective uncertainty about risk. Patient Educ. Couns. 2011;83(1).

12

Oncology Informatics: Behavioral and Psychological Sciences

David K. Ahern PhD[1,2,3], Ilana M. Braun MD[4], Mary E. Cooley PhD, RN, FAAN[5,6] and Timothy W. Bickmore PhD[7]

[1]Health Communication and Informatics Research Branch, Healthcare Delivery Research Program, National Cancer Institute, Bethesda, MD, United States [2]Program in Behavioral Informatics and eHealth, Department of Psychiatry, Brigham & Women's Hospital, Boston, MA, United States [3]Harvard Medical School, Boston, MA, United States [4]Dana-Farber Cancer Institute, Harvard Medical School, Boston, MA, United States [5]Phyllis F. Cantor Center, Research in Nursing and Patient Care, Dana-Farber Cancer Institute, Boston, MA, United States [6]College of Nursing and Exercise Health Science, University of Massachusetts-Boston, Boston, MA, United States [7]College of Computer and Information Science, Northeastern University, Boston, MA, United States

OUTLINE

12.1 Introduction	232	
12.1.1 Why Is Behavioral Informatics Relevant to Cancer Now?	232	
12.1.2 Background	232	
12.2 Role of Behavioral/Psychological Science in Advancing Informatics	232	
12.2.1 Theories and Models of Behavior Change	232	
12.2.2 Cognitive Processes and CDS	236	
12.2.3 Behavioral Measures in EHRs	237	
12.2.4 HIT Infrastructure	238	
12.2.5 Contribution to mHealth	238	
12.3 Definition and Role of Behavioral Informatics	239	
12.3.1 Behavioral Ontologies	239	
12.4 Applications of Behavioral Informatics Resources and Tools in Cancer Care	241	
12.4.1 Tobacco Use and Informatics-Based Interventions	241	
12.4.2 Physical Activity Promotion	242	
12.4.3 Screening and Intervention for Adverse Health Behaviors and Emotional Distress	243	
12.4.4 Implementing Psychosocial Screening: An Informatics-Based Approach	244	
12.4.5 Low Literacy Support	248	
12.5 Conclusions	248	
List of Acronyms and Abbreviations	249	
References	249	

B. Hesse, D. Ahern & E. Beckjord: Oncology Informatics.
DOI: http://dx.doi.org/10.1016/B978-0-12-802115-6.00012-4

12.1 INTRODUCTION

12.1.1 Why Is Behavioral Informatics Relevant to Cancer Now?

According to the American Society of Clinical Oncology (ASCO), there is a crisis in cancer care with gaps in care and discontinuities in information sharing both among providers and with patients. One reason for this crisis is the paucity of informatics approaches and solutions that connect disparate and disconnected oncology practices and which support a learning system, such as the Cancer Learning Intelligence Network for Quality (CancerLinQ) described in Chapter 1, "Creating a Learning Health Care System in Oncology" by Schilsky et al., to enable and support provider decision support and patient self-management. Another reason is that current solutions do not typically draw from the evidence base of behavioral science in their design or deployment. A major premise for this chapter is that behavioral informatics will contribute to the development, implementation, and ongoing evaluation of usable, effective, and efficient informatics solutions for providers (eg, advanced clinical decision support, CDS), patients (eg, actionable personal health records and mHealth apps), and health systems (eg, CancerLinQ) alike.

In this chapter, we address this integration opportunity and illustrate how cancer care, in particular, can benefit from behaviorally based, informatics solutions. We also contend that informatics solutions that do not take into account the knowledge base about behavior and its controlling factors, no matter how well designed or implemented, are likely to fail in adequately addressing the complexity of challenges facing the health care system today.

12.1.2 Background

The potential for informatics platforms and solutions to improve cancer care is well delineated in the previous section of this book *Informatics Support Across the Cancer Continuum*. In this section of the chapter we present the case for the critical role that behavioral, psychological, and cognitive sciences, hereafter condensed to behavioral sciences, play in realizing the future success of informatics in improving cancer care. Fundamental principles of the behavioral sciences, prevailing theories and models, and core elements of behavior change are described and illuminated. Informatics platforms and resources that draw from the behavioral sciences in the areas of tobacco control, physical activity promotion, and emotional distress screening are provided as exemplars in applied and clinical settings.

Behavioral science as applied to health and disease has a rich history and robust portfolio of evidence [1].

The discipline of behavioral medicine emerged in the mid-1970s and spawned the Society of Behavioral Medicine as the dominant national organization promoting research and clinical practice at the intersection of behavior, disease, and health [2]. The growth of behavioral medicine as a professional specialty of behavioral science applied to the study of behavior, health, and disease coincided with the evolution of the personal computer and technology revolution of the last 40 years. In many ways, both behavioral medicine and technology have matured to a point where there is a unique opportunity to integrate these two domains to help solve the complex and intractable societal problems, including the crisis in cancer care, that adversely impact the health of our nation.

12.2 ROLE OF BEHAVIORAL/ PSYCHOLOGICAL SCIENCE IN ADVANCING INFORMATICS

Researchers in the behavioral sciences have a long tradition of studying the effects of technology-mediated, eHealth interventions [3], with a particular interest in the computerization of messaging and the benefits of tailoring [4,5]. Over the last decade substantial attention and resources have been allocated to advancing the science of eHealth and technology-enabled, health behavior change interventions through funding from the Robert Wood Johnson Foundation [6], and the National Institutes of Health (NIH), with the National Cancer Institute (NCI) assuming a prominent role in fostering a broad portfolio of communication and informatics research initiatives [7].

12.2.1 Theories and Models of Behavior Change

Fundamental to the application of behavioral science principles to informatics is the formulation of theoretical models and approaches to behavior change that are incumbent to technology-mediated interventions. Theories and models are useful in predicting outcomes and explaining behavior changes from these interventions. They also can guide and enhance development through the selection of intervention components and aid in the evaluation process.

Pingree, et al. [8] explicate the value of theory for enhancing and understanding eHealth interventions. Theory can address the putative underlying causal mechanisms for observed changes in behavior and help determine the likely behavioral and psychological processes involved. Theory-based mediational analyses can help explain the "why" and "how" of intervention effectiveness. Self-Determination Theory (SDT) is proffered as a plausible and comprehensive theoretic approach to explaining the effects of complex, multilayered eHealth interventions. They use their well-established, evidence-based eHealth intervention, Comprehensive Health Enhancement Support System (CHESS) as an example and describe how, through mediation analysis [8], SDT aids in deconstructing the impact of its multiple, interactive components (see DuBenske et al., Chapter 10, "Advanced Cancer: Palliative, End of Life, and Bereavement Care" for further explication of CHESS and its impact in cancer). Pingree and colleagues conclude by arguing that having an explicit theoretic model provides a clear framework for the initial development process, and importantly the adaptation of an intervention over time. This latter point is crucial to the challenge of staying current with the rapid and iterative evolution of technology-mediated interventions.

Similarly, Hesse [9] provides a useful classification scheme for linking the key components of eHealth interventions to the three major constructs of SDT: (1) autonomy, (2) competence, and (3) relatedness. With respect to autonomy, the range of eHealth and informatics resources such as self-help apps, personal health records, and patient portals provide support. Competence is enabled by functional health literacy, tailored information prescriptions, and engagement techniques. Relatedness is engendered by social networks, shared knowledge repositories, and advocacy groups.

Historically, in addition to SDT, other prominent behavioral and psychological models such as the Transtheoretical Model (stages of change) [10], Social Cognitive Theory [11], and The Behavior Change Wheel for characterizing and designing behavior change interventions [12], among others, have served as the underlying foundation for technology-mediated, health behavior change interventions. Although useful for guiding overall design and informing selection of intervention components to facilitate and explain behavior change, these traditional models have been viewed as insufficient in accounting for rapidly evolving technology-mediated interventions [13]. This limitation is especially salient to the emergence of interventions delivered through mobile devices that require more flexible theories and models which can accommodate the dynamic and adaptive nature of real-time usage. Moreover, mobile technologies expand the range of inputs beyond self-report to include time/location parameters, psychophysiological state, activity level, history of behavior patterns, and social context [13]. Relevant to cancer prevention, studies of context-sensitive mobile technologies and apps targeting tobacco use and cessation are underway currently and promise greater adoption and use [14].

In response to the call for more flexible and contemporary models of health behavior change for the digital era, Mohr et al. [15] delineate the Behavioral Intervention Technologies (BITs) Model for eHealth and mHealth interventions. BITs are defined as subsets of eHealth and mHealth applications that employ a broad range of technologies including the web, mobile, and smartphones, and sensors to enable behavioral and cognitive modification across physical and mental health and wellness domains. According to the authors, the BIT Model represents a "broad hybrid framework" that includes both core behavioral principles with technological features that can serve as a bridge between the two disciplines of behavioral science and technology. In many ways the BIT Model provides a roadmap for conveying evidence-based behavioral science principles, in combination with human system design and engineering requirements, into technology-mediated interventions. One strength of this approach is the ability to generate testable hypotheses that can be subjected to multilevel analysis and evaluation.

The BIT Model is explicated by considering the areas of focus for development and deployment of BITs, namely (1) *Why*, (2) *How* (subdivided into conceptual and technical), (3) *What*, and (4) *When*. In their classification scheme, the "Why" refers to the primary intention of the developer of the BIT with respect to a clinical or usage goal. In most cases the BIT is created to achieve a clinical aim of health behavior change, such as promoting weight reduction, increased physical activity, or tobacco cessation. The intent of the developer in some instances may be more focused on the use of intervention or level of engagement. The "How" at the conceptual level is where the core evidence-based behavioral intervention strategies are delineated and incorporated into the intervention. Here the strategies include education/knowledge dissemination, goal setting, self-monitoring/tracking, feedback, and motivation enhancements. The technical "How" characteristics include the medium (text, audio, video); complexity of task requirements; esthetics; and degree of personalization and extent of machine learning. The "What" includes the core elements such as information delivery, notifications, logs, passive data sensing and collection, messaging elements, and end-user reports. Finally, the "When" represents the workflow or manner and timeframe for when and under what conditions BIT interventions are delivered in various settings or environments. Frequency, timing, and event-driven features are commonly part of the workflow design. Personalization can be achieved not only through initial tailoring to end-user characteristics and preferences but also through machine learning methods that can automatically adapt over time to meet changes in user needs and capabilities.

Taken together, features of the BIT Model extend other more current models for technology-enabled behavior change [3,16] and provide a useful map that can translate clinical goals into behavioral strategies for application development and evaluation. Furthermore, Mohr et al. [17] offer a novel methodological framework for the continuous evaluation of BITs given rapid iteration of technology-mediated solutions often not suitable for evaluation via traditional research designs and analytic methods.

Pagoto and Bennett [18] provide a compelling rationale for the critical role for behavioral/psychological science and behavioral medicine in advancing digital health and informatics. They propose five key areas in which behavioral/psychological science can impact digital health technologies: (1) research to determine which health technologies actually impact behavior and health outcomes; (2) evaluation studies to understand how evolving online social networks can be applied to health behavior change on a large scale; (3) emphasis on a team science approach to the developmental process of health technologies; (4) achieving a desirable balance between the fast pace of innovation and the slower pace of research; and (5) promoting the role of behavioral scientists as integral in informing the development of digital health technologies and their inclusion into the health care system. Central to their argument is that behavioral/psychological science adds value through demonstrating the most effective feedback strategies for tailoring, methods to improve participant engagement and utilization, creation of scientifically sound application rating systems, and enhancing the impact of digital health technologies through inclusion of evidence-based, behavioral strategies.

The evidence base from behavioral medicine provides an important resource to achieve "meaningful use" of Health Information Technology (HIT) within the health sector as promulgated by the Health Information Technology for Economic and Clinical Health Act of 2009 (HITECH). Hesse et al. [19] offer a rationale for leveraging behavioral medicine given the focus on user's behavior as the essential component to achieving meaningful use of HIT. The authors offer several ways that behavioral medicine can inform the necessary system redesign to support patients and providers including: (1) crafting a health services environment that optimizes communication among stakeholders, for example, building and evaluating a web-based interdisciplinary patient-centered plan of care [20]; (2) assisting providers and policy makers in the creation of "decisional architectures" for "nudging" desirable behavior change through the use of incentives; (3) promoting creation of understandable patient educational materials; (4) making the default decision the healthiest choice; (5) constructing positive feedback loops; and (6) enabling structured decision making.

Similarly, Ahern et al. [21] provide a framework for organizing patient-facing technologies into categories of meaningful use, and how these technologies can

improve health care quality, safety, and population health. Growing patient demands for information and "convenience services" has stimulated a variety of HIT-enabled functions designed to maximize patient participation, including services that allow patients to conduct health-related transactions, increase access to professionals and electronic health record (EHR) information, and support self-care management. As predicted by behavioral theory, those technologies that patients perceive as useful and which are effective in terms of sustained health behavior change in their target domain are likely to be adopted and used.

Although showing great promise, the design, development, and implementation of these patient-facing technologies require careful attention to myriad factors that impact their effectiveness, efficiency and patient-centeredness. Valdez et al. [22] offer an expanded framework for patient-facing technologies. They propose a multilevel analysis and approach that accommodates a broad array of patient, family, and environmental factors in design and deployment of these technologies, which they refer to as *consumer health informatics* (CHI) applications. The authors refer to "patient work" as the conceptual framework for organizing the various health-related activities that must be considered in formulating a full and accurate representation of the context for which a CHI is designed, developed, and deployed. Drawing from human factors engineering and medical social science as well as biomedical informatics, the authors contend that the "patient work" framework can help guide the user-centered design process in the creation of CHIs.

The authors recognize that existing behavioral theoretical models, such as the Transtheoretical Model and SDT, that are commonly used in the design and evaluation of CHI's need to be accommodated in the larger context of the patient work perspective. Clearly, further research on this framework is necessary and called for by the authors but their approach holds promise for supporting patients' self-management efforts.

Fortunately, research in behavioral science and behavioral medicine over the last two decades has contributed to a fundamental understanding of behavior, context, and its controlling factors [1]; and can help inform multilevel approaches to the creation of robust behavioral informatics platforms, tools, and resources.

There are strong multilayered connections between behavior, health, and disease. Table 12.1 illustrates the broad range of behavior-health linkages among major causes of death and in relation to cancer risk and development of the disease. As shown in the table, the three major risk factors (tobacco use, poor diet, and physical inactivity) both influence the development of cancers, and when addressed through behavior change interventions, can alter the onset and course of the disease. As an example, increasing evidence indicates that obesity

TABLE 12.1 Behavior-Health Linkages Among Major "Actual Causes" of Death and Cancer

Cause of death/disease	Behavior-health linkage
LINKAGE 1: BEHAVIORAL, ENVIRONMENTAL, AND GENETIC INFLUENCES MODERATE ONE ANOTHER	
Tobacco use	Both environmental and genetic factors influence onset and persistence of smoking
Poor diet	Environmental factors are more important than genetic influences in food preferences among older adults
Cancer	Nutrition and lifestyle intervention reduces prostate gene expression and tumorigenesis in men
LINKAGE 2: BEHAVIOR INFLUENCES HEALTH	
Tobacco use	Numerous Surgeon General's reports have concluded that smoking is a leading cause of cancer, cardiovascular and pulmonary disease, and premature death
Poor diet	Systematic reviews conclude that obesity contributes to hypertension, hyperlipidemia, diabetes, cardiovascular disease, and some cancers
Physical activity	Randomized trials and systematic reviews conclude that physical activity is associated with decreased all-cause mortality reduced risk for chronic diseases, and reduced risk of breast cancer
Cancer	Findings from systematic reviews, meta-analyses, large prospective studies, and randomized trials link risk for cancer with poor diet, physical inactivity, smoking, stress, and social involvement
LINKAGE 3: BEHAVIOR CHANGE INTERVENTIONS PREVENT DISEASE	
Tobacco use	A major multisite trial demonstrated that smoking-cessation programs substantially reduce mortality even when only a minority of patients stop smoking
Poor diet	Systematic reviews and randomized trials of interventions for childhood obesity show positive impacts on diet, weight gain trajectory, and weight loss maintenance, and on insulin resistance
Physical activity	Among overweight, previously inactive women at risk for type 2 diabetes, accumulating 10,000 steps/day for 8 weeks improved glucose tolerance and reduced both systolic and diastolic blood pressure
Cancer	In a number of large prospective longitudinal studies and meta-analyses, physical activity has been linked to reduced risk of colon cancer
LINKAGE 4: BEHAVIOR CHANGE INTERVENTIONS IMPROVE DISEASE MANAGEMENT	
Tobacco use	Self-management skills (eg, setting quit date, planning for coping with temptations to relapse) help individuals quit smoking
Poor diet	Randomized behavioral interventions show that peer nutrition education positively influences diabetes self-management in Latinos
Physical activity	Randomized clinical trials show that exercise training reduces HbA1c among those with diabetes
Cancer	Randomized trials of patients with cancer indicate that physical activity increases functional capacity during chemotherapy, improves marrow recovery and decreases complications during peripheral blood stem transplantation, and decreases fatigue and other symptoms associated with radiation therapy and chemotherapy
LINKAGE 5: PSYCHOSOCIAL AND BEHAVIORAL INTERVENTIONS IMPROVE QOL	
Tobacco use	Improved health-related QOL is a significant health outcome for ex-smokers compared to current smokers
Poor diet	In randomized trials, lifestyle interventions show improved nutritional status and QOL and less depressive symptoms and improved physical functioning
Physical activity	Randomized trials show physical activity improves QOL in older adults and improves QOL and fatigue in breast cancer survivors
Cancer	Randomized psychosocial interventions show decreased psychological distress, pain, and nausea secondary to treatment and improve QOL and immune system modulation
LINKAGE 6: HEALTH-PROMOTION PROGRAMS IMPROVE HEALTH OF POPULATION	
Tobacco use	Antismoking campaign in California that includes counter-media, youth prevention programs, cessation services, and tax increases reduced smoking and accompanying rates of cardiovascular disease and death rates from lung cancer

(Continued)

TABLE 12.1   Behavior-Health Linkages Among Major "Actual Causes" of Death and Cancer (Continued)

Cause of death/disease	Behavior-health linkage
Poor diet	Mass-media health education campaigns and policy and environmental supports can lead to substantial improvements in fruit, vegetable, and fat consumption in general populations
Physical activity	Community-wide walk-to-school programs increase walking and biking to school and walking and fitness trails increased physical activity in a rural African-American population
Cancer	In 2006, overall cancer death rates declined because of a 50% reduction in male smoking from 47% in the 1960s to less than 23%

Source: Adapted from Fisher E, Fitzgibbon M, Glasgow R, Haire-Joshu D, Hayman L, Kaplan R, et al. Behavior matters. Am J Prevent Med 2011;40(5):e15–e30, with permission.

is a major determinant of colorectal and breast cancer risk, among others. Given the substantial link between behavior and cancer, there are a number of effective interventions that focus on prevention, treatment, and survivorship. Interventions that incorporate behavioral components are both efficacious and cost-effective in terms of relative cost per Quality Adjusted Life Year (QALY) when compared to alternative treatments.

Behavioral and psychological research in cancer prevention and control has addressed a variety of key processes and outcomes across the cancer care continuum from prevention to end-of-life care [23]. Research designs and methods have been refined and evolved to evaluate the underlying behavioral, psychological, and cognitive processes that contribute to the persistence of adverse health behaviors, for example, tobacco use, as well as to promote positive outcomes in cancer control. Findings from this body of research have informed the importance of taking a multilevel approach to understanding the complex interplay among the biobehavioral and psychological, social and organizational, and environmental levels of influence.

12.2.2 Cognitive Processes and CDS

Behavioral and psychological research on cognitive processes of decision making is particularly salient to the development, impact, and evaluation of CDS tools and informatics resources. Fundamental cognitive processes, such as memory, language, attention, and motivation, are critical determinants of how the information delivered via CDS will be received, processed, and acted upon by patients [23]. In 2010, The Office of the National Coordinator for Health Information Technology (ONC) funded the Strategic HIT Advanced Research Projects (SHARP). SHARP addressed strategic cross-cutting themes, including patient-centered cognitive-support that is essential to promoting and optimizing the meaningful use of HIT (http://www.healthit.gov/policy-researchers-implementers/strategic-health-it-advanced-research-projects-sharp).

Three areas of investigation were pursued by the National Center for Cognitive Informatics & Decision Making in Healthcare funded under SHARP: (1) studies that examine the cognitive foundations for decision making, drawing from multiple disciplines, including cognitive and psychological sciences; (2) studies of methodologies that improve the efficacy and applicability of CDS by integrating patient and environmental-specific factors; and (3) construction of an interface that optimizes cognitive information design and visualization and that supports the integration of clinical understanding, decision making, and problem solving (http://www.healthit.gov/policy-researchers-implementers/national-center-cognitive-informatics-and-decision-making-healthcare).

One recent study from this work that illustrates the role of cognitive factors in CDS utilized qualitative and quantitative approaches to examine medical information-seeking among eight critical care physicians [24]. The physicians provided a verbal report of their cognitive processes as they performed a clinical diagnosis task. Measures included verbal descriptions of physician's activities, sources of information they used including electronic and paper records, time spent on each information source, and recordings of interactions with other clinicians. Results indicated that information-seeking behavior was both exploratory and iterative, and characterized by the contextual organization of the information. Information obtained by electronic records was classified into a higher level of knowledge structure as compared to information gleaned from paper records. In contrast, paper records provided an overall gestalt of the patient's condition and were easier to review the annotated written narrative than on electronic notes. The authors concluded that a process of *local optimization*, that is, the conventional approach for that setting and culture, drove information-seeking behavior and physicians' utilized information that maximized their gain even if it required greater cognitive effort. The authors recommend that enriching aspects of the electronic record to highlight key concepts may improve clinical reasoning and lead to quicker and more accurate

TABLE 12.2 Types of Evidence for Fuzzy-Trace Theory

Evidence for gist and verbatim representations

Encoded, stored, and retrieved independently

Data from many tasks, groups, countries, and different laboratories

Experiments: Counterintuitive hypotheses tested

Manipulation of causal factors (eg, representations) to observe whether predicted behavior change occurs

Modeled mathematically and tested for fit to real data

Estimates of independent contributions of gist and verbatim representations, as well as judgment processes, in a variety of tasks

Mathematical models combined with experiments

Individual gist and verbatim parameters are tested for fit with data and to see if they respond to experimental factors as predicted by theory

Neuroimaging and neuropsychological evidence

Different brain regions are activated when gist and verbatim representations are encoded and retrieved, and different patient populations show selective impairments for such representations

TABLE 12.3 Examples of Gist Representation and Retrieved Values Used in Medical Decision Making and Health

Representation	Value	Decision
Chemotherapy is poison	Poison is bad	Do not choose chemotherapy
Surgery removes the lump	The lump is bad	Choose surgery
Condom blocks fluids	Exchange of fluids is bad	Use condoms
Feel okay or take a chance on feeling okay or not okay	Better to feel okay	Do not screen
Screening detects disease early	Early is better	Choose screening

Source: From Reyna, VF. A theory of medical decision making and health: fuzzy trace theory. Med Decis Making 2008;28:850-65., with permission.

decisions. Here behavioral research on key attentional processes, such as cognitive load and stimuli saturation, can provide guidance in enhancing informatics platforms, tools, and resources [23].

In the cancer care literature, Reyna et al. [25] review the prevailing theoretical models and practical implications for optimizing decision making in the context of cancer prevention and screening, treatment, survivorship, and end-of-life care. They critique theoretical approaches to decision making that explain the roles of cognition and emotion, and their interaction. Historically, theoretical models of decision making have highlighted cognition while deemphasizing emotion as more disruptive than facilitative. In contrast, the authors contend that modern theoretical models, such as fuzzy-trace theory [26], are dual process: that is the models attempt to accommodate how cognition and emotion interact by emphasizing the bottom line or "gist" of options that can also incorporate relevant social and moral values in decision making. The types of evidence which support fuzzy-trace theory and examples of gist representations and retrieved values are shown in Tables 12.2 and 12.3.

The challenge facing decision making in cancer care is to translate and deliver evidence-based, behavioral interventions at population level that draw from the most current and rapidly advancing scientific evidence. The application of informatics is one potential solution to this challenge. With respect to cancer, examples are provided later in this chapter that illustrate how informatics approaches, applied to the prevalent and vexing problems of distress screening and health illiteracy, can be addressed and remediated.

12.2.3 Behavioral Measures in EHRs

One major challenge that has begun to be addressed is standardization of measurement of environmental, behavioral, and psychosocial factors which can be collected in the clinical encounter and documented within the electronic medical record (EMR) [27]. Recently, the Institute of Medicine (IOM) published a report entitled *Capturing Social and Behavioral Domains and Measures in Electronic Health Records—Phase 2* that represented the outcome of a two-phase study to identify social and behavioral domains that most strongly determine health, and then to evaluate the measures of those domains that can be used in EHRs [28]. This IOM report drew heavily from the recent work of behavioral scientists who conducted a systematic review and consensus process about identifying candidate measures that can be reliably measured, are feasible, and represent relevant socioeconomic and behavioral determinants of health [27]. Through this effort, 12 measures were identified and vetted for consideration to be included in EHRs. Combining these measures with other elements of the medical record will allow for a more comprehensive evaluation of risk status and greater precision in addressing health conditions and predicting future adverse health events. Further, incorporating these behavioral and psychosocial measures in the medical record supports the movement toward precision medicine whereby treatments can be targeted and tailored to individual genetic, biological, behavioral, and psychosocial characteristics (http://nih.gov/precisionmedicine).

Within the behavioral/psychological science and behavioral medicine community, considerable effort is underway to develop a behavioral ontology or structured vocabulary that enables consistent and reliable use of terms within the medical record and for supporting research evaluation [29]. A comprehensive behavioral ontology will complement the ontologies created within the biomedical informatics domain that support advanced CDS. With respect to research, ontology is critical for determining active components of effective interventions. Ontologies are described in more detail below.

12.2.4 HIT Infrastructure

The last 20 years has witnessed an explosion of health information resources attributable to the Internet and evolution of technology to deliver targeted communications. HITECH set in motion the rapid uptake in HIT infrastructures of EHRs/personal health records, has led to advances in connected health (telemedicine and telehealth), and created the architecture *to enable behavior change on a large scale* [19]. The deployment of EHRs in physician practices and hospitals, despite their widely recognized limitations, has contributed to advances in CDS at the point of care; improved health care quality; and reduced medical errors. Patient portals have begun to be offered by physician groups, albeit slowly, as part of electronic record systems to engage patients in their own care and provide them access to certain aspects of their medical record. Health Information Exchanges (HIEs) have sprung up in most states and regions to address the lack of interoperability of many of the current EHR systems and with the goal of seamlessly transmitting data across disparate health settings and to improve community health.

12.2.5 Contribution to mHealth

More recently there has been a rapid growth of mHealth tools and resources, leveraging the smartphone and tablet computer, and including a plethora of apps designed to address a wide range of health behaviors and conditions. Mobile phone messaging interventions for preventive health care is receiving increasing attention as well, although a Cochrane systematic review of randomized controlled trials (RCTs), and quasi-RCTs found only limited evidence of demonstrable impact across a range of health behaviors [30]. The evidence for smoking-cessation interventions, however, was deemed of high quality. Advances in sensor technology and the emergence of "wearable" devices has enabled the "quantified self" movement—groups of individuals interested in understanding their own personal health data and the role it can play in improving health. Collectively, these developments in mobile computing hold great promise in improving the health and well-being of individuals and populations if harnessed and implemented effectively.

With respect to cancer, there have been notable efforts to support cancer patients using mobile apps. Mirkovic

THE YOUNG ADULT PROGRAM AT THE DANA-FARBER CANCER INSTITUTE (YAP@DFCI)

S. Julie is a 22-year-old, single recent college graduate. At a time when her classmates all seemed to be moving to big cities and starting their careers, Julie found herself confronting a breast cancer diagnosis, forgoing her first job opportunity, and moving back into her parents' suburban home. Socially isolated, she began treatment at the Dana-Farber Cancer Institute. "Everyone in the waiting room seemed so much older than me... I felt like a fish out of water," she recalls. A social worker who met with her during her first chemotherapy infusion supplied her with a leaflet about YAP@DFCI, the young adult program at her hospital. That night, she signed up through the patient portal and was rewarded with a wealth of offerings: educational materials, from self-help modules on managing anxiety to advice around fertility preservation in the setting of cancer; feature articles written by patients facing similar developmental challenges; and, perhaps even more cathartic, a rich and supportive online community. Through frequent chat room exchanges, Julie befriended several other young adult cancer patients. At an annual YAP@DFCI conference, she connected in person with some of these online friends. In addition, she relished the many technological capabilities harnessed by the conference. In a nod to being age appropriate, the conference designers had Twitter feeds and Spotify playlists that conference attendees could contribute to through the day. "I'm in a technology-proficient generation and YAP@DFCI meets us where we are and where we need it most."

et al. [31] describe the usability design process and development approach for creating the Connect Mobile app, which enables remote access to the Connect system that is an online portal that supports cancer patients in managing health-related issues. Through this iterative evaluation of a high fidelity prototype, the authors tested seven patients with cancer on nine functional tasks of varying levels of complexity. From this observational study, the authors identified 27 design considerations and issues (13 for mobile apps and 14 for tablet apps) for mapping to source events, such as navigation, requests for assistance, and patient feedback. From these issues, the authors defined a set of general design recommendations that can be used when developing mobile apps for cancer. Useful design features that were highlighted include easy input and navigation prompts, good ergonomic and minimalistic design approaches (to avoid overengineering by including functions that are superfluous), and options to customize features and content placement.

The mHealth movement also has fostered an ecological monitoring approach to collecting patient-reported outcome (PRO) data more frequently, unobtrusively, and in near real time. Moreover, advances in sensor technologies embedded within mobile devices can index dynamical changes in context and behavior that are more consistent with current behavioral models that rely on intensive longitudinal data [32]. As one example, Min et al. [33] report on a feasibility study of an app for sleep disturbance-related data collection from patients with breast cancer undergoing chemotherapy. Thirty patients were given access to a smartphone app prior to their start of chemotherapy and queried via the app for self-report of sleep patterns, anxiety level, and mood changes on a daily basis for 3 months. A total of 2700 daily push notifications were sent to the 30 participants over the 3-month period. As a result, 1215 data elements on sleep disturbance were collected achieving an overall compliance rate of 45%, and the median value of individual compliance of 41.1%. Compliance dropped steadily over the trial with the low point of 13.3% at the end of 3 months. Despite the decline over time in compliance, these results indicate that use of a smartphone for behavior sampling in real-world settings is feasible even over a long period of time. Combined with a dynamical systems modeling approach, such data can provide greater understanding of changes in behavior patterns and can inform the development of more effective interventions in the future.

12.3 DEFINITION AND ROLE OF BEHAVIORAL INFORMATICS

Behavioral informatics is a subfocus of biomedical informatics which the American Medical Informatics Association (AMIA) defines as "the interdisciplinary field that studies and pursues the effective uses of biomedical data, information, and knowledge for scientific inquiry, problem solving, and decision making, driven by efforts to improve human health." Bernstam et al. [34] provide a higher level definition of biomedical informatics as the science of information as applied to or examined in the context of biomedicine. As a subdomain of biomedical informatics, behavioral informatics integrates behavioral/psychological science with computer science, engineering, cognitive science, and data science to quantify and interpret human behavior and communications. In this section, we explicate the core behavioral/psychological science principles underlying the design, development, deployment, and evaluation of HIT and informatics solutions. We begin with a

discussion of ontologies, which provide a methodology for codifying and representing knowledge from the field of behavioral medicine.

12.3.1 Behavioral Ontologies

An ontology is a description of the concepts in an application domain and the relationships among them. Ontologies are similar to, but more powerful than, terminologies, nomenclatures, or taxonomies. Terminologies and nomenclatures (also "controlled vocabularies") simply list the set of terms that are used to refer to the concepts in a given domain, similar to a dictionary [35]. Example terminologies include the International Classification of Diseases (ICD), currently maintained by the World Health Organization (WHO) for reporting mortality statistics, and the Diagnostic and Statistical Manual of Mental Disorders (DSM-5), maintained by the American Psychiatric Association, used by mental health professionals as a standard classification of mental disorders.

Taxonomies add classification hierarchies to "flat" terminologies, by introducing "is-a" relationships among concepts. For example, the process of considering behavior "pros and cons" is a kind of "comparison of outcomes" behavior change technique in which an individual is advised to identify and compare reasons for wanting (pros) and not wanting (cons) to change their behavior [36]. An example taxonomy is the *Behavior Change Taxonomy* developed by Michie et al. [36], in which 85 health behavior change techniques were clustered into a taxonomy of 16 categories by a group of experts. Fig. 12.1 shows an excerpt from this taxonomy.

Full ontologies further extend taxonomies by adding arbitrary relations among concepts, as well as a variety of additional information, such as allowed value ranges and relationship cardinality (the number of values a relationship may take on, for example "number of spouses" is generally constrained to zero or one). An example ontology of health behavior change concepts is shown in Fig. 12.2 [37]. In this ontology, constructs from the Transtheoretical Model (introduced above) of health behavior change as applied to exercise promotion are represented. This ontology not only has "is-a" taxonomic relationships (eg, "stage of change" is a kind of "therapeutic mental state"), but other kinds of relationships among concepts as well (eg, there is a "next" relation expressing the standard sequence of stages an individual goes through as they change their behavior).

Ontologies have three primary uses in behavioral informatics [37]: (1) they provide a formalism that can facilitate clarification and description of the concepts in behavioral medicine through consensus of experts (as in Michie's work [36]); (2) they can facilitate interchange of information among diverse systems by describing, at

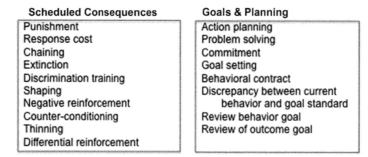

FIGURE 12.1 Excerpt from Behavior Change Taxonomy.

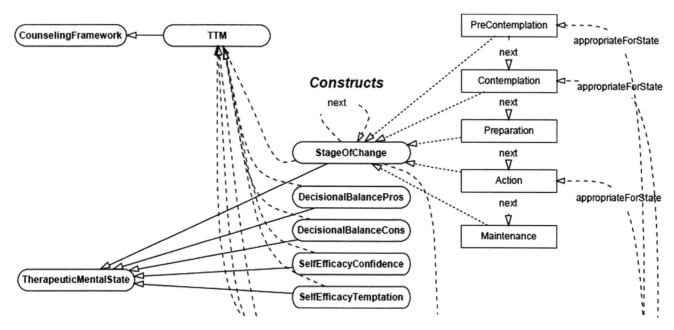

FIGURE 12.2 Excerpt from Behavior Change Ontology.

various levels of detail, the kinds of data entities that can be exchanged, independent of the particular names the entities are given in each system (the motivation for many of the terminologies in medicine, such as ICD and DSM-5); and (3) they can promote reuse of software components through the development of ontologies of the components themselves (descriptions of what the components do) and the data entities they operate on [37].

Facilitating interchange of information among disparate information systems will become increasingly important as behavioral informatics systems are developed to integrate into other parts of the medical infrastructure, for example, by integrating behavioral measures into EMRs, as noted above in the recent IOM report [28]. Ontologies are used in these exchanges to disambiguate different terms that are used in these systems to refer to the same underlying concepts. This disambiguation allows many people and institutions to share the work done by others [38], and is the motivation behind

standard interchange languages such as Health Level Seven International (HL7).

Just as importantly, ontologies can support reuse of software and knowledge in computerized health behavior change interventions in several ways. For example, many kinds of knowledge can be reused across interventions, such as which constructs are important to assess for a given health behavior change theory, which measures can be used to assess the constructs, and the specific actions the system should take to modify a given health behavior. Fig. 12.3 shows the kinds of knowledge that can be abstracted and reused in automated health behavior change interventions that interact with a user through dialog (simulated counseling conversations). Here, a Theory Model contains knowledge of the behavioral medicine theory the intervention is based on; a Behavior or BIT Model contains knowledge of how health behavior change theories are applied to a specific health behavior; a Protocol Model contains knowledge

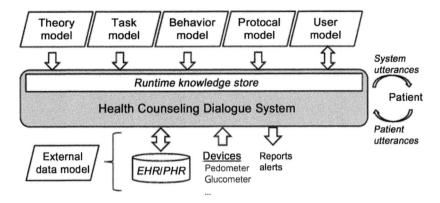

FIGURE 12.3 Reusable Knowledge in Health Counseling Dialog System.

about a particular behavior change intervention, including parameters such as duration of the intervention and expected number of user contacts per week, and ultimate behavioral criteria to be achieved; a User Model contains knowledge about a particular user, including fixed "tailoring" parameters that affect the intervention and messages, information about the user's medical condition, construct measures, and information that is dynamically updated over the course of an intervention; an External Data Model describes data inputs and outputs from the system; and finally a Task Model contains knowledge about how a health behavior change counseling system enacts the intervention, taking all of the other knowledge into account.

In one project in which a computational ontology was explicitly used to support software and knowledge reuse, an automated intervention to promote physical activity was designed using an ontology of health behavior change concepts and a suite of open-source software development tools [37]. Following a preliminary usability evaluation, the system was modified to promote fruit and vegetable consumption using only 9% of the calendar time and 4% of the person hours required to develop the initial physical activity promotion system, and demonstrated 98% reuse of the high-level software representations.

The resulting systems were evaluated in a four-arm randomized trial of a 2-month daily contact intervention comparing: (a) ACT—physical activity promotion intervention; (b) DIET—fruit and vegetable promotion intervention; (c) ACT+ DIET—both interventions; and (d) CONTROL—nonintervention control (both physical activity and fruit and vegetable consumption are associated with decreased cancer risk). A total of 122 participants were enrolled into the study and randomized among the four study arms, of which 113 (93%) completed the final 2-month assessment. Physical activity was assessed using daily pedometer steps (Omron) and the International Physical Activity Questionnaire (IPAQ) was administered at the start and end of the 2 months.

Daily servings of fruit and vegetables were assessed using the NIH/NCI self-report Fruit and Vegetable Scan (FVS). A linear mixed-effect model including effect of study day (time), study condition, and an interaction was fit to daily pedometer steps and indicated that participants in ACT increased their walking by 9.3 steps/day on average compared to CONTROL, while those in DIET decreased by 16.1 steps/day and those in ACT+ DIET decreased by 7.6 steps/day. There were no significant differences on IPAQ scores. At the end of the 2-month intervention participants in the DIET group consumed significantly more servings per day (+3.4, $p = 0.003$) of fruit and vegetables compared to those in the CONTROL group, and those in the ACT+ DIET consumed more servings per day (+2.2) compared to those in the CONTROL group (nearing significance, $p = 0.1$).

To conclude, as behavioral science matures, the architectures and ontologies for translation of the existing evidence base into the digital domain is well underway and promises to expand the reach and impact of behaviorally based interventions to improve health and health care [29,36,37].

12.4 APPLICATIONS OF BEHAVIORAL INFORMATICS RESOURCES AND TOOLS IN CANCER CARE

12.4.1 Tobacco Use and Informatics-Based Interventions

Smoking cessation enhances patient outcomes after cancer diagnosis. The most recent Surgeon's General Report on the Health Consequences of Smoking, "50 years of Progress," determined that there is sufficient evidence to conclude that continued smoking after the diagnosis of cancer is associated with adverse outcomes such as decreased survival and increased risk of second primary cancers [39]. Moreover, evidence suggests that continued smoking is associated with inferior response and increased toxicity from cancer treatments. This landmark report has shifted the paradigm of cancer care so that tobacco treatment is a necessary part of comprehensive cancer care. Unfortunately, tobacco treatment is rarely integrated into routine care despite the existence of evidence-based treatments. A US Public Health Service clinical practice guideline for tobacco dependence identifies combined use of pharmacotherapy and behavioral interventions as the best treatment for smoking cessation [40]. The effectiveness of physician counseling alone has an odds ratio (OR) for quitting of 2.2 [1.5–3.2] (95% CI) and a quit rate of 19.9% [13.7–26.2]; quit lines alone show an OR of 1.6 [1.4–1.8] and a quit rate of 12.7% [11.3–14.2]; and combination nicotine replacement therapies had an OR of 3.6 [2.5–5.2] and a quit rate of 36.5% [26.6–45.3]. Moreover, combining these therapies is more effective than individual components alone. Despite the fact that use of these interventions more than doubles cessation, there has been low uptake by clinicians and patients [41–43]. Common barriers include lack of a systematic approach to tobacco assessment and lack of knowledge related to the delivery and effectiveness of tobacco treatments [44,45].

Recent population-based analyses found that the prevalence of smoking among cancer survivors was 16–27% and 40% among those aged 18–44 years (as compared to 20.4% of the general population) [46]. Although cessation rates are high at the time of diagnosis, relapse back to smoking is common [47]. Thus, standardized and ongoing assessment is necessary to identify smokers who require assistance with their quit attempts. Systems-level interventions that use informatics resources have the potential to greatly enhance the reach and uptake of cessation interventions. Surprisingly, to our knowledge, there have only been two studies that have examined tobacco treatment interventions for patients with cancer using an informatics-based approach. Emmons et al. [48–50] developed and tested one of the only evidence-based informatics-based interventions, called the Partnership for Health (PFH) Study, that has shown efficacy to improve smoking-cessation rates among cancer survivors.

PFH is a theory-based, tailored peer-peer tobacco treatment intervention and consists of (1) print or web-based materials that provide information about the health risks of smoking in the context of cancer survivorship; (2) a report that provides feedback tailored to the interaction of smoking with risk perception, self-efficacy, motivation to quit smoking, and other topics of interest based on participant responses to an initial survey; (3) four phone calls from a peer counselor assigned to provide support during the cessation process; and (4) use of pharmacotherapy cessation aides. PFH led to a doubling in quit rates compared with usual care, and the intervention effect was sustained at 2–5 years. A second RCT was conducted to increase PFH's dissemination potential. The second PFH study compared a web and a print

format of the intervention and provided access to free pharmacotherapy. A key goal was to determine if the intervention outcomes in self-guided, scalable formats approximated those found with peer counseling. There were equivalent rates of cessation in the two PFH arms; the quit rates were equivalent to that found with peer counseling; and there were high rates of satisfaction with all of the conditions. These findings suggest that any of the PFH intervention formats could be recommended for use in practice to enhance cessation rates.

Warren et al. [51] evaluated an EMR-based intervention to determine whether automated assessment and referral could increase enrollment in a tobacco treatment program among patients being seen in a cancer care setting. The goal of this study was to design an evidence-based system that could be administered in an efficient and reproducible manner to large numbers of cancer patients. The intervention consisted of four components: (1) nurses asked patients specific standardized questions at the initial visit, during treatment and during follow-up after cancer and entered the answers into the EMR; (2) patients who reported tobacco use within the last 30 days and/ or were using a pharmacotherapy cessation aide were automatically referred to an institutional tobacco treatment program for cessation support that was generated by the EMR; (3) half of the participants received a mailing sent to their homes that discussed the benefits of cessation with an invitation to contact the tobacco treatment program; and (4) half of the participants received a telephone contact by the tobacco cessation program. Results from the study revealed that of the 1381 patients that received a mailed invitation, only 16 (1.2%) contacted the tobacco treatment program for assistance; whereas in the group that received telephone contact by the tobacco treatment program 1126 (81.4%) were contacted and of these 51 (4.5%) reported no current use of tobacco; 35 (3.1%) were medically unable to participate; and 30 (2.7%) declined participation. An important finding of the study was that three questions generated more than 98% of the referrals and 4 weeks appeared to be the optimal time for repeat tobacco assessment as this timeframe delayed referral in less than 1% of patients. Taken together, these findings suggest that tobacco treatment can be delivered to a large number of cancer patients using structured tobacco assessment and automated cessation referrals. However, contact through mail alone is insufficient for patients to engage in a tobacco treatment program.

12.4.2 Physical Activity Promotion

A number of automated interventions promote physical activity. There is clear evidence of an inverse, linear dose–response relationship between volume of physical activity and all-cause mortality rates for both men and women [52–55]. Epidemiological studies have found

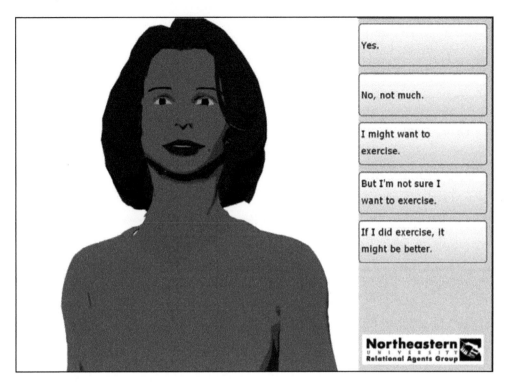

FIGURE 12.4 Virtual Exercise Coach.

reduced risk of breast, colon, and other cancers in more physically active or fit individuals [56–61]; as well as reduced mortality in individuals with cancer [62,63]. In one series of studies, "virtual coaches" have been successfully used to increase physical activity in sedentary adults, in which individuals have simulated counseling sessions with an animated counselor. In one effort, a virtual coach was linguistically and culturally tailored for a population of older, bilingual, Latino adults in either English or Spanish [64] (see Fig. 12.4). The intervention incorporated behavior change strategies based on Social Cognitive Theory and the Transtheoretical Model including self-assessment, motivationally tailored goal-setting, individualized feedback, positive reinforcement and support, and knowledge enhancement related to benefits of a physically active lifestyle. A two-arm, randomized, wait-list-control pilot evaluation study was completed. Forty participants (92.5% Latino) aged 55 and over were enrolled, half in each arm of the study. Those in the intervention group were asked to wear pedometers daily and check in three times a week for 4 months with an exercise promotion virtual coach set upon a touch screen computer in the computer room of a community center. Half of intervention group participants chose to conduct their counseling sessions in Spanish (selected by participants at enrollment time). Retention in the intervention group over the 4 months was 100%. Four-month increases in reported minutes of walking/week were greater in the virtual coach arm

(mean increase = 253.5 + 248.7 minutes/week) relative to health education (mean increase = 26.8 + 67.0 minutes/week; $p = 0.0008$). Walking increases in the virtual coach arm were substantiated via objectively measured daily steps (slope analysis $p = 0.002$).

12.4.3 Screening and Intervention for Adverse Health Behaviors and Emotional Distress

12.4.3.1 Screening for Emotional Distress and Unmet Needs

In 2008, the IOM published a report, "Cancer Care for the Whole Patient: Meeting Psychosocial Health Needs" [65]. Its authors argue that oncology's focus on extending life often comes at the expense of quality of life, and call for greater attention to patients' emotional distress, for instance, depression and anxiety, and unmet needs, for example, lack of resources or knowledge to manage illness. The IOM document fueled a then nascent psychosocial screening movement, which has since rapidly expanded, frequently on an electronic platform. In 2015, as a new requirement for accreditation, the American College of Surgeons (ACoS) Commission on Cancer (CoC) began requiring cancer centers to implement comprehensive screening programs for psychosocial distress, leaving many institutions unprepared to institute and universalize psychosocial screening, as well as the triage processes that follow from it.

TABLE 12.4 Common Screens for Emotional Distress in Oncology

Measure	Dimensions measured	Number of items	Permission needed to use	Available languages	Case finding capabilities
Distress Thermometer	*Distress	1	Yes	English, Bahasa Indonesian, Chinese, Greek, Korean, Polish, Spanish, Romanian, Swedish	No
GAD-7	*Anxiety	7	No	All major European; many Asian languages	Yes
HADS	*Anxiety *Depression	14	Yes	All major European languages; Arabic; Hebrew; Chinese; Japanese; Urdu; Farci	Yes
PHQ-9	*Depression	9	No	All major European languages; Mandarin; Oriya; Punjabi; Swahili; Tamil; Telugu; Thai; Turkish	Yes
PSSCAN	*Anxiety *Depression *Social support *Quality of life	21	No	English	Yes

Note: GAD-7, General Anxiety and Depression Scale 7-item; HADS, Hospital Anxiety and Depression Scale; PHQ-9, Patient Health Questionnaire-9; PSSCAN, Psychosocial Screen for Cancer.

At this time, clear consensus does not exist around the ideal screening instruments to use. Longer screens tend to maximize on comprehensiveness but add to patient burden. Shorter screens protect against survey fatigue but tend to lack diagnostic sensitivity and specificity [66].

In general, instruments querying emotional symptoms focus on the domains of anxiety and depression. Table 12.4 describes the most common instruments used in screening for emotional distress. Such tools include the Generalized Anxiety Disorder Symptom 7-item (GAD-7) with cutoff scores for general anxiety disorder as defined by the DSM-5; the Patient Health Questionnaire-9 (PHQ-9) with cutoff scores for major depressive disorder as defined by the DSM-5; and the Hospital Anxiety and Depression Scale (HADS) and Psychosocial Screen for Cancer (PSSCAN) in which case finds for both depression and general anxiety. By contrast, other instruments are designed to identify nonspecific "distress" rather than a DSM-5 psychiatric diagnosis. The most well-known is the one-item National Comprehensive Cancer Network (NCCN) Distress Thermometer. When such a screen is employed, additional evaluation to clarify diagnosis is warranted.

Because social stressors—financial, family, or work pressures—and physical symptoms, such as pain or dyspnea, often mediate emotional symptoms, other screens or components of screens query unmet needs. Perhaps the best known of these is the NCCN Problem List, which is a companion to the NCCN Distress Thermometer and covers family, practical, and spiritual concerns along with psychological and physical symptoms.

A variety of strategies to meet the psychosocial screening mandates and best serve the "whole patient" have been pursued. Some institutions rely on health providers to interview patients directly; others employ pen-and-pencil self-reports. However, because staffing is at

a premium and timely review of screens can be critical for the addressing of severe psychiatric distress or urgent unmet needs, electronic screen administration with instantaneous scoring is likely preferable to both options, particularly since several electronic systems now boast flagging of worrisome scores; tracking over time; automated triage capabilities; and provision of educational materials to providers and patients [66]. In recent years, several homegrown systems have been developed and a few commercial entities, for instance Polaris Health Solutions, have developed both screening platforms and applications.

12.4.4 Implementing Psychosocial Screening: An Informatics-Based Approach

As the mandate for psychosocial screening is implemented in centers throughout the country, it will be essential to have a plan in place to evaluate and treat distress. Studies have indicated that screening alone is not adequate for addressing sources of distress and improving patient outcomes [67,68]. Psychosocial screening needs to be part of a more comprehensive approach that includes further assessment and identification of the source of distress, referral to appropriate services, and initiation of evidence-based treatment [69,70].

Forsythe et al. [71] conducted a population-based study to identify how many cancer survivors discussed their psychosocial concerns with their health care providers and whether the survivors received psychosocial care services (defined as professional counseling or use of support groups). Results from this study identified that only 40% of patients reported discussion with their health care providers about their psychosocial concerns, 4.4% received psychosocial services only, and 8.9% reported both discussion with their health care providers and use of psychosocial services. Thus, this study provided important information about the implementation of psychosocial care on a population level.

As these services are implemented on a larger scale, a potential problem may be lack of an adequate number of qualified professionals to address patient psychosocial needs. Although most cancer care settings offer a range of psychosocial services to patients, many centers have fewer than three psychosocial providers [72] available to provide these services. Thus, innovative solutions are needed to prepare for the anticipated demand for services and to deliver high-quality, evidence-based psychosocial care to cancer patients. One potential partial solution is the use of evidence-based algorithms for nonbehavioral health providers to choose appropriate psychotropic medication for treatment of depression and anxiety in the oncology setting. Passik et al. [73] conducted a pilot study and demonstrated that oncologists can be empowered to recognize and treat depression with a "screen and intervene" approach using a paper-based algorithm for choosing an antidepressant treatment. Moreover, patients experienced improved mood and health-related quality of life.

Informatics-based approaches have a high potential to help fill the gap and create population-based approaches to augment delivery of psychosocial care. One example of an informatics-based system that has potential to enhance psychosocial and palliative care through CDS is the SAMI program. Cooley et al. [74] created computable algorithms for management of multiple symptoms, which included depression, anxiety, pain, fatigue, and dyspnea, based on national guidelines for use in an outpatient thoracic oncology setting. These algorithms were part of a web-based program that provided point-of-care CDS to health care providers to enhance symptom assessment and management.

The SAMI system comprises four components: (1) collection of patient-based symptom assessment data [PROs (depression, anxiety, pain, fatigue, dyspnea, comorbidities, laboratory values, prescribed medication) that were actually taken and their dose and frequency]; (2) guidelines in the form of algorithms that provide CDS for symptom management; (3) a web-service decision engine known as the System for Evidence-Based Advice through Simultaneous Transaction with an Intelligent Agent Across a Network (SEBASTIAN); and (4) a summary report for health care providers.

The *symptom assessment* component uses a web-based survey platform developed by Dana-Farber Cancer Institute for collecting PROs using validated instruments such as the PHQ-9. This application delivers questionnaires with the capacity for scoring weights and skip logic and stores the answers in a MySQL database. In the prototype, laboratory, medication, and comorbidity data are manually entered in a graphical user interface, but may be imported from an EMR in the future. The clinical decision logic is derived from guideline-based algorithms for symptom management that were adapted from national guidelines and then programmed into SEBASTIAN.

Decision rules were implemented in SEBASTIAN using an object-oriented computer programming language (Java). SEBASTIAN's web-services framework provides a scalable, system-agnostic approach to integrating knowledge into clinical practice. SEBASTIAN can receive requests for CDS capabilities from remote systems. In these requests, patient data are represented in eXtensible Markup Language (XML) format and encoded using standard terminologies. As a result, decision logic can be centralized in SEBASTIAN for use by many systems at different sites, which enables the sharing of computable knowledge across remote locations.

SYMPTOM ASSESSMENT AND MANAGEMENT (SAMI) CASE EXAMPLE

Mr Paul is a 58-year-old man diagnosed with stage III lung cancer. He currently smokes one pack of cigarettes per day and has smoked since age 12. He quit once about 5 years ago, and was able to maintain abstinence for about 6 months, but relapsed when his father died. He received chemotherapy and was scheduled to undergo surgical resection. He met with his oncologist and surgeon who both recommended that he quit smoking to improve his prognosis. Mr Paul agreed to pick a quit date, meet with a tobacco treatment counselor, and begin treatment with a 21 mg nicotine transdermal patch and 4 mg nicotine lozenge. He was scheduled to return for a follow-up visit in 3 weeks. Upon his return follow-up visit, Mr Paul completes the SAMI symptom tool and is found to have moderately severe anxiety. He quit smoking about 10 days before the visit and reported experiencing severe withdrawal symptoms. He was using the 21 mg nicotine transdermal patch but not using the lozenge related to taste aversion. He continued to smoke 2–3 cigarettes/day. He agreed to select another quit date and add bupropion to the combination nicotine replacement treatment and continue to meet with the tobacco treatment counselor to manage the nicotine withdrawal symptoms. Mr Paul's next follow-up appointment was in 3 weeks. Upon his return visit, SAMI reveals that he no longer has significant anxiety and his assessment scores were within normal range. Upon further assessment he reported that he has been tobacco free for the past 2 weeks and that his withdrawal symptoms have improved with the current pharmacotherapy regimen for tobacco control.

To generate care recommendations, four main steps are followed: (1) upon the clinician's request the SAMI client application retrieves the patient's symptoms, medications, and laboratory values from the patient database; (2) the patient data are transformed into the SEBASTIAN XML format [75]; (3) the client application submits a web-service request to a server that hosts an instance of SEBASTIAN; (4) SEBASTIAN executes a series of symptom management rules over the provided data and responds back to the client application with a set of recommendations also in XML format; and (5) the client application parses the XML recommendations and presents them to the clinicians in the SAMI user interface as a summary report consisting of text and graphics (see Fig. 12.5). As the figures show, SAMI provides tailored suggestions for evidence-based symptom management

(A)

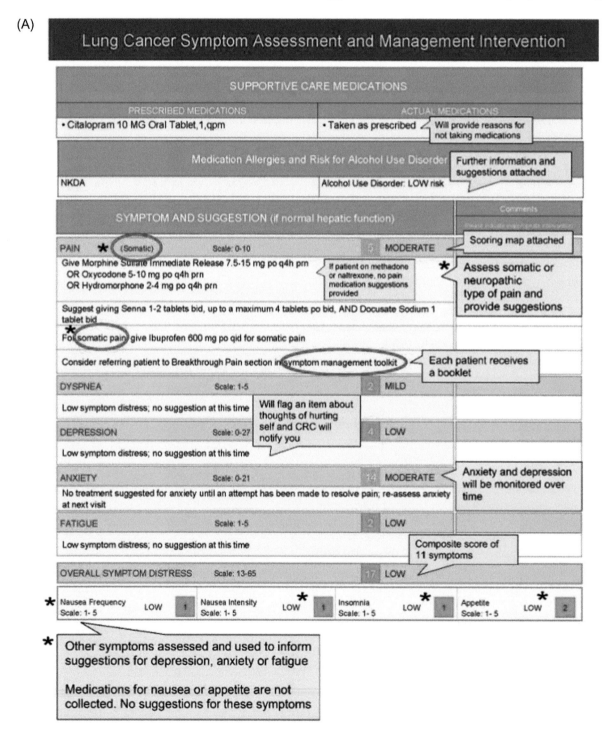

FIGURE 12.5   Lung Cancer Symptom Assessment and Management Intervention (SAMI) Report.

and a longitudinal summary of symptoms experienced over time.

SAMI was tested in a feasibility study in patients with advanced lung cancer and their clinicians and was found to be feasible [76]. Patients completed the symptom assessment at each clinic visit for 6 months and their clinicians received tailored suggestions for symptom management. Completion of assessment and delivery of reports were evaluated to assess feasibility. Patient completion of the symptom assessment was 84% (95%

CI, 81–87%) over time and delivery of the reports to clinicians was 90% (95% CI, 86–93%). Clinician adherence to the recommendations was 57% (95% CI, 52–62%). Cancer symptom management was assessed in 20 clinicians and their patients who were randomized to SAMI or usual care. A medical chart review was done to assess clinical management, defined as pharmacological management of the target symptom or use of supportive care referrals such as social work or palliative care consults, of the target symptoms [76]. Results of the study revealed that

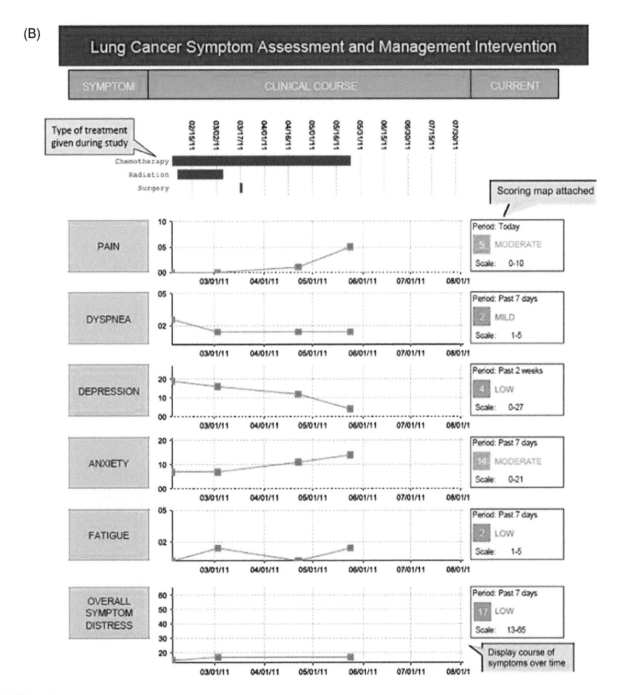

FIGURE 12.5 Continued.

the odds for clinical management of depression (1.6, 90% CI, 1.0–2.5); anxiety (1.7, 90% CI, 1.0–3.0); and fatigue (1.6, 90% CI, 1.1–2.5) were higher in the SAMI arm as compared to the usual care arm. Similarly, the odds of palliative care consults for pain (3.2, 90% CI, 0.7–13.4) appear to be higher in the SAMI arm as compared to usual care. Taken together, SAMI appeared to positively influence clinical management and increased palliative consults for pain.

12.4.5 Low Literacy Support

Oncology clinical trial protocols can be very complex, and their description, for example, in informed consent documents, can be very difficult for laypersons to understand, and almost impossible for individuals with low health literacy to fully comprehend and follow. Conversational agents—animated computer characters that simulate face-to-face conversation with a health provider—have been used to provide a medium that can be successfully deployed to help patients across the literacy spectrum understand these documents. In one series of studies, nurse–patient interactions were modeled in a conversational agent that could explain research informed consent documents to patients. In these studies, participants with inadequate health literacy had significantly higher levels of satisfaction with the agent compared to either a human research assistant explaining the document to them or a self-study condition ($F(1,14) = 5.0$, $p<0.05$) [77]. Follow-up studies characterized more details of nurse and research assistant behavior when explaining documents to individuals with different levels of health literacy, describing explanation strategies, hand gestures, and gaze behavior used, and how these varied for patients of varying health literacy levels [78].

A later study evaluated these mediums, demonstrating that study participants who had received an automated explanation of a research informed consent document by an agent had the same level of comprehension of the document compared to a group who received explanation by a human research assistant ($F(2,23) = 4.41$, $p<0.05$), regardless of health literacy level, and that all participants were more satisfied with the agent-based explanation ($F(2,23) = 4.78$, $p<0.05$) [79]. Qualitative interviews indicated that the increased satisfaction was due to participants feeling less pressured and less inferior in their interactions with the agent compared to those with a human.

Another series of studies evaluated a web-based conversational agent that helped cancer patients with low-literacy find cancer-related clinical trials of interest to them. Most cancer patients are unaware that there are clinical trials they can participate in [80], and other studies have demonstrated numerous barriers individuals face in finding trials they are eligible for Ref. [81]. Several web-based search engines have been developed to increase participation in clinical trials by allowing users to more easily find trials. However, these search engines may be difficult for individuals with low health and computer literacy to navigate. One study found that a state-of-the-art web-based search engine (NCI [82]) was unusable by participants with inadequate health literacy, who were only able to complete 0.43 of the three standardized tasks given on average (participants with adequate health literacy completed 1.17 tasks on average) [83].

To address these issues, a conversational agent interface was designed to interview cancer patients about their preferences and present candidate clinical trials to them in an incremental way, with numerous features to enhance understandability of the trial protocols. An evaluation study involving 87 cancer patients (26% inadequate health literacy) found that all participants were significantly more satisfied with the conversational agent-based search interface compared to the conventional search interface, and that low literacy participants exhibited better search performance and felt less pressure to enroll for studies when using the conversational agent [84].

12.5 CONCLUSIONS

The behavioral sciences offer a treasure-trove of systematic evidence that can be leveraged to advance oncology informatics and improve cancer prevention and control. The continued development of behavioral ontologies holds great promise in harmonizing disparate theories and models of behavior change with respect to determining the active components of interventions; reusing representations and resources in programming new applications; and promoting collaboration across disciplines of biomedical informatics, behavioral medicine, and computation linguistics [37]. One direct benefit of creating robust ontologies is the potential for embedding the formalisms as core elements of behavioral measures and metrics within EHRs. With respect to cancer prevention and treatment, health counseling dialog and symptom assessment and management systems can benefit from this integration and enable advanced decision support at the point of care. Sophisticated ontologies can represent actionable knowledge within the electronic record, support personalization processes at multiple levels, detect anomalous circumstances, such as missed diagnoses or comorbidities, that would require adjustment to standard interventions, and enhance health outcomes [85].

The emergence of more innovative research methods and designs is important for accommodating the rapidly evolving mHealth movement and approaches like the BIT Model offer a way to address major societal issues like tobacco cessation, obesity, and medication and treatment adherence for cancer control. A more "agile science" approach that is iterative and personalized is likely to meet the clarion call today for "precision medicine" that enables interventions that can be individualized and adapt to context, circumstances, and preferences (www.agilscience.org).

Consumer and patient-facing technologies that are built upon solid behavioral/psychological science principles and that take advantage of the burgeoning presence of mobile devices can go a long way to support informed and shared decision making [21]. The uptake of mobile technologies has accelerated in the last few years to where an estimated 64% of the US population owns a smartphone (http://www.pewinternet.org/fact-sheets/mobile-technology-fact-sheet/). This mobile platform is ideally suited for developing and deploying targeted apps with specific functionalities that address the challenges faced by patients with cancer. Recently, Apple announced the release of ResearchKit (https://www.apple.com/researchkit/) as an open-source platform and ecosystem for implementation of research studies that could revolutionize the ability to recruit and enroll patients into clinical trials at a rate and scale that is unprecedented. One such app that was included in the initial six released focuses on the recruitment of women who have survived breast cancer (http://sharethejourneyapp.org/). The *Share the Journey: Mind, Body and Wellness After Breast Cancer* app tracks five common issues related to breast cancer treatment: fatigue, cognitive difficulties, sleep disturbances, mood changes, and reduction in exercise performance. The overall purpose is to collect longitudinal information from these patients about variations in their symptoms over time to better understand the long-term effects of the disease. ResearchKit and other open-source platforms like it are the vanguard of new frameworks for hosting patient-centered tools and resources that enable participatory research, self-management, and decision support on a massive scale.

We have provided exemplars of informatics platforms and tools for tobacco cessation among cancer survivors, distress screening, physical activity promotion, and an automated approach for low literacy support. These are but a few examples of the promising application of behavioral/psychological science principles to the design, development, and evaluation of informatics solutions in oncology. The convergence of behavioral/psychological science and technology affords enormous opportunities to address the increasing burden of cancer prevention and control. The future success of oncology informatics is predicated on drawing from the best available scientific evidence from biomedicine and behavioral sciences as complementary resources.

LIST OF ACRONYMS AND ABBREVIATIONS

AMIA The American Medical Informatics Association
CHI Consumer health informatics
EHR Electronic health record
EMR Electronic medical record
HIE Health Information Exchange
HIT Health Information Technology
HITECH Health Information Technology for Economic and Clinical Health Act
IOM Institute of Medicine
NCI National Cancer Institute
NIH National Institutes of Health

References

[1] Fisher E, Fitzgibbon M, Glasgow R, Haire-Joshu D, Hayman L, Kaplan R, et al. Behavior matters. Am J Prevent Med 2011;40(5):e15–30.

[2] Medicine SoB. Field of behavioral medicine historical time-line: society of behavioral medicine; 2014. Available from: <http://www.sbm.org/UserFiles/file/Historyofbehavioral medicinetimeline4-18-14.jpg>.

[3] Ritterband LM, Thorndike FP, Cox DJ, Kovatchev BP, Gonder-Frederick LA. A behavior change model for internet interventions. Ann Behav Med 2009;38(1):18–27.

[4] Abrams DB, Mills S, Bulger D. Challenges and future directions for tailored communication research. Ann Behav Med 1999;21(4):299–306.

[5] Prochaska JO, DiClemente CC, Velicer WF, Rossi JS. Standardized, individualized, interactive, and personalized self-help programs for smoking cessation. Health Psychol 1993;12(5):399.

[6] Ahern DK, Patrick K, Phalen JM, Neiley JD. An introduction to methodological challenges in the evaluation of eHealth research: perspectives from the Health e-Technologies Initiative. Eval Program Plann 2006;29(4):386–9.

[7] Hesse BW, Beckjord E, Rutten LJF, Fagerlin A, Cameron LD. Cancer communication and informatics research across the cancer continuum. Am Psychol 2015;70(2):198.

[8] Pingree S, Hawkins R, Baker T, DuBenske L, Roberts LJ, Gustafson DH. The value of theory for enhancing and understanding e-health interventions. Am J Prevent Med 2010;38(1):103–9.

[9] Hesse B. Enhancing consumer involvement in health care. In: Parker JC, Thorson E, editors. Healthcare communication in the new media landscape. New York: Springer; 2008.

[10] Prochaska JO, Marcus BH. The transtheoretical model: applications to exercise Dishman RK, editor. Advances in exercise adherence. Champaign, IL: Human Kinetics; 1994. p. 161–80.

[11] Bandura A. Social foundations of thought and action. Englewood Cliffs, NJ: Prentice-Hall; 1986.

[12] Michie S, Van Stralen MM, West R. The behaviour change wheel: a new method for characterising and designing behaviour change interventions. Implement Sci 2011;6(42):11.

[13] Riley WT, Rivera DE, Atienza AA, Nilsen W, Allison SM, Mermelstein R. Health behavior models in the age of mobile interventions: are our theories up to the task? Transl Behav Med 2011;1(1):53–71.

[14] Baskerville NB, Struik LL, Hammond D, Guindon GE, Norman CD, Whittaker R, et al. Effect of a mobile phone intervention on quitting smoking in a young adult population of smokers: randomized controlled trial study protocol. JMIR Res Protoc 2015;4(1):e10.

[15] Mohr DC, Schueller SM, Montague E, Burns MN, Rashidi P. The Behavioral Intervention Technology model: an integrated conceptual and technological framework for eHealth and mHealth interventions. J Med Internet Res 2014;16(6):e146.

[16] A behavior model for persuasive designFogg BJ, editor. Proceedings of the fourth international conference on persuasive technology. New York: ACM; 2009.

[17] Mohr DC, Cheung K, Schueller SM, Brown CH, Duan N. Continuous evaluation of evolving Behavioral Intervention Technologies. Am J Prevent Med 2013;45(4):517–23.

[18] Pagoto S, Bennett GG. How behavioral science can advance digital health. Transl Behav Med 2013;3(3):271–6.

[19] Hesse B, Ahern D, Woods S. Nudging best practice: the HITECH act and behavioral medicine. Transl Behav Med 2011;1(1):175–81.

[20] Dykes PC, Carroll DL, Hurley A, Lipsitz S, Benoit A, Chang F, et al. Fall prevention in acute care hospitals: a randomized trial. JAMA 2010;304(17):1912–8.

[21] Ahern D, Woods S, Lightolwer M, Finley S, Houston T. Promise of and potential for patient-facing technologies to enable meaningful use. Am J Prevent Med 2011;40(5S2):S162–72.

[22] Valdez RS, Holden RJ, Novak LL, Veinot TC. Transforming consumer health informatics through a patient work framework: connecting patients to context. J Am Med Inform Assoc 2014. http://dx.doi.org/10.1136/amiajnl-2014-002826.

[23] Klein WMP, Bloch M, Hesse BW, McDonald PG, Nebeling L, O'Connell ME, et al. Behavioral research in cancer prevention and control: a look to the future. Am J Prevent Med 2014;46(3):303–11.

[24] Kannampallil TG, Franklin A, Mishra R, Almoosa KF, Cohen T, Patel VL. Understanding the nature of information seeking behavior in critical care: implications for the design of Health Information Technology. Artif Intell Med 2013;57(1):21–9.

[25] Reyna VF, Nelson WL, Han PK, Pignone MP. Decision making and cancer. Am Psychol 2015;70(2):105.

[26] Reyna VF. A theory of medical decision making and health: fuzzy trace theory. Med Decis Making 2008;28:850–65.

[27] Estabrooks PA, Boyle M, Emmons KM, Glasgow RE, Hesse BW, Kaplan RM, et al. Harmonized patient-reported data elements in the electronic health record: supporting meaningful use by primary care action on health behaviors and key psychosocial factors. J Am Med Inform Assoc 2012;19:575–82.

[28] Institute of Medicine Capturing social and behavioral domains and measures in electronic health records phase 2. Washington, DC: The National Academies Press; 2014.

[29] Michie S, Ashford S, Sniehotta FF, Dombrowski SU, Bishop A, French DP. A refined taxonomy of behaviour change techniques to help people change their physical activity and healthy eating behaviours: the CALO-RE taxonomy. Psychol Health 2011;26(11):1479–98.

[30] Vodopivec-Jamsek V, de Jongh T, Gurol-Urganci I, Atun R, Car J. Mobile phone messaging for preventive health care. Cochrane Database Syst Rev 2012;12:Cd007457.

[31] Mirkovic J, Kaufman DR, Ruland CM. Supporting cancer patients in illness management: usability evaluation of a mobile app. JMIR MHealth UHealth 2014;2(3):e33.

[32] Timms KP, Rivera DE, Collins LM, Piper ME. A dynamical systems approach to understanding self-regulation in smoking cessation behavior change. Nicotine Tob Res 2014;16(Suppl. 2):S159–68.

[33] Min YH, Lee JW, Shin YW, Jo MW, Sohn G, Lee JH, et al. Daily collection of self-reporting sleep disturbance data via a smartphone app in breast cancer patients receiving chemotherapy: a feasibility study. J Med Internet Res 2014;16(5):e135.

[34] Bernstam EV, Smith JW, Johnson TR. What is biomedical informatics? J Biomed Inform 2010;43(1):104–10.

[35] Gruninger M, Bodenreider O, Olken F, Obrst L, Yim P. Ontology summit 2007–ontology, taxonomy, folksonomy: understanding the distinctions. Appl Ontol 2008;3:191–200.

[36] Michie S, Richardson M, Johnston M, Abraham C, Francis J, Hardeman W, et al. The behavior change technique taxonomy (v1) of 93 hierarchically clustered techniques: building an international consensus for the reporting of behavior change interventions. Ann Behav Med 2013;46(1):81–95.

[37] Bickmore T, Schulman D, Sidner C. A reusable framework for health counseling dialogue systems based on a behavioral medicine ontology. J Biomed Inform 2011;44:183–97.

[38] Hammond W, Jaffe C, Cimino J, Huff S. Standards in biomedical informatics Shortliffe EH, Cimino J, editors. Biomedical informatics: computer applications in health care and biomedicine. New York: Springer; 2013. p. 211–54.

[39] Services USDoHaH The health consequences of smoking—50 years of progress: a report of the Surgeon General. Atlanta, GA: US Department of Health and Human Services, Centers for Disease Control and Prevention, National Center for Chronic Disease Prevention and Health Promotion, Office on Smoking and Health; 2014.17.

[40] Fiore M, Jaen CR, Baker T, Bailey W, Benowitz N, Curry S, et al. Treating tobacco use and dependence: 2008 update. Rockville, MD: Public Health Service; 2008.

[41] Warren GW, Marshall JR, Fau-Cummings KM, Cummings KM, Fau-Toll BA, Gritz ER, et al. Addressing tobacco use in patients with cancer: a survey of American Society of Clinical Oncology members (1935–469X (Electronic)).

[42] Cooley ME, Emmons Km Fau-Haddad R, Haddad R, Fau-Wang Q, Wang Q, Fau-Posner M, et al. Patient-reported receipt of and interest in smoking-cessation interventions after a diagnosis of cancer (1097–0142 (Electronic)).

[43] Emmons KM, Sprunck-Harrild K, Fau-Puleo E, Puleo E, Fau-de Moor J, de Moor J. Provider advice about smoking cessation and pharmacotherapy among cancer survivors who smoke: practice guidelines are not translating (1869–6716 (Print)).

[44] Duffy SA., Louzon Sa Fau-Gritz ER, Gritz ER. Why do cancer patients smoke and what can providers do about it? (1548–5315 (Print)).

[45] Sarna LP, Brown Jk Fau-Lillington L, Lillington L, Fau-Rose M, Rose M Fau-Wewers ME, et al. Tobacco interventions by oncology nurses in clinical practice: report from a national survey (0008–543X (Print)).

[46] Underwood JM, Townsend JS, Tai E, White A, Davis SP, Fairley TL. Persistent cigarette smoking and other tobacco use after a tobacco-related cancer diagnosis. J Cancer Surviv Res Pract 2012;6(3):333–44.

[47] Cooley ME, Sarna L, Kotlerman J, Lukanich JM, Jaklitsch M, Green SB, et al. Smoking cessation is challenging even for patients recovering from lung cancer surgery with curative intent. Lung Cancer 2009;66(2):218–25.

[48] Emmons KM, Puleo E, Fau-Mertens A, Mertens A, Fau-Gritz ER, Gritz Er Fau-Diller L, et al. Long-term smoking cessation outcomes among childhood cancer survivors in the Partnership for Health Study (1527–7755 (Electronic)).

[49] Emmons KM, Puleo E, Fau-Sprunck-Harrild K, Sprunck-Harrild K, Fau-Ford J, Ford J, et al. Partnership for health-2, a web-based versus print smoking cessation intervention for childhood and young adult cancer survivors: randomized comparative effectiveness study (1438–8871 (Electronic)).

[50] Emmons KM, Puleo E, Fau-Park E, Park E, Fau-Gritz ER, Gritz Er Fau-Butterfield RM, et al. Peer-delivered smoking counseling for childhood cancer survivors increases rate of cessation: the partnership for health study (0732–183X (Print)).

[51] Warren GW, Marshall JR, Cummings KM, Zevon MA, Reed R, Hysert P, et al. Automated tobacco assessment and cessation support for cancer patients. Cancer 2014;120(4):562–9.

[52] Hakim A, Petrovitch H, Brurchfiel C, Ross G, Rodriguez B, White L, et al. Effects of walking on mortality among nonsmoking retired men. N Engl J Med 1998;338:94–9.

[53] Hirvensalo M, Rantanen T, Heikkinen E. Mobility difficulties and physical activity as predictors of mortality and loss of independence in the community-living older population. J Am Geriatr Soc 2000;48:493–8.

[54] Kushi L, Fee R, Folsom A, Mink P, Anderson K, Sellers T. Physical activity and mortality in postmenopausal women. JAMA 1997;277:1287–92.

[55] Finucane P, Giles L, Withers R, et al. Exercise profile and subsequen mortality in an elderly Australian population. Aust J Public Health 1997;21:155–8.

[56] Carlons J, Ostir G, Black S, Markides K, Rudkin L, Goodwin J. Disability in older adults 2: physical activity as prevention. Behav Med 1999;24:157–68.

[57] Miller M, Rejeski W, Reboussin B, Ten Have T, Ettinger W. Physical activity, functional limitations, and disability in older adults. J Am Geriatr Soc 2000;48:1264–72.

[58] Huber H, Block D, Fries J. Risk factors for physical disability in an aging cohort: the NHANES I epidemiologic followup study. J Rheumatol 1993;20:480–8.

[59] Huang Y, Macera C, Blair S, Brill P, Kohl H, Kronenfeld J. Physical fitness, physical activity, and functional limitation in adults aged 40 and older. Med Sci Sports Exerc 1998;30:1430–5.

[60] Schmid D, Behrens G, Keimling M, Jochem C, Ricci C, Leitzmann M. A systematic review and meta-analysis of physical activity and endometrial cancer risk. Eur J Epidemiol 2015;30:397–412.

[61] Biswas A, Oh P, Faulkner G, Bajaj R, Silver M, Mitchell M, et al. Sedentary time and its association with risk for disease incidence, mortality, and hospitalization in adults: a systematic review and meta-analysis. Ann Int Med 2015;162:23–132.

[62] Otto S, Korfage I, Polinder S, van der Heide A, de Vries E, Rietjens J, et al. Association of change in physical activity and body weight with quality of life and mortality in colorectal cancer: a systematic review and meta-analysis. Support Care Cancer 2015;23(5):1237–50.

[63] Lahart I, Metsios G, Nevill A, Carmichael A. Physical activity, risk of death and recurrence in breast cancer survivors: a systematic review and meta-analysis of epidemiological studies. Acta Oncol 2015;54:635–54.

[64] King A, Bickmore T, Campero I, Pruitt L, Yin L. Employing 'Virtual Advisors' to promote physical activity in underserved communities: results from the compass study. Ann Behav Med 2011;41(Suppl. 1):S58.

[65] Adler NE, Page AEK. Cancer care for the whole patient: meeting psychosocial health needs. Washington, DC: The National Academies Press; 2008. 456 p.

[66] Bower JE, Bak K, Berger A, Breitbart W, Escalante CP, Ganz PA, et al. Screening, assessment, and management of fatigue in adult survivors of cancer: an American Society of Clinical oncology clinical practice guideline adaptation. J Clin Oncol 2014;32(17):1840–50.

[67] Carlson LE, Groff SL, Maciejewski O, Bultz BD. Screening for distress in lung and breast cancer outpatients: a randomized controlled trial. J Clin Oncol 2010. http://dx.doi.org/10.1200/JCO.2009.27.3698.

[68] Gilbody S, Bower P, Fletcher J, Richards D, Sutton AJ. Collaborative care for depression: a cumulative meta-analysis and review of longer-term outcomes. Arch Intern Med 2006;166(21):2314–21.

[69] Carlson LE, Waller A, Groff SL, Bultz BD. Screening for distress, the sixth vital sign, in lung cancer patients: effects on pain, fatigue, and common problems—secondary outcomes of a randomized controlled trial. Psychooncology 2013;22(8):1880–8.

[70] Lazenby M, Ercolano E, Grant M, Holland JC, Jacobsen PB, McCorkle R. Supporting Commission on Cancer-mandated psychosocial distress screening with implementation strategies. J Oncol Pract 2015;2014:002816.

[71] Forsythe LP, Alfano CM, Leach CR, Ganz PA, Stefanek ME, Rowland JH. Who provides psychosocial follow-up care for post-treatment cancer survivors? A survey of medical oncologists and primary care physicians. J Clin Oncol 2012;30(23):2897–905.

[72] Deshields T, Zebrack B, Kennedy V. The state of psychosocial services in cancer care in the United States. Psychooncology 2013;22(3):699–703.

[73] Passik SD, Kirsh KL, Theobald D, Donaghy K, Holtsclaw E, Edgerton S, et al. Use of a depression screening tool and a fluoxetine-based algorithm to improve the recognition and treatment of depression in cancer patients: a demonstration project. J Pain Symptom Manage 2002;24(3):318–27.

[74] Cooley ME, Lobach DF, Johns E, Halpenny B, Saunders T-A, Del Fiol G, et al. Creating computable algorithms for symptom management in an outpatient thoracic oncology setting. J Pain Symptom Manage 2013;46(6):911–24. e1.

[75] Kawamoto K, Lobach DF, editors. Design, implementation, use, and preliminary evaluation of SEBASTIAN, a standards-based web service for clinical decision support. In: AMIA Annual Symposium; 2005.

[76] Cooley ME, Blonquist TM, Catalano PJ, Lobach DF, Halpenny B, McCorkle R, et al. Feasibility of using algorithm-based clinical decision support for symptom assessment and management in lung cancer. J Pain Symptom Manage 2015;49(1):13–26.

[77] Bickmore T, Pfeifer L, Paasche-Orlow M. Health document explanation by virtual agents. In: 7th international conference on Intelligent Virtual Agents, Paris, September 17–19; 2007. p. 183–96.

[78] Bickmore T, Pfeifer L, Yin L. The Role of gesture in document explanation by embodied conversational agents. Int J Semant Comput 2008;2(1):47–70.

[79] Bickmore T, Pfeifer L, Paasche-Orlow M. Using computer agents to explain medical documents to patients with low health literacy. Patient Educ Couns 2009;75(3):315–20.

[80] Harris Interactive Misconceptions and lack of awareness greatly reduce recruitment for cancer clinical trials. Health Care News 2001;1:1–3.

[81] Ross S, Grant A, Counsell C, Gillespie W, Russell I, Prescott R. Barriers to participation in randomised controlled trials: a systematic review. J Clin Epidemiol 1999;52:1143–56.

[82] Atkinson N, Saperstein S, Massett H, Leonard C, Grama L, Manrow R. Using the Internet to search for cancer clinical trials: a comparative audit of clinical trial search tools. Contemp Clin Trials 2008;29:555–64.

[83] Utami D, Bickmore TW, Barry B, Paasche-Orlow MK. Health literacy and usability of clinical trial search engines. J Health Commun 2014;19(Suppl. 2):190–204.

[84] Bickmore T, Utami D, Matsuyama R, Paasche-Orlow M. Improving Access to Online Health Information With Conversational Agents: A Randomized Controlled Experiment. J Med Internet Res 2016;81(1).

[85] RiañO D, Real F, LóPez-Vallverdú JA, Campana F, Ercolani S, Mecocci P, et al. An ontology-based personalization of healthcare knowledge to support clinical decisions for chronically ill patients. J Biomed Inform 2012;45(3):429–46.

13

Communication Science: Connecting Systems for Health

Bradford W. Hesse PhD[1], Neeraj K. Arora PhD[2] and
William Klein PhD[3]

[1]Health Communication and Informatics Research Branch, Division of Cancer Control and
Population Sciences, National Cancer Institute, Rockville, MD, United States [2]Improving Healthcare
Systems, Patient-Centered Outcomes Research Institute, Washington, DC, United States
[3]Behavioral Research Program, Division of Cancer Control and Population Sciences,
National Cancer Institute, Rockville, MD, United States

O U T L I N E

13.1 The Communication Revolution   253
   13.1.1 Communication Science   254
   13.1.2 An Inventory of Informatics Tools for
      Improving Communication   255

13.2 Using Communication Science to Improve
   Quality of Cancer Care   260
   13.2.1 A Case Study of Communication Error
      in Oncology   260
   13.2.2 When Cancer Communication Goes Awry   261
   13.2.3 Ten Rules for Realigning Health Care   262

13.3 A Functional Approach to Patient-Centered
   Communication   263

13.3.1 Fostering Healing Relationships   263
13.3.2 Exchanging Information   264
13.3.3 Making Decisions   265
13.3.4 Enabling Self-Management   267
13.3.5 Coping With Emotions   269
13.3.6 Managing Uncertainty   270

13.4 Conclusion   271

List of Acronyms and Abbreviations   272

References   272

Those of us with multiple chronic conditions may consult many physicians in the course of a year. Last year, I saw 11. Not one of my doctors has ever communicated directly with another, despite the fact that some of them work in the same health system and have offices in the same building. I am the sole arbiter of who gets what information in what format and when. [1] **Jessie C. Gruman, President and Founder, Center for Advancing Health.**

13.1 THE COMMUNICATION REVOLUTION

In this chapter, we explore the intricacies of an informatics infused care system that is itself becoming a redesigned architecture for new patterns of communication in an era when oncology care is becoming more complex, integrated, demanding, and precise. We engage in this review at a time when a revolution in communication

B. Hesse, D. Ahern & E. Beckjord: Oncology Informatics.
DOI: http://dx.doi.org/10.1016/B978-0-12-802115-6.00013-6

technologies has been resculpting the foundations of a global economy [2], with new roles and communication patterns emerging across multiple industries as part of the digitally mediated information environment. We have watched as, one-by-one, these new communication technologies have augmented and enhanced social systems across many sectors of the economy. It is hard now to imagine what a global marketplace might look like without a global infrastructure for communications; or to picture a modern multinational airline industry that did not support users with individual access to electronic ticketing systems, reservation tools, and flight status information. It is hard to think of what a financial system might look like without quick and easy access to an interoperable network of automated teller machines and online account access, or how a restaurant might survive in this connected era without online advertising and computer-mediated reservation systems. These new capabilities have become the new normal in American life [3]. They also offer to revolutionize cancer oncology care [4].

At the same time, we recognize that any significant change in social processes and technology will most certainly bring with it a whole new spate of unexpected consequences [5]. The ease with which people can now communicate with each other using email, text-messaging, social media, and a host of other channels has led to an inundation of information through unwanted email (ie, spam), bewildering "friend requests," and a cacophony of mixed news messages. Not surprisingly, we've seen medical departments struggle with these same changes as email and electronic reminders clog the system before a new, compensated workflow is devised [6].

In 2001, at the height of the "dot.com" boom, we watched as the tech-heavy NASDAQ plunged and company after company fell by the wayside as their potentially innovative technologies failed to produce a viable business plan. Out of the ashes of the "dot.com implosion" we watched as a new slate of very successful companies began to thrive. What we saw was a transition from a Web 1.0 first version of the online economy based on traditional publishing and transactional models, to a new Web 2.0 version of online service centered on mass participation cultivated around norms of social trust. We have also watched the emergence of a Health 2.0 culture in which patient-engagement has become the new foundation upon which to base consumer-facing services [7], and we are watching as medical informaticists work diligently to bring health information technologies from their status as a "Gen 1" technology to "Gen 2" [6].

Our purpose throughout this review will be to identify the commensurate opportunities available to practitioners, insurers, policy makers, informaticists, and patients for improving the efficacy and reliability of their communication channels through informatics applications to serve the needs of a 21st-century oncology care system. Communication errors, as we will discover, are at the heart of many of the medical mishaps that cause negative consequences in care delivery for patients and the medical teams who care for them. Moreover, the sheer complexity of care in the new oncology environment coupled with the projected increases in volume means that it will be impossible to rely solely on traditional means of communication to cover the demands of the new oncology system. Anachronistic communication protocols, many of which are responsible for the current raft of error experienced throughout the system anyway, will likely fail to realize the Institute of Medicine's (IOM's) vision for safe, effective care [8]. In fact, under assumptions of increased demand, status quo habits may only compound the problem by perpetuating more errors, alienating patients, and demoralizing care teams. As with other topics covered by this book, the trick will be to create a new mix of technologies, people, and processes that as a whole achieve sustainable gains. This will take experimentation in new health care practices, informed by an awareness of how the science of communication can inform design.

13.1.1 Communication Science

Communication science, as it is used in this chapter, refers to the interdisciplinary mix of theory and empirical evidence that contributes to a more informed understanding of how humans convey information to each other across multiple channels, in multiple contexts, and in differing timeframes to achieve desired goals. In the context of health, communication assumes a vital role in "informing, influencing, and motivating individual, institutional, and public audiences about important health issues" [9]. Early models of health communication emphasized the role of mass media as a unidirectional channel for elevating awareness and motivating action. With the diffusion of Internet technologies, those models have expanded to encompass the one-to-one, one-to-many, many-to-many, and cognitively augmented capacities of computer-mediated communication channels [10,11]. Indeed, because of its centrality to health the US Office of Disease Prevention and Health Promotion included a separate objective within its Healthy People 2020 initiative on the topic of "health communication and health information technology."

One way to think about the process of communication in the context of an informatics-enabled health care system is to consider the interdefining attributes that comprise any instance of communication activity [12]. We illustrate this conceptualization in Fig. 13.1. From the figure, communication processes can be viewed as occurring within and across specific *environments*, as occurring between specific *people* or actors, and as

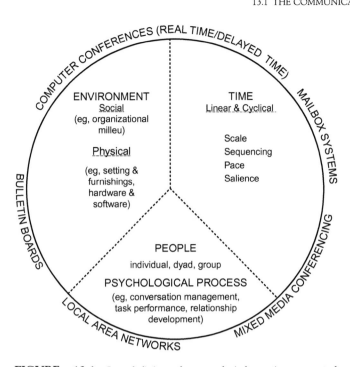

FIGURE 13.1 Interdefining facets of informatics-supported communication.

having identifiable *temporal* qualities. We consider each of those dimensions below.

- The *environments* in which cancer communication may unfold can include face-to-face conversations within the clinic or, in a mediated sense, can occur over a telephone or smartphone as one party engages in a virtual consultation with the other. An informatics intervention will usually allow health systems designers to reengineer the communication environment to achieve more effective care, or to save time and money by economizing on the use of expensive clinical settings. For some applications, the informatics structures may serve as the medium through which interaction occurs. In others, they may serve as a prompting mechanism to trigger face-to-face interactions as needed by the patient or patient's family.
- The *people* component of the communication may be restricted to the patient and oncologist, or the interaction could be broadened to include members of an interdisciplinary care team on the health care provider's side, or significant others and caregivers on the patient's side. We have included the psychological processes that govern behavior and decision making as an integral aspect of this people-related aspect of communication. As we shall see, many eHealth applications were designed using behavioral theory to augment the cognitive processes underlying effective decision making or to nudge behavior toward a desired, healthier goal.

- The *temporal* attribute of the framework is included to acknowledge that all communications unfold over time, and that time matters when it comes to thinking about disease processes and preemptive care. Temporal qualities include the *scale* of the interaction, expressed as a duration for interactions that occur over a short (eg, acute) or longer (chronic) timeframe; the *sequencing* of interactions over time, or the order in which events can or should unfold; the *pace* of the interaction, that is the slowness or rapidity of events; and the *salience* of past, present, or future activities embedded within the communication.

Informatics innovations support improvements to health care processes by offering solutions that reconfigure the profile of these interdefining facets in safer, more efficient, and effective ways [13]. For example, traditional medicine required providers and patients to be in the same space with each other to monitor vital signs or to examine a physical condition first hand. That would either necessitate a trip by the patient to a clinical facility for examination, an expensive proposition for someone living in a remote area, or it would require medical personnel to visit the patient onsite through a house call or emergency field visit. In the 1970s the carrying capacity of telecommunications expanded broadly enough to carry video signals, acoustically modulated computer signals, facsimile signals, and electronic messaging so that health care designers could begin experimenting with techniques for connecting patients in isolated, rural environments to medical practitioners living miles away [14].

Using the augmented capacities of the new telecommunications infrastructures, medical staff found that it was possible to obtain consults for remotely practicing physicians by linking their rural offices to urban facilities through video conferencing, faxing, and long-distance conversation. The innovation would serve to shorten the scale of communications by connecting the right people together across geographic distances without requiring either party to travel physically. It would save money, reduce the risks of a delayed diagnosis, and would extend capacity into otherwise underserved environments [15]. Of course, virtual visits would never be sufficient to support all of a patient's needs. Many of the patients' interpersonal trust and psycho-oncological needs would warrant face-to-face interactions. Programmatic research began emphasizing a balance, rather than a supplantation, of face-to-face and virtual visits as needed to meet patients' needs. Research on telemedicine was born.

13.1.2 An Inventory of Informatics Tools for Improving Communication

Much has been added to the armamentarium of oncology since the early days of telemedicine. The eHealth revolution of the 1990s placed an emphasis on exploiting Internet-related technologies to serve consumers' needs directly through web applications and computer apps. The mHealth revolution of the mid-2000s expanded geophysical access to information from home desk-top computers to the always-on, always-present ubiquity of mobile devices. Wireless sensors expanded support even further by offering the ability to transmit data from implanted medical devices (eg, implanted cardiac defibrillators) and at-home equipment (eg, blood glucose monitors) to support collaborative monitoring of patients' conditions remotely.

Meanwhile, the price of personal videoconferencing through smartphones and webcams has fallen. The *meaningful use* incentives from the Health Information Technology for Economic and Clinical Health Act (HITECH Act) have pushed for the adoption of health information technologies that would improve continuity of care and patient engagement, both of which have substantial communication components. In Table 13.1, we provide a list of just some of the types of informatics application that have begun to emerge in the marketplace. We consider each in terms of the environment in which they are commonly deployed; the supports they put in place for people; and the ways in which they alter the temporal fabric of communications.

Communication management systems. We begin at the top of the table with the notion of "communication management systems" as the first broad category afforded by fully functional informatics systems. As we introduce this concept, we refer to the capacities built into many fully functional electronic health record (EHR) platforms to keep track of the messages and required communications needed to ensure the efficient flow of information across the enterprise. Management systems are distinct, not because they host communications directly (though they may be responsible for issuing prompts and reminders), but because they offer the capability to assure *preemptively* that unsafe communication gaps *do not* occur.

Take as an example the use of administrative "dashboards"—the executive display systems that allow

TABLE 13.1　Informatics Enabled Communication Tools Expressed in Terms of Environment, People, and Temporal Attributes

Informatics application	Mechanism of action		
	Environment	People	Temporal
Communication management systems	• Multilevel tracking through reminders, dashboards, EHRs • Physician ordering systems assure electronic synchronization and error checking for orders	• Management support for patient navigators, physicians, hospitals • External memory aids—akin to "checklists"—for monitoring handoffs, communications	• Tracking algorithms enforce sequencing: eg, age-triggered or risk-triggered prompts • Emphasis is on effective workflow
Secure messaging	• Protected email • Virtual consultations • Text messages	• Patients, caregivers, & providers • Confidentiality promotes candor • Texts can be saved for reference	• Asynchronous, message anytime • Pace slower than face-to-face, but faster than phone tag
Patient portals	• Personal health information accessible by patients • Educational materials accessible in multiple formats	• Tool for patient empowerment • Relationship support for personal management of health care • Promotes self-determination	• Shortens scale for waiting; eg, lab reports, medication ordering • Life-spanning records allow for longitudinal tracking
Multiuser notes	• Health Systems: offers an editable record across providers • Open Notes for Patients	• Accessible by multiple users • Improves situational awareness • Improves quality control	• Asynchronous access to record • Record grows over time, preserving historical change
Medication adherence & remote physiological monitoring	• Cyberphysical support tools • Wearable technology • Interconnected, personal data can contribute to discovery	• Personal support tools for patients promote personal safety • Adaptive interventions conform to user responses	• Sequence-appropriate prompts support evidence-based timing • Real-time monitoring promotes prompt attention to abnormalities
Self-management & coaching tools	• Delivered through web, personal software, or mobile platforms • Decision architectures promote value congruence, personalization	• For use by health conscious consumers, patients, survivors • Adaptive interventions improve self-regulation skills	• Just in time support tools can be used as needed by patient • Automated customization reduces person-hour labor costs
Interactive conferencing	• Enables remote access for underserved environments • Saves money on office visits	• Makes optimal use of scarce medical personnel • Broad spectrum of personal cues	• Synchronous communications promote responsiveness • Allows for point-of-need care

health plan administrators to monitor outcomes across whole populations of patients. In the mid-2000s, Kaiser Permanente went through the meticulous process of integrating their health information technology (HIT) infrastructure to identify, and then address, gaps in care for every individual in their health plan across all population subgroups. System engineers coordinated the communication management systems with online Personal Action Plans for their patients. The online plans used health alerts, data visualizations, reminders, personalized content, and email to alert members when action was needed. Within 90 days of identifying a care gap, the system registered a 6-fold increase in completed pap screens, a 6-fold increase in completed mammograms, and a 10-fold increase in completed colorectal cancer screens. An academic review of this integrated approach revealed that the system was extremely effective in promoting equitable access to services across patient subpopulations when compared to a nonintegrated system in the same region [16].

In designing the attributes of a communications management system, the emphasis should be on creating an easy way to be sure that critical communications occur as needed across multiple levels of decision making and action—and that no vitally important communications are left uninitiated. Design follows much of the substantiated work from human factors psychology, made popular through the "checklist manifesto" [17] in medicine, noting that human decision makers are often blind to missing elements in their perceptual field (a phenomenon referred to as "inattentional blindness" by Horowitz and Rensink elsewhere in this book). Quite simply, human perception is guided neurologically through organizing frameworks, referred to as cognitive schemata. Schemata add meaning to incoming stimuli making it possible to act quickly on the myriad signals confronting the perceptual system in any moment. The problem is that these frameworks tend to fill in gaps with expectations of what might normally be present, which creates a blind spot for missing elements. The human factors solution is to structure decision support technologies to bring attention to those gaps preemptively, thus protecting the system from error. This is the reason why checklists have been shown to be effective in high-stakes fields such as aviation, and now in medicine; and is the way in which reminder systems or error-check routines within an informatics system can ensure thoroughness.

Secure messaging. We list secure messaging as the second broad class of utilities designed to support improved communication in health care settings. By secure messaging, we refer to protected email between patients and their care teams, virtual consults between patients and concierge providers, and text messaging. Data from the National Cancer Institute's (NCI) Health Information National Trends Survey (HINTS) have shown a slow but steady increase in the use of email by the general public for communicating with doctors or doctors' offices. In 2003, the first year of the survey, an estimated 7% of the adult population in the United States reported using the Internet to communicate with their physicians. That percentage rose to 9.6% in 2005, to 13.6% in 2007, to 18.9% in 2011, and up to 29.6% in 2013. GroupHealth, a health maintenance organization (HMO) headquartered in Washington State, reported hosting 2,264,761 email exchanges between members and clinical staff in 2014, compared to hosting 118,403 telephone visits and 351,690 calls to consulting nursing staff. The HMO reported hosting 28,633 virtual consultations, in which electronic images were exchanged and examined remotely by practitioners, for the same year.

For patients, secure messaging can be desirable because it can reduce barriers due to geography or incompatible work schedules. Because the exchanges are asynchronous, the patient or caregiver can send an email message ahead of—or instead of—a clinical visit. If a health plan can benefit from delivering patient-centered and value-driven care, as is the case in systems qualifying as "Accountable Care Organizations (ACOs)" for Medicare reimbursement, then these electronic exchanges can save money while improving patient satisfaction. Kaiser Permanente, for example, reported a 26.2% reduction in expensive office visits with support for patient access to messaging capabilities through an implementation of EHRs [18]. For physicians, the number of electronic messages will likely increase as EHRs with secure messaging features are deployed. Data covering a 10-year span of EHR implementation at a large academic hospital in Boston, MA showed a tripling of volume in electronic messages from patients to their physicians as enrollment in the systems' EHR portal climbed [19]. The increasing volume of electronic messages can be problematic for systems in which payment models have not been altered to support time consulting with patients online [20].

Patient portals. A patient portal is a secure online website that serves as a convenient 24-hour access to personal health information as well as to the administrative resources of the medical practice, such as scheduling, online ordering for medications, immunization records, secure messaging, and discharge summaries. In many respects, the patient portal can serve the same function on the patient side as communication management systems can serve on the provider side; that is, it can serve as a one-stop shop for patients to go to if they have any questions, or actions to perform, related to their care. If a health plan's member is experiencing a symptom or has set a resolution to live a healthier lifestyle, then the member can go to the plan's site to explore educational information or to pose a question through secure messaging to a provider. If the patient wants to explore information related to their condition, they can browse through a set of vetted educational materials as a type of "information prescription" [21]. The NCI's Physician Data Query (PDQ) database is an example resource containing up-to-date information on cancer that can be linked to from portal sites, or can be ingested electronically for delivery through the portal to cancer patients and their caregivers.

Portals have evolved to include functionality for setting up and checking on appointments, for ordering and checking on prescriptions, for viewing laboratory results, and for reviewing coverage and costs. All of these functions can put patients in the driver's seat for monitoring progress on their own conditions and for participating actively with service providers to ensure the best outcomes for their health and the health of loved ones [22]. Research from the behavioral sciences can be brought to bear on the design of these consumer-facing portals. In their work on a Comprehensive Health Enhancement Support System (CHESS) for cancer patients at the University of Wisconsin, for example, DuBenske and colleagues found utility in applying principles from self-determination theory to the design of an informatics system aimed at encouraging patient engagement [23]. We will explain more about how to use communication tools to support patients' sense of self-determination later in this chapter.

Multiuser notes. Experiments in portal functionality have produced observations of what may happen if barriers to information were removed through electronic means. One of the vanguard developments in this sense came from the "Open Notes" experiment funded through the Robert Wood Johnson Foundation's Pioneer Portfolio. In the initial study, conducted over three medical systems, 100 primary care physicians (PCPs) volunteered to open up their visitation notes to patients so they could review the content for accuracy, share it with others, and even contribute comments back for clarification. As might be expected, PCPs' initial reactions to this disruptive innovation were those of anxiety about disrupting workflow and causing undue worry to patients. Once the study was completed, though, most of the providers reported that their worries about workflow did not materialize. Granted, about 42% of PCPs still expressed concern over patients' worry at the end of the study, but data showed that only 7% of patients reported any concerns. Overall, a large majority of PCPs across the three systems (85%, 91%, and 88%, respectively) endorsed the idea of making notes available to patients after the visit as a good idea, citing improved patient relationships, trust, transparency, communication and shared decision making as positive outcomes [24].

Conceptually, the way in which the Open Notes platform worked was by providing a design that would improve the "collective intelligence" [25] of those directly involved in the patient's care. Research in the emerging area of "social computing," a priority for scientific research in the digital age according to the President's Council of Advisors on Science and Technology (PCAST) [26,27], describes the goal of system design as creating effective supports for "social" or "distributed" cognition. The idea is that shared decision making is necessarily a product of multiple perspectives and a combined, relevant knowledge base. The goal of system design in this regard is literally and figuratively to help put team members on the same page. In terms of patient safety, the goal is often discussed in terms of enhancing "situational awareness." Situational awareness can be thought of as giving team members knowledge of "what must be known to complete a particular task" [28]. This idea of creating a transparent space for immediate access to, and shared editing of, information is one of the more notable temporal innovations in computer science research. The temporal efficiency is embodied in the now common term "wiki," which takes its name from the "wiki-wiki" bus in Honolulu and is Hawaiian for "quick." Human factors experts have theorized that an EHR can serve in the same role as a wiki for complex patients; that is, it will represent a rapid, self-correcting repository of combined facts and knowledge about a patient's care to enhance situational awareness among stakeholders [29].

Medication adherence and remote physiological monitoring. When considering the role of communication science in oncology it is easy to restrict the discussion to instances involving direct or mediated communications between people. An expanded vision of communication is emerging, though, as scientists take into account the additive influence of wireless sensors, automated knowledge navigators (eg, Siri from Apple, and Watson from International Business Machines (IBM)), implanted biochips, and smart objects. This is a new class of application built on what many have referred to as the "Internet of Things"; that is, the network of connections enabled by embedding a computer chip and wireless signaling capability into objects. For example, a cancer survivor suffering from late term side effects from chemotherapy may suffer cardiac problems later in life and would then be required to receive an implantable defibrillator. New defibrillators customarily come with a built-in wireless capacity to send a constant stream of data. The data can in turn be read by the clinical team using a mobile visualization app on their smartphone or tablet computer. The shared signal could inherently become an electronic prosthesis for enhanced communications between patients and their care teams; unfortunately, that does not always happen. Arcane "data blocking" policies have sometimes prevented patients from getting access to their own data in meaningful ways [30].

Fortunately, the tide may be shifting in empowering patients with access to their own patient-generated data to enhance self-monitoring and to foster a collaborative, communicative spirit with health care providers and even researchers. Large consumer electronics companies, such as Apple, Garmin, Samsung, Fitbit, and others are entering the market with health and fitness apps and may be starting to fill that niche with consumer-facing displays. The "Share My Journey" app, for example, will allow breast cancer survivors to contribute data on the effects of their treatment through self-report combined with passive sensing [31]. Other applications should follow as an ecosystem of developers takes advantage of interoperable API's (Application Programming Interfaces) to enhance the flow between patient-generated data, patients, and the care team.

One way in which these new, automated communication aids can be utilized to improve results from cancer therapies is by serving as a clinical extender for oncologists and researchers. As we noted earlier, a movement toward oral chemotherapy regimens administered outside of the clinic may mean more risk for patients who are instructed to self-medicate at a time when stamina and vigilance are low, training is slim, and distractions abound [32]. The problem of medication nonadherence is pervasive across the entire health care system [33] with estimates by the New England Healthcare Institute that nonadherence accounts for $300 billion in avoidable costs annually [34]. David Rose, in his book "Enchanted Objects," illustrates how the use of a "smart object" can be used to enhance connections between the care team and patient and ultimately to improve adherence to treatment guidelines. In one particular illustration, he related his success in modifying the cap on a pill bottle with an embedded wireless chip and light emitting diode (LED) light. The cap would sense when the pill bottle had been opened and the patient had taken the prescribed medication. If the patient missed a dose, then the cap would respond by triggering a set of communications by phone, text, and an increasing glow in the cap to let the patient know it was time to take their next pill. The cap could also sense when supplies are near depletion and would send an automatic request for refill to the local pharmacy. Rose reported adherence rates up to 94% through use of the device, a rate that dramatically improves on rates of noncompliance reported in the safety literature [34].

Self-management and coaching tools. The field of health communication has produced a number of applications designed to support patients in achieving healthy behavior change, or in taking an active role in managing the many facets of their own care. Categorized under the general rubric of "eHealth," these applications typically take health communication theories and translate them into actionable behavioral supports for patients and their caregivers. They can include prevention tools, such as motivationally tailored applications to assist in smoking cessation, to control diet, or to guide an exercise regimen; and they can include condition management tools, such as applications designed to help patients monitor and control their pain or interventions designed to support informed decision making. The applications can extend the expertise of scarce, highly trained professionals to a broader group of individuals who can benefit from self-management, while reserving more expensive consultation times for those patients who need greater personal attention [35,36]. The approach is especially important as the biomedical enterprise shifts to a more proactive stance in keeping patients healthier longer, and will be an essential plank in public health policy as health systems around the world cope with extended needs of aging populations and the spread of chronic conditions [37,38].

Several behavioral theories underlie the construction of these eHealth applications—as described by Ahern, Braun, Cooley, and Bickmore elsewhere in the book—depending on the problems to which the applications are oriented to solve. The point in which communication science overlaps with a broader view of behavioral informatics is the point in which the application is intended to simulate or enhance communications. The University of Michigan, for example, experimented with techniques under funding from the NCI to simulate the communicative process of "motivational interviewing" within a computerized platform. Motivational interviewing is a counseling technique introduced in part by Miller and Rollnick [39] that works by reinforcing the intrinsic motivation of clients as they strive to make substantial changes in their health behaviors. The tailored coaching applications constructed by researchers at the University of Michigan mimicked the therapeutic process by helping patients engage in a behavioral change plan that is consistent with their values and goals, while identifying and avoiding environmental triggers [40–43].

Other applications have been designed to help patients gain a better understanding, or mental model, of the biologic processes underway with their particular cancer, and then to help them as they engage in the parallel work of coping emotionally with the disease while engaging in the precautionary behaviors needed to ensure compliance with evidence-based therapeutic recommendations. With the diffusion of smartphones and mobile devices, new theories are under development to strengthen the temporal responsiveness of the supportive application to the patient's dynamically changing internal motivations and contextual surroundings. Termed "adaptive interventions," these computationally sophisticated techniques are similar to precision therapeutics in that they utilize data models to personalize the coaching experience for patients relative to a targeted behavior [44].

Interactive conferencing. Once considered to be a high-end application of telemedicine, interactive conferencing

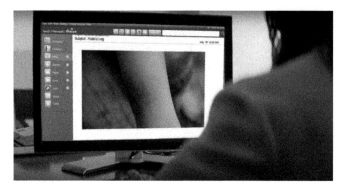

FIGURE 13.2 An excerpt from the Kaiser Permanente Thrive Campaign emphasizing their doctors' use of video conferencing with patients (see: http://share.kaiserpermanente.org/static/kp_annualreport_2014/).

is becoming a much more common and less expensive way to extend the reach of a limited number of professionals to patients in remote locations [45]. These capabilities are being made possible for a broader swath of patients through advances in the personal computer and mobile device markets. Personal computers are routinely shipped with a camera and microphone to make medium-fidelity videoconferencing readily available for little or no cost. Smartphones and tablets are similarly shipped with a camera, which at the very least can be used to send photographs but can also be used to support videoconferencing as needed (see Fig. 13.2 for an example). At the very least, the broad diffusion of cell phones both domestically and internationally is making it possible for more people in remote areas to connect with medical experts through voice-based teleconferencing.

What this broadening palette of interactive conferencing capabilities offers is the ability to broker communications in real-time with qualified professionals regardless of place. For example, medical ethicists have expressed concern over communicating genetic risk information for cancer directly to consumers without the necessary supports in place to interpret that information with professional help [46]. Oncology researchers have subsequently been experimenting with the use of telephone conferencing and video conferencing services to extend genetic counseling services from the cancer center by appointment into underresourced clinics. An initial implementation of a telephone conferencing protocol for communicating the results of *BRCA 1* and *BRCA 2* testing following a structure guided by the Self-Regulation Theory of Health Behavior resulted in a revision for clarified patient instructions, scheduled appointments, refined visual aids, expanded disclosure checklist items, and enhanced provider training [47]. Other examples of informatics-supported video conferencing include the use of imaging and videoconferencing capabilities for

a tissue-fluid biorepository [48]; the use of sensing and imaging technologies to support home care for patients with head and neck care [49]; development of a virtual tumor board among interdisciplinary contributors in a community setting [50]; and videoconferencing to support kidney cancer care in rural areas [51].

13.2 USING COMMUNICATION SCIENCE TO IMPROVE QUALITY OF CANCER CARE

In its 2001 *"Crossing the Quality Chasm: A New Health System for the 21st Century"* report [52] and again in its 2005 *"Building a Better Delivery System: A New Engineering/Health Care Partnership"* report [53], the IOM highlighted the importance of informatics technologies to address the errors that have seemed to permeate health care. Because medicine is essentially an information science, errors in the transmission of information can prove to be particularly problematic. Information and communication technology would be needed to improve the fidelity of transmission, and to ensure that the right information is delivered to the right person (or persons) at the right time to make a difference [10]. Information that is not delivered to the right person, at the right time, or that is miscommunicated through error in its conveyance, can lead to poorer outcomes. To understand how errors in communication can pose a threat to safety and quality improvement in oncology, consider the following case study.

13.2.1 A Case Study of Communication Error in Oncology

In its online case review at *Morbidity and Mortality (M & M) Rounds on the Web*, the Agency for Healthcare Research and Quality (AHRQ) presented the case of a 48-year-old man with a history of metastatic penile cancer who was admitted to an inpatient internal medicine service for a fourth round of chemotherapy. According to the case details, the patient had been admitted three times before—each time with a standard 3-day administration of paclitaxel, ifosfamide, and cisplatin without complication. The patient checked into the internal medicine service for a fourth round of administrations and went through a customary 3-day protocol with no incident. On day 4, he expected to be discharged. To his surprise, however, his nurse announced that he was scheduled to receive a fourth round of chemotherapy. Before receiving this additional dosage the patient asked to see a representative from the oncology care team responsible for directing his treatment. The oncology fellow arrived at his bedside and after talking with the patient and rechecking the orders discovered that there had been a serious error. Rather than ordering a 3-day regimen for penile cancer, the orders dictated a higher dose 5-day regimen of paclitaxel, ifosfamide, and cisplatin for germ cell cancer [54].

This case is instructive for two reasons. On the one hand, it shows what can happen when simple transcription errors interfere with an oncology team's intended treatment plan. This is a communication error. In the case of cancer care, which the AHRQ site describes as "*dangerous business [because] patients have a potentially life threatening disease and often require toxic therapies*," the consequences of these types of communication errors can have deadly effects—both to the patient as "first victim of medical error" but also to the oncology team who suffers as "the second victim of error" [55]. An accompanying commentary to the AHRQ article was quick to point out that this particular miscommunication could have been avoided if the oncology care team had been supplied with a functioning EHR to support its processes. As it turned out, a simple transcription error had occurred when hand-copying orders from the patient's chart to the nurse's duty roster. HIT has shown efficacy in ameliorating these types of transcription errors through the use of computerized physician ordering systems [56].

On the other hand, the case also illustrates just how essential the patient voice was in helping to alert the nurse that an error may have occurred in her orders and then to bring that error to the attention of the oncology team for immediate repair. The case embodies the notion that communication is a two-way process; and that when patient care is participatory [57] and patients are activated [58], the safety of the healthcare system can be enhanced through self-corrective communication processes [24]. The Cochrane Collaboration, a global independent network of professionals working to synthesize medical evidence into prescriptions for what works, emphasized this role of communication science in their review titled "*The Knowledgeable Patient: Communication and Participation in Health*." As the authors of the text explained it, consumer empowerment has become the policy focus of health systems and governments over the past 30–40 years. A focus on communication science within health care takes the execution of best practice away from personal intuition and puts it squarely "within the realm of evidence-based medicine" [32].

13.2.2 When Cancer Communication Goes Awry

It is not entirely clear what the true prevalence of communication errors—errors that occur in the meaningful transmission of information between one or more parties in either a unidirectional or bidirectional way—across the oncology spectrum might be. A seminal study of 4000 inpatients at two Boston hospitals reported that in-patient administration of antineoplastic agents accounted for about 7% of the overall tally of adverse drug events (ADE's) in the two hospitals and about 3–4% of all medication errors [59]. Studies in ambulatory settings, where most cancer care is delivered, placed medication error rates in a range between 0.3 and 5.8 errors per 100 visits. Those rates tend to be lower than for other specialty areas for inpatient and outpatient treatments. Speculations are that oncology care teams are highly cognizant of the potential dangers of highly toxic treatment modalities and remain especially vigilant to the demands of administering dose within semicontrolled settings [60]. As with any human system, though, human vigilance isn't perfect. Orders can still be misread, miscopied, or transmitted unclearly in a system of high stakes care [61].

The risk for error appears to go up considerably when treatment moves outside of the clinical setting altogether, as is the case for the rapid evolution of a new generation of oral chemotherapies administered in either a curative or adjuvant way. The types of errors identified from at least one sample of reported incidents included events associated with taking the wrong or extra dose (38.8% of documented cases), taking the wrong drug (13.6%), wrong number of days supplied (11.0%), and missed dose (10.0%). "With over 25 million doses administered annually," the authors of this particular study cautioned, the expansion of popularity for oral chemotherapy agents—whether taken as a monotherapy or in combination with other antineoplastic agents—has not been accompanied by a systematic adoption of protocols and prescription safeguards. From a 2006 survey, the authors found that only one in four US cancer centers had prescribing safeguards in place while less than one in five had measures in place to ensure safe administration and monitoring [32].

Going beyond a focus on chemotherapy, the Joint Commission on Accreditation, Health Care, and Certification presented data from its *Sentinel* database to describe the general prevalence of different types of medical errors across health systems. According to the Joint Commission's analysis, communication errors accounted for 63% of all reported mishaps in the Sentinel database. By communication errors, the Joint Commission was referring to instances in which information had been, or should have been, transmitted with fidelity from one party to another. They distinguished those errors from a category they referred to as "general human factors" errors, or instances in which the inadequacies of system design led to individuals making judgment errors on their own, making a mistake in course of action, or failing to take a necessary precaution. By their reckoning, the 63% prevalence of communication errors was second only to their notion of general "human factors" failings for the data recorded in 2013. When restricting analyses to "delays in treatment"—a mishap of egregious consequence in oncology—communication errors edged into first place as a root cause, accounting for 81% of all recorded errors in the Sentinel database [62].

The types of communication errors listed in the sentinel database included instances in which a provider was paged but the page was unanswered, cases in which a message was sent to the wrong individual, instances when parties were not able to connect by telephone over repeated tries (ie, "telephone tag"), as well as instances in which handwritten orders were misread or critical information was absent. A particular point of vulnerability in the communication process surrounded patient "handoffs," when one provider gave verbal details of a case to another. These customarily oral conversations are especially prone to miscommunication or flawed recollection after the fact [63].

To get a better sense of what types of errors might be occurring specifically in oncology care, Mazor and her colleagues conducted personal interviews with cancer patients across three clinical sites. Out of those interviewed, 28% of the reported mishaps were described as simply a breakdown in their care (eg, delays in diagnosis or in the treatment of their cancer) without ascribing a parallel problem in communication; 47% described a breakdown in communication as the sole determinant of reported mishap; and 27% described both a breakdown in communication and a serious breakdown in care as determinants. Most of the patients who had reported some type of serious breakdown in their care (20 of 22 patients, or 91%) believed that they had experienced physical harm as a result [64].

13.2.3 Ten Rules for Realigning Health Care

The IOM's *Crossing the Quality Chasm* report [52], along with a series of follow-up workshop and consensus reports, were oriented around six primary goals that would serve to guide the development of a safer, more effective healthcare system in the 21st century. Those goals included: (1) creating a system that is by its nature *safe*, and preemptive of error; (2) building a system that is *effective*, and based on scientific evidence; (3) orienting all aspects of the system to be truly *patient-centered*; (4) improving the system to deliver care to be *timely* in the way it responds to patient needs; (5) reducing waste and creating a system that is *efficient*; and (6) assuring that services are delivered in a way that is *equitable* across all populations. To achieve those overarching goals, the IOM proposed a set of 10 rules to bear in mind when

TABLE 13.2   Ten Rules for Improving Healthcare, From *Crossing the Quality Chasm: A New Health System for the 21st Century* [52]

1. *Care based on continuous healing relationships.* Patients should receive care whenever they need it and in many forms, not just face-to-face visits. This rule implies that the health care system should be responsive at all times (24 hours a day, every day) and that access to care should be provided over the Internet, by telephone, and by other means in addition to face-to-face visits.
2. *Customization based on patient needs and values.* The system of care should be designed to meet the most common types of needs, but have the capability to respond to individual patient choices and preferences.
3. *The patient as the source of control.* Patients should be given the necessary information and the opportunity to exercise the degree of control they choose over health care decisions that affect them. The health system should be able to accommodate differences in patient preferences and encourage shared decision-making.
4. *Shared knowledge and the free flow of information.* Patients should have unfettered access to their own medical information and to clinical knowledge. Clinicians and patients should communicate effectively and share information.
5. *Evidence-based decision-making.* Patients should receive care based on the best available scientific knowledge. Care should not vary illogically from clinician to clinician or from place to place.
6. *Safety as a system property.* Patients should be safe from injury caused by the care system. Reducing risk and ensuring safety require greater attention to systems that help prevent and mitigate errors.
7. *The need for transparency.* The health care system should make information available to patients and their families that allows them to make informed decisions when selecting a health plan, hospital, or clinical practice, or choosing among alternative treatments. This should include information describing the system's performance on safety, evidence-based practice, and patient satisfaction.
8. *Anticipation of needs.* The health system should anticipate patient needs, rather than simply reacting to events.
9. *Continuous decrease in waste.* The health system should not waste resources or patient time.
10. *Cooperation among clinicians.* Clinicians and institutions should actively collaborate and communicate to ensure an appropriate exchange of information and coordination of care.

engaging in any type of redesign effort. We include those rules for reference in Table 13.2.

The implications for creating an informatics solution that facilitates communication are implicit, if not explicit, throughout all ten of the IOM's explicit principles for improving care [65]. Rule #1, for example, explicitly refers to the use of Internet and telephone as adjuncts to the in-person visit; and alludes to the utility of asynchronous communications (eg, secure messaging, email, voice mail) to extend coverage to the point of need 24 hours a day, 7 days a week. Customization according to patients' needs and values, as embedded in Rules #2 and #3, implies a careful give-and-take of information between patients

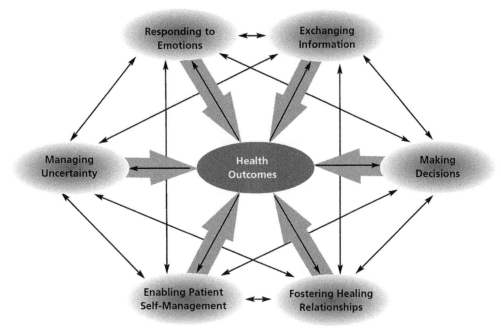

FIGURE 13.3 The six core functions of patient-centered communication from a review of the scientific literature.

and their providers taking into account patients' own needs for emotional resolution and a search for clarity in the face of uncertainty. That give-and-take can occur in real time through face-to-face encounters (the model of a traditional clinical visit), telephone, or videoconferencing (eg, Skype, Face Time); or it can occur in delayed time through secure email or through notes in an electronic chart. The same can be said for a call to promote "shared knowledge and the free flow of information" in Rule #4, a call for transparency in Rule #7, and a call for greater "cooperation among clinicians" in Rule #10. All will inherently require effective communication processes in order to be realized.

The IOM's follow-up activities have expanded further on the need for effective communication to support a high-quality health system as promoted through the other rules. The calls in Rule #5 to move medicine onto a foundation of scientific evidence and in Rule #8 to move toward a platform of predictive and precision medicine led to a series of activities through the IOM's Roundtable on Value and Science-Driven Health Care to improve the ways in which the medical system communicates data, probability, and evidence to patients. In its partnership with the National Academy of Engineering, the IOM repeatedly emphasized the importance of improving communication flows in order to create a system in which safety is perceived as an intrinsic property, as highlighted in Rule #6; and it emphasized that adjustments to communication protocols, assisted by technology, can be used to improve timeliness and reduce waste as emphasized in Rule #7.

13.3 A FUNCTIONAL APPROACH TO PATIENT-CENTERED COMMUNICATION

Picking up on the IOM's exhortation that a high-quality care system be "patient-centered," the NCI commissioned a thorough literature review in 2005 to understand more fully what patients' functional communication needs are *vis-à-vis* the evolving oncology care system. An underlying assumption of the review was that patient-centered care is best achieved when informed, activated patients and their families interact with an accessible, well-organized, and responsive health care system [66]. Authors of the report identified six broad areas of functional need as illustrated in Fig. 13.3. In this section, we examine each of those functional areas in detail.

13.3.1 Fostering Healing Relationships

Authors of the report began their discussion of the six functional domains with an area they termed "fostering healing relationships," an area that recapitulates the first of the ten rules for redesigning healthcare offered by the IOM. It also reinforces the point made by the organizational specialists Zuboff and Maxmin: that, in the age of the Internet, the successful companies are those who use the capacities of an enhanced communication environment to ensure a sense of "deep support" or "relationship" with their clients [67]. At first blush, it may not be obvious how an informatics system can be optimized to support this sense of a healing relationship.

When the NCI report's authors discussed the importance of "relationship building," they emphasized the idea that good provider-patient relationships "are characterized by trust and rapport," and that much of the work in establishing a good relationship is built on the give-and-take that allows patients to be keenly aware of what everyone's role should be in the healing process. "Healing relationships are more than sources of information and expertise; they also provide emotional support, guidance, and understanding," they argued [68]. This seems like a tall order for technology.

But it is not a tall order for sociotechnical systems. A highly effective sociotechnical system begins with a well-trained and competent workforce (people), and then gives them the capacity (technology) to extend their reach and effectiveness beyond historical environmental and temporal bounds. A good example in a nonhealth domain is one of the most successful information technology companies of the last 20–30 years: FedEx. Most people think of FedEx as a shipping company, made up of conscientious people who assure that a package will absolutely be delivered anywhere in the world, overnight if business demands it. That is completely true; but what made the business model of FedEx possible was its strategic use of information technology to log a parcel, arrange for pick-up and delivery, coordinate travel through an international supply chain of trucks and jets, and then guarantee delivery. The technology provided the conscientious employees with the wherewithal to build the company's competitive edge around two unbeatable dimensions: *trust* and *reliability*. Every aspect of customer communication, whether that means giving clients the facility to track their parcel or sending email notifications for delivery if requested, was engineered to keep the customer at the center of service. The technology is seamless and hidden behind the scenes.

The same can, and should, be said of healthcare. Just as FedEx uses its computer systems to keep track of every facet of a customer's long time history interacting with the company, honing its business focus on guaranteeing a reliable company experience, HIT can be designed to forge and protect a patient's relational trust with their care providers. Thus, when patients begin their journey, they can take heart knowing that a trusted medical professional will be just a mouse click, phone call, or personal appointment away [69,70]. If, as survivors, they want to review information from previous treatments in preparation for a visit to a new primary care doctor, they are confident in their abilities to access their own medical records instantaneously [22]. If parents worry about the side effects of an at-home treatment, they can take comfort knowing that it is possible to enter their concerns into a "clinician report" [59] alerting their care team—no matter what time of day or night [71]. Indeed, what the

missing link in healthcare reform might be, according to Tang and Lansky, is to use HIT as a mechanism for bridging the relational gap between patients and providers; that is, to give patients the controls that would allow them to become "copilots in their care" [65].

Notice that to support a healing relationship, the social and technical subsystems underlying hospital communications must be in synch. Imagine a patient portal designed to extend services such as appointment scheduling or medication ordering to patients through the Web or a mobile device. Now imagine what would happen if a patient thinks that an order for a medication refill has been successfully placed, only to find out that the order fell through and that no one bothered to call, text, or email. The consequences for not receiving the medication as expected could lead to serious health consequences if the patient is forced to become noncompliant. Just as importantly, a disconnected system may do irreparable damage to patients' trust in their provider, opening the system up to litigation, bad press, dissatisfaction, and loss in revenue. The communication system in this case is only as strong as its weakest link [72].

13.3.2 Exchanging Information

Of course one of the basic functions of communication, and a function that is most familiar to informaticists, is that of exchanging information. From a communication perspective, this implies getting data and information into the hands of the right person at the right time to influence care. From analyses of data from the NCI's HINTS, we know that nearly half (44.9%) of all adults 18 years and older living in noninstitutionalized settings in the United States in 2003 reported that they had looked for cancer information for themselves or a loved one. Of that group, though, 47.7% explained that the process of finding the information took a lot of effort, 41.3% expressed frustration, and 57.7% expressed concern over the quality of the information they found. A logistic regression analysis revealed that those who with negative experiences searching were two and a half times more likely to report that "almost everything causes cancer" (odds ratio (OR) 2.0, 95% confidence interval (CI) 1.5–2.6); were over two and half times more likely to report that "not much can be done to prevent cancer" (OR 2.7, 95% CI 1.9–3.8); and were over three times as likely to report that "it is hard to know which cancer recommendations to follow" [73].

From these data we know that many cancer patients and their loved ones appeared to be highly motivated to seek out credible information about cancer on their own, but that the process of getting the information they needed was frustrating and confusing. Looking further into where patients go when seeking information, the

HINTS survey revealed that an estimated 49% of the general US population would *prefer* to go to their healthcare provider as a first source of information as measured in 2003. That was not surprising given that an estimated 62.4% of Americans in 2003 listed their healthcare providers as their *most trusted* source for credible information relevant to their health. Interestingly, of those who actually reported looking for information about cancer only 10.9% reported going to their physicians first while an estimated 48.6% reported going to the Internet first. By 2008, the number of people *going online* first for cancer information rose to an estimated 54.9% while the number *going to their providers* first rose to 22.8%. Other sources—books, magazines, and newspapers—were being edged out. Trust in clinical providers actually rose during this period, with results showing that US adults were 1.29 times *more likely* to endorse physicians as their most trusted source of cancer information in 2008 as they were in 2003, while trust in online information went down (OR = 0.74). As Internet diffusion spread, looking for information online first became easier. At the same time, information seekers became more sagacious in their trust of online information and trust in care providers went up.

This trend, of relying both on physicians and the web to make sense of disease, appears to be a little different in health than it has appeared in other sectors. In other sectors, such as in the retail and travel industries, Internet technology has allowed consumers to bypass traditional intermediaries to acquire products or services directly from their source. Communication scientists refer to this phenomenon as *disintermediation* [74]. Health services researchers have introduced a new term, *apomediation*, to describe what appears to be happening in the healthcare industry. In healthcare, information may be seen as surrounding both patients and providers ("apo" means "apart from" as a Greek prefix). With barriers to medical information falling, patients are finding it easier to go online to find whatever information they can to give them a sense of predictive control over their condition. The quality of online content is uneven, however, and much of what patients find from the most credible sites is difficult to interpret by lay audiences [75]. Oncology teams—providers, nurses, and techs—offer an invaluable service in helping patients interpret what they find [76]. Recognizing this, sociotechnical system designers can support patients' information seeking needs by providing access both to well-written educational materials online and to oncology staff through secure messaging, telephone, or in-office visits.

One of the most critical vulnerabilities in patient care occurs at the point in which crucial information must exchange hands, say from one care provider to the next, or from the care provider to the patient. Errors have historically occurred at that vulnerable juncture when members of the care team completed their shift and then orally conveyed the details of their patients' conditions to the incoming team member [77]. They have also occurred as orders are shuffled between the many components of the medical enterprise to fill prescriptions, to order tests, to coordinate psychosocial services, to schedule treatments, to orchestrate surgery, and so on. Poor handwriting, misplaced requests, and missed telephone calls can all interrupt the vital flow of information from one member of the distributed care team to another. Coordinating the flow of that information is not trivial as illustrated by the multiple touch points in Fig. 13.4 both within and surrounding oncology care [78]. Coordination is further complicated when patients manifest with multiple comorbid conditions [79], or when patients transition from highly attentive oncology care back to the fragmented environment of posttreatment survivorship care [80,81].

Sociotechnical solutions can be deployed to prevent handoff errors in many ways. Communication management systems, such as those supporting patient-centered medical homes [82,83], can provide medical staff with an overview of handoffs to be sure that there are no gaps in service for either individuals or populations. Nurse navigators, medical staff, and others can be signaled with the appropriate reminder if a gap is detected through automated routines. Physician ordering systems can boost reliability by sending orders electronically from one component of the medical enterprise to the next, by reducing ambiguity over illegible writing, by catching errors at point of entry, and by preventing cross-system duplication through health information exchanges. Secure messaging can be used whenever the patient or other member of the distributed care team fails to receive an expected delivery. Multiuser notes can facilitate handoffs by documenting the details of a patient's treatment course in a commonly accessible space, to assist in shift change and to help coordinate care across multiple specialties. Representing the patient's voice in the record, perhaps through patient-reported outcomes (PROs) or comments provided through secure messaging, will help orient the team to the patient's values and preferences—a hallmark of patient-centered care.

13.3.3 Making Decisions

The health services trope of engaging patients as partners in their care is manifest critically in the area of *shared decision making*. The term "shared decision making" did not come first from interventional medicine, but was coined in 1982 by the President's Commission for the Study of Ethical Problems in Medicine and Biomedical and Behavioral Research. Its use was intended to underscore the important role of patients in shaping the course of their

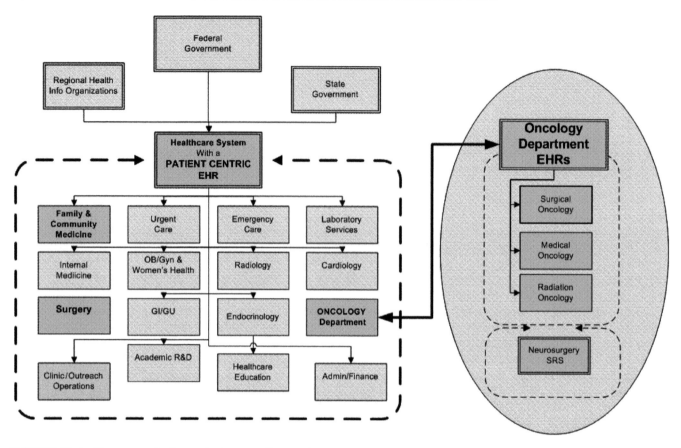

FIGURE 13.4   The communication context surrounding oncology care.

own treatment plans. Its explicit objective was to reform physician–patient communication and to improve the day-to-day implementation of informed consent in medical services [84]. From the perspective of shared decision making, a high-quality outcome requires that clinicians and patients integrate the best medical evidence available to them at the time with patients' values and preferences to develop a mutually agreed upon treatment plan [85].

One of the objectives of a high performance informatics system, then, is to create the decision support architecture [86] that will reinforce the communication process needed to reach a data-based decision in a timely fashion and in accordance with patient values. Some of that architecture will be focused on bringing together the data streams from different sources to support the best possible medical decision. As the consideration of evidence in predictive, preemptive, precise, and participative (ie, "4-P") medicine [87] becomes more complex, attention should be paid on adopting the best visualization tools available to reduce cognitive burden as outlined by Horowitz and Resink. Research from the decision sciences has begun to yield actionable design recommendations for how to present information in a way that is compatible with cognitive processes [88–92].

With data flowing throughout an informatics-enabled oncology system it is possible to envision how a high performance care system can be engineered to support collaborative decision making across multiple levels of action as illustrated in Fig. 13.5. Notice from the figure that medical decision-making can never be truly divorced from communication processes. In paper-based systems, an intake nurse might begin a patient's intake by taking certain physiologic measurements, and then recording those values in a chart. The PCP might pick up the chart, inquire as to the chief complaint, ask a few history questions, perform an initial examination, and then record the results of those activities on the chart. The primary care doctor might then place an order for laboratory tests, request a radiologic image, and perhaps suggest a specialty consult. As we have seen before, decision making will be impaired if there is a break anywhere in that chain. If handwriting is illegible on any area in the chart, or the subjective impressions of the patient's history or chief complaint is flawed, then those communication errors are likely to propagate [61].

An electronic system can address many of the problems inherent in health care's "crisis in communication," according to an eye-catching ad in the *Washington Post* by

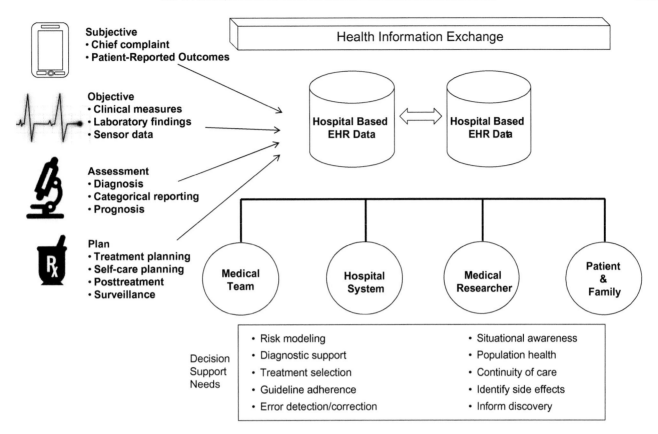

FIGURE 13.5 Decision support within a fully connected, data-driven environment of care.

Kaiser Permanente touting the importance of HIT before passage of the HITECH Act. Digital records can take away the guesswork resulting from illegible handwriting, while error-checking routines and encryption algorithms can preserve the fidelity and security of data flows across multiple layers of the organization. Multiuser access to medical data can ensure situational awareness for anyone involved in decision processes—including the patient and the patient's family. Decision support technologies can improve adherence to guidelines by communicating the results of vetted systematic reviews (eg, from the US Preventive Services Taskforce (USPST), the US College of Surgeons, or the Joint Commission), by structuring communications relevant to diagnosis and treatment, and by preemptively assuring that patients' values are included in the decision process.

13.3.4 Enabling Self-Management

As demographic shifts cause healthcare systems to move away from a limited focus on acute care, to a more proactive focus on prevention and chronic disease care, patient self-management becomes an essential tool in the healthcare systems armamentarium. Creating a culture of patient engagement, for example, has been central

to the healthcare modernization efforts of the United Kingdom's National Health Service. Directors acknowledged the importance of self-management as the best way to cope with an aging demographic and soaring medical costs [37]. It is more than just offloading costs (though studies have demonstrated cost savings from using remote monitoring technologies and well-designed patient portals to decrease visits to the emergency room, unnecessary visits to the clinic, and hospital admissions [18,93]); it also creates a reliable interface for empowered consumers to lead the way in applying medical evidence consistently within their own personal environments outside of the clinic [15,45,94]. The technologies supporting telemedicine, according to Donald Berwick, have "immense potential to revolutionize the reach of expertise and to reduce costs and inconveniences for patients, families, and clinicians." The communication capacity of the digital age will allow health systems to "move knowledge, not people," and will help create care that will "meet people where they are, literally" [95].

"Meeting people where they are" means more for patients than simply overcoming the inconveniences of geography; though that is certainly a huge problem in cancer treatment where patients may need to travel for to a high-quality cancer center for physical examination and in-patient treatment. It also means providing support to patients no matter where they are in their cancer journey. According to one survey, the most frustrating health care experiences for the online public comes from: (1) having to see their doctors in person to ask questions they could answer by telephone or email; (2) trying, but often failing, to get through to someone who can answer questions in a timely fashion; and (3) providing the same information over and over again each time the patient visits a physician's office [96]. An effectively designed patient portal can serve as a coordinating center for patients' self-management needs by facilitating communication through secure electronic messaging and/or providing lists of critical telephone numbers; by providing clinical summaries for easy digestion after office visits; by offering timely access to patient-specific educational resources as new questions arise; by giving patients and caregivers access to their biometric health data; and by utilizing patient reminders to encourage adherence in prevention, treatment, or follow-up care.

Enabling patient self-management goes beyond simple information management, though. Enabling self-management in this case means giving patients and their personal caregivers the skills to manage their own health proactively when away from the clinic, and to advocate for themselves when needed to acquire services or treatment [68]. DuBenske and colleagues demonstrated how the provision of an electronically collected Patient Reported Outcomes (e-PRO) measure helped patients stay ahead of negative symptomologies from their cancer treatments [97]. The e-PRO system enhanced the quality of patients' experience when visiting the clinic, resulted in greater caregiver involvement, and facilitated earlier interventions when compared against standard of care. Other studies have demonstrated how environments that support PRO's have been instrumental in encouraging better patient outcomes, of catching errors early before they lead to adverse consequences, and in relieving the stress of personal caregivers [98,99].

An important point to consider when designing electronic communication environments for patient engagement is the delicate touch needed to protect, and nurture, intrinsic motivation [100]. It can be touchy because health communication by design will be tinged with an element of exhortation, or in telling patients that "you should do this." Too much exhortation or demand by the system can create a sense of reactance or pushback from patients, especially if they feel that the system might be controlling them rather than supporting them. Informatics designers in oncology have been able to overcome this problem by orienting their user testing around three core principles from self-determination theory:

- *Nurture patient autonomy.* We have all experienced the frustration of working with commercial websites that seem to be operating on ulterior motives; that prevent us from performing actions of importance to us; that interrupt our attention with distracting pop-ups; or that force us to accept unalterable defaults. The experience creates the perception that the system is in control rather than the user, and in the commercial world can create a backlash among users. Contemporary principles in user-centered design can reverse those perceptions by aligning interface elements to convey a sense of service and deep support to patients as they pursue their health goals. User-centered design can help align the tone and content of textual components so that language is universally easy to understand. Data entry fields can be autopopulated from the EHR so that the user does not have to waste time on tedious data entry, while at the same time giving users the ability to enter corrections will not only help produce cleaner data but will give patients a sense of ownership for their own record. The Veteran's Administration's (VA) introduction of the "blue button initiative," encouraging patients to download their personal health information with a click of the mouse (on a blue button), reinforces an expectation that the patient is ultimately in control of their own health.

- *Enhance patient mastery.* Engaging patients entails providing them with the skills they need to monitor their condition, to self-administer medications as needed, to ameliorate negative side effects, and to self-advocate as needed. The goals of the user interface, as well as the system underlying it, should be to support patients as they hone the skills they need to enhance their own health. Clearly communicated prevention, treatment, and survivorship plans can help keep the patient on the same page as other members of the care team while they assume responsibility for self-management. Responsive feedback mechanisms can aid in self-monitoring and can shape behavior toward desirable health goals. The always on, always present, nature of health sensors is increasingly adding real-time biofeedback to the mix in helping patients maintain optimal body weight, to quit smoking and to monitor side effects from therapy.

- *Ensure connectedness.* Humans are social beings and derive motivation from connecting to others for hope, clarification, and support. The social media site "CaringBridge.org" is an example of an online platform offered by many hospitals to help connect patients in treatment to families, friends, and communities; as is the SmartPatients.com site described by Ziegler and Frydman elsewhere in this book. In the cancer realm, the Association of Cancer Online Resources (ACOR) has been a platform in which cancer patients could meet up online, learn from each other, and discuss ways of advocating collectively for cancer patients' needs. Berwick's exhortation that telemedicine technologies, including patient portals and online video conferencing capabilities, be made available to meet patients where they live strengthens the IOM recommendations that communication and informatics technologies be used to ensure a sense of connectedness with their healthcare provider.

13.3.5 Coping With Emotions

Cancer is a diagnosis loaded with intense emotion. Most cancer patients will experience a full gamut of emotional reactions—from experiencing despair to hope and everything in between—in varying intervals along their journey. Training programs for oncologists have done much to increase clinicians' attention to their patients' emotional cues, to navigate the difficult terrain of delivering bad news, to explore and validate patients' emotional responses, to empathize, and to offer tangible assistance in coping [68,101]. The importance for clinicians to be fully present during clinical interviews with their patients, to respond with compassion and empathy to the spectrum of emotions the patients and their families will be experiencing, cannot be overstated. In spite of that training, intense negative emotions can still spiral out of control in ways that are simply not perceptible from limited clinical interactions. In fact, data suggest that less than a third of emotionally compromised patients are recognized as such by their treating physicians. It is for this reason that the American College of Surgeons' Commission on Cancer passed a new Standard, *Standard 3.2*, in 2012 calling for cancer programs to screen patients diagnosed with cancer for psychological distress and to identify proactively the issues that may pose a threat to treatment and quality of life. The standard was slated to be fully implemented by January 1, 2015.

One of the goals of a patient-centered support system in oncology, then, is to ensure that the resources are in place to help patients cope with, and clarify, their emotional responses to the difficulties posed by their disease. The first step along this path is to be sure that clinicians, nursing staff, social workers, and psychologists are all operating "at the top of their license" in being fully cognizant of the patient's emotional needs. Operating "at the top of their license" is a phrase made popular in health systems design and means that highly trained professionals should be doing the work for which they are trained. In this case, that means paying attention to the emotional needs of patients and not being distracted by computer prompts or data-entry tasks. Examination rooms and workflows (environments and temporal qualities) should be designed to facilitate the professional,

face-to-face communication that will allow clinicians to use their training in helping patients work through their emotional responses. This may mean reconfiguring the arrangement of furniture in the clinician's office to allow for unobstructed eye contact, or hiring a scribe to take notes while the physician focuses on patients' interpersonal cues [6].

At a more general medical level, the IOM has recommended that EHR content should be expanded to include assessments of patients' psychosocial resources across care settings, precisely to serve as clinical input for clinicians to check routinely on patients' ongoing capacities to cope with the effects of disease and treatment [102]. The inclusion of psychosocial distress fields in the general record has allowed primary care doctors and specialists to be made aware of the ongoing needs that a cancer patient or cancer survivor may continue to experience over their life course [103]. Early feasibility studies suggest that it is possible to include patient-reported outcomes (PROs) as data elements to monitor other aspects of patient distress. Patient willingness to complete PRO measures was highest when instructed to do so in a face-to-face context in the clinic (61.4%) followed by telephone (48.8%) and letter (41.0%). The authors of the feasibility study speculated that engagement with electronically administered PROs may climb as patient-facing interfaces become more common and are engagingly designed [99].

Even without the presence of a structured set of PRO or assessment measures, the availability of digital communication channels may help patients as they navigate the unfamiliar environs of emotionally laden choices. Communication studies have revealed that it is often easier for people to reveal more online than they would in a face-to-face encounter, especially in a medical context when the social cues present from a doctor's office can be quite intimidating. When a patient hears bad news for the first time in a clinical encounter, it may be difficult to sort through their emotions in real time and then to reach a life-influencing decision. Such deliberations will likely take time to process. Patients who can reach back to their care team through secure email can afford to ask questions at a time when they are more emotionally available, and have begun to process the implications of what their decisions may mean for their relationships with significant others. Going online with one of the many electronic discussion groups available to cancer patients can allow patients to interpret their own emotions in light of what other cancer patients may have experienced, and may derive a strong sense of social support from these virtual communities.

Emotions can also interfere with sound decision making or assertive health behaviors [104]. Too much fear could lead to emotional blunting, which might prevent a cancer survivor from staying consistent with routine checkups or could lead to lapses in oral chemotherapy regimens [105]. A bias toward unrealistic optimism may nudge patients and their oncologists to seek unrealistically aggressive treatment options, or to avoid discussions about palliation or end-of-life care [106]. Structured decision-making architectures, powered at the backend by a robust communication management system, can anticipate those likely errors and then nudge the communications needed to improve outcomes for the patients' benefit in spite of what would be considered by anyone as a sensitive and emotional time. A reliable, sociotechnical system engineered to include opportunities for face-to-face communications backed by a reliable way to assess distress when it may not be obvious and to answer questions as needed, should help oncology teams create the kind of practice that will nurture patients' resilience during emotional times.

13.3.6 Managing Uncertainty

After reviewing the concept of uncertainty in the medical literature, Han and colleagues [107] found it useful to distinguish between different sources of uncertainty in practice. Using the context of breast cancer treatment, they distinguished between conceptual notions of: (1) *probability*, or the indeterminancy of future outcomes (eg, 20% probability of benefit from a specified treatment); (2) *ambiguity*, or the confusion that arises from imprecision or conflict in evidence (eg, 10–30% probability of benefit from a treatment, or "the jury is out on protocol x"); and (3) *complexity*, or the difficulties associated with communicating a multiplicity of causal factors (eg, 20% probability of long-term remission from treatment in patients with localized disease). Authors of the Patient-Centered Communication report suggested that the role of the delivery system is to reduce uncertainty wherever possible; but when it persists, to help patients manage the uncertainty in healthful ways. It is worth examining each of the three facets of uncertainty described by Han and colleagues to explore how an oncology informatics system may be deployed to meet both of these goals.

Uncertainty in terms of probability: As a scientific enterprise, medicine is built on an evidentiary foundation that is statistical in nature. Most, if not all, of medical decision making is based on a probabilistic understanding of the facts. "Uncertainty is endemic," explained Robert Wachter in his book *The Digital Doctor: Hope, Hype, and Harm at the Dawn of Medicine's Computer Age*, "… so the 'correct' answer [in diagnosis and treatment] is often a surprisingly probabilistic notion … and unfolds over time" [6]. Fortunately, communication science has made significant strides in creating charts and data visualizations that are generally comprehensible by the lay and professional publics. The news industry, for example,

has created a multimillion dollar enterprise in taking meteorological data collected through the aegis of the National Oceanic and Atmospheric Administration (NOAA) and converting those data into usable probabilities for the day's and week's forecasted weather. Similarly, the financial industry has long exploited the real-time data streams from equity markets and government collected econometric data to inform professionals, individual investors, and the general public of probabilistic trends. Today, consumers can review these probabilistic data in print form through daily deliveries of newspapers, they can go online, or they can tap on a downloaded app to their mobile smart device.

These same techniques are being applied with some success in public health and medicine. Researchers working within the Surveillance, Epidemiology, and End Results (SEER) program convert cancer statistics into highly usable trends reports to inform decision making in cancer control and prevention. The decisions made by policy makers, preventive oncologists, and public health officials are probabilistic in nature, guiding allocation of resources and serving as a coordinating tool for community cancer control efforts. Efforts have also been underway to convert those, and similar, data into individually based "risk calculators" for use by PCPs and patients. User testing within cognitive laboratories has helped guide the presentation of probability statistics to reduce the public's sense of uncertainty with respect to their own personal risk, and to inform decisions to adopt the necessary precautions [108]. With more powerful data visualization techniques coming online, the interfaces created to portray the probabilistic nature of medical evidence should serve well as a common architecture to support shared decision-making and collaborative care in oncology [90].

Uncertainty in terms of ambiguity: Ambiguity, as described by Han and colleagues, tends to represent the harder problem to solve in terms of managing uncertainty. Ambiguity arises when medical evidence is in conflict or when the metrics underlying data-based decision making are imprecise. The problem is often exacerbated when early scientific research is portrayed by the news or advertising media as a "new, scientific breakthrough," or when commercial interests purposely seek to muddy the waters by selling doubt in scientific consensus (as the Tobacco Companies did in the 1970s) [109]. Again, medicine has evolved best practices for weighing the evidence and reaching suggested recommendations for standards of care in the midst of uncertainty. Guideline building bodies have been especially important in helping to inform best practice. Examples include the US Preventive Services Task Force, the American College of Surgeons Commission on Cancer, the American Society of Clinical Oncology, and the National Committee for Quality Assurance along with others. It has long been a vision in informatics research that EHR structures and

HIT-supported workflows would help instantiate a consistent portrayal of evidence-based guidelines. A capacity to provide nimble updates electronically to *Clinical Decision Support* (CDS) tools, which can be transparently presented to patients, should help put all of the parties in a shared decision-making activity on the same page without forcing them to search through 1.2 million new records added to the National Library of Medicine's Medline database each year on their own.

As before, patient portals will be the likely vehicle to help disambiguate recommendations for patients by conveying the cancer system's standards in easy-to-comprehend language. Putting information up on the Web will probably not be sufficient; patients will likely want to discuss what they find online with a trained healthcare provider. It will be the provider's role to help interpret the strength of the evidence underlying one approach or another, and to offer a professional assessment of which approach appears to be superior. In those instances when the evidence base around treatment options is truly unsettled, the physician will want to work with patients to cope with the uncertainty of the choices before them and to select a path forward, however tentative, based on other parameters relevant to the decision. The patient may be encouraged to acquire a second opinion if the stakes are high, and the physician may even make the referral to speak to another provider through the hospital's scheduling system.

Uncertainty in terms of complexity: Another source of uncertainty stems from understanding treatments or medical protocols that are complex in nature. This is a significant issue in oncology. Under the penumbra of precision medicine, indications for effective treatment will be highly conditionalized on a complex protocol of genomically informed risk assessments, molecular pathways, and even a patient's own unique physiological and behavioral history. Implementing the full vision of precision medicine *without* the aid of computational technology would seem almost impossible.

Complexity can also be manifest in the meticulous attention needed to administer cancer treatments for patients undergoing care, and for helping postcare survivors stay adherent to recommendations to monitor for recurrence, to stay vigilant for new occurrence, to deal with potentially delayed adverse reactions from treatment, and to stay adherent to recommendations for diet and exercise. Gone are the days of "silver bullet" thinking in oncology, or the hope of a "one-and-done" treatment. Adherence to contemporary therapies for patients means rethinking the scripts of daily living. This is one of the reasons why treatment and survivorship care plans have been considered to be important by the IOM [110]. The problem is that a paper-based care plan is static and can be misplaced. Alternatively, an informatics supported care plan can be made accessible

to all parties with a stake in the patient's long term care, and can evolve over time [111]. The new objective is to create a record that is life-sensitive, and that can reduce complexity in spite of a change in environment or even a change in scientific knowledge [80].

13.4 CONCLUSION

Productivity gains in an era of electronic connectivity have been substantial across many sectors of the global economy, with expectations that further connectivity in areas such as health care, energy, transportation, and fundamental science will go even further on tackling significant societal problems [26,27]. One way of conceptualizing those gains in health care—and to identify gaps in need of further scaffolding—is to take a systems analytic perspective [112] on the ways in which information is flowing throughout the sector; and to ask one significant, but fundamental question. Is information flowing to the right people, at the right time, in a way that is usable and understandable, to support the evolution of a care system that is safe, effective, patient-centered, timely, efficient, and equitable?

This is the question that communication science can assist in answering. In this chapter, we have reviewed the ways in which communication engineering has begun to address some of the fundamental threats to quality in a system that is expanding in complexity, while becoming more precise in its choice of treatments for individual patients. We began with an inventory of some of the most promising informatics solutions designed to improve communication outcomes in cancer care. Innovations included executive management systems to keep track of needed communications across the enterprise; secure messaging systems to promote timely responses to patients' questions; patient-portals as a trusted, one-stop-shop for personal needs; multiuser notes to keep all parties on the "same page" for collaborative care; wireless sensors and medication adherence tools to support remote care; self-management and personal coaching tools; and interactive video and telephone conferencing.

The strategic use of these tools, we argued, should serve the overarching objectives and rules governing healthcare redesign according to principles published through the IOM's *"Crossing the Quality Chasm"* workshop series. Moreover, to be truly patient-centric, the informatics-enabled communication system should be engineered to assist in meeting the functional needs of cancer patients. Those needs, as culled from a comprehensive literature review published by the NCI, not only included information exchange (the classic communication need), but in fostering *healing relationships* between patients and providers, in supporting *decision-making,* enabling *self-management*, coping with *emotions*, and managing *uncertainty*.

At first blush, it may seem paradoxical to think that informatics solutions can resolve communication weaknesses in the oncology enterprise; after all, when patients think about good communication they pay particular attention to the observed or inferred affections of their providers. Did the provider team listen carefully to patients' questions, and did they do so with a good "bedside manner" showing sympathy and respect? Do patients report a general feeling of trust and reliance in their care system or do they report an ineffable, general sense of frustration or isolation? These are the questions that are especially important to patients and their caregivers, and no amount of technology could possibly make up for a surly clinician's attitude or a soulless administrative bureaucracy. Nevertheless, from a sociotechnical perspective informatics solutions can serve to augment the communication skills of a well-trained and professional workforce. They can extend the oncologist's reach beyond the walls of the clinic and the temporal constraints of an already crowded workday. Engineered correctly, they can serve to broaden the bandwidth through which virtual members of the extended healthcare and patient team engage in one of the most essential of human activities: *communication*.

LIST OF ACRONYMS AND ABBREVIATIONS

ACO Accountable Care Organization
ACOR Association of Cancer Online Resources
ADE Adverse drug events
AHRQ Agency for Healthcare Research and Quality
API Application Programming Interface
CDS Clinical Decision Support
CHESS Comprehensive Health Enhancement Support System
CI Confidence interval
EHR Electronic health record
HINTS Health Information National Trends Survey
HIT Health information technology
HITECH Health Information Technology for Economic and Clinical Health
HMO Health maintenance organization
IBM International Business Machines
IOM Institute of Medicine (now referred to as National Academy of Medicine)
LED Light emitting diode
M&M Morbidity and Mortality
NCI National Cancer Institute
NOAA National Oceanic and Atmospheric Administration
OR Odds ratio
PCAST President's Council of Advisors on Science and Technology
PCP Primary care physician
PDQ Physician Data Query
PRO Patient reported outcome
SEER Surveillance, Epidemiology, and End Results
USPST US Preventive Services Taskforce
VA Veteran's Administration

References

[1] Gruman JC. Making health information technology sing for people with chronic conditions. Am J Prev Med 2011;40(5 Suppl 2):S238–40.

[2] Friedman TL. Rev. pbk. ed. The world is flat: a brief history of the twenty-first century. New York, NY: Picador; 2007.

[3] Fox S, Rainie L. The web at 25 in the U.S Center PR, editor. Internet and American life. Washington, DC: Pew Research Center; 2014.

[4] Viswanath K. Science and society: the communications revolution and cancer control. Nat Rev Cancer 2005;5(10):828–35.

[5] Berwick DM. Taming the technology beast. JAMA 2008;299(24):2898–9.

[6] Wachter, RM. The digital doctor: hope, hype, and harm at the dawn of medicine's computer age. New York, NY: McGraw-Hill Education; 2015. p. 71–92.

[7] Hesse BW, Hansen D, Finholt T, Munson S, Kellogg W, Thomas JC. Social participation in health 2.0. IEEE Comput 2010;43(11):45–52.

[8] Hesse BW, Shneiderman B. eHealth research from the user's perspective. Am J Prev Med 2007;32(5 Suppl):S97–103.

[9] Parrott R. Emphasizing "communication" in health communication. J Commun 2004;54(4):751–87.

[10] Kreps GL. Health communication SAGE benchmarks in communication. Los Angeles, CA: SAGE; 2010.

[11] Kreps GL, Neuhauser L. Artificial intelligence and immediacy: designing health communication to personally engage consumers and providers. Patient Educ Couns 2013;92(2):205–10.

[12] Hesse BW, Werner CM, Altman I. Temporal aspects of computer-mediated communication. Comput Hum Behav 1988;4(2):147–65.

[13] Hesse BW, Suls JM. Informatics-enabled behavioral medicine in oncology. Cancer J 2011;17(4):222–30.

[14] Shortliffe EH, Cimino JJ. Biomedical informatics: computer applications in health care and biomedicine Health informatics series, 3rd ed. New York, NY: Springer; 2006. xxvi, 1037 pp.

[15] Frist WH. Connected health and the rise of the patient-consumer. Health Aff (Millwood) 2014;33(2):191–3.

[16] Rhoads KF, Patel MI, Ma Y, Schmidt LA. How do integrated health care systems address racial and ethnic disparities in colon cancer? J Clin Oncol 2015;33(8):854–60.

[17] Gawande A. The checklist manifesto: how to get things right, 1st ed. New York, NY: Metropolitan Books; 2010. x, 209 pp.

[18] Chen C, Garrido T, Chock D, Okawa G, Liang L. The kaiser permanente electronic health record: transforming and streamlining modalities of care. Health Aff (Millwood) 2009;28(2):323–33.

[19] Crotty BH, Yamrat Y, Mostaghimi A, Safran C, Landon BE. Patient-to-physician messaging: volume nearly tripled as more patients joined system, but per capita rate plateaued. Health Aff (Millwood) 2014;33(10):1817–22.

[20] Dixon RF. Enhancing primary care through online communication. Health Aff (Millwood) 2010;29(7):1364–9.

[21] Kemper DW, Mettler M. Information therapy: prescribed information as a reimbursable medical service, 1st ed. Boise, ID: Healthwise, Inc; 2002. xii, 248 pp.

[22] Krist AH, Woolf SH. A vision for patient-centered health information systems. JAMA 2011;305(3):300–1.

[23] Pingree S, Hawkins R, Baker T, DuBenske L, Roberts LJ, Gustafson DH. The value of theory for enhancing and understanding e-health interventions. Am J Prev Med 2010;38(1):103–9.

[24] Delbanco T, Walker J, Bell SK, Darer JD, Elmore JG, Farag N, et al. Inviting patients to read their doctors' notes: a quasi-experimental study and a look ahead. Ann Intern Med 2012;157(7):461–70.

[25] Hesse BW, O'Connell M, Auguston EM, Chou WYS, Shaikh AR. Realizing the promise of web 2.0: engaging community intelligence. J Health Commun 2011;16(Suppl 1):10–31.

[26] President's Council of Advisors on Science and Technology. Designing a digital future: federally funded research and development in networking and information technology, Executive Office of the President, editor. Washington (DC): Executive Office of the President of the United States; 2010.

[27] President's Council of Advisors on Science and Technology. Designing a digital future: federally funded research and development in networking and information technology, Executive Office of the President, editor. Washington (DC): Executive Office of the President of the United States; 2013.

[28] Karsh B-T. Clinical practice improvement and redesign: how change in workflow can be supported by clinical decision support. Rockville, MD: Agency for Healthcare Research and Quality; 2009.

[29] Naik AD, Singh H. Electronic health records to coordinate decision making for complex patients: what can we learn from wiki? Med Decis Making 2010;30(6):722–31.

[30] The Office of the National Coordinator for Health Information Technology (ONC). Report on health information blocking, in report to congress, Department of Health and Human Services, Editor. Washington (DC): Department of Health and Human Services; 2015.

[31] Nasr R. "Share the journey" app boost data collection in cancer fight. Englewood Cliffs, NJ: CNBC; 2015.

[32] Weingart SN, Toro J, Spencer J, Duncombe D, Gross A, Bartel S, et al. Medication errors involving oral chemotherapy. Cancer 2010;116(10):2455–64.

[33] Osterberg L, Blaschke T. Adherence to medication. N Engl J Med 2005;353(5):487–97.

[34] Rose D. Enchanted objects: design, human desire, and the Internet of things. First Scribner hardcover edition. ed. vol. xiii. New York, NY: Scribner; 2014. p. 304.

[35] Hesse BW, Cole GE, Powe BD. Partnering against cancer today: a blueprint for coordinating efforts through communication science. J Natl Cancer Inst Monogr 2013;2013(47):233–9.

[36] Frieden TR. A framework for public health action: the health impact pyramid. Am J Public Health 2010;100(4):590–5.

[37] Cayton H. The flat-pack patient? Creating health together. Patient Educ Couns 2006;62(3):288–90.

[38] Noar SM, Harrington NG. eHealth applications: an introduction and overview Noar SM, Harrington NG, editors. eHealth applications: promising strategies for behavior change. New York, NY: Routledge; 2012. p. 3–16.

[39] Miller WR, Rollnick S. Meeting in the middle: motivational interviewing and self-determination theory. Int J Behav Nutr Phys Act 2012;9:25.

[40] Alexander GL, McClure JB, Calvi HH, Divine GW, Stopponi MA, Rolnick SJ, et al. A randomized clinical trial evaluating online interventions to improve fruit and vegetable consumption. Am J Public Health 2010;100(2):319–26.

[41] Resnicow K, Davis R, Zhang N, Saunders E, Strecher V, Tolsma D, et al. Tailoring a fruit and vegetable intervention on ethnic identity: results of a randomized study. Health Psychol 2009;28(4):394–403.

[42] Strecher VJ, McClure JB, Alexander GL, Chakraborty B, Nair VN, Konkel JM, et al. Web-based smoking-cessation programs: results of a randomized trial. Am J Prev Med 2008;34(5):373–81.

[43] Woolford SJ, Clark SJ. Tailored mobile phone text messages as an adjunct to obesity treatment for adolescents. J Telemed Telecare 2010;16(8):458–61.

[44] Lin PH, Intille S, Bennett G, Bosworth HB, Corsino L, Voils C, et al. Adaptive intervention design in mobile health: intervention design and development in the Cell Phone Intervention for You trial. Clin Trials 2015;12(6):634–45.

[45] Kvedar J, Coye MJ, Everett W. Connected health: a review of technologies and strategies to improve patient care with telemedicine and telehealth. Health Aff (Millwood) 2014;33(2):194–9.

[46] Mackenzie A, Patrick-Miller L, Bradbury AR. Controversies in communication of genetic risk for hereditary breast cancer. Breast J 2009;15(Suppl 1):S25–32.

[47] Patrick-Miller LJ, Egleston BL, Fetzer D, Forman A, Bealin L, Rybak C, et al. Development of a communication protocol for telephone disclosure of genetic test results for cancer predisposition. JMIR Res Protoc 2014;3(4):e49.

[48] Butler WE, Atai N, Carter B, Hochberg F. Informatic system for a global tissue-fluid biorepository with a graph theory-oriented graphical user interface. J Extracell Vesicles 2014;3:1–16.

[49] Peterson SK, Shinn EH, Basen-Enqquist K, Demark-Wahnefried W, Prokhorov AV, Baru C, et al. Identifying early dehydration risk with home-based sensors during radiation treatment: a feasibility study on patients with head and neck cancer. J Natl Cancer Inst Monogr 2013;2013(47):162–8.

[50] Stevenson MM, Irwin T, Lowry T, Ahmed M, Walden TL, Watson M, et al. Development of a virtual multidisciplinary lung cancer tumor board in a community setting. J Oncol Pract 2013;9(3):e77–80.

[51] Alanee S, Dynda D, LeVault K, Mueller G, Sadowski D, Wilber A, et al. Delivering kidney cancer care in rural Central and Southern Illinois: a telemedicine approach. Eur J Cancer Care (Engl) 2014;23(6):739–44.

[52] Institute of Medicine (U.S.) Committee on quality of health care in America Crossing the quality chasm: a new health system for the 21st century. Washington, DC: National Academy Press; 2001. xx, 337 pp.

[53] Reid PP, Compton WD, Grossman JH, Fanjiang G. Building a better delivery system: a new engineering/health care partnership. Washington, DC: National Academies Press; 2005. xiv, 262 pp.

[54] Jacobson JO, Weingart SN. Right regimen, wrong cancer: patient catches medical error. web M&M: morbidity & mortality rounds on the web 2013 May 2013 [cited 2015 February 20, 2015]; Available from: <http://webmm.ahrq.gov/case.aspx?caseID=299>.

[55] Edrees HH, Paine LA, Feroli ER, Wu AW. Health care workers as second victims of medical errors. Pol Arch Med Wewn 2011;121(4):101–8.

[56] Buntin MB, Jain SH, Blumenthal D. Health information technology: laying the infrastructure for national health reform. Health Aff (Millwood) 2010;29(6):1214–9.

[57] Hill S, Cochrane Collaboration The knowledgeable patient: communication and participation in health Cochrane handbook. Chichester: John Wiley & Sons; 2011. p.

[58] Greene J, Hibbard JH, Sacks R, Overton V. When seeing the same physician, highly activated patients have better care experiences than less activated patients. Health Aff (Millwood) 2013;32(7):1299–305.

[59] Gandhi TK, Bartel SB, Shulman LN, Verrier D, Burdick E, Cleary A, et al. Medication safety in the ambulatory chemotherapy setting. Cancer 2005;104(11):2477–83.

[60] Walsh KE, Dodd KS, Seetharaman K, Roblin DW, Herrinton LJ, Von Worley A, et al. Medication errors among adults and children with cancer in the outpatient setting. J Clin Oncol 2009;27(6):891–6.

[61] Kohn LT, Corrigan J, Donaldson MS. To err is human: building a safer health system. Washington, DC: National Academy Press; 2000. xxi, 287 pp.

[62] The Joint Commission Sentinel Event Data: Root Causes by Event Type 2004–2013; 2014.

[63] Giardina TD, King BJ, Ignaczak AP, Paull DE, Hoeksema L, Mills PD. Root cause analysis reports help identify common factors in delayed diagnosis and treatment of outpatients. Health Aff (Millwood) 2013;32(8):1368–75.

[64] Mazor KM, Roblin DW, Greene SM, Lemay CA, Firneo CL, Calvi J, et al. Toward patient-centered cancer care: patient perceptions of problematic events, impact, and response. J Clin Oncol 2012;30(15):1784–90.

[65] Tang PC, Lansky D. The missing link: bridging the patient-provider health information gap. Health Aff (Millwood) 2005;24(5):1290–5.

[66] Clauser SB, Wagner EH, Aiello Bowles EJ, Tuzzio L, Greene SM. Improving modern cancer care through information technology. Am J Prev Med 2011;40(5 Suppl 2):S198–207.

[67] Zuboff S, Maxmin J. The support economy: why corporations are failing individuals and the next episode of capitalism. New York, NY: Viking; 2002. xvii, 458 pp.

[68] Epstein R, Street RJ. Patient-centered communication in cancer care: promoting healing and reducing suffering. Bethesda, MD Bethesda, MD: National Cancer Institute; 2007 2007. Patient-centered communication in cancer care: promoting healing and reducing suffering. Bethesda, MD Bethesda, MD: National Cancer Institute; 2007.

[69] Abernethy AP, Hesse BW. Information technology and evidence implementation. Transl Behav Med 2011;1(1):11–14.

[70] Turvey C, Klein D, Fix G, Hogan TP, Woods S, Simon SR, et al. Blue Button use by patients to access and share health record information using the Department of Veterans Affairs' online patient portal. J Am Med Inform Assoc 2014;21(4):657–63.

[71] Madhavan S, Sanders AE, Chou WY, Shuster A, Boone KW, Dente MA, et al. Pediatric palliative care and eHealth opportunities for patient-centered care. Am J Prev Med 2011;40(5 Suppl 2):S208–16.

[72] CRICO Strategies. Malpractice risks in communication failures: 2015 Annual Benchmarking Report. Boston, MA: Harvard University Press; 2016.

[73] Arora NK, Hesse BW, Rimer BK, Viswanath K, Clayman ML, Croyle RT. Frustrated and confused: the American public rates its cancer-related information-seeking experiences. J Gen Intern Med 2008;23(3):223–8.

[74] Eysenbach G. From intermediation to disintermediation and apomediation: new models for consumers to access and assess the credibility of health information in the age of Web2.0. Stud Health Technol Inform 2007;129(Pt 1):162–6.

[75] Berland GK, Elliott MN, Morales LS, Algazy JI, Kravitz RL, Broder MS, et al. Health information on the Internet: accessibility, quality, and readability in English and Spanish. JAMA 2001;285(20):2612–21.

[76] Hesse BW, Nelson DE, Kreps GL, Croyle RT, Arora NK, Rimer BK, et al. Trust and sources of health information: the impact of the Internet and its implications for health care providers: findings from the first Health Information National Trends Survey. Arch Intern Med 2005;165(22):2618–24.

[77] Starmer AJ, Sectish TC, Simon DW, Keohane C, McSweeney ME, Chung EY, et al. Rates of medical errors and preventable adverse events among hospitalized children following implementation of a resident handoff bundle. JAMA 2013;310(21):2262–70.

[78] Hesse BW, Hanna C, Massett HA, Hesse NK. Outside the box: will information technology be a viable intervention to improve the quality of cancer care? J Natl Cancer Inst Monogr 2010;2010(40):81–9.

[79] Tinetti ME, Fried TR, Boyd CM. Designing health care for the most common chronic condition—multimorbidity. JAMA 2012;307(23):2493–4.

[80] Alfano CM, Smith T, de Moor JS, Glasgow RE, Khoury MJ, Hawkins NA, et al. An action plan for translating cancer survivorship research into care. J Natl Cancer Inst 2014;106(11):1–9.

[81] Beckjord EB, Reynolds KA, van Londen GJ, Burns R, Singh R, Arvey SR, et al. Population-level trends in posttreatment cancer survivors' concerns and associated receipt of care: results from the 2006 and 2010 LIVESTRONG surveys. J Psychosoc Oncol 2014;32(2):125–51.

[82] Sprandio JD. Oncology patient-centered medical home. J Oncol Pract 2012;8(Suppl. 3):47s–9s.

[83] Bauer AM, Thielke SM, Katon W, Unutzer J, Arean P. Aligning health information technologies with effective service delivery models to improve chronic disease care. Prev Med 2014;66:167–72.

[84] Alston C, Berger Z, Brownlee S, Elwyn G, Fowler FJ, Hall LK, et al. Shared decision-making strategies for best care: patient decision aids Evidence communication innovation collaborative of the IOM roundtable on value and science-driven health care. Washington, DC: Institute of Medicine; 2014. 43 pp.

[85] Politi MC, Street Jr. RL. The importance of communication in collaborative decision making: facilitating shared mind and the management of uncertainty. J Eval Clin Pract 2011;17(4):579–84.

[86] Hesse BW. Decisional architectures. In: Dieffenbach MA, Miller SM, Bowen D, editors. Handbook of health decision science. New York (NY): Springer Verlag; [In Press].

[87] Shaikh AR, Butte AJ, Schully SD, Dalton WS, Khoury MJ, Hesse BW. Collaborative biomedicine in the age of big data: the case of cancer. J Med Internet Res 2014;16(4):e101.

[88] Ancker JS, Chan C, Kukafka R. Interactive graphics for expressing health risks: development and qualitative evaluation. J Health Commun 2009;14(5):461–75.

[89] Ancker JS, Senathirajah Y, Kukafka R, Starren JB. Design features of graphs in health risk communication: a systematic review. J Am Med Inform Assoc 2006;13(6):608–18.

[90] Shneiderman B, Plaisant C, Hesse BW. Improving healthcare with interactive visualization. IEEE Comput 2013;46(5):58–66.

[91] Brewer NT, Gilkey MB, Lillie SE, Hesse BW, Sheridan SL. Tables or bar graphs? presenting test results in electronic medical records. Med Decis Making 2012;32(4):545–53.

[92] Nelson DE, Hesse BW, Croyle RT. Making data talk: Communicating public health findings to journalists and the public. New York, NY: Oxford University Press; 2009. 323 pp.

[93] Coye MJ, Haselkorn A, DeMello S. Remote patient management: technology-enabled innovation and evolving business models for chronic disease care. Health Aff (Millwood) 2009;28(1):126–35.

[94] Ahern DK, Woods SS, Lightowler MC, Finley SW, Houston TK. Promise of and potential for patient-facing technologies to enable meaningful use. Am J Prev Med 2011;40(5 Suppl 2):S162–72.

[95] Berwick DM, Feeley D, Loehrer S. Change from the inside out: health care leaders taking the helm. JAMA 2015;313(7):1707–8.

[96] Wilson EV. Asynchronous health communication. Commun ACM 2003;46(6):79–84.

[97] Dubenske LL, Chih MY, Dinauer S, Gustafson DH, Cleary JF. Development and implementation of a clinician reporting system for advanced stage cancer: initial lessons learned. J Am Med Inform Assoc 2008;15(5):679–86.

[98] Chih MY, DuBenske LL, Hawkins RP, Brown RL, Dinauer SK, Cleary JF, et al. Communicating advanced cancer patients' symptoms via the Internet: a pooled analysis of two randomized trials examining caregiver preparedness, physical burden, and negative mood. Palliat Med 2013;27(6):533–43.

[99] Basch E, Artz D, Iasonos A, Speakman J, Shannon K, Lin K, et al. Evaluation of an online platform for cancer patient self-reporting of chemotherapy toxicities. J Am Med Inform Assoc 2007;14(3):264–8.

[100] Deci EL, Ryan RM. Self-determination theory in health care and its relations to motivational interviewing: a few comments. Int J Behav Nutr Phys Act 2012;9:24.

[101] Kissane DW, Bylund CL, Banerjee SC, Bialer PA, Levin TT, Maloney EK, et al. Communication skills training for oncology professionals. J Clin Oncol 2012;30:1242–7.

[102] Institute of Medicine. Capturing social and behavioral domains and measures in electronic health records: phase 2. pages cm. Washington, DC: National Academies Press; 2015.

[103] Chiang AC, Buja Amport S, Corjulo D, Harvey KL, McCorkle R. Incorporating patient-reported outcomes to improve emotional distress screening and assessment in an ambulatory oncology clinic. J Oncol Pract 2015;11(3):219–22.

[104] Ferrer RA, Klein WMP, Lerner JS, Reyna V, Keltner D. Emotions and health decision making: Extending the Appraisal Tendency Framework to improve health and health care. In: Roberto C, Kawachi I, editors. Behavioral economics and public health. Cambridge, MA: Harvard University Press; 2016. p. 101–31.

[105] Cameron LD, Leventhal H. The self-regulation of health and illness behaviour. London, NY: Routledge; 2003. xii, 337 pp.

[106] Klein WM, Bloch M, Hesse BW, McDonald PG, Nebeling L, O'Connell ME, et al. Behavioral research in cancer prevention and control: a look to the future. Am J Prev Med 2014;46(3):303–11.

[107] Han PK, Klein WM, Arora NK. Varieties of uncertainty in health care: a conceptual taxonomy. Med Decis Making 2011;31(6):828–38.

[108] Han PK, Klein WMP, Lehman T, Killam B, Massett H, Freedman AN. Communication of uncertainty regarding individualized cancer risk estimates: effects and influential factors. Med Decis Making 2011;31(2):354–66.

[109] Hesse BW, Beckjord EB, Rutten LF, Fagerlin A, Cameron LD. Cancer communication and informatics research across the cancer continuum. Am Psychol 2015;70(2):198–210.

[110] Hewitt ME, Ganz PA. From cancer patient to cancer survivor: lost in transition: an American Society of Clinical Oncology and Institute of Medicine Symposium. Washington, DC: National Academies Press; 2006. vi, 189 pp.

[111] Beckjord EB. The need for focus on outcomes and the role of informatics (Commentary). J Oncol Pract 2014;10(2):e93–4.

[112] President's Council of Advisors on Science and Technology. Better health care and lower costs: accelerating improvement through systems engineering. Washington (DC): The White House; 2014. p. 55.

III. SCIENCE OF ONCOLOGY INFORMATICS

Cancer Surveillance Informatics

Lynne T. Penberthy MD, MPH[1], Deborah M. Winn PhD[2] and Susan M. Scott MPH[1]

[1]Surveillance Research Program, Division of Cancer Control and Population Sciences, National Cancer Institute, Rockville, MD, United States [2]Office of the Director, Division of Cancer Control and Population Sciences, National Cancer Institute, Rockville, MD, United States

OUTLINE

14.1 Background on Cancer Surveillance	277	14.3.3 Clinical Trials Case Identification in Real Time	283
14.2 Current Status and Opportunities for Informatics in Cancer Surveillance: NLP, Automation, and Linkages	280	14.3.4 Expanded Ability to Assess Quality of Care	283
14.2.1 Automation Through NLP	280	14.3.5 Expanded Ability to Make Sense of Cancer Patterns and Trends	283
14.2.2 Expanding on Data Linkages for Surveillance	280	14.4 Conclusion	284
14.3 New Areas for Cancer Surveillance Supported Through Informatics	282	List of Acronyms and Abbreviations	284
14.3.1 Biorepositories	282	Acknowledgments	284
14.3.2 A National Virtual Registry	283	References	284

14.1 BACKGROUND ON CANCER SURVEILLANCE

Cancer surveillance is the collection of data on cancer cases to provide population-based trends and outcomes for cancer, typically representing a complete census of all cases within a defined geographic region, such as a state. Traditional functions of cancer surveillance include reporting incidence, prevalence, survival, and mortality trends for populations covered. The purposes of cancer surveillance systems may include monitoring the magnitude of and trends in the burden of cancer in the population and using that information to inform cancer prevention and control efforts.

Surveillance data are used by a variety of stakeholders, including medical and public health professionals, researchers, policymakers, and the general public. In the United States, the Centers for Disease Control and Prevention (CDC) supports the National Program of Cancer Registries (NPCR), and the National Cancer Institute (NCI) supports the Surveillance, Epidemiology, and End Results (SEER) Program. The SEER Program has been funded by NCI since 1973 and was established as a result of the National Cancer Act of 1971, which mandated that the NCI "...collect, analyze, and disseminate all data useful in the prevention, diagnosis, and treatment of cancer..." [1]. Together, SEER and NPCR collect data from state cancer registries from the

B. Hesse, D. Ahern & E. Beckjord: Oncology Informatics.
DOI: http://dx.doi.org/10.1016/B978-0-12-802115-6.00014-8

50 states, the District of Columbia, Puerto Rico, and the US Pacific Island Jurisdictions, enabling the compilation and reporting of national surveillance statistics.

As cancer care has become more complex, the value of cancer surveillance data to support research on cancer has grown in importance. Reporting by health care providers of all cancer cases, treatment, and outcomes is mandated by regulation in all states in the United States. That requirement enables cancer surveillance data to be used as a sampling frame in research studies, providing a study sample of cancer patients that is representative of a particular geographic area. A second feature of cancer surveillance that facilitates research is that, because the reporting and maintenance of Protected Health Information (PHI) is necessary to perform longitudinal follow-up for each patient and to link data from various reporting sources, the use and disclosure of this information for research purposes is permitted, with certain stipulations, according to the Health Insurance Portability and Accountability Act (HIPAA) Privacy Rule. This means that it is possible to utilize research data sets—deidentified in accordance with the standards set by the HIPAA Privacy Rule—based on registry data representing the entire population of cancer cases followed longitudinally (ie, over time) [2]. Because the data are longitudinal, researchers can conduct studies that investigate such questions as whether the diffusion of a new cancer therapy with demonstrated success in clinical trials improves survival in the general population.

Traditionally, cancer surveillance data have been captured primarily from hospital-based cancer registries. Hospital-based registries collect data only about patients in that facility. Therefore, the data are not population-based (ie, the data are not representative of the population) and are often incomplete, as only a portion of the care and diagnostic evaluation may be conducted in the hospital and accessible to the hospital registrar. These data are then consolidated and adjudicated from across multiple reporting entities (including hospitals, pathology laboratories, and physician offices) by the state or central cancer registry to form a complete depiction of the cancer burden and characterization of each cancer in the population covered by that state or registry. Data collection from these reporters has been primarily manual, with a registrar abstracting data from medical records and entering the data into a common, structured cancer abstract format.

The clinical service location where patients are diagnosed and treated is becoming more and more diverse and includes settings that are beyond what have been traditionally accessed by hospital cancer registrars. These sources include community oncology practices, specialty laboratories, and private industry (eg, pharmacies), among others, as shown in Fig. 14.1.

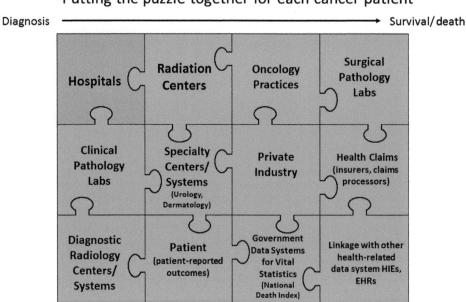

Cancer surveillance: Where do we need to go?
Putting the puzzle together for each cancer patient

FIGURE 14.1 Sources of cancer surveillance data. The wide spectrum of health care settings that provide data about a cancer case, from diagnosis through long-term survival or death from cancer, is shown. Hospitals (shown in green) are the traditional data source. HIEs, health information exchanges; EHRs, electronic health records.

For example, patients today may receive a cancer diagnosis based on information from an independent pathology laboratory, and they may be treated in a dermatology physician practice. The same patients may then receive radiation therapy at a freestanding radiation facility. That diversity of services, combined with the growing duration and complexity of treatment and other elements required to correctly characterize the cancer case (see Fig. 14.2), make it necessary for registries to capture data in categories not traditionally included in the cancer abstract. Such data include subsequent therapy, orally administered treatment received at a pharmacy, or testing for genetic mutations that would indicate susceptibility to a targeted therapy. These new categories also mean that manual data collection from hospital facilities is no longer sufficient to provide a complete description of the disease course for each patient.

Further, tumor characterization is no longer sufficient with only anatomic descriptors such as histology, stage, grade, and tumor size. It must also include progressively more sophisticated molecular and genetic information to describe the tumor in the context of prognosis and therapeutic response. For example, mutations in the *BRAF* gene are common in melanomas, and drugs that target this mutation have been developed to treat patients with

such mutations [3]. This is just one of many new molecular tests that have implications for how a patient's cancer is treated. As precision medicine becomes ever more important to the diagnosis and treatment of each case, it is critical for cancer surveillance to be able to provide trends and rates specific to each of these important and more clinically relevant categories represented by molecular characterization.

The molecular characteristics of a patient's cancer may not be accessible to the hospital registrar and/or may require clinical interpretation, thus risking missing or incorrect data. The greater complexity, coupled with the increased absolute number of necessary data elements, the amplified number of cases in an aging population, and the correspondingly higher burden on registrars, necessitates the development and use of informatics tools. These include data linkages to information maintained by diverse data stewards and reliance on natural language processing (NLP) to enable capture of data that are both more clinically relevant and essential to understanding trends in cancer incidence, prevalence, and mortality. Using these types of approaches and methods will provide the flexibility and agility required to maintain relevancy of the data in cancer surveillance.

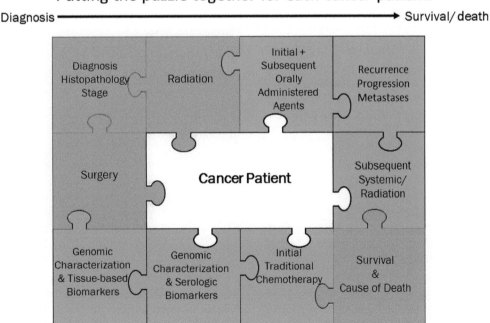

Cancer surveillance: What do we need to collect?
Putting the puzzle together for each cancer patient.

FIGURE 14.2 Cancer surveillance data domains. Information that has traditionally been captured by registries is shown in green. Shown in blue are information categories for which efforts are underway to begin collecting data or to enhance and expand upon existing collection.

14.2 CURRENT STATUS AND OPPORTUNITIES FOR INFORMATICS IN CANCER SURVEILLANCE: NLP, AUTOMATION, AND LINKAGES

14.2.1 Automation Through NLP

According to the Centers for Medicare & Medicaid Services (CMS), the Medicare and Medicaid Electronic Health Record (EHR) Incentive Programs provide financial incentives for the meaningful use of certified EHR technology to improve patient care [4]. While "meaningful use" is an opportunity for discrete data extraction and reporting from hospitals and physician providers to cancer registries, there has been limited implementation of the complex software modifications required by vendors to provide this reporting. Further, the current lack of interoperable EHRs (also called electronic medical records), even for the same vendor across different institutions, represents a challenge to automated reporting from EHRs in the immediate future. Thus alternative solutions are needed that can bridge the gap and provide a platform for future automated reporting.

Given the pressing need for automation, the surveillance community has been developing systems for automated collection of data sources that can be leveraged using informatics tools and processes. The first such opportunity is the capture of electronic pathology (e-path) reports. Many cancer registries have been receiving e-path reports in near real time since 2004. Currently, the NCI SEER registries receive e-path reports covering about 80% of their cancer cases directly from hospitals and freestanding pathology laboratories. The reports received include both the initial report and subsequent reports or addenda that contain important information about the tumor. Currently, the automated processing of e-path reports in the registry community is limited and consists of autoconsolidation of all of the reports with existing cancer records, automated selection of probable diagnosis [based on International Classification of Diseases for Oncology (ICD-O) histology codes], and increasingly sophisticated viewing capabilities that permit more efficient manual review.

The unstructured data in the e-path reports represent additional opportunities for data enhancement, as they are a rich source of information critical to the case report; such data include anatomic and, more and more frequently, molecular characterization of the tumor, notably providing information on tissue-based biomarker data. As precision medicine becomes even more relevant to the diagnosis and treatment of each cancer case, cancer surveillance must be able to provide trends and rates by these important and more clinically relevant categories represented by molecular characterization. Despite the potential availability of structured formats in pathology reports based on the College of American Pathologists (CAP) Synoptic checklist [5], these reports are typically sent in unstructured text in a variety of formats. Thus, interim tools to optimize the use of these unstructured data are necessary to meet the needs of data collection for cancer surveillance.

Examples of data currently being collected manually or available in the e-path reports for automated extraction include the molecular markers *ER/PR/Her2neu/ki67* for breast cancer, *EGFR/ALK/BRAF* for lung cancer, and *KRAS/BRAF/MSI* for colon cancer. Because of the expanding capacity of laboratories nationwide to test for these markers and the issuance of clinical guidelines calling for routine testing for them [6], capturing this information is critical for understanding the quality of care (ie, compliance with guidelines), estimating the potential for response to therapy, and understanding cancer at the population level—outside the clinical trial setting. The growing availability of NLP tools provides a solution for capturing and extracting data from unstructured text [7,8]. Using these techniques for processing e-path reports would enable extraction of this information without continued reliance on manual processes.

NCI's SEER Program is working with registries, investigators, and commercial entities to optimize the extraction of this information automatically from existing data sources such as e-path reports, mainly by using NLP tools. When that objective has been accomplished, the same technology and methods can be applied to other data sources, such as radiologic imaging reports, clinical notes, and discharge summaries [9,10]. Beyond using NLP and automation to extract critical information about individual tumors, tapping into "agile technology" (ie, technology developed to meet the time pressures of a real-world operating environment) [11] to modify NLP processes would also provide information to assess the dissemination of new technologies over time at the population level.

14.2.2 Expanding on Data Linkages for Surveillance

In addition to leveraging NLP and automation for extracting data from free text, other automation sources and methods are necessary to provide complete surveillance representation of each cancer case. These other sources (Fig. 14.1) provide key information categories (Fig. 14.2) that are critical to cancer surveillance and that may not be captured in the EHR (at least in the hospital setting) or in free text documents such as e-path reports. To enable registries to more completely characterize and follow each patient longitudinally, a second major methodologic approach to cancer surveillance informatics is underway. The goal is to identify large population-based data sets that can be linked at the patient level to cancer registry cases. These direct linkages would provide complete information on certain data categories, reduce the effort required by registrars, and reduce errors associated with interpretation or data entry. Registries have a long history of linking with external data sources to supplement information already captured from existing sources; the potential supplemental sources include Medicare claims data, the National Death Index, and the Department of Motor Vehicle databases (to track residential changes and monitor survival status), among others [12–14]. Such linkages provide important information about individual cases to the registry in a secure environment, and registries are legally mandated to collect health data about the cancer cases and monitor them indefinitely for vital status.

When assessing and planning potential data linkages to supplement existing cancer surveillance information, the key criteria are: (1) importance of the data to understanding cancer; (2) potential for population reporting/representativeness (ie, whether the data cover most, if not all, of the population); and (3) opportunity to leverage standardized data reporting formats or nomenclature that can be scaled or generalized.

Orally administered antineoplastic agents represent one example of a key data category that could be enhanced through linkages. Increasingly, antineoplastic drugs are being administered orally instead of by more invasive methods such as infusion. In addition, because they usually are not administered in hospitals or prescribed through a hospital pharmacy, they are often missing from cancer surveillance data collected from hospitals. Moreover, while electronic prescribing of such drugs captures which have been ordered, that information may not reflect whether the prescriptions were actually filled or whether the patient took them as ordered.

A second example of a key data category are specific tests such as Oncotype DX used in subsets of breast cancer patients to predict the benefit of chemotherapy. This 21-gene assay test is currently performed by one company (Genomic Health) and, beginning in 2008, has been included in one of the National Comprehensive Cancer Network (NCCN) guidelines for breast cancer treatment decision making—specifically, for women with hormone receptor-positive, HER2-negative tumors that are 0.6 to 1.0 cm and moderately/poorly differentiated or with unfavorable features, or larger than 1 cm [15]. Often the test results are provided directly to the oncologist and may not be recorded in the hospital record that is accessible to the cancer registrar. Thus this information may not be available to the central registry through the usual reporting sources. A third example is infusion chemotherapy. Much of the intravenously administered chemotherapy is given in the outpatient setting, including the community oncology practice; thus the information

is not accessible to the hospital registrar. Additionally, no detail on the specific agents and doses for this more traditional treatment modality is captured by cancer registries, even for the initial course, and no information is captured on subsequent courses of treatment. This lack of detail and limited focus represents a gap in the data at the case level, which in turn limits understanding cancer care and its outcomes in populations.

Examples of current and planned linkages that address these gaps include use of claims data, data from industry partners, and secondary sources that capture data not readily available to the registry community.

14.2.2.1 Claims Data

Linkage with claims data has been ongoing within the SEER Program, with registry data linking to Medicare data at the individual person level since the late 1990s [16]. The linked data have been used extensively to support health services research and outcomes analyses, as well as to assess quality of care. While this linkage is of great value to research endeavors, it includes only patients 65 years of age and older, and there are certain restrictions on using the data to supplement registry information on treatment. For example, only the more generic information, such as none, one, or more than one chemotherapy agent used, is permitted to be used for supplementing SEER treatment information. Several studies evaluating the benefit of automated software that processes claims data from physician practices have demonstrated significant improvement in the completeness and accuracy of treatment capture [17–19]. Therefore, linkages with claims other than Medicare, such as from oncology practices, may be an important additional component to supplementing treatment and is being evaluated [20]. For example, on a state level, automated reporting of cancer and its treatment directly from oncology practices to cancer registries has been initiated in the Florida Cancer Data System, which is the state registry.

The Florida registry offered physicians the opportunity to meet their legal cancer case reporting requirement by submitting the standardized 837 formatted claims common for all insurance billing to the central registry via a secure server. Once submitted, software extracts the key information on demographics, diagnosis, and treatment and stores it in a database. The database maintains complete information on detailed treatment based on Healthcare Common Procedure Coding (HCPC) codes. On a scheduled basis, the software links with existing cancer cases in the registry that have been captured from hospitals and other sources, creates an automated abstract in the standardized format, and permits consolidation of this information with existing data. This system continues to be developed; to date, more than 9 million claims have been submitted by more than 1200 oncology physicians in the state. This mechanism permits automatic capture of detailed treatment information that is unlikely to be accessible to the hospital registrar but will provide critical information to support research. Capturing this detailed data is critical for many analyses, and will enable researchers to better understand the disparate outcomes among cancer patients. Without detailed and complete treatment information, it is not possible to know why these differences occur.

14.2.2.2 Data From Industry Partners

Other types of linkages would focus on key data sets that may be incompletely available to the more traditional hospital-based reporting sources. Such linkages would include data from industry partners who perform critical genomic tests, such as Genomic Health, Inc. for Oncotype DX, or collaborating with key specialty EHR vendors (eg, oncology specialty providers such as radiation oncology machine manufacturers). Because a single or small number of specialty vendors capture all or most of the data on cancer patients across the United States, these types of linkages would ensure complete capture of information on all patients. Linkages with commercial partners are essential because, as mentioned above, the test results may not be included in the hospital record, but instead are sent directly to the physician provider. The information would therefore be missing from the hospital cancer abstract. Similarly, linkages with specialty providers (radiation oncology or medical oncology) would supplement the information on cancer cases, as detailed diagnosis and treatment data are being collected and stored with greater frequency in these outpatient facilities, who often may not report directly to the registry [17–20]. Notably, reporting from these various providers to the individual state registries is required by law in every state. Therefore, automating this process would streamline the reporting providers' roles while simultaneously enhancing the completeness and accuracy of the reported cancer case information.

14.2.2.3 New Challenges to Surveillance Data Quality Raised by Informatics

As these new surveillance methods are put in place, new methods for evaluating and ensuring the quality of what is captured will need to be developed. New statistical methods for assessing the quality of linkages are needed to ensure that the correct individuals are being linked. Considerations for how to impute data from a population subset may be required, as some data may be available only for a limited subset, and it will be necessary to understand how that subset represents the larger population. As new NLP processes are implemented, statistical and other tools must be in place to

ensure accuracy in interpreting the extracted information. Finally, with multiple linkages, registries will need to assure patient confidentiality. While as mentioned above, reporting to state central cancer registries is HIPAA exempt and registries must maintain PHI, ongoing linkages will require secure measures to protect the confidentiality of the linked information.

14.3 NEW AREAS FOR CANCER SURVEILLANCE SUPPORTED THROUGH INFORMATICS

14.3.1 Biorepositories

Population-based cancer registry systems currently utilize annotation including detailed and structured histopathologic and anatomic tumor characterization, and all SEER registries collect initial course of cancer-directed treatment information and patient demographics. Many SEER registries already have developed methods to access residual tumor tissue from cancer patients in their coverage area through formal arrangements with pathology or hospital laboratories. Such an arrangement could enable an organizational entity to serve as an honest broker for multiple registries and researchers, linking researchers who lead projects requiring tissue with the pathology laboratories who hold the residual tissue. A model that has been used successfully in several of the SEER registries is for the registry to serve as an honest broker to deidentify the tissue specimens and linked annotation, thereby protecting subject identity. The Institutional Review Boards (IRBs) for the registries serving as honest brokers do not consider use of deidentified tissues and associated data in this manner to be research involving human subjects. The research supported by these population-based tissue specimens could have far-reaching implications and, unlike results from many biobank studies, is generalizable to the entire population [21–24].

A centralized process would permit one-stop shopping [25] within a large-scale potential biorepository. This will allow investigators to work with only one entity, specify the types of cases and tumor tissue needed for a project, and eliminate the need to interact directly with multiple registries. The researchers could receive the tumor tissue and the rich, extensive annotation about the cancer and the patient, enabling them to conduct their research. Informatics is vital for implementing such an efficient system, which crosses cancer registries, links to disparate sources of tumor tissue, helps to deidentify data, and matches the researcher to the specific types of patients who are needed for the project and have tissue material available. Using informatics tools to upload and link deidentified information from the cancer abstract to a deidentified set of pathology reports would provide a rich source from which investigators could select specimens representing unusual cancers, outcomes, or population subsets. Such a scaled virtual biorepository, supported through the informatics tools and methods discussed above, would serve as an invaluable resource to support a variety of research not readily supported by traditional biobanks. Leveraging automation including NLP searches would increase efficiency for investigators who study tissue categories that have rarely been available within single institution-based biorepositories or even across geographic regions.

14.3.2 A National Virtual Registry

As described above, each central cancer registry collects and maintains data according to individual state laws. Registry data are often used to provide information on cancer cases, including outcomes such as survival and cause of death, for a variety of research enterprises including cohort studies, clinical trials, and postmarketing surveillance for drugs that demonstrate a potential for increased risk of cancer. All of these types of research require information from cancer registries about which of their study participants have developed a cancer, the specific details of that cancer, and often the outcomes and cause of death for participants. State laws typically prohibit the cancer registry from pooling its registry data with data from other registries or permitting any other organizational entity to control the use of their data. Current practice requires an investigator to approach each registry, obtain IRB approval there, and then perform the linkage, often requiring many months but identifying no matches for their targeted patients. This is especially problematic for researchers whose study participants reside in multiple states or move to different states over a prolonged follow-up period.

With the availability of new informatics techniques for matching and new security protocols, a more efficient, centralized process is in development that permits "virtual" pooling of data from multiple registries and does not yield control by the registry regarding use of the data. Pilot studies have demonstrated that a virtual registry is an efficient and effective method for identifying patients within registries who match specific study participant lists. Developing this type of automated process will not only increase efficiency, but will also improve accuracy by permitting routine linkage with a larger number of registries. At the same time, it will require minimal effort by the investigator and the registry. In addition, routine use of this virtual national registry linkage would enhance deduplication of cancer cases within registries that do not routinely match their data, thereby improving the accuracy of surveillance data in reporting trends over time.

14.3.3 Clinical Trials Case Identification in Real Time

Although the complete abstract for a cancer case is not available in real time, as described above, the e-path report and potentially other documents and data linkages are available in near real time. The e-path report is received at the registry at the same time that it is submitted to the physician or hospital record. Using this data source, many registries are already performing real-time case ascertainment to identify patients who are potentially eligible for a clinical trial or other study. As new NLP tools are applied to perform additional automated data extraction, the capacity to use registry data for screening patients based on specific clinical trial eligibility requirements will be enhanced. Consequently, such tools will likely improve the number of patients who are rapidly screened for potential eligibility [26–29]. The ability to prescreen large patient populations is becoming more critical as clinical trial requirements become more specific and restrictive, resulting in lower and slower accrual and often causing trials to close due to poor accrual [30].

14.3.4 Expanded Ability to Assess Quality of Care

As described above, surveillance data have the capacity to provide population-based estimates of compliance with some clinical guidelines for cancer diagnosis and treatment, even given current limitations with respect to their level of treatment detail. As additional data are added, including expanded capture of tumor biomarkers and other molecular characterizations, surveillance data have the potential to better support population-based monitoring of the quality of cancer care. With the advent and implementation of automation and NLP tools that permit agile and flexible adaptation of registry data collection, the data also can be used to assess dissemination of new technologies and practices within the population as a whole and within geographic, racial, and ethnic subgroups. Collaboration of other entities such as ASCO's CanceLinQ with these enhanced surveillance systems could serve to efficiently expand the capacity of such organizations to perform quality control.

14.3.5 Expanded Ability to Make Sense of Cancer Patterns and Trends

As noted in the introduction to this chapter, the fundamental purpose of cancer surveillance systems is to monitor the magnitude of and trends in the burden of cancer in the population and use that information to inform cancer prevention and control efforts. In addition to using novel informatics methods in surveillance to enhance research, the surveillance community is moving toward presenting surveillance data in more relevant categories to better address the mandate for reporting of trends. For example, breast cancer as an organ site provides information on the overall burden, but it is more important to patients and physicians to provide the data according to the molecular subgroups, such as triple negative or hormone receptor positive, for them to understand an individual's prognosis. Other examples of opportunities to more clearly define the cancer burden include esophageal cancer, which is largely represented by squamous cell and adenocarcinoma and for which the two major histologies have differing trends over time. Leveraging the more sophisticated reporting through more refined reporting of the data will be an important step for cancer surveillance.

14.4 CONCLUSION

Surveillance systems serve as a foundation for research in populations and are the source for understanding trends in cancer incidence, prevalence, and mortality. Data captured through national surveillance systems such as the SEER Program provide a critical infrastructure that can support a wide variety of research areas and questions. However, the changing landscape of how cancer care is provided, coupled with the mounting complexity of cancer diagnosis and treatment, requires new surveillance tools and methods that will maintain and expand research infrastructure and provide trends for clinically relevant categories.

Informatics tools and applications represent a promising set of solutions to the challenges facing cancer surveillance in this era of precision medicine. The need to acquire and link data from multiple sources, as described in the examples above, highlights the need to establish collaborative partnerships with a variety of organizations involved in diagnosing and caring for cancer patients. Without such collaboration and the integration of sophisticated informatics tools, it will be impossible to understand the larger picture of cancer trends and quality of care. Thus, it is essential to not only enhance the data sources from which surveillance information is collected, but also increase the categories of relevant information and develop new and expanded partnerships with organizations who are the data stewards. These objectives will be feasible only through broadening and intensifying existing informatics efforts, including automation and linkages.

LIST OF ACRONYMS AND ABBREVIATIONS

CAP College of American Pathologists
CDC Centers for Disease Control and Prevention
CMS Centers for Medicare & Medicaid Services
e-path Electronic pathology
HCPC Healthcare Common Procedure Coding
EHR Electronic Health Record
HIPAA Health Insurance Portability and Accountability Act
ICD-O International Classification of Diseases for Oncology
NCCN National Comprehensive Cancer Network
NCI National Cancer Institute
NPCR National Program of Cancer Registries
PHI Protected Health Information (also called Personal Health Information)
SEER Surveillance, Epidemiology, and End Results

Acknowledgments

The authors thank Ms Jessica Boten for assistance with graphics.

References

[1] National Cancer Institute. Office of Government and Congressional Relations. National Cancer Act of 1971. [cited July 16, 2015] Available from: <http://legislative.cancer.gov/history/phsa/1971>.

[2] National Cancer Institute. SEER Program. Research repositories, databases, and the HIPAA privacy rule. NIH Publication Number 04-5489; January 2004. [cited April 15, 2015] Available from: <http://seer.cancer.gov/biospecimen/hipaa_research_repositories_final.pdf>.

[3] Spagnolo F, Ghiorzo P, Orgiano L, Pastorino L, Picasso V, Tornari E, et al. BRAF-mutant melanoma: treatment approaches, resistance mechanisms, and diagnostic strategies. OncoTargets Ther 2015;8:157–68.

[4] Centers for Medicare & Medicaid Services. 2014 Definition stage 1 of meaningful use. CMS Web site. [cited March 31, 2015] Available from: <http://www.cms.gov/Regulations-and-Guidance/Legislation/EHRIncentivePrograms/Meaningful_Use.html>.

[5] College of American Pathologists. Cancer protocol templates. CAP Web site. [cited March 31, 2015] Available from: <http://www.cap.org/web/home/resources/cancer-reporting-tools/cancer-protocol-templates?_afrLoop=506603857187688#%40%3F_afrLoop%3D506603857187688%26_adf.ctrl-state%3Deq2setzv5_4/> .

[6] National Comprehensive Cancer Network (NCCN). Guidelines for treatment of cancer by site. NCCN Web site. [cited July 30, 2015] Available from: <http://www.nccn.org/professionals/physician_gls/f_guidelines.asp#site/>.

[7] Friedman C, Hripcsak G. Evaluating natural language processors in the clinical domain. Methods Inf Med 1998;37(4–5):334–44.

[8] Buckley JM, Coopey SB, Sharko J, et al. The feasibility of using natural language processing to extract clinical information from breast pathology reports. J Pathol Inform 2012;3:23.

[9] Petkov VI, Penberthy LT, Dahman BA, Poklepovic A, Gillam CW, McDermott JH. Automated determination of metastases in unstructured radiology reports for eligibility screening in oncology clinical trials. Exp Biol Med (Maywood) 2013;238(12):1370.

[10] Patrick J, Asgari P, Li M, Nguyen D. Using NLP to identify cancer cases in imaging reports drawn from radiology information systems. Stud Health Technol Inform 2013;188:91–4.

[11] Agile Alliance. What is Agile Software Development; June 8, 2013. [cited July 5, 2015] Available from: <http://www.agilealliance.org/the-alliance/what-is-agile/>.

[12] Hernandez MN, Voti L, Feldman JD, Tannenbaum SL, Scharber W, Mackinnon JA, et al. Cancer registry enrichment via linkage with hospital-based electronic medical records: a pilot investigation. J Regist Manage 2013;40(1):40–7.

[13] Lin G, Ma J, Zhang L, Qu M. Linking cancer registry and hospital discharge data for treatment surveillance. Health Inform J 2013;19(2):127–36.

[14] Bradley CJ, Penberthy L, Devers KJ, Holden DJ. Health services research and data linkages: issues, methods, and directions for the future. Health Serv Res 2010;45(5 Pt 2):1468–88.

[15] National Comprehensive Cancer Network. NCCN updates breast cancer guidelines; January 22, 2008. [cited April 16, 2015] Available from: <http://www.nccn.org/about/news/newsinfo.aspx?NewsID=127/ > .

[16] Healthcare Delivery Research Program. National Cancer Institute. SEER-Medicare. [cited April 15, 2015] Available from: <http://healthcaredelivery.cancer.gov/seermedicare/>.

[17] Hernandez MN, MacKinnon JA, Penberthy L, Bonner J, Huang YX. Enhancing central cancer registry treatment data using physician medical claims: a Florida pilot project. J Regist Manag 2014;41(2):51–6.

[18] Penberthy LT, McClish D, Agovino P. Impact of automated data collection from urology offices: improving incidence and treatment reporting in urologic cancers. J Regist Manag 2010;37(4):141–7.

[19] Penberthy L, Petkov V, McClish D, Peace S, Overton S, Radhakrishnan S, et al. The value of billing data from oncology practice to supplement treatment information for cancer surveillance. J Regist Manag 2014;41(2):57–64.

[20] Penberthy L, McClish D, Peace S, Gray L, Martin J, Overton S, et al. Hematologic malignancies: an opportunity to fill a gap in cancer surveillance. Cancer Causes Control 2012;23(8):1253–64.

[21] Goodman MT, Hernandez BY, Hewitt S, Lynch CF, Cote TR, Frierson Jr HF, et al. Tissues from population-based cancer registries: a novel approach to increasing research potential. Hum Pathol 2005;36:812–20.

[22] Chaturvedi AK, Engels EA, Pfeiffer RM, Hernandez BY, Xiao W, Kim E, et al. Human papillomavirus and rising oropharyngeal cancer incidence in the United States. J Clin Oncol 2011;29:4294–301.

[23] Takikita M, Altekruse S, Lynch CF, Goodman MT, Hernandez BY, Green M, et al. Associations between selected biomarkers and prognosis in a population-based pancreatic cancer tissue microarray. Cancer Res 2009;69:2950–5.

[24] Sy MS, Altekruse SF, Li C, Lynch CF, Goodman MT, Hernandez BY, et al. Association of prion protein expression with pancreatic adenocarcinoma survival in the SEER residual tissue repository. Cancer Biomark 2011;10:251–8.

[25] Altekruse SF, Rosenfeld GE, Carrick DM, Pressman EJ, Schully SD, Mechanic LE, et al. SEER cancer registry biospecimen research: yesterday and tomorrow. Cancer Epidemiol Biomarkers Prev 2014;23(12):2681–7.

[26] Beauharnais CC, Larkin ME, Zai AH, Boykin EC, Luttrell J, Wexler DJ. Efficacy and cost-effectiveness of an automated screening algorithm in an inpatient clinical trial. Clin Trials 2012;9:198–203.

[27] Embi PJ, Jain A, Clark J, Bizjack S, Hornung R, Harris CM. Effect of a clinical trial alert system on physician participation in trial recruitment. Arch Intern Med 2005;165:2272–7.

[28] Weng C, Batres C, Borda T, Weiskopf NG, Wilcox AB, Bigger JT, et al. A real-time screening alert improves patient recruitment efficiency. AMIA Annu Symp Proc 2011:1489–98.

[29] Penberthy LT, Dahman BA, Petkov VI, DeShazo JP. Effort required in eligibility screening for clinical trials. J Oncol Pract 2012;8(6):365–70.

[30] Schroen AT, Petroni GR, Wang H, Gray R, Wang XF, Cronin W, et al. Preliminary evaluation of factors associated with premature trial closure and feasibility of accrual benchmarks in phase III oncology trials. Clin Trials 2010;7:312–21.

15

Extended Vision for Oncology: A Perceptual Science Perspective on Data Visualization and Medical Imaging

Todd S. Horowitz PhD[1] and Ronald A. Rensink PhD[2]

[1]Behavioral Research Program, Division of Cancer Control and Population Sciences, National Cancer Institute, Rockville, MD, United States [2]Departments of Computer Science and Psychology, University of British Columbia, Vancouver, BC, Canada

OUTLINE

15.1 Introduction   287

15.2 How Vision Works (and How It Can Fail)   288
   15.2.1 Preattentive System   288
   15.2.2 Attentional System   289
   15.2.3 Nonattentional Systems   290
   15.2.4 Coordination of Systems   291

15.3 Visualization and Data Exploration   292
   15.3.1 Visualization as Extended Vision   293
   15.3.2 Visual Variables   293
   15.3.3 Attentional Control   293

15.4 Example 1: Human Number Perception and Quantitative Data   294

15.5 Example 2: Visual Attention and Medical Images   294
   15.5.1 The Prevalence Effect   296
   15.5.2 Subsequent Search Misses   298

15.6 Frontiers of Perceptual Science and Oncology Informatics   299
   15.6.1 Foraging for Cancer   299
   15.6.2 Strategies for Volumetric Search   300

15.7 Conclusions   300

List of Acronyms and Abbreviations   300

References   301

The gap between human information needs and the capabilities of our information technology is at the heart of informatics. Human beings are best at constructing and processing meaning; whereas computers are best at processing data ... Although this gap presents a problem, it also means that human beings and computers are naturally complementary.
Bernstam et al., 2010 [101]

15.1 INTRODUCTION

Recent years have seen an explosion in the use of medical informatics, the application of computing power to medicine. This development has created great opportunities for improving the science and practice of oncology and cancer care, as illustrated in many other

B. Hesse, D. Ahern & E. Beckjord: Oncology Informatics.
DOI: http://dx.doi.org/10.1016/B978-0-12-802115-6.00015-X

chapters in this volume. In principle, getting more information faster should let us make better, more timely decisions. However, any such system faces a critical bottleneck: the human being who must make sense of this information. An oncology informatics system typically presents information visually—for example, in the form of a dashboard, a graph, or a digital mammogram. But the nature of this bottleneck—the limitations of the human observer—is often not well understood, and so often is not adequately considered when designing a medical informatics system. This can cause problems.

In this chapter, we start with the view that any system for processing information is incomplete unless the human observer—the person supposed to explore, analyze, and ultimately use the information—is taken into account. We do not pretend that this is a new insight. There is a considerable body of work on improving the effectiveness of systems to convey quantitative information visually. To date, however, this has been a fairly empirical tradition. In contrast, we suggest here that oncology informatics could be substantially improved by drawing on basic research in visual perception to offer a better understanding of how best to present data and images. To this end, we begin with an introduction to the functional properties of the human visual system. We follow this with a general discussion of how knowledge of vision science can be applied to the field of visualization, which is concerned with developing effective ways of conveying information visually. Then, to illustrate how this approach can be applied to the design of improved informatics systems, we discuss in detail two specific examples: the effective display of quantitative data, and the effective display of medical images.

15.2 HOW VISION WORKS (AND HOW IT CAN FAIL)

When looking at the world, we generally have an impression that we immediately see everything in front of us. This has led to several commonly held beliefs about how vision works: (1) because the "picture" we experience is unitary, visual perception must involve a single, undifferentiated system; (2) because our experience is immediate, this system must be extremely fast and simple; and (3) because our experience is so full of apparent detail, this system must describe everything in sight. However, recent work in vision science has shown that each of these beliefs is wrong: (1) several distinct systems are involved rather than one; (2) they have far more intelligence than previously believed; and (3) instead of providing a complete, detailed description of the world in front of us, perception creates a dynamic "just-in-time" representation of only what is needed

at the moment, a representation that is sensitive to what the viewer knows and the goals they have at that moment.

If the older—and still prevalent—view about visual perception guides the design of an informatics system, significant problems can arise in using human vision to explore datasets and communicate results. But if the newer view is embraced, the possibility arises to develop systems that can seamlessly extend human vision, effectively "amplifying" its innate intelligence. To provide a better feel for the issues at stake, this section provides a brief overview of this emerging view of visual perception, focusing on the characteristics of the major perceptual systems involved (for further details, see Palmer [1].)

15.2.1 Preattentive System

We begin our discussion of the human perceptual system with a description of the events that occur in the first hundred milliseconds (ms) or so of encountering a visual stimulus, even before cognitive attention has been allocated. When light enters the eye, it strikes the retina and is transformed into an array of neural signals that travel along the optic nerve, maintaining the original spatial organization. The next stage is characterized by processes that are spatially parallel (ie, operating locally on each point of the input) and rapid (ie, completed within 100–200 ms). These are believed to operate automatically, without any need for attention, and are therefore often referred to as *preattentive processes* [2].

15.2.1.1 Visual Features

Preattentive processes are believed to create a set of *visual features* at each point in the representation of an image; these are essentially the primitive elements of perceptual experience. Information about their nature has been largely obtained via experiments on three kinds of phenomena: texture perception, perceptual organization, and visual search. Studies of texture perception investigate the properties supporting the effortless segmentation of an image into regions of similar texture (Fig. 15.1A). Related to this is the study of perceptual organization, which focuses on properties that govern grouping (Fig. 15.1B). Studies on visual search attempt to determine the properties governing the speed at which a given target item can be found in an image. Here, basic features are identified by their ability to immediately "pop out" of a display (or become salient) if they are unique (Fig. 15.1C). These features are believed to be the basic elements available to attention, and upon which it operates. As we will see later in the chapter, an understanding of preattentive processes can help guide the development of computer-assisted screening and diagnostic tools in oncology.

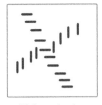 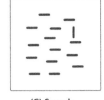

(A) Texture   (B) Organization   (C) Search

FIGURE 15.1 Phenomena providing insights into preattentive processing. (A) Texture perception, where the image spontaneously segments into regions of different textures. Here, segmentation is done on the basis of orientation. (B) Perceptual organization, where items are spontaneously perceived as belonging to particular groups. Here, the center item of the "X" is seen as belonging with other items of the same orientation. (C) Visual search, where an item with a unique property can immediately "pop out" of a set of items with different properties. Here, the vertical item among horizontal ones is noticed almost immediately.

15.2.1.2 Simple Properties

The studies described above suggest that the features at preattentive levels include a number of simple properties [2,3], such as

- orientation in the plane,
- curvature,
- color,
- contrast,
- width,
- length, and
- motion.

All of these properties can be computed by the brain on the basis of the limited information in the neighborhood about each point, allowing them to be processed rapidly and in parallel across the image. Most models of the underlying processes posit an initial stage of linear filtering, followed by various local nonlinear operations [1]. Texture segmentation appears to be based exclusively on the outputs of these feature analyzers, with regions determined via the density of features over space. Importantly, combinations of these properties do not appear to be formed at this level nor is there access to their precise spatial position. In a similar fashion, visual search appears to rely on a series of neural maps, each the output of an array of analyzers describing the distribution of each feature in the image [2].

15.2.1.3 Complex Properties

Although many visual features are simple, the structures they describe can be complex. For example, although a figure in a display will pop out if it has a distinctive length, this "length" is that of the entire figure; the length of the component lines is irrelevant [4]. Grouping of this kind indicates a fair degree of visual intelligence at this level, even in the absence of attention. Another example is the ability to compensate for occlusion. If a line is

partly occluded by a cube, say, its visible portions will be linked, reflecting the fact that they correspond to the same object in the scene [5]. As such, the final output of the early visual system might be best characterized as an array of measurements on a set of *proto-objects*, localized precursors of objects with at least some degree of structure. Among other things, these proto-objects appear to form the basis of estimates of image clutter.

Importantly, preattentive processes also appear capable of inferring several properties of the scene itself [6]. For example, visual search can be affected by three-dimensional orientation, surface convexity/concavity, direction of lighting, and the presence of shadows, with these estimates made on the basis of "quick and dirty" assumptions that are usually—but not always—true in the real world (eg, an assumption of lighting from above). More generally, the goal of this stage of visual processing appears to be a viewer-centered description of the world in which scene properties are represented in a fragmented way, a description that then serves as the input to all subsequent processes, including object perception and scene perception [7].

15.2.2 Attentional System

Performance in any task—including those supported by an informatics system—is governed by a factor within the observer that enables certain operations to be carried out, but which is limited in capacity. For example, when keeping track of several signals on a medical monitor, only a small number of signals can be handled simultaneously; if more are attempted, performance begins to fail. This limited factor is generally referred to as *visual attention*. Models of attention include a "spotlight" that travels around the image, enabling operations in the "illuminated" zone [2], or a "hand" that "grasps" particular proto-objects to knit them into a coherent visual object [8]. Such mechanisms are believed to act on structures already formed at preattentive levels. Furthermore, most of the effects of attention are believed to be relatively transient, lasting only as long as attention is being given to the relevant proto-objects [9].

15.2.2.1 Involvement in Perceptual Experience

Attention appears necessary for several aspects of conscious perception [10]. For example, if an observer's attention is somehow diverted, they can often miss unexpected objects and events, even when these are large and potentially relevant, a phenomenon known as *inattentional blindness* [11]. This can easily occur in everyday life—for example, inattentional blindness can cause automobile accidents, due to the attentional distraction resulting from cell phone use [12]. It can also occur in "heads-up" displays where two or more images are superimposed: an event shown in the unattended image can often be missed, even when the observer is gazing directly at it [13]. Inattentional blindness may also be the culprit when too many reminders or medical alarms are triggered simultaneously within an electronic health record (EHR) system [14].

Another kind of failure—possibly reflecting a different kind of attention—involves the integration of visual features. Attention is believed to be necessary for the perception of combinations (or conjunctions) of preattentive features. The absence (or incomplete engagement) of attention can therefore yield "partial perception," where features are seen, but not correctly combined, a phenomenon known as *illusory conjunction* [2]. For example, an observer might briefly glance at a display and see a red bottle with a blue label, when in reality there is a blue bottle with a red label.

Finally, an observer can also fail to see changes in a display, even when these are large and anticipated. This is known as *change blindness*, and is believed to indicate that attention is needed to see change [15]. Results suggest that no more than three to four items can be attended at a time, a limit that remains even after extensive practice. A related phenomenon is *change simultanagnosia*, the inability of an observer to see more than one distinct change among the attended items; essentially the change signals are pooled together, resulting in considerable cross-talk [16]. Compounding all these effects is *change blindness blindness*, a lack of awareness of the existence of these deficits in everyday life [17].

15.2.2.2 Precise Estimation of Number

When observing an array of fewer than five objects, we can apprehend the number in a glance, whereas larger numbers require effortful counting. This phenomenon is referred to as *subitizing* [18]. If we ask observers to count an array of objects, the plot of reaction time (also known as response time, or RT) as a function of number exhibits a characteristic elbow around 5: it takes very little more time to report that there are 4 objects than to report that there are 2, but there is a large difference between reporting 8 and 6.

While subitizing is fast and may feel immediate, it is not preattentive. For example, when observers busy with an unrelated task were presented with an unexpected array of items, they could not enumerate more than one or two items; if they expected the array, accuracy substantially improved [19]. These effects are specific to small numbers: under conditions of high attentional load performance for small numbers degrades, while performance for larger numbers does not [20].

15.2.2.3 Control

To minimize perceptual failures of the kinds described above, attention (including eye movements) must be carefully controlled. In everyday life, this is done via several interacting subsystems. The most basic of these relies on *exogenous control*, in which attention is allocated on the basis of the physical properties in the image; the beliefs and goals of the observer are largely irrelevant. Allocation priority is determined by salience, a scalar property that takes into account several different considerations [21]. One is the presence of visual features that are distinctive in the image (eg, a unique color or orientation); this is the basis of the pop-out described above. Others include the level of detail in the item, and whether it is illuminated. Intersections of long lines in an image can be salient as well [6]. Computer interface designers often take advantage of exogenous control by designing systems with the elements to be attended made salient by, for example, having them blink off and on, or placing them in a highlighted area.

To take advantage of knowledge about the world, attentional allocation also employs *endogenous control*, which incorporates higher-level factors such as the viewer's interest in a particular object at a particular moment, or their expectations about it. "Interest" is difficult to define, but in part involves features that are unexpected in the given context [22]. More generally, endogenous control depends on an awareness of the situation at hand, and therefore requires processes that are more sophisticated and time-consuming [23]. But although endogenous control is slower than its exogenous counterpart, it can take advantage of the observer's knowledge to predict events. This is why technical training and practice can be effective in helping, say, radiologists detect certain textures in mammograms that may signal a malignant tumor. The exact way the two types of control interact is not completely known; however, endogenous control can override exogenous considerations when interest is sufficiently high [24].

15.2.3 Nonattentional Systems

Although visual attention is often believed to be a "gateway" through which all visual processing must pass, recent results point to the existence of systems that operate concurrently with—and largely independent of—any kind of attentional processing. Several of these cognitive systems have a degree of visual intelligence that shows considerable sophistication, even in the complete absence of a conscious visual picture.

15.2.3.1 Statistical Summaries

Human vision can rapidly create *statistical* (or *ensemble*) *summaries* of sets of briefly presented items [25]. For example, within 50 ms, observers can determine the mean size of a group of disks as accurately as they can an individual disk [26]. This ability extends to other visual properties, from simple features like color and orientation to the center of mass of a set of items to sophisticated properties such as facial expressions [25]. Other kinds of summary measures are also possible, such as correlation in a scatterplot [27].

15.2.3.2 The Approximate Number System

Believed to be a form of ensemble summary perception, the approximate number system allows us to grasp the numerosity of any set of items almost immediately. The estimate is a noisy one; it would be easy to distinguish between 30 and 50 items, for example, but difficult to distinguish between 45 and 50 items. More generally, the standard deviation of the distribution of these estimates are proportional to the mean; discriminating between 100 and 120 items is just as difficult as discriminating between 10 and 12 items. This is *Weber's Law*, a principle which holds true for many psychophysical quantities, such as brightness, line length, and duration [28]. The ratio of the standard deviation to the mean is known as the *Weber fraction*, and is a measure of the precision of whatever system is making the discrimination. For adults, the average Weber fraction for numerosity is about 0.11 [29].

This system yields similar results when using arrays presented visually or auditorally [30]. It appears to be innate in humans, not a product of mathematical training or language. Indeed, other primates [31] show the same capacities, suggesting that the approximate number sense is part of our evolutionary heritage, rather than a cultural product of mathematical training. And unlike the precise estimation of number, approximate estimation does not require focused attention, or the intention to enumerate.

15.2.3.3 Scene Gist

Another faculty possibly related to summary statistics is the ability of observers to rapidly determine the abstract meaning (or gist) of the image of a scene, whether it is of a city, kitchen, or harbor. This can be done within 100ms, a time insufficient for attending to more than a few items [32]. Gist can also be extracted from blurred images—indeed, two different gists can be determined simultaneously [33].

An intriguing study [34] suggests that specialists in oncological imaging may be able to identify the "abnormal gist" in medical images. They showed mammograms and cervical micrographs to, respectively, radiologists and cytologists, as well as naïve observers, for only 250 to 2000ms. Naïve observers (who received a brief tutorial on what to look for) were at chance at the 250ms duration, though they managed to do better than chance by 1000ms. Unsurprisingly, experts performed better than naïves at the longer durations. But they also performed better at exposures of only 250ms, indicating that radiologists and cytologists have some information about abnormalities in a single glance, without necessarily focusing their eyes on the abnormality. If we could identify the information the experts exploited in these experiments, we might be able to enhance it to speed reading times, or use it to train new radiologists and cytologists more effectively.

15.2.3.4 Layout

Another nonattentional process is the determination of *layout*—the spatial arrangement of objects in a scene [35]. Layout also appears to contain a coarse, partial description of the size, color, and orientation of these objects. Some layout information appears to be extracted almost immediately, and some within several seconds of viewing—likely via eye movements or attentional shifts. In any event, once layout information has been extracted, it can be maintained for several seconds, apparently without the need for attention [36].

15.2.3.5 Sensing

When looking at—but not seeing—a change in an image, some observers report that they can "feel" or "sense" it happening, even though they do not have a visual picture of it [37]. This phenomenon is still poorly understood, and there is some disagreement as to how to interpret it. However, the effect itself has been replicated in several studies, with some indicating that nonattentional processes are likely involved [38]. Sensing may also explain reports by some radiologists that they could immediately detect the presence of an abnormality in an image, even before consciously seeing it [39].

15.2.4 Coordination of Systems

Although the perceptual limits described above can be severe, failures of visual perception do not seem to be common in everyday life. This suggests that we may not represent everything that is in front of us, but only what we need at any particular moment. In this view, perception is not about *accumulating* information over time, but about *managing* the component systems so that detailed, coherent representations (requiring attention) can be formed exactly when needed for the task at hand.

15.2.4.1 Virtual Representation

To account for the impression that we can see everything in front of us, it has been proposed that our perception is based on a virtual representation, in which attention is given to the right object in a "just-in-time" fashion [8]. This architecture is dependent on an effective coordination of attention, as follows (Fig. 15.2):

- Processes in the preattentive system provide a constantly regenerating array of proto-objects that provide the "basic stuff" of perception, representing those properties visible to the observer.

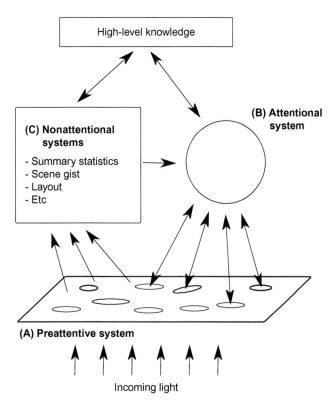

FIGURE 15.2   Coordination of interacting systems. (A) Preattentive system creates volatile proto-objects from the incoming light. (B) Attentional system "grabs" selected proto-objects and forms them into an object with both temporal and spatial structure; this lasts as long as attention is being allocated to it. (C) Nonattentional processes determine quantities such as gist and layout; these enable access to long-term memory about what might be expected in the scene. This in turn guides the allocation of visual attention to verify understanding. Control of attention is based on this along with exogenous control of attention based on physical properties, so as to handle unexpected events.

- Nonattentional processes use these proto-objects to determine gist and layout, which help access long-term knowledge—in the form of a scene schema—about the general kind of scene encountered. This knowledge (along with layout information) can help guide visual attention to important items in the image.
- Attention verifies the current schema by focusing on just a few items at a time. Consistent items are briefly checked, but need not be maintained in detail afterwards. Inconsistent items receive further processing to determine their identities, or even cause a reevaluation of the schema. Unexpected objects can be handled via exogenous control, using salient properties at the preattentive level.

According to this view, then, a complete representation of the scene is never created—only a small number of coherent objects ever exist in the visual picture we experience at any one time. Because the representation of any object of interest is created whenever needed, all

objects in a scene will appear to be in it simultaneously (as in fact, is usually the case in the external world). The key point is that at any one time we only experience a small number of visual objects—items that are coherent. It is still possible that fragments of different colors, shapes, and sizes are concurrently experienced as "background" over the entire visible area [10].

15.2.4.2 Implications

Given that the visual picture we experience is a dynamic one, the result of a great deal of processing, a number of implications follow. To begin with, our experience of what is in front of us does not reflect "raw" reality, but incorporates existing beliefs and goals [40]. Since individuals differ in their background knowledge and goals, different people can literally see the same thing differently. Indeed, because consistency is not explicitly checked, an individual observer may not even be consistent in their interpretation from moment to moment as their goals (and perhaps knowledge) evolve.

More generally, this view also suggests that visual perception involves a partnership between observer and environment: rather than internally recreating the incoming image in all its detail, the observer treats the world as an external memory, a memory that can provide detailed information whenever requested. This interactive interrogation of a scene by our visual system is much like the operation of computer network browsers; it may even explain why browser use can feel quite natural. In any event, note that such interaction need not be limited to memory: the world could, for example, also be used as an external processor of information [41]. Thus, if an informatics system can manage the relevant perceptual mechanisms sufficiently well, it could enable a completely seamless extension of human abilities and experience to the visualization of completely new realms, with the resulting experience remaining as effortless and natural as simply seeing the world around us.

15.3 VISUALIZATION AND DATA EXPLORATION

An increasingly important way of analyzing data is the use of visualization to explore large, messy datasets [42]. This approach originated with the use of graphs and charts, which allowed analysts to more easily perceive unexpected trends and outliers in datasets [43]. More recent developments have allowed visualizations to become more complex (eg, networks) and interactive, so that analysts can obtain overviews and drill down on selected items whenever required [42]. In the oncological domain, data that can be analyzed in this way range from mammograms to genomic datasets to the complete medical records of everyone in a community. Such a system could, for example, enable an analyst to explore the incidence of a particular cancer in terms of factors such as genotype, geographical location, and social networks. An appropriate visualization could also enable the effective communication of the results to nonspecialists.

15.3.1 Visualization as Extended Vision

At the most general level, visualization can be described as "using vision to think" [44]. More precisely, a visualization system translates the problem at hand into graphical form, ideally enabling the most appropriate visual mechanisms to be engaged on the task. If this is done well, the viewer and the visualization system form an "extended" visual system that can enable an analyst to perceive structure in a given dataset much as they would perceive structure in a real-world scene when using "basic" vision [27]. Because consideration is no longer restricted to the physical world, however, unfamiliar and nonintuitive patterns are encountered much more often, pushing visual mechanisms to their limits. A solid knowledge of visual perception is therefore essential for these systems to function well.

Several kinds of visualization are in current use [43]: data visualization (scientific data); information visualization (abstract data); biological visualization (specialized display of genomic data); and visual analytics (interactive visualization that engages higher levels of cognition, as described by Onukwugha et al. in Chapter 11: "Data Visualization Tools for Investigating Health Services Utilization Among Cancer Patients"). Older forms include statistical graphics (statistical data) and maps (geographical data). All, however, rely on many of the same visual mechanisms, and so can benefit from many of the same design principles.

15.3.2 Visual Variables

A central element of visualization is the assignment of numerical values or categories to visual properties—or visual variables—in an image. The right mapping can enable the visual system of an analyst to find structure in an abstract dataset (eg, groups or outliers) in the much same way as it finds structure in the real world. For example, if color is used to represent the temperature of a patient, the representation of patients with similar temperatures will group together, and outliers will become immediately apparent. Because such groups are also the basic elements of attentional selection, any of these can then be selected for further processing. And because the rapid estimation of summary statistics can be based on color, this representation could also support the immediate estimation of average temperature, and possibly its variance as well. Indeed, properties such as size, color, and orientation carry information in various tasks, supporting

functions such as the perception of trends and the rapid perception of correlation [27]. In general, then, the most effective mappings involve visual variables that are preattentive features [45]. Note that these can be easily changed in different mappings, providing the analyst with different "views" of the same dataset.

If preattentive features are used as visual variables, it is also possible to display several data dimensions simultaneously. For example, temperature, age, and blood pressure could be represented by color, orientation, and size, respectively, allowing their interactions to be explored. Although it is currently unclear how much intelligence the visual system has, it is at least possible that it could successively compare pairs (or perhaps even triples) of such features in an image. It is worth noting that not all properties can be selected independently of each other; those that can—such as color and orientation—are termed separable, while those that cannot—such as width and height—are referred to as integral [46].

Finally, mapping of values in a data set need not be limited to scalars. For example, each member of a set of categories (days of the week, say) could be associated with a different color. In such cases, the values used in the mapping must be such that they can be rapidly discriminated from each other, effectively forming distinct categories. As a rule of thumb, about four distinct values (two bits) should be used for each spatial dimension, and about eight values (three bits) for features such as orientation and color [45].

15.3.3 Attentional Control

Another important element in visualization—and indeed, in any visual task—is the control of visual attention. Given that attention is needed for various aspects of conscious experience, a failure to adequately manage it could result in an analyst failing to notice important items or events in a display, or at the very least noticing them only after a delay. To minimize the chance of this occurring, the attention (and thus the viewing experience) of the analyst must be controlled. Ideally, if control is done well, the analyst would notice nothing unusual, and the required information would simply appear to them, as if by magic.

Techniques for attentional management exist that are both powerful and fairly natural. These rely on a variety of approaches. A first set of techniques relies on exogenous control—for instance, the use of unique visual features that are highly salient (eg, brightness, color, length, or motion), automatically attracting attention to their location. Assigning such properties to items or events considered relevant for the task effectively highlights them, and thus makes them less likely to be overlooked. Related techniques include using a literal highlight (via illumination), and increasing the level of detail (or sharpness) of the relevant item. A second set of techniques for attentional control is based on the use of *directives*—symbols that depend on learned associations such as arrows or the direction of gaze of the eyes in a face; such symbols can automatically send attention in the direction indicated. Finally, a third set of techniques involves manipulating the high-level interests of the analyst—for example, assigning a high value to particular items, so as to ensure that attention is given to them more often [6].

15.4 EXAMPLE 1: HUMAN NUMBER PERCEPTION AND QUANTITATIVE DATA

As a concrete example of how knowledge of human vision can influence the design of an oncology informatics system, consider the display of quantitative data. Whether we are looking at a patient's medical record, surveying the variability of cancer rates in primary care operations, or trying to convey the risks and benefits of cancer screening, conveying quantitative information is perhaps the most important task of such a system. While a great deal of effort has gone into trying to improve the display of such information, most of the research has been from the perspective of decision making (eg, [47]). However, we argue that the displays involved could be improved by understanding and exploiting relevant research in basic vision science and cognitive psychology. Here we sketch out an account of this might be done via an understanding of the human number sense.

The ability to estimate number appears to be innate in humans (and indeed, in several species), comprising two core systems: a limited-capacity, attention-demanding precise number system which can subitize up to four objects at a glance (see Section 15.2.2.2), and a nonattentive approximate number system which provides rapid estimates, subject to the limitations of Weber's Law (see Section 15.2.3.2). How do these number systems interact in practice? The approximate number system can operate across all numerosities, while the precise number system is useful only for small numerosities [20]. To get high precision above the subitizing range, it is necessary to count, which requires effortful shifting of the precise number system from one group to the next [48].

Communication of quantitative information should be tailored to the limitations of these core systems. For example, icon arrays have been proposed as a way to more effectively present to patients the success rates of different treatments [47]. Icon arrays convert numerical information (eg, a 75% cure rate) into a pictorial representation (an array of, say, 100 circles, with 75 of them shaded to indicate cured patients). This can help reduce the influence of anecdotal information [47] and reduce denominator neglect [49] (see Fig. 15.3A,B).

The perception of icon arrays depends on the interplay between the approximate and precise number systems. For example, Garcia-Retamero et al. [49] asked people to compare the risk of dying from heart disease without an imaginary drug (50/500) and with it (2/100). In this case, the number of deaths in the second array is perceived much more precisely than in the first array, since it is below the subitizing limit. In general, numerical perception will be more accurate if a ratio can be translated into something in the subitizing range. Instead of showing 75 out of 100 patients successfully cured [47], it might be more effective to show 3 out of 4. Indeed, icon arrays are perceived to have more "truth value," and are preferred by participants, when using fewer items, such that the size of the subset falls into the subitizing range [50] (Fig. 15.3C,D). In addition, icon arrays may not improve performance when the difference between conditions falls below a patient's Weber fraction. Since the Weber fraction varies with age [51], different strategies may be appropriate for young adults and the elderly (Fig. 15.3E,F). On the other hand, icon arrays should be well suited for a variety of different populations, since numerosity perception does not seem to depend on education or cultural background.

More broadly, when designing a visualization system, we should think of numerosity as an important visual variable (see Section 15.3). When we pick a color scheme for a graph or chart, we would ensure that adjacent colors were easily discriminable. Similar care should be taken when presenting numerical information, so that observers (whether patients viewing an icon array or physicians trying to interpret data summarize across EHRs) are not asked to distinguish quantities that can only be discriminated through time-consuming and error-prone counting.

15.5 EXAMPLE 2: VISUAL ATTENTION AND MEDICAL IMAGES

Another example of using knowledge about human perception for design involves the display of medical images. Medical image interpretation plays a critical role in cancer detection and diagnosis. Many screening and diagnosis protocols involve a highly trained observer interpreting a complex image, such as a mammogram, chest radiograph, or CT scan. Colorectal cancer screening involves a visual "fly-through" of the colon, while the widely used Papanicolaou (Pap) screening test for cervical cancer requires a cytologist to visually inspect thousands of stained cells. Such images are both complex and unnatural, and the signs of cancer can be relatively subtle. Radiologists, cytologists, and pathologists

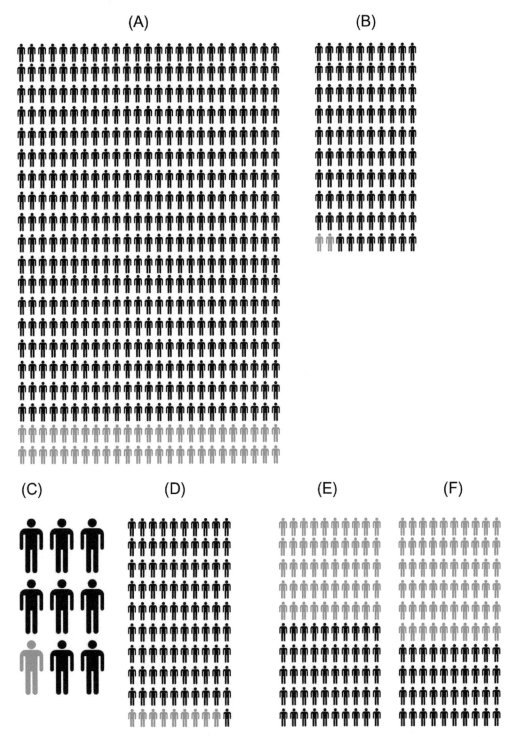

FIGURE 15.3 Icon arrays and human number perception. Icon arrays present ratios in graphic form. In these examples, blue figures represent the proportion of people who will experience a given outcome (eg, side effects, mortality/survival). Given a verbal description of probabilities, people often neglect the denominator; they tend to compare absolute numbers rather than dividing the number of events by the number of people involved. For example, if 50 out of 500 people who do not take a hypothetical drug die (A), compared to 2 out of 100 people who do take the drug (B), the drug reduces the risk of death by 80%. Given this information verbally, people are likely to overestimate the effectiveness of the drug, because 50 is so much larger than 2. If people are presented icon arrays, such as those shown here, they are much more accurate [49]. We suggest that this is because the icon array allows us to offload the mathematical computations onto the visual system, in particular the approximate number system. When possible, it may be more effective to use the precise number system; people are more likely to perceive the data in (C) as valid than the data in (D), even though the proportions are the same [50], probably because the number of blue elements in (C) is below the subitizing limit and can be apprehended more easily. However, above the subitizing limit, the utility of icon arrays will be limited by the precision of an individual's approximate number system. For example, which panel, (E) or (F) shows a greater proportion of blue figures? This difference (Weber fraction = 0.20) will be easily discriminable by college-age adults [29], but many older adults cannot discriminate Weber fractions below 0.25 [51].

are of course highly trained and experienced observers, but they are still subject to the perceptual and attentional limitations outlined in Section 15.2. Here we discuss relevant research in vision science that bears on the problems faced by these expert observers. In particular, we discuss two major, long-standing problems in the field of medical image perception, the prevalence effect and satisfaction of search, and then sketch some future directions for this emerging field of research.

15.5.1 The Prevalence Effect

One area of application concerns the effect of prevalence on disease detection. Here we refer not to the incidence of a disease in the general population, but to the frequency of signs of the disease in the images seen by the observer. Prevalence is typically high in training contexts, to give trainees an adequate sample of what they are looking for. But in the clinic prevalence is usually low: For example, in lung cancer screening it is 1.1% [52], while breast cancer screening is characterized by a prevalence of 0.5% [53]. Does this matter? It has long been known that the *positive predictive value* (the proportion of true positives out of all positive responses) necessarily decreases with prevalence, when holding disease detectability constant [54]. The interesting scientific and practical question is whether prevalence has an influence on an observer's performance at the case level.

How can we measure performance at the case level? Sensitivity and specificity are not independent quantities. The mathematical relationship between these two quantities is expressed in signal detection theory (SDT, see Macmillan and Creelman [55] for an excellent introduction). Briefly, SDT allows us to transform sensitivity and specificity into *detectability* and *criterion*. Detectability (often denoted as d') refers to the observer's ability to detect the presence or absence of a target (ie, disease), while criterion (often denoted as c) describes the balance between sensitivity and specificity. Low detectability means that the observer will make relatively more errors overall, while a liberal criterion means that the observer will make more false positives (and fewer misses) than with a conservative criterion. From an SDT point of view, we can ask whether prevalence influences detectability.

There is some evidence from field studies that low prevalence may actually improve detectability. Kundel [56] compiled data from 12 lung cancer screening studies (encompassing a total of 2,132,207 cases) with prevalence ranging from 0.09% to 47.6%. He found that d' increased as prevalence decreased. However, he pointed out that experimental studies in which the same readers are tested at both low and high prevalence would be necessary to make a valid comparison. Two small laboratory studies [57,58], using between 40 and 72 cases, showed evidence for declines in detectability at low prevalence. The most extensive laboratory study was conducted by Gur et al. [59], who recruited 14 observers (including radiology faculty, fellows, and residents) to read 1632 chest radiographs for five different types of abnormalities (nodules, pneumothorax, interstitial disease, alveolar disease, and rib fracture) under prevalence levels ranging from 2% to 28%, and found no effect whatsoever of prevalence on detectability.

The answer to the question from the laboratory thus seems to be very different from what was observed in the field data. While detectability declined with prevalence in Kundel's [56] field data, Gur et al. [59] saw no evidence for any effect of prevalence on detectability under controlled conditions in the laboratory. This heroic study seemed to set to rest any fears that prevalence could have a noticeable impact on performance at the case level.

However, recent studies in the basic vision science literature have provided new insights, using variants of the *visual search* task. In visual search, the observer is asked to look for a target item in an image (see Sections 15.2 and 15.2.1). There are many variants of this task: the target may be known in advance or not; there may be multiple potential targets; the task might be to discriminate target present from target absent, to distinguish which target is present, or to enumerate the targets in the image. The task is thus a fairly good laboratory analog for the radiological observer's task (Fig. 15.4). However, prevalence is typically 50% in visual search studies. In 2005, Wolfe et al. [62] varied prevalence from 1% to 50% and found fairly dramatic effects on search performance. Low prevalence substantially increased false negatives, and true negative RTs became faster than true positive RTs, a striking reversal of the usual pattern. Later studies showed the converse pattern at very high prevalence [63]. When targets are present on 99% of trials, false negatives become rare and there is an excess of false positives, accompanied by extremely slow true negative responses.

Generally speaking, excessive false negatives at low prevalence can reflect three basic error types: (1) motor errors, where the observer recognizes the target but makes the wrong response; (2) early search termination errors, where the observer decides that no target is present before having seen the target; and (3) perceptual errors, where the observer has seen the target but not recognized it. Both early termination errors and motor errors can be eliminated by using multiple target types with different frequencies, setting overall prevalence to 50%. Under these conditions, rare targets are still missed more often than common targets [64]. Indeed, target frequency (in the context of 50% overall prevalence) is logarithmically related to false negative errors all the way down to frequencies of 0.078% [65]. These findings demonstrate a critical role for perceptual errors.

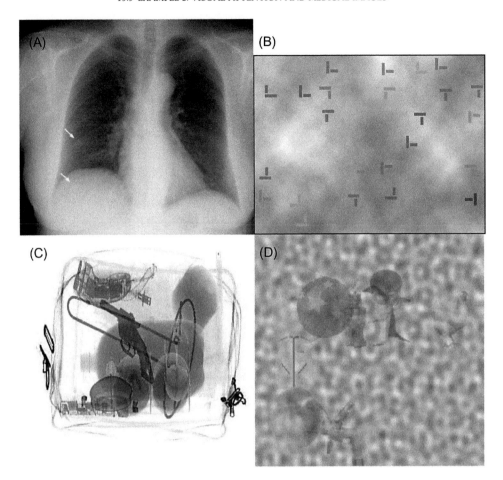

FIGURE 15.4 Visual search displays. Panel (A) shows a posteroanterior chest radiograph displaying two nodules in the right lung (arrows) (reprinted with permission from Ref. [60]). These manifestations of lung cancer would be more difficult to find in a low-prevalence screening context than in the high-prevalence diagnostic context (prevalence effect). Furthermore, detecting one nodule would make detection of the second nodule less likely, relative to a radiograph that contained only second nodule (SSM). The prevalence effect and SSM are the result of basic cognitive processes and have been studied using complex, but more easily controlled stimuli. Panel (B) illustrates stimuli designed to study SSM. There are two targets (T-shapes) in this image, embedded in distractors (L-shapes) and obscured with gray noise. The high salience target (lower right) is likely to be found first, reducing the chance of detecting the low salience target (upper right), relative to an image which contains only a low salience target (reprinted with permission from Ref. [61]). The prevalence effect has been studied with stimuli such as simulated baggage X-rays (find the weapon) (C) and objects in noise (find the tool) (D). *Reprinted with permission from Wolfe JM, Horowitz TS, van Wert MJ, Kenner NM, Place SS, Kibbi N. Low target prevalence is a stubborn source of errors in visual search tasks. J Exp Psychol Gen 2007;136(4):623–38.*

In the SDT terms introduced above, changing prevalence does not affect the observer's ability to detect the target, but only alters their criterion [64]: high prevalence leads to liberal criteria, low prevalence leads to conservative criteria. In fact, prevalence shifts two independent decision criteria, or thresholds [63]. Any extended search task (one that cannot be resolved in a single glance) actually consists of a series of decisions. A potential target (eg, lung nodule) is identified, and attention is shifted to that location. At this point, the observer has to decide whether or not the attended item is a target, and this decision has a threshold attached to it. At low prevalence, more evidence is required for the visual system to classify an item as a target, relative to high prevalence; in other words, the same set of pixels will look less like a nodule when nodules are rare. If the item is deemed

not to be a target, a second decision must be made: is it time to quit and declare the image free of targets, or keep on looking? This decision also has a threshold, which is lowered when targets are rare. With this theoretical account in mind, we can take a second look at the data from medical image perception studies. In this literature, the debate has been about whether there is an effect on d', so many studies have failed to report c. However, it is possible to compute c for the studies reported in Kundel's survey of lung cancer screening in the field [56], and this analysis shows that criterion clearly becomes more conservative as prevalence decreases. Gur et al. [66] reported a similar trend in their laboratory study. Both field and laboratory data from the medical image perception field, then, are consistent with the criterion shift account of the prevalence effect. More recently, the criterion shift account has been directly tested in both breast cancer [67] and cervical cancer screening [68] contexts. Both studies showed clear evidence for a shift to a more conservative criterion at low prevalence.

Armed with an account of the mechanism driving the prevalence effect, researchers have begun to test potential "cures." For example, observers' criterion settings can be affected by the costs and benefits of different outcomes, known as the *payoff matrix*. If I pay you $500 for each correct detection and subtract only $1 for false positives, you will start making many more positive responses, and your criterion will become extremely liberal. Changing the payoff matrix is an obvious route for changing the behavior of medical observers. However, we do not understand how the payoff matrix interacts with prevalence. In visual search experiments, it is typically assumed that the payoff matrix is neutral in that false positives and false negatives are equally undesirable, but this has not been empirically measured. One study tested payoff matrices explicitly designed to shift criterion at low prevalence in a more liberal direction, with mixed results [69]. When the experimenters changed the structure of the experiment so that observers were competing against each other so that the highest scorer in the experiment won a bonus, they observed large (and economically optimal) criterion shifts. The implicit payoff matrix in the radiology suite (or other oncology imaging setting) is unknown, but presumably not neutral. Both types of errors have potentially severe real-world consequences for the patient, but it is unknown how this translates into the payoffs for the radiologist. False negatives are of great concern in the United States due to litigation concerns. Making the payoff matrix more explicit may help to shift behavior toward false positives and away from false negatives, if that is seen as desirable. A competitive system might not be practical for professional medical observers, but the approach is promising.

The simplest solution, of course would be to simply increase prevalence to 50% (or whatever level is desired to bring about the optimal ratio of false negatives to false positives). This could be done by enriching the radiologists' caseload with known positive cases. However, that is obviously not practical. In addition to the cost of having highly remunerated professionals read fake cases, there is a danger that radiologists would learn the perceptual characteristics of the fake cases, and this would make it more difficult to find the real cases. However, it might be possible to alter *perceived* prevalence, by either explicit or implicit means.

Several studies have tried explicitly cueing observers about the probability of a target on an upcoming trial, to mixed results [70,71]. One study showed that providing false feedback (ie, on 20% of true negative trials, observers were informed that they had missed a target)

could successfully shift observers' criteria in the desired direction; they found more targets, and made more false positives, without changing overall detection rates [72]. Again, such a manipulation might not be entirely practical for oncological settings, but it is promising that feedback can meaningfully change behavior. The clinical setting rarely provides immediate case-by-case feedback, a fact likely to exacerbate the prevalence effect [64].

One approach that might be more practical is to enrich the caseload for a brief duration. Recent experience on the order of 40–50 trials [63], or even 10 trials [71] can alter criterion. Wolfe et al. [64] exploited this property and inserted brief high prevalence "bursts" into a long series of low prevalence trials. Critically, during low prevalence trials, observers did not receive feedback, while immediate (and veridical) feedback was provided during the bursts. These bursts had a carryover effect on subsequent low prevalence trials. Such a system might be adapted to a clinical setting. Radiologists could sit down and do a brief, high prevalence "refresher" session before turning to their regular caseload. There is tentative evidence that such a procedure can be effective in the baggage screening context [73].

Computer-aided detection (CAD) systems can provide online assistance to medical observers. The vision science literature provides some cautionary notes for the design of such systems, in the context of the prevalence effect. It is well known that false negative errors can be reduced when the color of the target is known in advance (in a display of multicolored items) [74]. However, this does not attenuate the effects of low prevalence [75]; in fact, if the target happens to show up in the wrong color (invalid cueing), the prevalence effect is exacerbated. Similar effects are observed for spatial cueing (ie, narrowing the physical area of search).

15.5.2 Subsequent Search Misses

In laboratory search tasks, observers are usually given a specific target to look for, and there is typically a single instance of that target present in the display. In cancer screening and other medical search tasks, however, there can be multiple target types (eg, calcifications, architectural distortions, masses), and multiple instances in the same image. We will first discuss the problems associated with multiple targets in the stimulus, and then issues around searching for different types of targets.

It has been known for a long time that detecting one abnormality interferes with the detection of others in the same image [76]. This phenomenon was originally termed "satisfaction of search," based on the hypothesis that the observer is searching in order to assign meaning to the image. Once the meaning has been established as "abnormal," the observer is "satisfied" and likely to discontinue searching [76]. This explanation was later disproved by evidence that observers do not stop searching after identifying the first target [77]. Adamo et al. [78] have therefore suggested renaming the problem "subsequent search misses" (SSM), which we will adopt here.

What is the cause of SSM, if not satisfaction of search? Berbaum et al. [79] suggested instead that SSM might reflect either a strategy to reduce false positive errors, or a "perceptual set" effect; when an abnormality of one type is found, the observer keeps searching for that type, and thus is more likely to miss a subsequent abnormality of a different type.

As with the prevalence effect, studying SSM in a basic vision science context has yielded new insights. SSM is observed whether the targets are identical or drawn from different categories, indicating that the "perceptual set" explanation is not sufficient [80]. While nonexpert laboratory observers may not be as motivated as trained professionals, adding monetary incentives for accuracy did not reduce the effect. While SSM can be seen without explicit time pressure [81], fewer SSM errors were made when observers were given more time.

Perhaps the most intriguing suggestion to come out of this line of work is that SSM might reflect a shortage of cognitive resources, specifically working memory [61], so that radiologists can look right at a lung nodule, yet fail to recognize it [82]. This explanation suggests that SSM might be minimized through the use of cognitive prostheses, such as providing a method to "mark off" already detected abnormalities, or encouraging observers to reexamine locations that were fixated soon after detecting an abnormality.

Search is based on a target template held in memory. When searching for a single target type, template is well-defined, and the visual system can use the target feature set to guide attention to items that are likely to be targets [83]. In other words, instead of scrutinizing every object in a scene (or every part of a radiograph) the visual system can use target features to narrow down the search space and improve search efficiency. With multiple targets (eg, searching for nodules and lobular masslike opacities in the lung), one must either maintain multiple target templates, or use a broad, less useful template [84]. The evidence suggests that only one target template is typically active [85]; maintaining two at once is possible, but costly [86]. These findings suggest that there might be utility in having observers specialize in different target types, rather than having a single observer simultaneously search for multiple target types [84].

In oncological contexts, however, there may be not just two potential target types, but many, such as calcifications, architectural distortions, masses, and enlarged lymph nodes in mammography. How does the size of this "memory set" influence search? Recent work has examined this issue using relatively complex and heterogeneous stimuli (photorealistic objects) and larger set sizes. The RT functions appear to be a logarithmic function of memory set size, up to at least 100 targets [87]. These results are also observed at low (1%) prevalence [88], when observers memorize verbal descriptions of objects [88], or a set of target categories [89]. In general, searching for more than one category of abnormality incurs two types of performance costs: reduced guidance to targets, and increased memory search time. However, the marginal costs of adding additional target categories to the memory search decreases; the largest costs are going from single- to dual-target searches.

15.6 FRONTIERS OF PERCEPTUAL SCIENCE AND ONCOLOGY INFORMATICS

The application of basic vision science to the problems of oncological image perception (and medical image perception in general) has led to major progress on well-established problems such as the prevalence effect and satisfaction of search. The cross-fertilization of these two fields will no doubt yield new insights into expert perception, and ways to improve the accuracy of cancer screening and diagnosis. Major areas of future innovation include the application of new theoretical tools imported from population ecology, the study of 3D imaging, and understanding the contribution of nonfocal vision to medical image interpretation.

15.6.1 Foraging for Cancer

The strategic aspects of visual search, particularly in the oncology context, may be subsumed under a more general class of *foraging* problems. The study of foraging originally developed in behavioral ecology, to explain the behavior of animals searching for food [90]. Optimal foraging theory posits that an organism should seek to maximize its intake of nutrients, while minimizing expenditures, such as time and energy [91]. For example, a key principle in optimal foraging is the Marginal Value Theorem (MVT) [92], which states that the optimal time to leave a patch is when the instantaneous local rate of return drops below the average rate of return in the environment. These concepts turn out to be applicable to a wider set of problems, from understanding how we search for information on the Internet [93], to how criminals choose their targets [94].

Optimal foraging theory provides a potential solution to a major theoretical problem in visual search: the quitting time problem [95]. If the observer knows in advance the number of targets in a display, she can quit after finding all of them. However, certainty about the number of targets present is rare. Even in simple laboratory search tasks, there might be zero or one targets; how long should an observer search before giving up and declaring that the target is not present? In the context of cancer screening, for example, the problem is far more complex: typically there is no target present, but there might be several targets, and they can be of different categories, appearing with different frequencies. Furthermore, there are time costs. A radiologist cannot spend all day scrutinizing a single mammogram to ensure that every single possible mass or calcification is caught. These problems are isomorphic with many of the issues faced by animals foraging for food in a patchy environment: Should I try to catch more fish from this pond, or should I move on to the next? If I pick more berries from this bush, will the calories I extract compensate for the risk of being caught by a predator?

The application of optimal foraging principles to visual search is in its infancy, and has not yet reached the oncology context. In laboratory search tasks, observers behave like optimal foragers at 50% prevalence, but diverge from optimal when prevalence is more extreme (either high or low) [96]. These data emphasize the importance of understanding observers' *priors*; their assumptions about target prevalence coming in to the experiment.

The distribution of patch quality (the likelihood of targets in a single patch, or case) is also important [97]. Given uniform patch quality, observers behave optimally. Introducing variability in patch quality produces departures from optimal foraging behavior. When observers can estimate patch quality (the likelihood of targets) using preattentive information (see Sections 15.2.1.2 and 15.2.3) such as color, behavior is driven more strongly by item color than by instantaneous rate of return. When color information was eliminated, observers coarsely categorize patches into "good" or "bad," exhaustively clicking through the good patches and quickly leaving the bad patches.

These two studies mark the beginning of a new direction for the study of visual search behavior, and suggest new avenues of exploration for medical image perception. What priors do radiologists and pathologists bring to the clinic? How variable is the "patch quality" of mammograms or cytopathology slides? How might we alter digital oncology images to better convey the likelihood of abnormal findings? How might the workflow of the clinic be optimized to reduce the cost of switching to a new patch (case)?

15.6.2 Strategies for Volumetric Search

A major challenge in the study of perception of oncological images is the switch from 2D to 3D imaging. The classical medical image perception literature is rooted in the study of the perception of 2D film. However, 3D modalities are becoming more common, and they appear to be more effective than their 2D counterparts [98]. In part, this is because 3D imaging allows the observer to avoid or disambiguate artifacts caused by overlapping tissues [99]. However, very little is known about how observers interact with these new imaging modalities, and what the optimal strategies might be.

For example, chest CTs are organized into virtual stacks of horizontal slices, so the observer sees an axial cross-section of the lung, and can scroll up or down to reach other slices. Eye tracking data show that individual radiologists adopt one two strategies: "drilling" and scanning [100]. Drilling involves focusing on a small portion of the lung at a time while scrolling up and down; scanning involves covering the entire horizontal slice before moving on in the depth direction. When searching for lung nodules, drilling seemed to be a more effective strategy; drillers covered more of the lung and found more nodules. Drillers also made more recognition errors; they looked at nodules but failed to recognize them. Nevertheless, even the drillers covered less than 75% of the lung, presumably leading to many false negative errors. These findings may reflect the difficulty of remembering where one has already looked in a volumetric space; one solution might be to utilize eye tracking as a cognitive prosthesis.

15.7 CONCLUSIONS

The critical element in any informatics system is the human observer, the one who has to make sense of the relevant information and put it to use. Visualizations of various sorts, from simple charts to virtual colonography, are often the most efficient way to communicate information to and from this observer, as well as having them detect patterns such as trends and outliers. In fact, when done properly, the informatics system can be considered an extension of the human visual system, allowing us to apply our powerful native perceptual capabilities to new problems. To achieve this end, however, we have to keep the nature of the perceptual system in mind. The aim of this chapter has been to give the reader an idea of those abilities and limitations, along with some idea of the experimental techniques used by perception scientists to elucidate them. We hope that this introduction provides a useful guide for allowing us to use our extended visual systems to solve many of the problems posed in other chapters in this volume.

LIST OF ACRONYMS AND ABBREVIATIONS

CAD Computer-aided detection
ms Milliseconds
RT Response time, or reaction time

SDT Signal detection theory
SSM Subsequent search misses

References

[1] Palmer SE. Vision science: photons to phenomenology, 1st ed. Cambridge, MA: The MIT Press; 1999, p. 832.

[2] Treisman A. Features and objects: the fourteenth Bartlett memorial lecture. Q J Exp Psychol A 1988;40(2):201–37.

[3] Wolfe JM, Horowitz TS. What attributes guide the deployment of visual attention and how do they do it? Nat Rev Neurosci 2004;5(6):495–501.

[4] Rensink RA, Enns JT. Preemption effects in visual search: evidence for low-level grouping. Psychol Rev 1995;102(1):101–30.

[5] Rensink RA, Enns JT. Early completion of occluded objects. Vision Res 1998;38(15–16):2489–505.

[6] Rensink RA. The management of visual attention in graphic displays Human attention in digital environments. New York: Cambridge University Press; 2011, p. 63–92

[7] Marr D, Poggio TA, Ullman S. Vision: a computational investigation into the human representation and processing of visual information. Cambridge, MA: The MIT Press; 2010, p. 432.

[8] Rensink RA. The dynamic representation of scenes. Vis Cogn 2000;7(1/2/3):17–42.

[9] Wolfe JM, Klempen N, Dahlen K. Postattentive vision. J Exp Psychol Hum Percept Perform 2000;26(2):693–716.

[10] Rensink RA. Perception and attention. In: Reisberg D, editor. Oxford handbook of cognitive psychology. New York: Oxford University Press; 2013. p. 97–116.

[11] Mack A, Rock I. Inattentional blindness. Cambridge, MA: MIT Press; 2000, p. 273.

[12] Strayer DL, Drews FA, Johnson W. Cell phone induced failures of visual attention during simulated driving. J Exp Psychol Appl 2002;9(1):23–32.

[13] Haines RF. A breakdown in simultaneous information processing. In: Obrecht G, Stark LW, editors. Presbyopia research. New York: Springer; 1991, p. 171–5.

[14] Cvach M. Monitor alarm fatigue: an integrative review. Biomed Instrum Technol Assoc Adv Med Instrum 2012;46(4): 268–77.

[15] Rensink RA, O'Regan JK, Clark JJ. To see or not to see: the need for attention to perceive changes in scenes. Psychol Sci 1997;8(5):368–73.

[16] Rensink RA. Change blindness: implications for the nature of visual attention. In: Jenkin M, Harris L, editors. Vision and attention. New York: Springer; 2001, p. 169–88.

[17] Levin DT, Momen N, Drivdahl SB, Simons DJ. Change blindness blindness: the metacognitive error of overestimating change-detection ability. Vis Cogn 2000;7(1/2/3):397–412.

[18] Kaufman EL, Lord MW, Reese TW, Volkmann J. The discrimination of visual number. Am J Psychol 1949;62(4):498–525.

[19] Railo H, Koivisto M, Revonsuo A, Hannula MM. The role of attention in subitizing. Cognition 2008;107(1):82–104.

[20] Burr DC, Turi M, Anobile G. Subitizing but not estimation of numerosity requires attentional resources. J Vis 2010; 10(6):20.

[21] Itti L. Models of bottom-up attention and saliency. In: Tsotsos JK, Itti L, Rees G, editors. Neurobiology of attention. Burlington, MA: Academic Press; 2005, p. 576–82.

[22] Bruce N, Tsotsos J. Saliency based on information maximization. In: Weiss Y, Schölkopf B, Platt JC, editors. Advances in neural information processing systems. Cambridge, MA: MIT Press; 2006, p. 155–62.

[23] Yarbus AL. Eye movements and vision. New York: Plenum Press; 1973.

[24] Egeth HE, Yantis S. Visual attention: control, representation, and time course. Annu Rev Psychol 1997;48(1):269–97.

[25] Alvarez GA. Representing multiple objects as an ensemble enhances visual cognition. Trends Cogn Sci 2011;15(3):122–31.

[26] Chong SC, Treisman AM. Representation of statistical properties. Vision Res 2003;43(4):393–404.

[27] Rensink RA. On the prospects for a science of visualization. In: Huang W, editor. Handbook of human centric visualization. New York: Springer; 2014, p. 147–75.

[28] Treisman M. Noise and Weber's law: the discrimination of brightness and other dimensions. Psychol Rev 1964;71(4):314–30.

[29] Halberda J, Feigenson L. Developmental change in the acuity of the "Number Sense": the approximate number system in 3-, 4-, 5-, and 6-year-olds and adults. Dev Psychol 2008;44(5):1457–65.

[30] Feigenson L, Dehaene S, Spelke E. Core systems of number. Trends Cogn Sci 2004;8(7):307–14.

[31] Brannon EM, Terrace HS. Ordering of the numerosities 1 to 9 by monkeys. Science 1998;282(5389):746–9.

[32] Thorpe S, Fize D, Marlot C. Speed of processing in the human visual system. Nature 1996;381(6582):520–2.

[33] Oliva A. Gist of the scene. In: Tsotsos JK, Itti L, Rees G, editors. Neurobiology of attention. Burlington, MA: Academic Press; 2005, p. 251–6.

[34] Evans KK, Georgian-Smith D, Tambouret R, Birdwell RL, Wolfe JM. The gist of the abnormal: above-chance medical decision making in the blink of an eye. Psychon Bull Rev 2013;20(6):1170–5.

[35] Hochberg JE. Perception, 2nd ed. Englewood Cliffs, NJ: Prentice Hall; 1978, p. 256.

[36] Tatler BW. What information survives saccades in the real world? The brain's eye: neurobiological and clinical aspects of oculomotor research. Amsterdam: Elsevier; 2002, p. 149–63.

[37] Rensink RA. Visual sensing without seeing. Psychol Sci 2004;15(1):27–32.

[38] Busch NA, Fründ I, Herrmann CS. Electrophysiological evidence for different types of change detection and change blindness. J Cogn Neurosci 2009;22(8):1852–69.

[39] Kundel HL, Nodine CF. Interpreting chest radiographs without visual search. Radiology 1975;116(3):527–32.

[40] Johansson P, Hall L, Sikström S, Olsson A. Failure to detect mismatches between intention and outcome in a simple decision task. Science 2005;310(5745):116–9.

[41] Clark A. Natural-born cyborgs: minds, technologies, and the future of human intelligence, 1st ed. New York: Oxford University Press; 2004, p. 240.

[42] Thomas JJ, Cook KA, editors. Illuminating the path: the research and development agenda for visual analytics. Los Alamitos, CA: National Visualization and Analytics Ctr; 2005.

[43] Rensink RA. Visual displays. Encyclopedia of perception. Thousand Oaks, CA: SAGE Publications, Inc.; 2010, p. 1072–6.

[44] Card SK, Mackinlay JD, Schneiderman B. Information visualization Readings in information visualization: using vision to think. San Francisco, CA: Morgan Kaufman; 1999, p. 1–34.

[45] Ware C. Information visualization. Perception for design, 3rd ed. Waltham, MA: Morgan Kaufmann; 2012, p. 536.

[46] Garner WR. The processing of information and structure. Oxford: Lawrence Erlbaum; 1974, p. 203.

[47] Fagerlin A, Wang C, Ubel PA. Reducing the influence of anecdotal reasoning on people's health care decisions: is a picture worth a thousand statistics? Med Decis Making 2005;25(4):398–405.

[48] Trick LM, Pylyshyn ZW. Why are small and large numbers enumerated differently? A limited-capacity preattentive stage in vision. Psychol Rev 1994;101(1):80–102.

[49] Garcia-Retamero R, Galesic M, Gigerenzer G. Do icon arrays help reduce denominator neglect? Med Decis Making 2010;30(6):672–84.

[50] Schapira MM, Nattinger AB, McAuliffe TL. The influence of graphic format on breast cancer risk communication. J Health Commun 2006;11(6):569–82.

[51] Halberda J, Ly R, Wilmer JB, Naiman DQ, Germine L. Number sense across the lifespan as revealed by a massive Internet-based sample. Proc Natl Acad Sci 2012;109(28):11116–20.

[52] The National Lung Screening Trial Research Team Results of initial low-dose computed tomographic screening for lung cancer. N Engl J Med 2013;368(21):1980–91.

[53] Breast Cancer Surveillance Consortium. BCSC Screening Performance Benchmarks: Sensitivity and Specificity (2009 Data) [Internet]; 2015. Available from: <http://breastscreening.cancer.gov/statistics/benchmarks/screening/2009/tableSensSpec.html>.

[54] Kundel HL. Disease prevalence and radiological decision making. Invest Radiol 1982;17(1):107–9.

[55] Macmillan NA, Creelman CD. Detection theory: a user's guide. Mahwah, NJ: Lawrence Erlbaum Associates; 2005, p. 526.

[56] Kundel HL. Disease prevalence and the index of detectability: a survey of studies of lung cancer detection by chest radiography. In: Proceedings of SPIE; 2000, p. 135–44.

[57] Egglin TP, Feinstein AR. Context bias: a problem in diagnostic radiology. JAMA 1996;276(21):1752–5.

[58] Ethell SC, Manning D. Effects of prevalence on visual search and decision making in fracture detection. In: Proceedings of SPIE; 2001, p. 249–57.

[59] Gur D, Rockette HE, Armfield DR, Blachar A, Bogan JK, Brancatelli G, et al. Prevalence effect in a laboratory environment. Radiology 2003;228(1):10–14.

[60] Katsuragawa S, Doi K. Computer-aided diagnosis in chest radiography. Comput Med Imaging Graph 2007;31(4–5):212–23.

[61] Cain MS, Mitroff SR. Memory for found targets interferes with subsequent performance in multiple-target visual search. J Exp Psychol Hum Percept Perform [Internet] 2012. Available from: <http://doi.apa.org/getdoi.cfm?doi=10.1037/a0030726>.

[62] Wolfe JM, Horowitz TS, Kenner NM. Rare items often missed in visual searches. Nature 2005;435(7041):439–40.

[63] Wolfe JM, van Wert MJ. Varying target prevalence reveals two dissociable decision criteria in visual search. Curr Biol 2010;20(2):121–4.

[64] Wolfe JM, Horowitz TS, van Wert MJ, Kenner NM, Place SS, Kibbi N. Low target prevalence is a stubborn source of errors in visual search tasks. J Exp Psychol Gen 2007;136(4):623–38.

[65] Mitroff SR, Biggs AT. The ultra-rare-item effect: Visual search for exceedingly rare items is highly susceptible to error. Psychol Sci 2014;25(1):284–9.

[66] Gur D, Bandos AI, Fuhrman CR, Klym AH, King JL, Rockette HE. The prevalence effect in a laboratory environment: changing the confidence ratings. Acad Radiol 2007;14(1):49–53.

[67] Evans KK, Birdwell RL, Wolfe JM. If you don't find it often, you often don't find it: why some cancers are missed in breast cancer screening. PLoS ONE 2013;8(5):e64366.

[68] Evans KK, Tambouret RH, Evered A, Wilbur DC, Wolfe JM. Prevalence of abnormalities influences cytologists' error rates in screening for cervical cancer. Arch Pathol Lab Med 2011;135(12):1557–60.

[69] Navalpakkam V, Koch C, Perona P. Homo economicus in visual search. J Vis 2009;9(1):31.

[70] Reed WM, Ryan JT, McEntee MF, Evanoff MG, Brennan PC. The effect of abnormality-prevalence expectation on expert observer performance and visual search. Radiology 2011;258(3):938–43.

[71] Ishibashi K, Kita S, Wolfe JM. The effects of local prevalence and explicit expectations on search termination times. Atten Percept Psychophys 2012;74(1):115–23.

[72] Schwark J, Sandry J, Macdonald J, Dolgov I. False feedback increases detection of low-prevalence targets in visual search. Atten Percept Psychophys 2012;74(8):1583–9.

[73] Wolfe JM, Brunelli DN, Rubinstein J, Horowitz TS. Prevalence effects in newly trained airport checkpoint screeners: trained observers miss rare targets, too. J Vis 2013;13(3):33.

[74] Egeth HE, Virzi RA, Garbart H. Searching for conjunctively defined targets. J Exp Psychol Hum Percept Perform 1984;10(1):32–9.

[75] Russell NCC, Kunar MA. Colour and spatial cueing in low-prevalence visual search. Q J Exp Psychol 2012;65(7):1327–44.

[76] Tuddenham WJ. Visual search, image organization, and reader error in roentgen diagnosis. Radiology 1962;78(5):694–704.

[77] Berbaum KS, Franken EA, Dorfman DD, Rooholamini SA, Coffman CE, Cornell SH, et al. Time course of satisfaction of search. Invest Radiol 1991;26(7):640–8.

[78] Adamo SH, Cain MS, Mitroff SR. Self-induced attentional blink: a cause of errors in multiple-target search. Psychol Sci 2013;24(12):2569–74.

[79] Berbaum KS, Franken Jr EA, Dorfman DD, Rooholamini SA, Kathol MH, Barloon TJ, et al. Satisfaction of search in diagnostic radiology. Invest Radiol 1990;25(2):133.

[80] Fleck MS, Samei E, Mitroff SR. Generalized "satisfaction of search": adverse influences on dual-target search accuracy. J Exp Psychol Appl 2010;16(1):60–71.

[81] Berbaum KS, Schartz KM, Caldwell RT, Madsen MT, Thompson BH, Mullan BF, et al. Satisfaction of search from detection of pulmonary nodules in computed tomography of the chest. Acad. Radiol. 2013;20(2):194–201.

[82] Berbaum KS, Franken EA, Dorfman DD, Miller EM, Caldwell RT, Kuehn DM, et al. Role of faulty visual search in the satisfaction of search effect in chest radiography. Acad Radiol 1998;5(1):9–19.

[83] Wolfe JM. Guided search 2.0: a revised model of visual search. Psychon Bull Rev 1994;1(2):202–38.

[84] Menneer T, Barrett DJK, Phillips L, Donnelly N, Cave KR. Costs in searching for two targets: dividing search across target types could improve airport security screening. Appl Cogn Psychol 2007;21(7):915–32.

[85] Olivers CNL, Peters J, Houtkamp R, Roelfsema PR. Different states in visual working memory: when it guides attention and when it does not. Trends Cogn Sci 2011;15(7):327–34.

[86] Barrett DJK, Zobay O. Attentional control via parallel target-templates in dual-target search. PLoS One 2014;9(1):e86848.

[87] Wolfe JM. Saved by a log: How do humans perform hybrid visual and memory search? Psychol Sci 2012;23(7):698–703.

[88] Guild EB, Cripps JM, Anderson ND, Al-Aidroos N. Recollection can support hybrid visual memory search. Psychon Bull Rev 2013;21(1):142–8.

[89] Cunningham CA, Wolfe JM. Lions or tigers or bears: oh my! Hybrid visual and memory search for categorical targets. Vis Cogn 2012;20(9):1024–7.

[90] Emlen JM. The role of time and energy in food preference. Am Nat 1966;100(916):611–7.

[91] Pyke GH, Pulliam HR, Charnov EL. Optimal foraging: a selective review of theory and tests. Q Rev Biol 1977:137–54.

[92] Charnov EL. Optimal foraging, the Marginal Value Theorem. Theor Popul Biol 1976;9(2):129–36.

[93] Pirolli P, Card S. Information foraging. Psychol Rev 1999;106(4):643.

[94] Eck JE. If the fox knows many ways to forage, the modeller cannot be a hedgehog: reflections on the use of wildlife foraging models to understand criminal target search. Leg Criminol Psychol 2014;19(2):211–4.

[95] Chun MM, Wolfe JM. Just say no: how are visual searches terminated when there is no target present? Cognit Psychol 1996;30(1):39–78.

[96] Cain MS, Vul E, Clark K, Mitroff SR. A Bayesian optimal foraging model of human visual search. Psychol. Sci. 2012;23(9):1047–54.

[97] Wolfe JM. When is it time to move to the next raspberry bush? Foraging rules in human visual search. J Vis 2013;13(3):10.

[98] Andriole GL, Crawford ED, Grubb RL, Buys SS, Chia D, Church TR, et al. Prostate cancer screening in the randomized prostate, lung, colorectal, and ovarian cancer screening trial: mortality results after 13 years of follow-up. J Natl Cancer Inst 2012; 104(2):125–32.

[99] Park JM, Franken EA, Garg M, Fajardo LL, Niklason LT. Breast tomosynthesis: present considerations and future applications. RadioGraphics 2007;27(suppl. 1):S231–40.

[100] Drew T, ML-H Vo, Olwal A, Jacobson F, Seltzer SE, Wolfe JM. Scanners and drillers: characterizing expert visual search through volumetric images. J Vis 2013;13(10):3.

[101] Bernstam EV, Smith JW, Johnson TR. What is biomedical informatics? J. Biomed. Inform. 2010;43(1):104–10 {quote from p. 106-107}.

PART IV

ACCELERATING PROGRESS

16

Crowdsourcing Advancements in Health Care Research: Applications for Cancer Treatment Discoveries

Emil Chiauzzi PhD, Gabriel Eichler PhD and Paul Wicks PhD

PatientsLikeMe, Inc., Cambridge, MA, United States

OUTLINE

16.1 Introduction	307		16.4.1 Methodological Issues	320
16.1.1 Clinical Trial Challenges	308		16.4.2 Ethical Issues	321
16.1.2 Overview of This Chapter	308		16.4.3 Data Privacy	322
			16.4.4 Conflicts of Interest and IP	323
16.2 The Crowdsourcing Concept	308			
16.2.1 Definition	308		16.5 The Future of Crowdsourcing	323
16.2.2 A Brief History of Crowdsourcing	308		16.5.1 Patient Partnership in Clinical Research	323
16.2.3 Parameters of Crowdsourcing	309		16.5.2 Biomarker Discovery	324
			16.5.3 Phenomics	324
16.3 Crowdsourcing in Health Care	312		16.5.4 Real World CER	325
16.3.1 Crowdsourcing for Diagnostics and Drug			16.5.5 Phase IV Surveillance, Adverse Event	
Discovery	312		Detection and Drug Safety	325
16.3.2 Crowdsourcing for Optimizing Treatment	314			
16.3.3 Crowdsourcing for Health Care Delivery			16.6 Conclusion	326
Improvements	314		List of Acronyms and Abbreviations	326
16.3.4 Patient as Researcher	315			
			Acknowledgments	326
16.4 Methodological and Ethical Issues in				
Crowdsourcing	320		References	326

16.1 INTRODUCTION

According to the 2014 American Society of Clinical Oncology (ASCO) Report *State of Cancer Care in America*, cancer will be our greatest health challenge. There will be 45% more new cancer cases in the United States by 2030, cancer will become the nation's leading cause of death [1], and a recent in-depth evaluation indicated that the quality of cancer care is "in crisis" [2]. Fear of medical liabilities has led physicians and health care institutions to overtreat, order unnecessary tests, and be slow to embrace proven, novel approaches to care [3]. The nature of the challenge is changing too, as there are currently 13.7 million cancer survivors [4], a number

B. Hesse, D. Ahern & E. Beckjord: Oncology Informatics.
DOI: http://dx.doi.org/10.1016/B978-0-12-802115-6.00016-1

likely to increase as these patients live longer and so the scope evolves from one of tumor control to one of living life well—*survivorship*.

With the increased availability of diagnostic biomarkers, imaging, and genetic sequencing, a vast array of data is now available for analysis to help address the cancer burden; however, these techniques often do not lend themselves easily to automated processing and analysis and require large sample sizes to produce reliable estimates. *Crowdsourcing* is a potentially promising methodology that might overcome this rate-limiting step and facilitate the development of novel medical technologies in the fight against cancer. Crowdsourcing is based upon principles of enabling a widely distributed group of individuals to work independently (but in coordination) to solve complex problems.

16.1.1 Clinical Trial Challenges

An important methodology in the fight against cancer is the clinical trial. While traditional clinical trial methodologies are likely to remain the gold standard for some time to come, current practice has been subject to broad criticism from a variety of stakeholders, some of which might be addressable by crowdsourcing. Today, fewer than 5% of adult cancer patients participate in clinical trials [5]. One in five trials sponsored by the National Cancer Institute (NCI)-sponsored trials fails to enroll a single patient, and only half of all cancer trials result in analyzable data [6]. These limitations are driven by multiple factors including patients' distrust of the medical establishment, fearing that they will be treated "like a guinea pig"; be subject to adverse side effects of experimental treatment; or have concerns about logistics and study procedures (eg, randomization, the demands of the protocol, the inclusion of placebo or no-treatment conditions, and inconvenient follow-up visits) [7].

Attempts by trial designers to improve recruitment and retention have been disappointing, with efforts to develop innovative improvements hindered by regulatory or ethical concerns [8]. Meanwhile, patients themselves are participating increasingly in a "consumer culture" characterized by data sharing and social media, in which customers can interact directly with brands, voters can connect with politicians, and citizens are as likely to be producers of content, as they are consumers. These changing dynamics in health care suggest that it is time for new research paradigms that recognize and integrate the more involved contributions of patients [9]. Creative methodologies that leverage patient-centered data collection based on social media content, biometric sensors, digital technologies, and patient-reported outcome (PRO) measures will need to be devised, validated, and incorporated into standard practice [10]. By harnessing crowdsourcing effectively, more patients might be encouraged to participate in more engaging cancer clinical trials with more relevant outcomes, lower burden, and better participant retention than the studies we have today.

16.1.2 Overview of This Chapter

This chapter will explore the history of crowdsourcing, its potential, and limitations. The chapter begins with a definition and brief history of crowdsourcing, with examples from both medical and nonmedical applications. Because the number of examples in cancer are sparse, we then describe case studies of how diagnostics, drug discovery, development, and delivery are being impacted by crowdsourcing approaches and the promise they bring in other serious diseases, aspects of which could be applied to cancer. Because medical privacy, intellectual property (IP), and strict regulatory environments complicate this environment, we will also consider methodological concerns, ethical challenges, commercial conflicts of interest, and data privacy. Finally, the chapter concludes with a discussion of the future opportunities and frontiers for crowdsourcing in oncology.

16.2 THE CROWDSOURCING CONCEPT

16.2.1 Definition

Distributed problem-solving projects have existed for nearly 300 years, but the term "crowdsourcing" was first introduced in 2006 in a *WIRED* Magazine article, which noted the shift from reliance on employees to perform tasks, to outsourcing tasks through an open call to an undefined network of people [11]. Most definitions utilize three components: (1) a problem-solving or production model; (2) an online mechanism for engagement; and (3) a distributed set of participants [12,13]. Based on prior published work, we define crowdsourcing for the purpose of this chapter with the following working definition [12,13]:

> …the creation of new data, information, knowledge or innovations that result from the engagement of a crowd of individuals through a call for achieving a specific objective for potential rewards of personal development, recognition, personal satisfaction, and/or monetary awards.

16.2.2 A Brief History of Crowdsourcing

In 1707, during the War of Spanish Accession, the British Navy suffered a catastrophic loss of life when four British warships were lost not to enemy fire, but by the rocks of the Isles of Scilly, due to their inability to accurately navigate. The British Parliament enacted the Longitude Act in 1714, creating a prize-based competition that resembled modern crowdsourcing. Prizes were awarded based on the precision of the method devised—from £10,000 for determining accuracy within one degree, to £20,000 for accuracy within 30 minutes of arc. There were also prizes for furthering progress toward the goals of the prize. Some of the first attempts at solving the problem were submitted by the Swiss mathematician, Leonhard Euler; the British watchmaker, Larcum Kendall; and surveyor, Charles Mason (of "Mason-Dixon line" fame), exemplifying the diversity of participants often credited with generating creative solutions [14]. Although the largest award was made in 1776 to John Harrison for his work on chronometers that kept precise time, which enabled the use of celestial navigation, the main prize was (contentiously) never awarded.

In the 250 years that followed, there have been dozens of distributed work projects and prize-based competitions, including the creation of the Oxford English Dictionary in 1884, and the design of the Sydney Opera House in 1957 [15]. However, such activities were still relatively obscure and inaccessible to the general public. This state of affairs changed in 2001, when Jimmy Wales and Larry Sanger launched Wikipedia, "an encyclopedia anyone can edit." Today, Wikipedia contains more than 34 million articles in 287 languages (http://en.wikipedia.org/wiki) and has overturned many misconceptions about the quality and accuracy of crowdsourced knowledge, though some expert groups remain skeptical [16]. Beginning in 2008, Google Flu trends began to geotag millions of symptom searches from members of the public in order to identify possible outbreaks of influenza and other infections (https://www.google.org/flutrends/us/#US).

In 2009, in celebration of its 40th anniversary, the United States Defense Advanced Research Projects Agency (DARPA) published its $40,000 Network Challenge, which invited teams to locate 10 red balloons placed at randomly selected locations throughout the United States [17]. DARPA originally thought that solving the challenge would take days or weeks, but the winning team from Massachusetts Institute of Technology (MIT) identified the locations of all 10 balloons within just 9 hours. Their multilevel marketing approach used social media networks, such as Facebook and Twitter, to distribute money prizes to individuals who found balloons and the chain of individuals who invited the finders to participate. This provided an incentive for individuals to either spot the balloon or to recruit potential balloon reporters in a viral fashion. Any excess prize money was to be donated to charity and the team's organizers explicitly allotted themselves no prize money. While each of these examples of crowdsourcing arguably solve far simpler problems than those of health care, they each exhibit parameters that could be brought to bear in health challenges.

16.2.3 Parameters of Crowdsourcing

Characteristics of crowdsourcing activities can be divided into four domains: (1) task characteristics; (2) participant characteristics; (3) task motivational structure; and (4) data characteristics. *Task characteristics* are described in Table 16.1 and are based on Brabham's [18] typology. Knowledge discovery and management describes a top-down process in which an organization mobilizes an online community to organize existing information. Distributed human intelligence tasking is the least creative of crowdsourcing types, as it breaks up large data processing tasks into small, piecework tasks completed by a group. Broadcast search involves casting a wide net in the hope of finding an individual who can produce the right answer to a problem. In peer-vetted creative production, an organization issues a creative challenge to an online community, allowing individuals to propose solutions and evaluate peer submissions so that the best submission can be identified.

Crowdsourcing to advance health care science and research and development typically fall within categories

TABLE 16.1 Types of Crowdsourcing

Task characteristics/ type of crowdsourcing	Description	Well-suited problems	Poorly suited problems
(A) Knowledge discovery and management	Crowd is tasked with finding and assembling accessible information	Collecting and organizing a set of broadly accessible information resources	Cases where data cannot be easily obtained validated or manipulated
(B) Distributed human intelligence tasking	Crowd is tasked with processing, structuring, or analyzing problems with large-scale data sets	Problems requiring solutions that can be obtained more efficiently through a crowd than computer analysis	Contexts in which the data or information is proprietary, requires deep domain knowledge, or requires computer analysis
(C) Broadcast search	Crowd is tasked with solving an empirical problem	Concretely defined problems with a clear definition of success or correctness	Ill-defined, subjective, or possessing poor definitions of success
(D) Peer-vetted creative production	Crowd is tasked with identifying creative solutions to a problem	Artistic or design solutions based on subjective or aesthetic impressions	Problems in which there are concrete definitions of a useful solution

Adapted from Brabham DC. Crowdsourcing. Cambridge, MA: MIT Press; 2013.

A, B, or C of Table 16.1. More specifically, tasks such as annotating genomic variants via a crowd-based set of contributors (A), interpreting CT scans of diseased colons (B), and the Prize4Life's Biomarker Challenge (C) demonstrate these parameters [19–21]. Typically, these endeavors require a scale of work and massive effort paired with a level of human judgment, perception, innovation, and evaluation that cannot be replicated by existing computing technologies. A less often encountered form of crowdsourcing in health care is peer-vetted creative work (D). Through rare, one example is the patient-led design of medical devices, for example, working with crowds of customers (patients) to identify and prototype new products or improvements to existing colostomy bags [22]. Some problems remain out of reach from crowdsourcing efforts, such as those that have ill-defined definitions of success, are inaccessible to a broad population of participants, or have proprietary/intellectual property (IP) limitations that preclude the distribution of the problem to a group.

Participant characteristics vary by the nature of their interaction (active vs passive) and their expertise (expert vs layperson). For example, InnoCentive's crowdsourcing marketplace (see Section 16.3.1) attracts experts who, by and large, volunteer their time and effort to solve well-defined innovation *Challenges* in exchange for the opportunity to win prize money. Active crowds knowingly participate in the crowdsourcing initiative and usually must commit time, or resources to address the task at hand. Conversely, passive forms of crowdsourcing gather data without the awareness or constant attention of participants. For example, the mobile traffic data feature of Google Maps (maps.google.com) and Waze (www.waze.com) collect the location and speed of mobile devices to infer traffic patterns. An active component of Waze allows drivers to add descriptions of road conditions or potential road hazards.

The type of *crowd* can be based on a variety of backgrounds and features (eg, perspectives, skills, resources, or capabilities) required to complete the requested task or activity. Research suggests that the most likely persons to solve a crowdsourced initiative have backgrounds tangentially related to the challenge [14]. In other words, a synthetic chemist specializing in plastics might be more likely to bring a successful approach to a challenge in medicinal chemistry than a geologist or an architect, because they bring an approach that is grounded in practicalities, while offering a fresh perspective.

Expert crowds usually contain technical or well-versed domain experts familiar with the context of the problem and can often contribute to its solution. Experts have experience working in the domain of the problem, or have worked in similar related domains. For example, the aforementioned Longitude Prize relied upon the expertise of skilled surveyors and chronographers to innovate

on new solutions. A 2014 review of the crowdsourcing literature found that 64% of articles are published by academics alone, 18% by professionals working in various industries, and 18% by both [23]. These researchers generally work in the information sciences, management sciences, communications, or information technology fields [23].

Nonexpert crowds include individuals who may not have a specific expertise, as evidenced by a lack of certifications, educational degrees, or experience in a particular area of inquiry. For example, there is much potential in patient crowds taking an active role in crowdsourcing—a logical evolution of the tradition of disease advocacy—in serious conditions such as cancer. By 2024, there will be 19 million cancer survivors, offering a large pool of potential advocates and patient stakeholders who can collaborate on studies and be involved in crowdsourcing initiatives [1]. With increasing proportions of the population completing higher education, the widespread availability of high-quality information resources to the public, and the increasing recognition that patients bring a different kind of expertise than their physicians, patients themselves represent an underutilized resource with a great deal of potential. In recent years, research has increasingly been influenced by patient advocacy in the allocation of research funding, research team participation, clinical trial implementation, translation of findings with researchers and the public, and even the oversight of research and policy [24]. Because cancer survivors have shown an ability to make scientific judgments, the patient of the future will be actively engaged in shared decision making, be an assertive driving force in research, and interact with personal health data as much or more than the researchers who collected it. These developments will translate into more opportunities for collaboration and leadership of cancer patients to collaborate in crowdsourcing efforts as peers and experts in their own right.

The *task motivational structure* for participants in crowdsourcing studies varies greatly. Often, the winners of crowdsourcing competitions invest many hours toward the development of their solution. For every successful solution found, there may be hundreds of others whose efforts are wasted. This level of commitment of time and resources requires that crowdsourcing competitions carefully consider how they incentivize the crowd to participate—whether it is financial reward, recognition, good will, gamification, or some combination of these.

Some crowdsourcing studies pay out *financial rewards* to one or more top participants to stimulate engagement. Financial motivation may not be limited to cash payments, but may take the form of retention of IP rights, yielding potential greater rewards in the long term [25]. Due to the global nature of many Internet-based pursuits, prize money (often a key feature of publicity about the contest) can be viewed very differently by participants coming from outside the United States or other advanced economies. For example, reward levels may need to be higher for US workers compared to workers in other parts of the world due to perceptions of what represents reasonable compensation.

In some crowdsourcing tasks, nonmonetary rewards such as recognition and goodwill are reward enough. Some crowdsourcing competitions attract such a large swell of fanfare and publicity that winning can lead to considerable benefits, such as new rewarding job opportunities or status within a peer group. It is not uncommon for winners of crowdsourcing competitions to include that accomplishment on their curriculum vitae or to be prominently featured on major media stories [26]. Similarly, some initiatives, such as those run by the popular crowdsourcing website, Kaggle, provide exclusive access to jobs and consulting opportunities for winners or top performers. In addition, companies such as GoodCrowds harness the goodwill of motivated participants toward the goal of the nonprofit or nongovernmental organization (NGO) entities (www.goodcrowds.com). GoodCrowds offers consulting services to help nonprofits or NGOs apply crowdsourcing-based approaches to advance their missions.

As a means of nonmonetary engagement, gamification has been used in crowdsourcing efforts to turn tasks into a fun, enjoyable experience. For some participants, the competition to collect points and compete with other game players is enough of a motivator to invest significant effort. Consequently, many computational crowdsourcing tasks feature a leaderboard and social signals, such as virtual badges. Nonmonetary factors can benefit the crowdsourcing effort up to a point; however, if the organizer appears to be profiting financially from the crowdsourcing endeavor, then recognition, goodwill, or gamification is rarely a sufficient reward in and of themselves [27]. Participants tend to find such a scheme to be inequitable, and the most skilled participants choose not to engage. No matter what motivating factors are applied in a crowdsourcing initiative, it must be fair to garner deep and engaged participation by a large crowd. Therefore, a critical dimension of crowdsourcing is careful consideration of the mixture of motivations for participants.

There are two perspectives in the consideration of *data characteristics*—the source and type of data. Crowdsourcing activities in health care often involve either preexisting or crowd-generated data. For example, the Moffit Cancer Center and Ohio State University Comprehensive Cancer Center founded a network of cancer patient data, the Oncology Research Information Exchange Network (ORIEN), to establish a rich data resource for research. This resource brings together data from more than 100,000 consenting patients and links many of them to clinical specimens to enable informatics-based research. In this case, the input and data are created by the crowd and become a preexisting asset for future research. Another example of patient-reported data is gathered by the Patient Powered Research Network (PPRN) PatientsLikeMe (PLM), which represents PRO data on patients' conditions, treatments, and symptoms. The data can be aggregated and enables academic, commercial, and patient-generated research [28]. PLM is discussed in greater detail below.

Swan [29] describes big data streams—traditional data, "-omics" data, and the Quantified Self. *Traditional data streams* include patients' personal and family health history, prescription history, current and past lab results, demographic data, and standardized questionnaire data [30]. This data may be quantitative, for example, medications, lab values, assays, medical claims, and diseases and treatments based on standardized nomenclature such as the Current Procedural Terminology (CPT), the Systemized Nomenclature of Medicine (SNOMED), the International Statistical Classification of Diseases and Related Health Problem, 10th Revision (ICD-10), and others. Or the data may be qualitative such as clinical notes, medication diaries, and even data generated in social media (eg, Facebook/Twitter/blog posts) [31].

The *-omics data streams* include genomics, proteomics, metabolomics, single-cell analysis, phenotyping, microfluidics, and imaging data that will enable the development of more informed treatments based on disease stratification, disease progression, and patient treatment response [32]. Each patient has the potential to generate billions of data points (data clouds) that can not only be used to treat disease in an individualized manner, but may even predict illness while the patient is still well [32].

Quantified self-data streams are generated by patients using sensors and trackers to generate health data for personal use [33]. A recent Pew Internet and American Life survey found that 69% of US adults track weight, diet, symptoms, or health routines through various methods, including smartphone health applications [34]. However, among the 100,000+ available apps there is little physician guidance on their safe and appropriate usage [35]. Existing device research focuses on informing or assisting patients with their conditions in the context of nonclinical use [33]. With the advent of US Food and Drug Administration (FDA) guidance and regulation on mobile apps, more rigorous testing is likely to escalate as manufacturers seek labeling claim or medical device approval [36].

Nontraditional data streams arise from a variety of data sources, for example, food purchases, health club memberships, and number of speeding tickets. Many nonhealth industries (eg, finance) have found ways to gain insights and make transformations by integrating data from heterogenous data sources at the level of an individual person [31]. Although the integration of these diverse data sets present obvious privacy issues in health, they suggest the potential for a more holistic picture of disease and wellness.

Technology will enable the continued expansion of data available for crowdsourcing. "P4 medicine" is based on principles of systems medicine and envisions the integration of patient social networks and medical big data networks to build a health care system that is *predictive, preventive, personalized,* and *participatory* [32]. Because data clouds will be developed while people are still healthy, insights about health and wellness may begin before they receive a diagnosis. The availability of platforms will allow expert crowds (eg, researchers) and patient crowds to share, analyze, and interpret this data. Networks of patients and crowdsourcing will drive the acceptance of this vision ushering in important advances in cancer diagnostics, drug discovery, and the development of treatments [32].

16.3 CROWDSOURCING IN HEALTH CARE

This section explores a series of case studies of how crowdsourcing has been applied to health care including the *ALS Prize4Life Biomarker Challenge, Novel Molecule Challenges* on the InnoCentive platform, *FoldIt,* and 23andMe. In this nascent phase of medical crowdsourcing, there are few robust examples in oncology, but it is hoped that lessons learned from adjacent areas may be informative. In addition, it should be noted that many uses of crowdsourcing are not derived from academic research but across a broad array of industries. As a result, the evidence base within the field has not matured and is still growing.

16.3.1 Crowdsourcing for Diagnostics and Drug Discovery

Challenges. InnoCentive (www.innocentive.com) is a crowdsourcing company that has completed more than 2000 *Challenges* with its global community of more than 350,000 volunteer *Solvers.* Challenges have included identifying optional routes of molecular synthesis, assay development, and bio-molecular informatics. The Novel Molecule Challenge (NMC) addresses a key problem in the early stages of developing new therapies—building a diverse library of potential molecules that share core physical characteristics (eg, a particular subcomponent of the molecule), but also vary in other attributes, such as their overall size, attached subcomponents, or moieties. This library is then screened against an assay to determine their likely effect and properties inside of cells.

NMCs provide solvers with the core characteristics of the sought after molecule, and then, invite proposals for other molecules that contain the core characteristics and vary in other ways. InnoCentive's client then has the opportunity to select the most interesting molecules, which can then be synthesized and supplied by the Solver who proposed them. IP surrounding the molecules and their applications are transferred to the client so they can continue to invest in the molecule's development, a process that InnoCentive has completed for tens of thousands of molecules. As the construction of drug screening libraries for anticancer drug development continue to demand new and innovative molecules, crowdsourcing approaches such as the NMC may enhance the diversity and scale that can be achieved through the integration and innovation of tens or hundreds of contributing chemists. Beyond small molecule drugs, this approach has been applied to noncommercial chemical compounds, proteins, extracts, polymers, and DNA sequences.

Another example of crowdsourcing diagnostics was conducted with Amyotrophic Lateral Sclerosis (ALS), a rare and lethal disease for which no effective therapies exist. In 2006, the *ALS Prize4Life Biomarker Challenge* was established to fund a prize-based crowdsourcing effort to develop new measures of disease progression [37] on the basis that a more precise measure of disease progression would enable shorter, faster, cheaper clinical trials. *Prize4Life* paid out multiple prizes that represented progress toward the goal and furnished a $1 million prize for anyone who could accomplish the complete goal of measuring ALS disease progression. A handful of "thought prizes" and "progress prizes" were paid out to promising participants in 2007 and 2009. Because the economic potential of a biomarker for ALS is far greater than the $1 million top prize, the winner would retain IP rights to develop and commercialize their technology further. More than 1000 Solvers from 20 countries participated. Even more, two-thirds of participants were outside the ALS research domain, suggesting that the problem attracted a diverse crowd of potential Solvers. For example, one progress prizewinner was Dr Harvey Arbesman, a dermatologist who observed skin differences between disabled ALS patients and similarly disabled quadriplegics, and designed a means for quantifying disease progression dermatologically [37]. In 2011, the Chief of Neuromuscular Disease, Seward Rutkove, in the Department of Neurology at Harvard Medical School's Beth Israel Deaconess Medical Center, captured the full $1 million prize for his application of electrical impedance myography to patients with ALS, a concrete and commendable success for proponents of crowdsourcing in health care [37].

Gamification. While the human cost of illness is high and altruism can serve as a powerful motivator, some projects have used gamification to make complex analytical tasks seem like fun. One such project dealt with the concept of protein folding. Understanding the three dimensional folding structure of proteins is important because drugs interact with their structure. Typically, stable and properly folded proteins remain at the lowest possible energy configuration. But because proteins can contain hundreds or thousands of amino acids with hinge regions, the number of possible folding configurations can be astronomical. Therefore, the task of estimating the optimal folded structure of a protein through computations is extremely difficult because there are so many possible configurations. This is analogous to deducing the folding process that created a piece of folded origami containing 1000 creases.

In 2008, an innovative approach to solving this problem called FoldIt was created by Seth Cooper at the Center for Game Science at the University of Washington, in collaboration with the University's Department of Biochemistry. The platform utilizes gaming to enable individuals to "fold" a digital representation of a protein by manipulating the amino acid configuration piece by piece. Players of the game receive points for making folds that leave the protein in a lower energy state. Slowly, many players working together as a team identify the optimal folded configuration of the protein. The performance on this platform was based on the work of 57,000 FoldIt players and achieved successful protein folding results that rivaled or surpassed some computational approaches [38]. A similar system, known as *Phylo*, provides a similar game-based approach to solving multispecies nucleic acid sequence alignments [39]. It should be noted that complicated tasks such as protein folding attract thousands of participants, but only a very limited number of individuals exhibit the skill required to produce the most significant breakthroughs. It is likely that the game component of these platforms may act as a gateway for recruiting the most talented and expert problem solvers.

Human Intelligence Tasking. Services such as Amazon's Mechanical Turk (www.mturk.com/mturk/welcome), Crowdflower (www.crowdflower.com/), TopCoder (www.topcoder.com/), Turkit (http://groups.csail.mit.edu/uid/turkit/), and Crowdforge (http://smus.com/crowdforge) manage this type of crowdsourcing task. Participants are paid to work on *Human Intelligence Tasks* (*HITs*)—single, self-contained tasks that require a response and offer small amounts of money (typically about $0.50) per completion. The crowds have a large number of college educated individuals, but they do not possess any particular technical training, so the HITs must be simple enough for an untrained worker to engage and perform the expected task.

The potential range of tasks varies tremendously including biomedical image analysis, drug indication annotation, genomic variant annotations, structured annotations of clinical trial descriptions, and complex sequence alignments. Scientific data curation and annotation efforts can also be completed as HITs. These labor-intensive efforts require structuring and annotating the volumes of free-text generated by medical science. It has been estimated that there are more than 10,000 publications that associate genomic differences with phenotype or disease annually [19]. Annotation of such data is extremely expensive and time-consuming. This flow of constant discovery and new knowledge, while promising, is only as valuable as the degree in which data is integrated within a common framework and annotation system to store and manage all of these small discoveries. Overall, these studies frequently report superior economic and speed performance, while maintaining or exceeding existing performance thresholds [40–42]. Though these examples may not be specific to cancer R&D, they could also, quite naturally, be applied to advance cancer-related research or clinical trials, since the crowd itself is agnostic to differences between diseases.

Consumer Genetic Testing Services. Direct to consumer genetic testing services, such as 23andMe (www.23andme.com), Navigenics (www.navugenucs.com), and DeCode (www.decode.com), have capitalized on the decreasing price of genetic testing. Using data donated and shared by individual consumers, these services can potentially crowdsource new associations between genes and phenotypes without the intermediary of a geneticist or physician. The principle behind these services was described by 23andMe's cofounder, Anne Wojicki, when discussing the relatively small data sets upon which medical discoveries are based: "I don't want to bet [my health] on the people or system that is currently in place today. I want to learn from the crowd." First launched in 2007, the company offer personalized online genetic testing reports based on saliva samples submitted by customers. The reports describe a variety of ancestral and health-related traits, based on published studies of associations between traits and single nucleotide polymorphism (SNP) data. To obtain a critical mass of samples (around 10,000 individuals), disease-specific and underrepresented groups such as Parkinson's disease patients (www.23andme.com/pd/) and African Americans (www.23andme.com/en-gb/roots/), respectively, were offered free or reduced-price testing.

There are three forms of crowdsourcing at work here. The first is distributed data collection—anyone can submit their DNA sample and complete surveys on their medical history and phenotypic traits, leading to the rapid development of research studies with traditional formats, but executed with greater speed. For example, the company has published conference abstracts and high-impact, peer-reviewed scientific papers (www.23andme.com/for/scientists/) in fields as diverse as motion sickness, rosacea, asthma, Parkinson's disease, myopia, and alopecia, while also maintaining a degree of reflexive self-study to the ways in which members react to receiving their own information. However, this first set of crowdsourcing activity is driven mostly by the company's own scientists or their collaborations with academic institutions. A second, less formal class of crowdsourcing that 23andMe enables is made possible because members can choose to download their SNP data as a text file and then manually upload it anywhere they choose.

Finally, the third and least formal activity of crowdsourcing takes place at an individual level, where members of the site read and interpret health and trait findings, discuss the results with others in forums or on blogs, and attempt to make changes to their lifestyle or treatment to improve their outcomes. For example, Sergei Brin, the cofounder of Google and ex-husband of 23andMe founder, Anne Wojicki, found out he had a *LRRK2* Parkinson's gene, indicating a significantly higher risk of developing Parkinson's disease. In a media interview, it was revealed that he is drinking caffeine regularly because other people who go on to have Parkinson's disease have been shown in some studies to have a lower premorbid caffeine intake.

16.3.2 Crowdsourcing for Optimizing Treatment

Patients seeking to find answers for undiagnosed illnesses endure multiple visits to physicians, diagnostic work-ups and impressions, treatment tests, medical costs, and most of all, the emotional turmoil of this uncertain journey. Jared Heyman's 18 year-old sister, Carly, began experiencing extreme weight gain, hormonal problems, and depression. She was treated by 24 physicians before finding her solution through a multidisciplinary medical team at the NIH Undiagnosed Diseases Program who finally arrived at a diagnosis of fragile X-associated primary ovarian insufficiency, which was successfully treated with a hormone replacement patch [43].

Heyman recognized the power of "crowds" to solve complex diagnostic challenges and founded *CrowdMed* (www.crowdmed.com/), a crowdsourcing website devoted to helping patients find solutions to their undiagnosed medical problems. The average patient who joins CrowdMed has seen eight physicians over 8 years of illness and has spent $50,000 in medical costs along the way (https://www.crowdmed.com/faqs). CrowdMed enlists "medical detectives" who may have experience in health care (physicians, nurses, etc.), but also include lay people and patients who have experienced similar medical problems. Patients begin by posting case information about their symptoms, treatments, and health

history. Medical detectives then suggest potential diagnoses and assign confidence points to the resulting diagnoses, which is entered into an algorithm that analyzes this data and creates a report for the patient highlighting the top three diagnostic possibilities. As individual detectives solve cases, they build their status in the CrowdMed community and may also receive payment (when offered by patients) for correct diagnoses.

Despite anecdotal reports that 50% of patients posting cases have reported progress in obtaining a diagnosis, the effectiveness of CrowdMed has still not been established [44]. There is no clear peer-reviewed data documenting the sensitivity and specificity of this methodology in identifying correct diagnoses. Patients who list cases are required to sign a liability waiver that offers no recourse if the information that they receive results in a negative medical outcome. It should also be noted that crowdsourcing websites aggregating patient rare disease cases may find it difficult to protect user's privacy [45].

Like many other segments of the population, physicians are increasingly using social media sites like Facebook and Twitter [46]. Perhaps the best known physician community is the medical community *Sermo* (www.sermo.com). This community consists of 300,000 members with verified credentials, accounting for 40% of US physicians and doctors of osteopathy (http://sermo.com/what-is-sermo/faq). Sermo provides a platform for physicians to share questions and feedback about medical questions and difficult cases. Their peers can ask follow-up questions, advice, or vote on the best strategies to address the question. Members can also respond to/post surveys or join focus groups that are sponsored by pharmaceutical companies, medical device firms, and biotech companies.

16.3.3 Crowdsourcing for Health Care Delivery Improvements

The *ONC i2 Initiative* of the Office of the National Coordinator for Health Information Technology (ONC), called the Investing in Innovations Initiative, uses competitions and prizes to accelerate HIT innovation (www.health2con.com/devchallenge/). The competitions target projects that allow secure sharing of individual health information through social networks; health data exchange with consumer control over privacy settings; connections between individuals during emergencies and natural disasters; and information access for patients, health care providers, and caregivers. Challenges typically last 3–6 months, and teams submit software and hardware solutions such as web and mobile applications, visualizations, sensor systems, and data models (http://www.health2con.com/devchallenge/). Successful submissions are offered financial support and potential partnership opportunities to further the development and commercialization of the application. The sponsors include health collaboratives, as well health insurance, pharmaceutical, and high technology companies.

The "Crowds Care for Cancer: Supporting Survivors Challenge" is an example of a successful cancer challenge that was presented by ONC in conjunction with the NCI. This 2013 challenge offered a $25,000 prize for the development of information management tools that would help cancer survivors manage the transition from specialty to primary care treatment. The winner was Medable (www.medable.com), a secure online platform that allows communication that's compliant with the Health Insurance Portability and Accountability Act (HIPAA), collaboration, and data sharing between patients and providers. Their "Together" mobile application allows patients and caregivers to communicate with multiple members of their care team; integrates home monitoring and wearables data (eg, FitBit); adds additional big data sources such as 23andMe genomic information; and formulates Health Level Seven International (HL7)-compliant personal health monitoring reports. Other projects have focused on the use of the "Blue Button" medical data sharing standard to share personal health data, the assessment of pressure ulcers, and tools to schedule timely follow-up appointments following hospital discharge.

Kaggle (www.kaggle.com) is a community of thousands of PhD-level data scientists from the computer science, statistics, econometrics, mathematics, and physics fields. Members of Kaggle compete with each other to solve quantitative problems in a wide variety of industries, for example, life sciences, financial services, energy, information technology, and retail. The 2012 Heritage Health Prize (sponsored by the Heritage Health Network) challenged entrants to predict how many days patients would spend in the hospital. The ultimate goal was to help providers reduce emergencies and unnecessary hospitalizations through the creation of proactive care plans. Contestants were given two sets of anonymized data—a "training set" consisting of 2 years of patient health data (including the number of days spent in hospital) and a "validation set" consisting of a third year of health claims data for the same patients (which did not include hospitalization days) (www. heritagehealthprize.com/c/hhp/rules). Although a $500,000 progress prize was awarded in June 2013, the $3 million top prize remains unclaimed [47].

Clear Health Costs (http://clearhealthcosts.com/) and *NewChoiceHealth* (www.NewChoiceHealth.com) are examples of crowdsourcing websites devoted to health care pricing transparency. Although the rate of spending growth has slowed somewhat over the past few post-recession years, the United States spends almost $9000 per person annually on health care, for a total of almost $3 trillion [30]. One of the contributing factors is the lack of transparency in costs to the consumer seeking health care services or treatments, allowing the noncompetitive inflation of hospital, physician, and drug manufacturer list prices [48]. More than half of US health consumers believe that providers charge similar prices for the same services (which they do not) or did not know how pricing worked [49]. About 70% felt that a website showing price comparisons between doctors would help them monitor their health care spending.

Crowdsourcing of pricing has already reached many other industries. Travelers are now able to quickly compare and review prices of airline flights, restaurants, hotels, and other services (eg, TripAdvisor, Trulia, Kayak). Several for-profit companies, nonprofit organizations, and state governments provide online price information for health consumers for services, lab tests, devices, and other health care costs, but less than 20% of the public use these services [49].

Clear Health Costs, launched by New York Times reporter Jeanne Pinder, combines crowdsourcing and reporting and allows consumers to share prices through an interactive widget. These prices include diagnostic imaging, women's and men's health consultations, blood tests, walk-in services, dental, and cosmetic services. Users may search across states, mileage radius, and zip code. A visit to this website shows broad variations in pricing such as a range of $50–607 for a mammogram in New York City. Clear Health Costs is collaborating with the radio station KQED in San Francisco, CA on an initiative called Price Check (http://blogs.kqed.org/stateofhealth/2014/06/23/share-your-bill-make-health-costs-transparent-in-california), in which consumers can report total charged price, insurance payments, and out-of-pocket expenses. Consumers may also share their experiences with health services. A price check on mammograms in San Francisco and Los Angeles indicates that they range between $128 and $694 [50].

NewChoiceHealth allows entry of self-pay and insurance prices across procedures, cities, and facilities. For example, selecting a location reveals a list of price ranges for common procedures, consumer reviews, and quality scores. In Washington, DC, for example, colonoscopies range between $470 and $1550. Consumers can request a quote, which might one day lead to the unusual scenario of providers bidding for a patient's business rather than assuming that, through the power of an insurance network, the patient is "locked in."

16.3.4 Patient as Researcher

There is a long tradition of self-experimentation in scientific discovery. Scientists and physicians have exposed themselves to infectious diseases, radioactivity, medical procedures, and vaccines, hoping to understand disease mechanisms or confirm the safety and efficacy of certain treatments [51]. Salk and Sabin administered polio vaccines to themselves, their wives, and their children before testing the vaccines in field trials [51]. Despite their risk, their efforts have led to major medical breakthroughs. As institutional ethical review has taken hold, these potentially risky efforts have receded in favor of much larger, closely controlled, and tightly regulated clinical trials. While developed with an appropriate emphasis on preventing abuse of participants, this risk aversion may have become too extreme, slowing the pace of discoveries and contributing to a power imbalance between researcher and subject.

In an article entitled *Subjects No More: What Happens When Trial Participants Realize They Hold the Power?* Wicks et al. [52] describe the outcomes of the unbalanced social contract between patients and researchers in clinical trials [53]. Patients have taken to the Internet to assert control by unblinding themselves, reviewing the scientific literature on their own, and as described above, conducting their own studies. This may be a response to traditional research studies, which tend to adopt one-way relationships with participants, thus obviating incentives for participants to remain truly fully engaged.

There are multiple points of contact for patient participation in research. Mullins et al. [54] have proposed the concept of "continuous patient engagement," which describes a 10-stage process in which patients are active throughout the research continuum, from idea conception, to data collection and execution, and dissemination of results [54]. As can be seen in Table 16.2, all of these steps require the participation of both patients and researchers so they may complement each other, as researchers offer technical expertise while patients offer "real-world" expertise. The tasks indicated in the table reflect realistic expectations of patients as collaborators [55].

Rather than taking on the role of "subjects," patients can take an active role in the conduct of research, particularly as it affects their care. In fact, "citizen scientists" have in some cases taken matters into their own hands, by generating their own clinical data, conducting comparative effectiveness test of treatments, and then sharing findings [56]. Participant-led research (PLR) is often not encumbered by the oversight of an institutional review board (IRB) or the pressure to publish. As Roberts [57] states about the self-experimentation related to his sleep, mood, and weight, "I had the subject-matter knowledge of an insider, the freedom of an outsider, and the motivation of a person with the problem."

In an effort to add rigor to participant-led studies, crowdsourced health research platforms have been developed by companies to help citizen scientists develop study ideas and methodologies, recruit participants, and contribute personal data. Two of these efforts, DIYGenomics (www.diygenomics.org) and Genomera

(www.genomera.com), help people wishing to explore linkages between their genomic data and phenotypic characteristics to design and conduct studies with other participants. For example, DIYGenomics offers studies investigating the relationships between genetic and microbiome profiles with aging, sleep, cognition, and vitamin deficiencies. A third company, Althea Health (www.altheahealth.com), connects patients to raise funds for research, involve professionals, and participate in studies that will ultimately lead to pharmaceutical partnerships developing new therapies. These communities gather data through leveraging smartphones, connected health devices, electronic medical records (EMRs), and personal social network data to advance research in rare diseases.

PatientsLikeMe. PLM is one of the largest and most established patient crowdsourcing platforms, with over 300,000 registered patients. Launched in 2004, PLM was born out of a desire to help chronic disease patients share their experiences with life-threatening diseases. Brothers Ben and Jamie Heywood founded the company with Jeff Cole, a lifelong friend, after struggling to assist their brother Stephen Heywood, who was diagnosed with ALS. They realized that many patients have questions about their treatments, disease course, and self-management, and designed an open online patient registry that allows patients and caregivers to share personal data and experiences in real time. The platform began as an ALS-specific community, but has now expanded to more than 2000 conditions. In keeping with a patient-centered philosophy, the key core values of PLM are "putting patients first," promoting transparency, and fostering openness among members.

PLM is termed a "patient-powered research network" that assists patient in answering the question, "Given my current status, what is the best outcome that I can hope to achieve and how do I get there?" To help patients answer these questions, PLM helps members to: (1) find information about living with and treating disease; (2) connect with others who have the same condition (patients like me); and (3) input, track, and share real-world data on their conditions, including treatment history, side effects, hospitalizations, symptoms, disease-specific functional scores, mood, and quality of life.

As the mission of PLM is to conduct research that helps patients understand their conditions, while promoting scientific advances, patients are encouraged to share their personal medical data on the PLM website (www.patientslikeme.com). Data about patients' condition(s) (primary/secondary, comorbidities); symptoms; treatments (start/stop dates, indications, outcomes, effectiveness, side effects, adherence, treatment burden); hospitalizations; and laboratory tests are collected systematically and presented in graphical form. Patients may supplement this data with free text narratives about

TABLE 16.2 Steps in Continuous Engagement

Steps in continuous engagement	Purpose of patient engagement	Researcher activities	Patient activities
Topic solicitation	Define potential research topics that are relevant to patients	Gather information through literature reviews, consultations with experts, and meetings with patients Determine where gaps exist in the evidence base	Contribute real-world research questions Provide input on challenges/facilitators in patient disease journey that require further investigation
Prioritization	Determine relative importance of potential topics	Assess feasibility and public health impact of research question	Determine topics of greatest urgency and impact on patients Determine questions that have greatest impact in patients' daily lives
Framing the question	Define research questions with a "real-world perspective"	Address questions that can generate testable hypotheses or guide data exploration	Structure questions in the voice of the patient so that real-world impact is addressed
Selection of comparators and outcomes	Determine treatment comparators and outcomes that match real-world research questions	Work with patient representatives to help finalize research questions	Act as patient representatives to help finalize research questions Assure inclusion of real-world outcomes Determine most realistic treatment comparisons (re: affordability, access, and burden)
Creation of conceptual framework	Determine potential hypotheses and research questions	Conduct literature review Gather expert input	Gather peer perspectives Communicate on social media Review proposed research questions and suggest possible factors and barriers that might affect results
Analysis plan	Determine the data sources most likely to deliver real-world patient perspectives	Select data sources, eg, registries, claims reporting, patient-reported outcome measures, laboratory tests, interviews, focus groups, etc. Define statistical procedures.	Provide input on importance of key factors and variables Assist in determining who is eligible for participation Assist in selection of valid measures that reduce participant burden Review of informed consent materials for comprehension and burden. Provide feedback on logistics of study to reduce patient burden
Data collection	Determine sources and methods of data collection	Develop recruitment and data collection plan	Assist is defining potential real-world data sources Pilot testing measures and surveys Assist in recruitment Craft study name and materials to reduce stigma Serve on data safety monitoring board
Reviewing and interpreting results	Determine meaningful results	Perform statistical analyses	Input on relevance of findings Provide feedback on believability of results
Translation	Define results with highest impact for professional and patient audiences	Determine message for professional audience	Integrate the patient voice in linking findings to real-world experience Assist in development of dissemination plan
Dissemination	Distribute findings to professional and patient communities	Develop and participate in academic/clinical publishing and presentation	Create plain language summaries Participate as authors on publications and presentations

Adapted from Mullins CD, Abdulhalim AM, Lavallee DC. Continuous patient engagement in comparative effectiveness research. J Am Med Assoc 2012;307:1587–8 and PCORI. PCORI Engagement Rubric; 2015. <http://www.pcori.org/sites/default/files/PCORI-Engagement-Rubric-with-Table.pdf>.

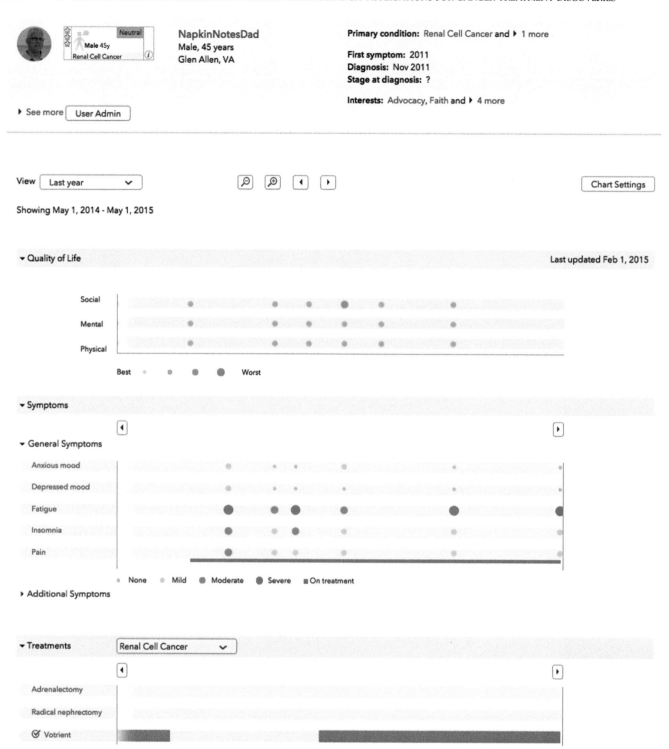

FIGURE 16.1   A profile of a PLM renal cell cancer patient.

their disease journeys. This information allows patients to build updatable and sharable visual tracking profiles that help them understand their disease course and learn about the relationships between their conditions, symptoms, and treatments. Patients can also find and contact others with similar profiles. Fig. 16.1 depicts a profile of a PLM renal cell cancer patient.

As can be seen from the profile, treatments, symptoms, and medical data can be viewed along a timeline, allowing an individual to detect trends. When viewed in aggregate form across patients, researchers can conduct data mining studies and compare patient cohorts across conditions, symptoms, treatments, etc. Patients join PLM knowing that research and scientific advancement are important missions. Because the data is observable to members, there are opportunities for both researchers and patients to conduct studies. This is especially valuable when patients are suffering from rare conditions or there is a desire among patients or researchers to understand the potential effectiveness of emerging treatments.

ALS Study. The best-known participant-led study on PLM involved ALS patients [58]. In 2007, a group of ALS participants translated an Italian conference abstract into English and found that an ALS research group in Pisa was claiming that lithium carbonate slows disease progression. A patient in Brazil and a US caregiver (with a PhD in geology) started encouraging other patients to ask their doctors to prescribe lithium off-label and submit their data on a Google Spreadsheet. The Italian group's findings were published in the *Proceedings of the National Academy of Sciences (PNAS)* with the title "Lithium delays progression of amyotrophic lateral sclerosis" [59]. Against such a brief prognosis, many patients started taking lithium and crowdsourcing their data online.

In response, PLM upgraded their data capture systems to collect information about lithium dosage, blood levels, side effects, and longitudinal ALS Functional Rating Scale (Revised) (ALSFRS-R) scores. The original Italian study was small, with just 16 lithium-treated participants and 28 controls. By contrast, more than 160 participants started taking lithium off-label and tracking their data online, with many times that number being available as a historical control group. Both participant groups and researchers from PLM conducted their own analyses of the data. The participant group used rudimentary inferential statistics to look at differences in progression rate between self-treating participants and a random sample of control participants. They quickly realized that lithium did not seem to have a strong effect on progression. A more rigorous statistical analysis by PLM researchers used a carefully matched set of control participants and published their findings in peer-reviewed literature, along with a deidentified copy of the data set to allow replication. Like the participant group, they could find no effect of lithium on progression. While the participant-lead study generated a great deal of interest outside the field, traditional academic researchers still went ahead with a number of randomized double-blind placebo-controlled trials, all of which also failed to find an effect of lithium on progression or were halted prematurely. Although the data collected through participant-generated registries can be rapid and useful, today traditional methods still remain the preferred approach for specific hypothesis-testing.

Open Research Exchange. Another form of PLM research involving both participant collaboration and leadership relates to the development of PRO measures, which refers to information gathered directly from the patient, typically through questionnaires or surveys, without intermediate interpretation or filtering by health professionals. PROs may be used clinically to determine level of function and changes over time (such as a mood measure in depression), in research to describe populations (such as the quality of life across asthma patients with different levels of access to care), or as an endpoint in a clinical trial (such as the level of pain and disability experienced in rheumatoid arthritis). Increasingly PROs also find themselves used in "*n*-of-1" studies and self-tracking activities. Since their first appearance in the medical literature in the mid-20th century, there are probably several thousand PROs in existence; although they vary dramatically with regards to their quality, reliability, and appropriateness for use in different settings, and the degree to which they have been updated for modern times. For instance, many widely used measures of activities of daily living attempt to grade patients' ability to function in the world by their ability to do grocery shopping, balance a checkbook, or participate in social activities, when the modern world allows groceries to be delivered, banking to be conducted online, and social activities to take place at a computer screen rather than in person. Because developing a PRO has traditionally required psychometric expertise and a means of distribution, development has been slow. However, the use of online social networks and the increased availability of open source tools and open access scientific publications means more patients can get involved in the process of developing and using PROs.

The Open Research Exchange (ORE) is a PRO development platform funded by the Robert Wood Johnson Foundation and hosted by PLM. Using the tool, researchers can engage with a selected group of patients to query them directly on what matters to them and should be measured in PROs from the convenience of their own homes rather than traditional methods, which involved face-to-face interviews. The psychometric process consists of five steps, including concept elicitation, in which PLM users comment on how they experience the illness in question. Draft items are then developed and undergo a second phase of online cognitive evaluation by patients. Patients provide quantitative and qualitative feedback on the clarity, relevance, and adequacy of response options of items. After items have been reviewed and organized into an instrument, the last three phases of test, retest, and follow-up evaluation occur. Researchers are able to view results in real time at the item, person, and group levels. Completed instruments are then available via Open Access through a Creative Commons license. The ORE allows for input from hundreds of patients rather than dozens and takes place over a period of hours rather than years [60]. To date, 12 instruments covering a range of diseases (diabetes, hypertension, Parkinson's disease) and treatment constructs (treatment burden, medication adherence, palliative care) have been created using this platform.

There have also been a small number of cases where patients themselves have even developed their own PROs to address gaps they perceived in the literature. For instance, Cathy Wolf, a woman living with ALS, who is quadriplegic and dependent on a ventilator to breathe, was frustrated by the widely used ALSFRS-R when she scored at the floor level, despite living (in her view) an active mental and social life thanks to technology that allowed her to communicate, albeit slowly [61]. She used her online community to develop and validate a set of extension items to the ALSFRS-R, identifying the ability to show emotion in the face or manipulate technology with the fingertips as being an important extension of communication beyond speech or using a pen. The ALS Functional Rating Scale (Extension Items) (ALSFRS-EX) were psychometrically validated, translated into other languages and have been used in a number of scientific studies including the Veterans Administration's (VA) Brain Biobank Repository [62,63]. Although cases like Cathy Wolf's are unusual, they show the potential of more rapidly crowdsourcing measures that matter to patients in a timely manner [64].

In a second example, a multiple sclerosis (MS) patient wanted to create a pain measure that would be more patient-centered than standard pain rating scales. Although the symptoms of MS created some difficulties in task completion, this patient was able to navigate the entire ORE process with support, including concept elicitation, item selection and refinement, and test-retest evaluation. The resulting instrument, called Impact of Pain Scale, is available on the ORE website. It should be noted that the value in such patient-led efforts is not limited to the resulting research, but in the educational and therapeutic aspects of participation:

> I had never heard of "patient-led research" so when it was explained to me, a hobbyist researcher but in no way a formal researcher, I was a bit in awe of the whole process… I also did not anticipate the ways this project would grow and sprout off other ideas for potential research, which I hope we see picked up and looked into… I would absolutely recommend other patients jump at any chance to work on a project that is "patient led." Who better to give insight than the patients, themselves?!
>
> *Tamara M.*

Although the research developments of PLM did not develop the much-wanted cure for Stephen Heywood, who died in 2007, it has produced more than 65 scientific studies in the peer-reviewed literature and strives to bring patient-centric values to the research enterprise.

Quantified Self Studies. The term "quantified self" was coined in 2007 by Gary Wolf and Kevin Kelley, editors at *WIRED* Magazine [65]. This term describes behaviors conducted routinely by many people every day— weighing themselves, tracking their calories, running miles, or recording their blood pressure. Quantification of health has traditionally been a paper-and-pencil exercise, viewed on pedometers, or managed on spreadsheets. With the advent of technology that is wearable, easy to use, and linked to smartphones and computers, people can record their activities and various biological functions virtually all day long. Aggregation of this data on infographics and dashboards allows easy tracking of progress for personal data analysis. Increasingly, self-tracking devices and applications are being integrated to form larger data sources. This will allow quantified selfers to share and compare findings, and perhaps generate new insights about their personal health.

Because of the sheer number of individuals contributing data, the quantified self movement offers the opportunity for rich data sources that can be aggregated into crowdsourced databases.

There is a burgeoning quantified self movement in which individuals track personal health and lifestyle data and share their findings about diet, exercise, sleep, chronic disease symptoms, etc. at "meet-ups" around the country. However, the most personally detailed quantified self study has been conducted by Larry Smarr, director of the California Institute for Telecommunications and Information Technology in La Jolla, California [66]. In more than 10 years of personal data collecting, Smarr has tracked his personal activity, sleep, heart rate, ultrasound and MRI imaging, biomarkers in blood and stool samples, and gut microbiomes [66]. In the course of losing weight, getting healthier, and tracking this data, Smarr discovered changes in C-reactive protein and lactoferrin that ultimately led to his diagnosis with Crohn's disease [67,68]. This case highlights the extent of individual data clouds as described by "P4 medicine" and suggests the potential for aggregating data from large numbers of patients to affect populations, as well as individuals. If such n-of-1 trials can be coordinated and continuous data gathered, the potential to change the course of evidence-based and personalized medicine could be vast [69].

16.4 METHODOLOGICAL AND ETHICAL ISSUES IN CROWDSOURCING

16.4.1 Methodological Issues

The large-scale cohorts participating in crowdsourced studies can accelerate scientific discoveries, but the levels of scientific rigor across studies can vary greatly [13].

One of the primary concerns is sampling bias due to self-selection of participants [70]. By definition, crowdsourcing studies target an unselected groups of people, resulting in a high likelihood of attracting individuals who are interested in such studies and who may therefore be systematically biased. Indeed, an examination of Mechanical Turk studies found that they tend to attract younger, more highly educated female participants than the general population [71]. Because crowdsourcing involves computer-based tasks, individuals with low literacy or limited computer access may be underrepresented, thus limiting the generalizability of crowdsourcing methodologies [72]. In many cases, crowdsourcers may not even know the composition of their sample due to anonymous participation. Published crowdsourcing studies rarely report sample demographics, size of cohorts, logistics of data collection, and motivations for participation, despite the fact that reporting standards would assist readers in comparing studies [73]. This makes it difficult to compare and generalize samples to other clinical populations. Another concern is that the blending of the participant and researcher roles, which has been termed "apomediation," renders blinding difficult in intervention studies [44]. Participants may consciously or unconsciously introduce bias into their self-reported data by failing to follow protocols correctly or even falsifying data.

Organizations that engage in multiple streams of crowdsourcing face nuanced problems. For instance, a challenge for 23andMe is that while the data collection of its population-level SNP analysis and surveys follow a clear scientific method and robust ethical underpinning (IRBs), its less formal activities, such as crowdsourced discovery, are led mostly by volunteers who operate with less oversight and likely less scientific rigor. While the company's scientific research is peer-reviewed and evaluated by experts in the context of a wider literature, individual users of the service might choose to make significant health decisions on the basis of interpretations of data they provide, such as changing their diet or even their medication regimen. A similar criticism could apply to PLM, who on the one hand conducts scientific research with classically conducted studies through a virtual interface, but on the other hand, also allow n-of-1 interpretation and insights that are less controlled and more subject to bias.

Even within its most stable area of scientific certainty, 23andMe has been criticized by researchers who have found inconsistencies in some genetic results provided by the company, identified biases in the types of users registering on the site, and have cautioned against, "their speculative and often contradictory lifetime risk estimates for complex diseases derived from genome-wide association studies" [74]. This criticism culminated in 2013 when the FDA sent a tersely worded warning letter ordering 23andMe to stop disclosing health results to members of its system, citing amongst other things concerns about the company's failure to engage with the regulator.

Looking to the future, however, it seems likely that 23andMe's approach will endure, even if the company must change strategy in the short term. At the time of this book's publication, members cannot receive health results as they once could, though 23andMe is working through the issues of identifying each condition to the FDA's standard, starting with Bloom's syndrome and working their way through sequentially.

Although criticized as upstarts by the traditional research establishment, both PLM and 23andMe have three advantages in their favor. First, as companies with technology, rather than academic medicine roots, they are in the habit of iterating and pivoting their model fluidly in a matter of weeks rather than decades; they have both shown themselves capable of adapting rapidly. Secondly, they benefit from advances in information and genetic technologies funded by others to a degree that no brick-and-mortar health facility could ever do. Finally, the increased push within health care and the insatiable curiosity of increasingly connected individuals to "know themselves" means that this form of crowdsourcing is likely to remain with us and become more central over the coming years.

16.4.2 Ethical Issues

The FDA as we now know it was borne out of tragedy. The FDA began as the Bureau of Chemistry and was tasked with monitoring the ingredients in new foods and drugs rather than approvals based on safety and efficacy [75]. In 1937, the S.E. Massengill Company began selling a new drug called Elixir Sulfanilamide, which was thought to treat a variety of conditions, including gonorrhea and sore throat. More than 100 people died after taking this medication, which led Congress to empower the FDA to monitor drug safety, and ultimately, require proof of medication efficacy [76]. Given the history of drug experimentation in the United States, for example the rampant use of patent medicines in the 18th and 19th centuries, it is no wonder that the rise of self-experimentation and PLR has sounded ethical alarms [77], especially the need to protect research participants by gaining their informed consent.

Informed consent is based on the "Common Rule," a procedure developed before the age of Internet research. This rule states that research participants must be informed of scope of the research, as well as the study's risks and benefits. They then sign a consent form that creates a legal agreement to proceed with the research. However, research models, such as crowdsourcing, have created ethical concerns that revolve around three issues: (1) the opaque nature of transactions; (2) evolving definitions of "research"; and (3) threats to the objectivity of the research and safety of participants due to organizational incentive structures or peer dynamics among participants. First, consider the traditional relationship between researcher and participant. The researcher designs a study, determines the characteristics of the study sample, and recruits through a number of means that involve a 1:1 relationship—direct advertisement, telephone, face-to-face, email, mail, etc. The relationship is direct and the control of the information flow between can remain private and confidential. Online recruitment of the crowd adds greater complexity, opaqueness, and uncertainty about control over the transactions between researcher and participant [78]. The parties involved in the transaction are much less identifiable and all transactions are subject to data capture, dissemination, and aggregation [78]. In apomediated research, individuals recruiting and being recruited share the risk, but the risk is shared by participants in a larger group, increasing threats to privacy [79]. This increases the potential for unauthorized disclosure and loss of participant confidentiality, particularly when the researcher and formal ethical oversight are removed from the equation in participant-led or crowdsourced data sharing research.

Second, participants may not even know that they are participating in research. A recent example of this was Facebook's "emotional contagion study," in which members of this online network were exposed to manipulations of the rate of presentation of positive and negative emotional content in their news feeds, which led to a public outcry [80]. Some researchers might argue that the application of traditional informed consent procedures to research in social computing environments may stifle potentially valuable research, and so creative solutions tailored for the online social networking and crowdsourcing environment are needed. However, burying often arcane consent language in website user agreements certainly does not fulfill the spirit of informed consent and consumers will need to be cautious to ensure their consent is not taken for granted.

The fluid and dynamic nature of crowdsourced and PLR studies have forced a reconsideration of the research review and informed consent process [81]. Vayena and Tasiloulas [82] envision three categories of ethical oversight of PLR: (1) government institutions, government-recognized institutions, or profit-making organizations would be subject to standard ethics review procedures; (2) if there is no institutional sponsorship, but there is more than minimal risk involved, then ethics review is required; and (3) if there is no institutional sponsorship and less than minimal risk involved, then ethics review is not required [82]. Option 1 would likely engage existing formal IRB structures. Option 2 might involve formal IRBs or perhaps an open protocol review

group [13]. This proposal leaves open major questions such as the determination of minimal risk, balancing of a bottom up approach to research with the formality of review, and the structure of alternative review bodies.

The subject of ethical review relates to changing notions of informed consent. Given the changing nature of the participant–researcher relationship and the way that data is collected and reused, biomedical ethicists have begun reconsidering the way in which informed consent is structured. One example is the Portable Legal Consent (PLC) developed by the Consent to Research project (http://sagecongress.org/WP/wp-content/uploads/2012/04/PortableLegalConsentOverview.pdf). This type of consent is framed for research contexts that require or promote data sharing. Participants agree to give up control over personal health and genomics data that they upload to an online database. In return, the data is limited to open access research, patient data cannot be reidentified, and any researcher reusing the data must agree to these conditions. Patients may remove their data at any time. As part of the process, patients view a video presentation describing the consent. To make the consent process easier for participants to understand, Sage Bionetworks (2015) has recently released a Participant-Centered Consent (PCC) toolkit (http://sagebase.org/pcc/participant-centered-consent-toolkit/). This user-centered toolkit was developed for researchers who are seeking to improve comprehension about consents in a more visual and interactive style. The toolkit includes icons and animations to help participants understand complex issues such as privacy and data sharing, design assets, and informed consent templates. The PCC toolkit lets its users create visual summaries of consent forms, mapped to key underlying text, for use in software or print. Overall, the PLC offers a promising means of avoiding a laborious reconsent process, while providing a transparent solution with clear requirements for researcher data access and use.

16.4.3 Data Privacy

There are numerous privacy and ethics concerns related to aggregating data in a public manner. Half of online Americans don't know what a "privacy policy" is, thinking that it ensures confidentiality of information that is collected [83]. A recent survey of individuals tracking health for themselves or a loved one found that about 70% of respondents were agreeable to data sharing with academic researchers, and for about 30% of the sample, privacy was not a concern with regard to data sharing. However, 57% reported that they needed an assurance of privacy with regard to their dominant shared condition [84]. More than 90% reported that any shared health and physical activity data should be anonymized.

Unfortunately, deidentification is difficult as almost 90% of the US population can be identified based on only three pieces of data: the 5-digit zip code, gender, and date of birth [53]. Researchers at the Data Privacy Lab at Harvard utilized the same data points and were able to identify between 84% and 97% anonymous profiles in the Personal Genome Project database [85]. Particularly when combined with GPS technology, patients may have significant concerns about data that reveals sensitive personal activities. Patients will feel more comfortable with data sharing if the nature, use, user(s), legal protections, and potential compensation are clearly spelled out [13]. Developing a clear value proposition for patients to share such data will be necessary to realize a vision of broad data aggregation. Organizations engaging in crowdsourced research will need to make privacy policies less opaque. Participants are likely to feel more comfortable when the reasons for accessing or sharing personal data are clear [86].

16.4.4 Conflicts of Interest and IP

Because much crowdsourcing takes place within a commercial environment, there is potential for incentives or motivations that do not promote the best interests of participants [82]. Organizational influences, lack of equipoise, profit motives, or peer pressure among participants may affect the objectivity (and ultimately safety) of the research. Because of the nature of relationships among participants who have an incentive to find treatments that work for debilitating conditions, there may be potential to lose objectivity and suppress dissenting opinions. In the language of clinical trials, there may be a lack of "equipoise" (genuine uncertainty about the efficacy of the proposed treatment) among participants leading the research. The same motivations may result in biased interpretations of the risk–benefit ratios in conducting certain treatments [82]. The same tendencies may arise in organizations or companies that have a financial incentive for positive outcomes with a treatment.

One of the challenges in developing a business model for commercially funded crowdsourcing websites is to navigate potential conflicts of interest. For example, pharmaceutical companies pay fees to Sermo to elicit, track, and analyze physician sentiments; identify key opinion leaders; and disseminate messaging [87]. These activities raise the possibility of conflicts of interest, resulting in calls for more regulated or self-regulated disclosures [46]. When physicians offer clinical recommendations through crowdsourcing for a particular posted case, those receiving this information may not be aware of the potential conflicts of interests at work. Clear links, statements, or electronic tags indicating conflicts of interest in Facebook posts, Twitter entries, online consultations, and blog posts would allow users to make informed decisions about the value of information presented [46].

One hurdle to all research and development investments is ensuring that confidential information and IP are properly managed. Ongoing investment in promising technologies or products requires a firm IP foundation such that ownership and usage rights of IP can be assured to the funders of future development efforts. Most crowdsourcing projects involving innovation or creating new IP must address the questions of how IP ownership and usage rights are managed upfront. Does the definition of the problem require the disclosure of information or data that are sensitive or valuable—such as, for example, health records or potentially reidentifiable medical information? There are a plethora of other questions that must be answered ahead of time, prior to the start of the crowdsourcing activity. Should the organizers retain the rights to the IP? What IP rights flow to the individuals or organizations providing the incentive? Failure to properly structure and address these issues can lead to very negative consequences and invalidate the crowdsourcing effort or IP all together. An in-depth discussion of these matters is beyond the scope of this chapter, but it is an important dimension of crowdsourcing that cannot be overlooked.

16.5 THE FUTURE OF CROWDSOURCING

16.5.1 Patient Partnership in Clinical Research

The engagement of patients in health research has been intensifying in recent years, and this trend is likely to continue. Key governmental, policy, and health care organizations are recognizing the centrality of patients in researching the treatments that may ultimately affect the course of their care. The Patient-Centered Outcomes Research Institute (PCORI), the FDA, and Institute of Medicine (IOM) have defined a much more proactive role for patients through shared decision making, research partnerships, and big data.

PCORI has formed 18 PPRNs to address key challenges in engaging patients in clinical research and promoting comparative effectiveness research (CER) [88]. Diverse and representative groups of patients and caregivers will be involved a wide variety of research-related activities—governance, data infrastructure design, data sharing and privacy, prioritizing the research agenda, and determining ways to enhance sustainability. The key takeaway is that research planning and implementation cannot occur in PCORI grants without core patient engagement and oversight.

The FDA Patient-Focused Drug Development Initiative is a provision of the Prescription Drug User Fee Act fifth authorization (PDUFA V), which collect industry fees for the drug development process. To maximize patient safety, this process identifies risks and benefits of available treatments. The patient perspective is critical in this determination, which led to inclusion of the Patient-Focused Drug Development in PDUFA V. Many stakeholders view this effort as an important shift toward patient-centered product development in the pharmaceutical industry [58]. This initiative will gather patients' perspectives on 20 different disease areas and produce "Voice of the Patient" reports that will be presented to patients at public meetings. These reports are enlightening and have major implications for clinical trial endpoints, patient treatment decision making, and treatment delivery. For example, a report on lung cancer was published in December 2013 (http://www.fda.gov/downloads/ForIndustry/UserFees/PrescriptionDrugUserFee/UCM379698.pdf). Patient feedback was gathered through a live webcast and polling questions. The "mixed effectiveness" that patients experience in the use of medication prescribed for treatment and side effects often leads them to seek nondrug alternatives (eg, acupuncture, yoga, supplements). The symptoms of lung cancer and the side effects of treatment are difficult to disentangle. Fatigue and breathing difficulties are the most impactful symptoms. The decision to accept or reject treatment is particularly wrenching due to pressure from family, friends, and providers. Although the qualitative data generated derived from discussions with a relatively small group of people, one cannot but wonder how universal these reactions are.

The growth of data sharing technologies and social networking now allow patients to become true partners and ultimately active investigators in PLR and crowdsourcing efforts. The patient-centered shift will open new avenues and possibilities for the future discovery, development, and delivery of new cancer treatments. Crowdsourcing offers a truly democratic means of enhancing partnerships, particularly for patients. As can be seen from the above discussion, discoveries are not exclusive to researchers—patients and other participants in crowdsourced studies can make group and individual discoveries in cancer and other diseases. With the availability of powerful online search tools, widely disseminated scientific literature, and social media, interested and engaged patients (and other interested stakeholders) will increasingly expect to have primary research roles rather than passive or secondary roles. And though there is little rigorous published data on the effectiveness of these efforts, the increasing development of tools that enable patient participation in research suggests that crowdsourcing implementation will become increasingly efficient and cost-effective.

16.5.2 Biomarker Discovery

Biomarker discovery relies on the collection of large specimen collections that have been molecularly profiled. Specimen libraries must also be associated with the disease characteristics of interest such as disease subtype, prognosis, or drug response versus nonresponse. Through careful analysis, the correspondence of one or more molecular markers may be associated with the sample characteristic of interest. In theory, crowdsourcing has the opportunity to augment the search for new biomarkers as a source of new or rare specimens or innovative analytical techniques to biomarker discovery.

Sources of New or Rare Specimens. Whether by active participation through the donation of tissue samples or blood, or via a more passive participation approach, when patients consent to research on the specimen that results from a surgical procedure on their tumor, the *patient crowd* is the main source of biospecimens. As PPRNs such as 23andMe or PLM become larger, the collection of samples from these patient populations becomes more feasible and powerful.

Innovative Analytical Techniques. As described earlier in the chapter, the crowd's ability to bring fresh and innovative approaches to computational problems has been well documented. As biomarker identification projects require the creation of new analytical techniques or serial deployment of multiple techniques, the crowd can help find the solution.

16.5.3 Phenomics

An emerging concept under study in biomedical science is the study of the state and course of complex disease. This concept, coined as *Phenomics*, was touched upon by several pieces of work focused on research to complement the newly arriving genomic era [89]. Though the field remains nascent and still a somewhat undefined area of research, it's clear that some disciplines, such as, for example, neuroscience, benefit from the systematic collection of disease experience since diseases in this space can be so complex. Furthermore, studies on patient crowds can provide some inputs into the patient-reported elements of the phenotype including, for example, immeasurable attributes of disease such as pain, nausea, fatigue and the psychological impacts of disease, such as anxiety and depression [90]. Some concrete examples of patient crowds participating in phenomics studies can be found in the literature, such as studies of yawning in ALS patients [91].

Others have published work explaining the concept of performing phenome-wide association studies, which somewhat invert the philosophy of genome-wide association studies by exploring the breadth of phenotypes associated with a single genetic variant [92]. This concept has been the subject of much attention through the rash of recent work being done on exceptional cancer responders, which seeks to characterize the patients who exhibit uncommonly rare, efficacy of an anticancer therapy [93]. The notion of starting with a rare, but important phenotype (eg, uncommonly good responses to a therapy) and then exploring the molecular underpinnings of that phenomenon has a real promise to uncover new biology and opportunities for new treatments. Patient crowds and large populations of patients serve as a cornerstone to these types of studies since the sought after events are uncommonly rare. It is not impossible to imagine that as patients continue to battle the psychological impact of oncology care, exceptionally strong willed and psychologically robust patients who maintain their psychological health through the trials of a cancer diagnosis and treatment may one day form a cohort for another exceptional responder study based on the phenomics of cancer.

16.5.4 Real-World CER

Although double-blind, placebo-controlled randomized clinical trials (RCTs) are the most robust means available for testing specific hypotheses, they have a number of limitations when it comes to generalizing their findings to "the real world." RCTs typically take place in highly selected samples, free of the comorbidities and complications that are commonplace in the broader population. Most RCTs are also set up to test new treatments against placebo or standard of care, and in a well-developed market there might be dozens of potential treatments (in a multitude of combinations) in widespread clinical use. A more pragmatic approach to generating evidence from the much messier "real world" is CER, which the IOM defines as "the generation and synthesis of evidence that compares the benefits and harms of alternative methods to prevent, diagnose, treat, and monitor a clinical condition or to improve the delivery of care." In their review of available data sources and methods, Meyer and colleagues emphasize the use of traditional medical data sources, such as claims data, EMRs, observational studies, registries, and hybrids that link unrelated data sets to boost power and close data gaps [94]. Basch emphasizes that the unanswerable questions most frequently fielded to him as an oncologist are not about mortality ratios or Kaplan–Meier curves, but rather "How did patients like me feel with this treatment?" a question unanswerable through traditional data sources [95]. Although early

days, it seems likely that these are the sorts of questions that might be effectively crowdsourced using PROs and patient treatment evaluations to present a new form of experiential data to supplement the traditional focus on efficacy and side effects.

16.5.5 Phase IV Surveillance, Adverse Event Detection and Drug Safety

In much the same way that RCTs provide only a narrow window on efficacy and representativeness, the traditional phase I–III architecture can provide false levels of confidence as to the safety profile of drugs that will be used in quite different ways in clinical practice. High profile issues with the antiinflammatory Cox-2 selective inhibitors Vioxx and Celebrex, which were recalled due to an increased risk of myocardial infarction, occurred in part because the phase I–III trials took place amongst a group of patients living with severe arthritis, but their use in the real world was in a much broader group of patients who differed substantially from trial enrollees [96]. Adverse event (AE) reporting is highly dependent on the limited time of health care professionals, who may find it challenging to prioritize completing and submitting complex forms for all but the most serious AEs.

Crowdsourcing AEs from Internet communities and social media discussion forums has been suggested numerous times and the FDA has even held hearings on the best way to process the data and incorporate it into its traditional data sets. However, to date, the issues of data quality and regulators have appeared unwilling to be flexible in considering the ways in which these new forms of data (such as a 140-character Tweet) must be reconciled with a 40-minute paper-based reporting process in generating high-quality actionable data. AEs detected through PROs, so-called PRO-AEs, have been proposed as another potential method of broadening and deepening the surveillance net after a new product has been introduced to the market [97]. Challenges remain, however, in terms of the biases and quality of data gathered, and in particular, a major challenge remains how to mix new sources with traditional sources without damaging the delicate balance of letting potent drugs remain on the market where they are needed and protecting the public.

At its most libertarian extreme, it has even been suggested that instead of the current process of regulatory approval to prove safety and efficacy before marketing authorization, with the right surveillance systems in place drug approval could function as a "free to choose medicine" market with every patient deciding what they want to take and the free flow of information being crowdsourced to determine, in near real time, its true efficacy, safety profile, and therefore, deserved price [98]. While we do not endorse this approach, with the current tools available it provides an interesting thought experiment and provokes the status quo.

16.6 CONCLUSION

As we have seen throughout this chapter, much of the research in crowdsourcing has taken place outside of the field of medicine and the studies devoted to cancer are limited. For crowdsourcing to gain acceptance as a methodology and as a driver of discoveries, those interested in crowdsourcing must strike a careful balance between a legacy that challenges established methodologies and delivering insights in a meaningful, actionable manner. Patients participating in their own research may drive the shift away from a traditional disease cure focus toward a personalized preventive care approach.

The acceptance of crowdsourcing in mainstream medicine will be dependent on several developments. First, the components of crowdsourcing must be better delineated and understood—recruitment processes, careful description of samples, rigor of procedures, and analytical methods. Greater standardization in reporting research methods and procedures will allow for better comparison between studies and generalization across diseases and populations. Second, the expansion of genomic, EMRs, quantified self, and nontraditional data sources will help accelerate the crowdsourcing research process. Future research must establish the value of these data sources across diseases, as well as investigate patients' privacy concerns in sharing such data. However, the notion that participants will someday share their nontraditional data sources, such as grocery loyalty card data or credit card data, to health researchers may not be so far-fetched. Third, strategies to diversify and expand populations of patients participating in crowdsourcing should be identified. Targeting crowdsourcing for the populations most at risk, for example, the elderly, disadvantaged, and minority populations, will be the true measure of its value. Fourth, as described above, new models of ethics review and informed consent that address the complexities of online data sharing will need to be developed. Fifth, crowdsourcing increases the potential for creative patient-researcher partnerships that follow the principles of continuous patient engagement. Expanding expert and patient crowds throughout the research process can assist in defining key research questions, implementing research protocols, and disseminating findings. Finally, much of the discussion about the value of crowdsourcing focuses on applications in medicine, for example, the development of new medications. Because many medical problems are exacerbated by unhealthy behaviors, crowdsourcing research may also provide a means for developing behavioral interventions for health promotion and disease prevention. Taken together, such potential suggests that crowdsourcing has already changed the discovery and development conversation to encourage a more personalized and inclusive approach to health care.

LIST OF ACRONYMS AND ABBREVIATIONS

AE Adverse event
ALS Amyotrophic Lateral Sclerosis
ALSFRS-EX ALS Functional Rating Scale (Extension Items)
ALSFRS-R ALS Functional Rating Scale (Revised)
ASCO American Society of Clinical Oncology
CER Comparative effectiveness research
DARPA Defense Advanced Research Projects Agency
EMR Electronic medical record
FDA Food and Drug Administration
HIPAA Health Insurance Portability and Accountability Act
HITs Human Intelligence Tasks
HL7 Health Level Seven International
IOM Institute of Medicine
IP Intellectual property
LRRK2 Leucine-rich repeat kinase 2
MRI Magnetic resonance imaging
NCI National Cancer Institute
NIH National Institutes of Health
NMC Novel Molecule Challenge
ONC Office of the National Coordinator
ORE Open Research Exchange
PCC Participant-Centered Consent
PCORI Patient-Centered Outcomes Research Institute
PDUFA Prescription Drug User Fee Act
PLC Portable Legal Consent
PLM PatientsLikeMe
PLR Patient-led research
PPRN Patient Powered Research Network
PRO Patient-reported outcome
RCT Randomized clinical trial
SNP Single nucleotide polymorphism

Acknowledgments

We would like to acknowledge the contribution of patients who share and learn from crowdsourced data at PatientsLikeMe and other online research networks. In particular, we are grateful to NapkinNotesDad for sharing his profile in this chapter.

References

[1] American Society of Clinical Oncology The state of cancer care in America, 2014: a report by the American Society of Clinical Oncology. J Oncol Pract 2014;10:119–42.

[2] Levit L, Balogh E, Nass S, Ganz PA, editors. Delivering high-quality cancer care: charting a new course for a system in crisis. Washington, DC: National Academies Press; 2013.

[3] Marchant GE, Campos-Outcalt DE, Lindor RA. Physician liability: the next big thing for personalized medicine? Per Med 2011;8:457–67.

[4] American Cancer Society. Cancer facts and figures 2014; 2014. <http://www.cancer.org/acs/groups/content/@research/documents/webcontent/acspc-042151.pdf>.

[5] Nass SJ, Moses HL, Mendelsohn J. A national cancer clinical trials system for the 21st century: reinvigorating the NCI cooperative group program. Washington, DC: National Academies Press; 2010.

[6] Kurzrock R, Pilat S, Bartolazzi M, Sanders D, Van Wart Hood J, Tucker SD, et al. Project Zero Delay: a process for accelerating the activation of cancer clinical trials. J Clin Oncol 2009;27:4433–40.

[7] Manne S, Kashy D, Albrecht T, Wong YN, Lederman Flamm A, Benson AB, et al. Attitudinal barriers to participation in oncology clinical trials: factor analysis and correlates of barriers. Eur J Cancer Care 2015;24:28–38.

[8] Brueton VC, Tierney JF, Stenning S, Meredith S, Harding S, Nazareth I, et al. Strategies to improve retention in randomised trials: a Cochrane systematic review and meta-analysis. BMJ Open 2014;4:e003821.

[9] Weisfeld N, English RA, Claiborne AB, editors. Envisioning a transformed clinical trials enterprise in the United States: establishing an agenda for 2020: workshop summary. Washington, DC: National Academies Press; 2012.

[10] Sanders J, Powers B, Grossman C, editors. Digital data improvement priorities for continuous learning in health and health care: workshop summary. Washington, DC: National Academies Press; 2013.

[11] Howe J. The rise of crowdsourcing. WIRED 2006;14:1–4.

[12] Estellés-Arolas E, González-Ladrón-de-Guevara F. Towards an integrated crowdsourcing definition. J Inf Sci 2012;38:189–200.

[13] Swan M. Crowdsourced health research studies: an important emerging complement to clinical trials in the public health research ecosystem. J Med Internet Res 2012;14:e46.

[14] Lakhani KR, Jeppesen LB, Lohse PA, Panetta JA. The value of openness in scientific problem solving. Harvard Business School Working Paper Number: 07-050. Cambridge, MA: Harvard University; 2007.

[15] Dawson R, Bynghall S. Getting results from crowds: the definitive guide to using crowdsourcing to grow your business. San Francisco, CA: Advanced Human Technologies Inc.; 2012.

[16] Hasty RT, Garbalosa RC, Barbato VA, Valdes PJ, Powers DW, Hernandez E, et al. Wikipedia vs peer-reviewed medical literature for information about the 10 most costly medical conditions. J Am Osteopath Assoc 2014;114:368–73.

[17] Tang JC, Cebrian M, Giacobe NA, Kim H, Kim T, Wickert D. Reflecting on the DARPA Red Balloon Challenge. Commun ACM 2011;54:78–85.

[18] Brabham DC. Crowdsourcing. Cambridge, MA: MIT Press; 2013.

[19] Burger JD, Doughty E, Khare R, Wei CH, Mishra R, Aberdeen J, et al. Hybrid curation of gene–mutation relations combining automated extraction and crowdsourcing. Database (Oxford) 2014 2014, bau094.

[20] Nguyen TB, Wang S, Anugu V, Rose N, McKenna M, Petrick N, et al. Distributed human intelligence for colonic polyp classification in computer-aided detection for CT colonography. Radiology 2012;262:824–33.

[21] Innocentive. Prize4Life awards $1 million prize for major milestone in ALS research; 2011. <http://www.innocentive.com/prize4life-awards-1-million-prize-major-milestone-als-research>.

[22] Eisenberg I. Lead-user research for breakthrough innovation. Res Technol Manag 2011;54:50–8.

[23] Zhao Y, Zhu Q. Evaluation on crowdsourcing research: current status and future direction. Inf Syst Front 2014;16:417–34.

[24] Perlmutter J, Bell SK, Darien G. Cancer research advocacy: past, present, and future. Cancer Res 2013;73:4611–5.

[25] Woolhandler S, Ariely D, Himmelstein DU. Why pay for performance may be incompatible with quality improvement. Br Med J 2012;345:e5015.

[26] Lohr S. The invention mob, brought to you by Quirky; 2015. <http://www.nytimes.com/2015/02/15/technology/quirky-tests-the-crowd-based-creative-process.html?_r=027>.

[27] Muhdi L, Boutellier R. Motivational factors affecting participation and contribution of members in two different Swiss innovation communities. Int J Innov Manag 2011;15:543–62.

[28] Brownstein CA, Brownstein JS, Williams DS, Wicks P, Heywood JA. The power of social networking in medicine. Nat Biotechnol 2009;27:888–90.

[29] Swan M. The quantified self: fundamental disruption in big data science and biological discovery. Big Data 2013;1:85–99.

[30] California Healthcare Foundation. Health care costs 101: slow growth persists; 2015. <http://www.chcf.org/~/media/MEDIA%20LIBRARY%20Files/PDF/H/PDF%20HealthCareCosts14.pdf>.

[31] Weber GM, Mandl KD, Kohane IS. Finding the missing link for big biomedical data. J Am Med Assoc 2014;311:2479–80.

[32] Hood L, Friend SH. Predictive, personalized, preventive, participatory (P4) cancer medicine. Nat Rev Clin Oncol 2011;8:184–7.

[33] Chiauzzi E, Rodarte C, DasMahapatra P. Patient-centered activity monitoring in the self-management of chronic health conditions. BMC Med 2015;13:77.

[34] Fox S, Duggan M. Tracking for health. Pew Research Center's Internet and American Life Project; 2013. <http://www.pewinternet.org/2013/01/28/tracking-for-health>.

[35] Aitken M, Gauntlett C. Patient apps for improved healthcare from novelty to mainstream. IMS Institute for Healthcare Informatics; 2013. <http://www.imshealth.com/deployedfiles/imshealth/Global/Content/Corporate/IMS%20Health%20Institute/Reports/Patient_Apps/IIHI_Patient_Apps_Report.pdf>.

[36] Food and Drug Administration Mobile medical applications: guidance for industry and Food and Drug Administration staff. Rockville, MD: Food and Drug Administration; 2013.

[37] Prize4Life. Biomarker Prize; 2014. <http://www.prize4life.org/page/prizes/biomarker_prize>.

[38] Khatib F, DiMaio F, Foldit Contenders Group Foldit Void Crushers Group Cooper S, Kazmierczyk M, et al. Crystal structure of a monomeric retroviral protease solved by protein folding game players. Nat Struct Mol Biol 2011;18:1175–7.

[39] Eiben CB, Siegel JB, Bale JB, Cooper S, Khatib F, Shen BW, et al. Increased Diels-Alderase activity through backbone remodeling guided by Foldit players. Nat Biotechnol 2012;30:190–2.

[40] Khare R, Burger JD, Aberdeen JS, Tresner-Kirsch DW, Corrales TJ, Hirchman L, et al. Scaling drug indication curation through crowdsourcing. Database (Oxford) 2015 2015, bav016.

[41] Lakhani KR, Boudreau KJ, Loh PR, Backstrom L, Baldwin C, Lonstein E, et al. Prize-based contests can provide solutions to computational biology problems. Nat Biotechnol 2013;31:108–11.

[42] Wang S, Anugu V, Nguyen T, Rose N, Burns J, McKenna M, et al. Fusion of machine intelligence and human intelligence for colonic polyp detection in CT colonography. In: Symposium on biomedical imaging: from nano to macro, ISBI Chicago, IL; 2011.

[43] Crocker T. Mining the masses with medical crowdsourcing. MD News; 2015. <http://www.mdnews.com/news/2015_04/mining-the-masses-with-medical-crowdsourcing.aspx>.

[44] Eysenbach G. Medicine 2.0: social networking, collaboration, participation, apomediation, and openness. J Med Internet Res 2008;10:e22.

[45] Arnold C. Can the crowd solve medical mysteries? Nova Next; 2014. <http://www.pbs.org/wgbh/nova/next/body/crowdsourcing-medical-diagnoses/>.

[46] DeCamp M. Physicians, social media, and conflict of interest. J Gen Intern Med 2013;28:299–303.

[47] Conn J. Heritage Health competition awards interim prize; 2013. <http://www.modernhealthcare.com/article/20130603/NEWS/306039952>.

[48] Kyle MK, Ridley DB. Would greater transparency and uniformity of health care prices benefit poor patients? Health Aff 2007;26:1384–91.

[49] Public Agenda. How much will it cost? 2015. <http://publicagenda.org/files/HowMuchWillItCost_PublicAgenda_2015.pdf>.

[50] Aliferis L. Variation in prices for common medical tests and procedures. JAMA Intern Med 2015;175:11–12.

[51] Weisse AB. Self-experimentation and its role in medical research. Tex Heart Inst J 2012;39:51–4.

[52] Wicks P, Vaughan T, Heywood J. Subjects no more: what happens when trial participants realize they hold the power? Br Med J 2014;348:g368.

[53] Sweeney L. Simple demographics often identify people uniquely. Carnegie Mellon University, Data Privacy Working Paper 3; 2000. <http://dataprivacylab.org/projects/identifiability/paper1.pdf>.

[54] Mullins CD, Abdulhalim AM, Lavallee DC. Continuous patient engagement in comparative effectiveness research. J Am Med Assoc 2012;307:1587–8.

[55] PCORI. PCORI Engagement Rubric; 2015. <http://www.pcori.org/sites/default/files/PCORI-Engagement-Rubric-with-Table.pdf>.

[56] Swan M, Hathaway K, Hogg C, McCauley R, Vollrath A. Citizen science genomics as a model for crowdsourced preventive medicine research. J Participatory Res 2010;2:e20.

[57] Roberts S. The unreasonable effectiveness of my self-experimentation. Med Hypotheses 2010;75:482–9.

[58] Perfetto EM, Burke L, Oehrlein EM, Epstein RS. Patient-focused drug development: a new direction for collaboration. Med Care 2015;53:9–17.

[59] Wicks P, Vaughan TE, Massagli MP, Heywood J. Accelerated clinical discovery using self-reported patient data collected online and a patient-matching algorithm. Nat Biotechnol 2011;29:411–4.

[60] Tran VT, Harrington M, Montori VM, Barnes C, Wicks P, Ravaud P. Adaptation and validation of the Treatment Burden Questionnaire (TBQ) in English using an internet platform. BMC Med 2014;12:109.

[61] Cedarbaum JM, Stambler N, Malta E, Fuller C, Hilt D, Thurmond B, et al. The ALSFRS-R: a revised ALS functional rating scale that incorporates assessments of respiratory function. J Neurol Sci 1999;169:13–21.

[62] Abdulla S, Vielhaber S, Körner S, Machts J, Heinze HJ, Dengler R, et al. Validation of the German version of the extended ALS functional rating scale as a patient-reported outcome measure. J Neurol 2013;260:2242–55.

[63] Brady CB, Trevor KT, Stein TD, Deykin EY, Perkins SD, Averill JG, et al. The Department of Veterans Affairs Biorepository Brain Bank: a national resource for amyotrophic lateral sclerosis research. Amyotroph Lateral Scler Frontotemporal Degener 2013;14:591–7.

[64] Wicks P. Commentary: measuring what matters: the case for patient generated PROMS. Br Med J 2015;350:h54.

[65] Wolf G. What is the quantified self? 2011. <http://quantifiedself.com/2011/03/what-is-the-quantified-self>.

[66] Smarr L. Quantifying your body: a how-to guide from a systems biology perspective. Biotechnol J 2012;7:980–91.

[67] Bowden M. The measured man; 2012. <http://www.theatlantic.com/magazine/archive/2012/07/the-measured-man/309018>.

[68] Cohen J. The patient of the future; 2012. <http://www.technologyreview.com/featuredstory/426968/the-patient-of-the-future>.

[69] Lillie EO, Patay B, Diamant J, Issell B, Topol EJ, Schork NJ. The n-of-1 clinical trial: the ultimate strategy for individualizing medicine? Per Med 2011;8:161–73.

[70] Janssens AC, Kraft P. Research conducted using data obtained through online communities: ethical implications of methodological limitations. PLoS Med 2010;9, e1001328.

[71] Paolacci G, Chandler J, Ipeirotis PG. Running experiments on Amazon Mechanical Turk. Judgment Decis Making 2010;5:411–9.

[72] Turner AM, Kirchhoff K, Capurro D. Using crowdsourcing technology for testing multilingual public health promotion materials. J Med Internet Res 2012;14:e79.

[73] Ranard BL, Ha YP, Meisel ZF, Asch DA, Hill SS, Becker LB, et al. Crowdsourcing—harnessing the masses to advance health and medicine, a systematic review. J Gen Intern Med 2014;29:187–203.

[74] Angrist M. The audacity of interpretation: protecting patients or piling on? Appl Transl Genomics 2014;3:68–9.

[75] Akst J. The Elixir tragedy, 1937. The Scientist Magazine; 2013. <http://www.the-scientist.com/?articles.view/articleNo/35714/title/The-Elixir-Tragedy—1937>.

[76] Ballentine C. Taste of raspberries, taste of death: the 1937 elixir sulfanilamide incident. FDA Consumer 15; 1981. <http://www.fda.gov/aboutfda/whatwedo/history/productregulation/sulfanilamidedisaster/default.htm>.

[77] Graber MA, Graber A. Internet-based crowdsourcing and research ethics: the case for IRB review. J Med Ethics 2012;39:115–8.

[78] Curtis BL. Social networking and online recruiting for HIV research: ethical challenges. J Empir Res Hum Res Ethics 2014;9:58–70.

[79] O'Connor D. The apomediated world: regulating research when social media has changed research. J Law Med Ethics 2013;41:470–83.

[80] Kramer AD, Guillory JE, Hancock JT. Experimental evidence of massive-scale emotional contagion through social networks. Proc Natl Acad Sci 2014;111:8788–90.

[81] Mello MM, Francer JK, Wilenzick M, Teden P, Bierer BE, Barnes M. Preparing for responsible sharing of clinical trial data. N Engl J Med 2013;369:1651–8.

[82] Vayena E, Tasioulas J. Adapting standards: ethical oversight of participant-led health research. PLoS Med 2013;10, e1001402.

[83] Smith A. What Internet users know about technology and the Web; 2014. <http://www.pewinternet.org/2014/11/25/web-iq>.

[84] Health Data Exploration Project. Personal data for the public good; 2014. <http://www.rwjf.org/ content/dam/farm/reports/reports/2014/rwjf411080>.

[85] Sweeney L, Abu A, Winn J. Identifying participants in the personal genome project by name. Cambridge, MA: Harvard University Data Privacy Lab; 2013. White Paper 1021-1. Available from: <http://privacytools.seas.harvard.edu/files/privacytools/files/1021-1.pdf?m=1372350219>.

[86] Lin J, Amini S, Hong JI, Sadeh N, Lindqvist J, Zhang J. Expectation and purpose: understanding users' mental models of mobile app privacy through crowdsourcing. In: Proceedings of the 2012 ACM conference on ubiquitous computing; 2012, p. 501–10.

[87] Landa AS, Elliott C. From community to commodity: the ethics of pharma-funded social networking sites for physicians. J Law Med Ethics 2013;41:673–9.

[88] PCORnet PPRN Consortium Daugherty SE, Wahba S, Fleurence R. Patient-powered research networks: building capacity for conducting patient-centered clinical outcomes research. J Am Med Inform Assoc 2014;21:583–6.

[89] Bilder RM, Sabb FW, Cannon TD, London ED, Jentsch JD, Parker DS, et al. Phenomics: the systematic study of phenotypes on a genome-wide scale. Neuroscience 2009;164:30–42.

[90] Jacobsen PB, Andrykowski MA. Tertiary prevention in cancer care: understanding and addressing the psychological dimensions of cancer during the active treatment period. Am Psychol 2015;70:134–45.

[91] Wicks P. Excessive yawning is common in the bulbar-onset form of ALS. Acta Psychiatr Scand 2007;116:76.

[92] Monte AA, Brocker C, Nebert DW, Gonzalez FJ, Thompson DC, Vasiliou V. Improved drug therapy: triangulating phenomics with genomics and metabolomics. Hum Genomics 2014;8:16.

[93] Kaiser J. Rare cancer successes spawn 'exceptional' research efforts. Science 2013;340, p. 263.

[94] Meyer AM, Carpenter WR, Abernethy AP, Stürmer T, Kosorok MR. Data for cancer comparative effectiveness research. Cancer 2012;118:5186–97.

[95] Basch E. Toward patient-centered drug development in oncology. N Engl J Med 2013;369:397–400.

[96] Timbie JW, Fox DS, Van Busum K, Schneider EC. Five reasons that many comparative effectiveness studies fail to change patient care and clinical practice. Health Aff 2012;31:2168–75.

[97] Banerjee AK, Okun S, Edwards IR, Wicks P, Smith MY, Mayall SJ, et al. Patient-reported outcome measures in safety event reporting: PROSPER consortium guidance. Drug Saf 2013; 36:1129–49.

[98] Conko G, Madden BJ. Administrative law and regulation; 2014. <http://www.fed-soc.org/library/doclib/20140130_FTCM. pdf>.

CHAPTER

17

Patient-Centered Approaches to Improving Clinical Trials for Cancer

Roni Zeiger MD, MS[1,2] and Gilles Frydman BSc[1,3]

[1]Smart Patients, Mountain View, CA, United States [2]Santa Clara Valley Medical Center, Santa Clara, CA, United States [3]Association of Cancer Online Resources, Mountain View, CA, United States

OUTLINE

17.1 While Trials Are Important, Trial Participation Rates Are Dismal 331

17.2 Barriers to Trial Participation 332
17.2.1 Randomization and in Particular Fear of Receiving a Placebo 332
17.2.2 Fear of Side Effects 332
17.2.3 Distrust of the Research Process 332
17.2.4 Perceived Complexity of the Protocol 333
17.2.5 Lack of Awareness of Trials 333
17.2.6 Fear of Jeopardizing the Relationship With Their Physician 333
17.2.7 Inconvenience and Expense of Frequent Travel to Trial Site 333

17.3 Patients Searching for Trials Online 333

17.4 Current Use of the Internet and Online Cancer Communities 334

17.5 How the Internet Shaped Online Cancer Communities, and Vice Versa 334

17.6 What Do Patients Talk About in Online Cancer Communities? 336

17.7 Impact of Online Patient Communities 336

17.8 Participatory Research 337

17.9 Borrowing From Silicon Valley and User-Centered Design 337

17.10 Participatory Clinical Trial Design 338

17.11 What If Trial Participants Discuss the Trial in Online Communities? 339

17.12 Challenges and Next Steps 339

List of Acronyms and Abbreviations 339

References 340

17.1 WHILE TRIALS ARE IMPORTANT, TRIAL PARTICIPATION RATES ARE DISMAL

Since the first double-blind controlled trials of the 1940s, clinical trials have become the cornerstone upon which we base our clinical knowledge [1]. Trials are now more important than ever as we are in the midst of a paradigm shift in how cancers are defined and treated, with a rapidly growing number of questions that need to be answered with rigorous science. Yet trial participation rates among US adults remain at 2–3% and less than one-third of trials meet their recruitment goals [2–5].

While many have bemoaned this apparent disconnect, there is no evidence that these rates are improving. Clearly, as a clinical and scientific community, we are

B. Hesse, D. Ahern & E. Beckjord: Oncology Informatics.
DOI: http://dx.doi.org/10.1016/B978-0-12-802115-6.00017-3

doing an inadequate job of recruiting subjects into trials. Part of the problem may be the very language itself: the idea of being recruited as a subject does not seem to be attractive to many patients or their families.

An instructive exception exists in the domain of pediatric oncology. Trial participation rates for children with cancer are over 50%, approximately 20 times that of adult cancer patients! [6] This may be due in part to the fact that research has improved cure rates for pediatric cancers as a whole from 10% to well over 70% since the 1950s [7] and thus the importance of research was instilled in the broader community from early on. A related fact is that most pediatric oncology centers are part of the Children's Oncology Group, or COG, which is the evolution of cooperatives that started in the 1950s [8].

How might we help bring the same culture to all of oncology, including adults? Before attempting to answer this question, let us better understand the current barriers to trial participation.

17.2 BARRIERS TO TRIAL PARTICIPATION

As mentioned above, overall clinical trial participation rates among adults in the United States are approximately 2–3%. The figures for participation in adult cancer trials are only slightly better, if at all, even though we might expect more people to consider experimental therapies when faced with a poor cancer prognosis.

The outlook is worse for minorities. For example, while Blacks have the highest cancer rates in the United States, Blacks and Hispanics have a participation rate of only 1.3% in clinical trials for cancer. Fortunately, the exception of the pediatric oncology world appears to apply to minority children, as 60% of minority cancer patients younger than age 15 are enrolled in trials [9].

Unfortunately, participation is very low for young adults, for reasons that are not clear. Among adolescents aged 15–19, only 10% take part in cancer clinical trials [10]. Also underrepresented are women, rural residents, the elderly, and lower income patients [11,12].

Trial recruitment is already a critical bottleneck for the development of needed therapies for patients and families suffering from cancer. This new era of personalized medicine will require a much larger number of smaller cohorts with more stringent requirements, further complicating trial recruitment [13].

Several important barriers to trial participation from the patient perspective are frequently discussed, including:

- randomization and in particular fear of receiving a placebo

- fear of side effects
- distrust of the research process
- perceived complexity of the protocol
- lack of awareness of trials
- fear of jeopardizing the relationship with their physician
- inconvenience and expense of frequent travel to the trial site

Let's consider each in turn.

17.2.1 Randomization and in Particular Fear of Receiving a Placebo

Although patients often are not very open about their concerns, fear of having one's treatment chosen randomly by a computer is high on the list [14]. When considering several potential barriers to clinical trials, randomization and fear of receiving a placebo were ranked highly by patients as well as oncologists [15]. The placebo issue is especially worthy of discussion because it is one of communication, or rather, miscommunication. It is a requirement that patients who join cancer trials are either given the best treatment available for their specific cancer (standard of care) or receive a new treatment being investigated [16]. Indeed, in 99% of cancer trials, if a placebo is used, it is given in conjunction with a standard therapy [17].

17.2.2 Fear of Side Effects

In one study, patients identified fear of side effects as the greatest barrier to participation in clinical trials [15]. For many people, their only knowledge of cancer is the visible and uncomfortable side effects of chemotherapy—hair loss, nausea and vomiting, wasting, and the like—so this fear should not be surprising.

17.2.3 Distrust of the Research Process

While most relevant to the Black community, any discussion about distrust of the research process should include the lasting after-effects of the Tuskegee syphilis experiments, arguably "the most infamous biomedical research study in US history" [18]. Note that these experiments ended only in 1972, when many of the patients diagnosed with cancer today were already adults. Such distrust is reinforced by a health system which is perceived to continue to discriminate against those of lower socioeconomic status [19]. Lack of knowledge and misconceptions about use of placebos also go hand-in-hand with distrust.

17.2.4 Perceived Complexity of the Protocol

Lengthy trials and extensive testing during trials have been cited as factors that most correlate with lack of patient participation [14]. Our experience with cancer patients, discussed further below, also suggests that unclear descriptions of trials in public sources such as clinicaltrials.gov also contribute to perceptions of complexity. In many cases, lack of clarity may be worse than complexity itself.

17.2.5 Lack of Awareness of Trials

Some data suggest that only one-third of US adults are aware of clinical trials in general [20]. This, in turn, is at least in part because only 6% of patients report that their physicians have ever suggested they consider participating in a clinical trial [21]. This should not surprise us given the increasing pressure on physicians for efficiency and the ever-increasing challenge of keeping up with new scientific developments, including relevant clinical trials. Financial disincentives also exist for physicians whose practices or institutions do not participate in trials, as they risk losing patients by referring their patients to trial sites.

17.2.6 Fear of Jeopardizing the Relationship With Their Physician

Since most physicians do not suggest clinical trials as options, patients may feel that asking about trials is somehow akin to asking if they might get their care from someone different than the physician.

17.2.7 Inconvenience and Expense of Frequent Travel to Trial Site

Patients in our online communities often discuss clinical trials and many wish to participate in them. Frequently, however, they share that they struggle with the degree to which joining a trial would disrupt their lives. Even if they are physically able to travel to a trial site and can afford to do so financially, they carefully weigh the burden with the perceived benefit the trial may provide them. This burden may affect trial enrollment as well as trial retention, as patients may drop out of studies if they decide after joining that the commitment is too much.

Finally, we will add an item to the list of barriers that is rarely discussed. In our experience building and managing online communities for cancer patients and caregivers, a more subtle challenge often interferes with effective communication about clinical trials and exacerbates many of the above factors: while researchers generally frame trials as experiments, cancer patients considering trials tend to think about them as treatment options. While clinical trials are of course both experiments and treatment options, the perceived distinction is one that must be addressed. Part of the challenge lies in the legal limitations that trial sponsors have in promoting their (unapproved) therapies as treatment options. While such restrictions are appropriate, many patients want to learn more about trials and have trouble finding sources to answer their questions.

Learning more about clinical trials in general and about specific trials of interest is one of many reasons patients have turned more to the Internet and to each other over the last two decades.

17.3 PATIENTS SEARCHING FOR TRIALS ONLINE

The traditional model of informing patients about potentially appropriate clinical trial opportunities via their physicians is not working adequately, as we have seen. More recently, the Internet has made it easier for patients to find and research such opportunities on their own.

From our experience with managing online cancer communities—particularly for rarer cancers—patients frequently teach each other about the value of clinical trials in general and about the relevance of specific trials of interest to one or more of the community members. Note that this does not require a majority of a community's members to be scientifically literate. It takes only a few "micro-experts" in a given area to lead and direct discussions that are accessible to the broader group, who frequently ask clarifying questions. This results in a constant process of peer-driven improvements in health and science literacy.

Patients are increasingly using the Internet to find trials they wish to join. While many sites provide the ability to search for trials, their functionality and content vary greatly and searchers need specific skills to use them successfully [22]. Searching a database for clinical trials is obviously more complex than many other types of online searches. This is further complicated by the fact that trial details at the most commonly used trial search engine, clinicaltrials.gov, are not written in lay language and details such as inclusion and exclusion criteria are inconsistently described from one trial to another.

While this public resource is intended both for health professionals and for patients, the primary source of the content is trial sponsors themselves [23]. Inspection of trial descriptions readily demonstrates that even multiple trials from a single sponsor can vary greatly in the way in which trials are described. A readability analysis showed that most trial descriptions are written at an 11th grade level, significantly higher than most would recommend [22]. Beyond reading level, limitations of clinicaltrials.gov and other available databases include the need for significant knowledge about one's diagnosis and treatment history, difficulty in assessing how inclusive the underlying database is, and ease of use. Equally challenging is that patients in particular expect trial search tools to function like Google and other web search engines, where simple unstructured queries lead to results where the best results are listed first. Trial search engines often require structured queries that filter the underlying database and do not intend to imply that a trial listed above another is necessarily better. Indeed, users of these tools must have "perseverance to sift through search results" [22]. On the other hand, a searcher who adds too many parameters might find zero results, with no "Did you mean…" or other hints about how to proceed.

Attempts have been made to build a better trial matching service by analyzing the eligibility criteria listed in clinicaltrials.gov, in order to build systems that could either be more intuitive for patients or could automatically match patient records in electronic health record systems to relevant trials. Unfortunately, one study demonstrated that approximately 90% of trial listings contained significant barriers to automatic eligibility interpretation [24].

Other problems with trial listing data may be even more problematic for patients. Nearly 25% of trials listed as recruiting also showed a study completion date in the past. Perhaps worst of all, over 30% of the trial coordinators were not reachable at their listed phone number or email [24].

We seem to be at a challenging moment in history, where many patients are ready to explore research opportunities on their own but the research establishment has not yet provided the tools to do so easily. As we might expect, when patients aren't finding useful answers from the traditional experts, they go online and turn to each other.

17.4 CURRENT USE OF THE INTERNET AND ONLINE CANCER COMMUNITIES

While professionals have struggled to recruit patients to trials, patients have been organizing themselves into online communities. Before turning to how we can build upon this phenomenon to improve cancer trials, let's look more deeply at how patients use the Internet to find health information and, increasingly, to find each other.

Eighteen percent of Internet users have gone online to find others affected by issues similar to theirs [25]. Those with chronic and rare conditions are even more likely to look for peers online [25]. More than a quarter of Internet users have read or watched someone else's experience about health issues in the last 12 months [26].

While clinicians are still the top source of health information, when US adults were asked who they turned to the last time they had a serious health issue, the results were as follows: [26]

- 70% got information, care, or support from a doctor or other health care professional.
- 60% got information or support from friends and family.
- 24% got information or support from others who have the same health condition.

Today, online communities serving cancer patients include ACOR (the Association of Cancer Online Resources) [27], Cancer Survivors Network [28], Facebook groups, Inspire.com [29,30], PatientsLikeMe [31], Smart Patients [32], and many regular disease-specific Twitter chats or tweetchats [33].

17.5 HOW THE INTERNET SHAPED ONLINE CANCER COMMUNITIES, AND VICE VERSA

Nearly a half century ago in 1969, ARPANET, the forerunner of the Internet, used packet switching instead of circuitry to link host computer nodes in four locations and thus created the first long-distance computer network. It is likely that this pre-Internet was used to discuss personal health information not long after electronic mail was introduced in 1972 [34].

However, before the Internet reached home users, the first real online tool for collaboration—and for the exchange of health information—was the bulletin board system or BBS. A bulletin board linked local users to a central computer, originally via cumbersome manual modems. While the system was designed for users to read and post messages, this led to the creation of forums in which users could communicate about specific topics of mutual interest. BBSs grew in popularity and also became easier to use. In 1994 over 60,000 BBSs operated in the United States alone, 16 years after the first BBSs opened in Chicago [35]. One of them evolved into The WELL, often regarded as the birthplace of the modern online community [36]. Other proprietary systems grew in the 1980s and 1990s, including Compuserve and AOL. Together these services helped create thousands of online communities of interest, including many dealing with medical issues.

In 1986 an engineering student in Paris developed software for the automated LISTSERV email discussion lists. This allowed individual users to email a group of people all at the same time to discuss their common interest. Email could be sent to the group address or to other individual users in private conversations. The software provided tools for the list owner (administrator) to manage the group without the burdensome effort of manually maintaining and running an email list [37].

In 1994 the faster, more user-friendly, and globally-connected Internet prevailed in most areas of the world. By that time there were already 3 million host sites on the Internet compared with about 60,000 local BBSs in the United States [38]. Many Internet service providers incorporated aspects of BBSs by creating their own service-specific message boards and live chats. Some had predetermined topics while others had topics set by the participants. It was natural that some of these forums, user groups, email discussion lists, chat rooms, and email exchanges would center on cancer, especially driven by patients and family members unsatisfied by information they could find elsewhere. Many such groups have disappeared while others continue to prosper.

In 1994, most of the Internet provided a passive experience of receiving information from static websites that might occasionally be updated. Email, bulletin boards, message boards, chat rooms, and USENET groups offered users a living exchange of messages and information, creating their own content and interacting with one another.

In 1995, experienced Internet user Gilles Frydman found himself frustrated at being unable to find information about breast cancer, which would help his recently diagnosed wife. The lack of information led him to create ACOR. This nonprofit coalition united many volunteer-managed email groups, growing quickly to span a wide spectrum of cancers. ACOR used L-Soft's LISTSERV(R) list management software with list hosting generously donated by L-Soft [39]. At that time, universities were the main adopters of L-Soft's services. Thus, many of the groups that joined ACOR were accustomed to thoughtful, evidence-based, high level discussions of cancer research and treatment options. This set the tone for the high-quality communities for which ACOR is known.

At its peak, ACOR included approximately 150 mailing lists and delivery of more than 1,500,000 email messages per week [40]. In ACOR's interactive cancer communities, patients and caregivers exchanged email messages of information and emotional support on the individual topic of the email list. Members interested in a specific topic joined a separate list for that topic, which might be a type or subtype of cancer, a particular approach to care, or psychosocial aspects.

At first email lists were an innovative and effective means of communicating. People became skilled at searching the ACOR archives that contained every post of a list. Many longtime users were satisfied with the system and were unaware of the richer functionality available elsewhere on the web. Others remained with

ACOR despite these limitations because of the information and emotional support they received from their community. But as years passed, many ACOR users and list owners began to see email lists as overly demanding, limited in features, and antiquated. They began to turn to web-based communities such as Facebook, Inspire, and PatientsLikeMe.

Even as email participation was decreasing, the level of information shared by ACOR list members continued to advance. Experienced patients and caregivers quickly brought new members up to speed with information needed to cope with their diagnosis or the situation confronting a loved one. People were coached at their own information level, with many members serving as "translators" between the more sophisticated users and the less scientifically literate. ACOR members have served as board members and active participants in national and international patient organizations, as speakers at hearings before Congress and the Food and Drug Administration (FDA), and as patient representatives on professional committees.

Challenges with ACOR, however, included increasing email spam and phishing and unsustainable demands on the list owners, who were typically nontechnical volunteers. As membership of ACOR plateaued, Gilles Frydman and other list owners also recognized a new challenge. Traditional communities, including ACOR's email lists, were essentially silos with respect to one another. That is, members who wanted information about a different cancer had to join another email list. Patients with different cancers often face similar issues such as chemotherapy side effects, frequent computed tomography (CT) scans to check for recurrence, and emotional issues affecting the patient and family members.

The emergence of targeted therapies for cancer magnified this issue. An increasing number of people were being treated based on mutation status instead of the traditional organ-based definition of their cancers. Of course, the email lists were defined in the traditional manner, for example, lung cancer versus kidney cancer. As targeted therapies were typically initially developed in one cancer group, the knowledge accumulated by that patient community was not organically shared with the next community that was going through clinical trials for their cancer.

With a deepening understanding that information was not being shared with all of those who wanted or need it, ACOR's founder Gilles Frydman made contact with members of Google's health team. While the collaboration he intended did not materialize, he connected with Google's Roni Zeiger who subsequently left the company to join Frydman in creating a new web-based system for online patient communities, Smart Patients, in 2012. Many of the communities from ACOR have migrated to Smart Patients.

17.6 WHAT DO PATIENTS TALK ABOUT IN ONLINE CANCER COMMUNITIES?

Any given community can take on its own personality, which in our experience depends in large part on its initial membership, how it is managed, and characteristics of the disease or of its treatments.

An analysis of the 15 largest Facebook communities focused on type 2 diabetes was done in 2011 [41]. Researchers coded the most recent posts in each of these communities, with the results shown in Table 17.1.

Different results were found in an analysis of themes discussed across 10 cancer communities on ACOR in 2007, as shown in Table 17.2. (GF was one of the authors of this analysis.)

Our experience with cancer communities at Smart Patients is similar to that in the above ACOR communities, as we might expect given that several of those communities moved from ACOR to Smart Patients.

We should add, however, that we see increasing discussion about the emerging science underlying targeted therapies and about specific clinical trials, especially those for targeted therapies. As alluded to above, patients are asking each other for information about trials of interest, whether they learn about them by searching online, from their clinicians, or elsewhere. Regarding clinical trials, one of the most common issues discussed is which trial sites are recruiting and what is the correct contact information for a given trial site. This should not be a surprise given the data discussed above about how often this data is inaccurate or out-of-date on clinicaltrials.gov and other trial search tools.

TABLE 17.1 Coded Categories of Facebook Posts From Popular Type 2 Diabetes Communities, in Descending Order of Frequency

Categories of Facebook posts in type 2 diabetes communities
Providing information
Support
Advertisements
Requesting information
Irrelevant

Adapted from Greene J. Online social networking by patients with diabetes: a qualitative evaluation of communication with Facebook. J Gen Intern Med 2011; 26(3):287–92.

TABLE 17.2 Coded Categories of ACOR Posts From 10 Cancer Communities, in Descending Order of Frequency

Categories of ACOR posts in cancer communities
Specific treatments
Communicating with health care providers to obtain good care
Problem management strategies
Coping with cancer recurrence

Adapted from Meier A, Lyons E, Frydman G, Forlenza M, Rimer B. How cancer survivors provide support on cancer-related internet mailing lists. J Med Internet Res 2007;9(2):e12.

17.7 IMPACT OF ONLINE PATIENT COMMUNITIES

Online communities are popular among patients and family caregivers. In addition, studies have shown that online communities can provide effective support, reduce feelings of depression and isolation, and help patients effectively manage their cancer care.

The best data on the clinical impact of online patient communities comes not from the cancer world but in type 2 diabetes, where multiple randomized studies have suggested that hemoglobin A1c can be lowered by exposure to online peer support [42–44]. Regarding emotional issues, a study of family caregivers of dementia patients found that after using an online forum for 12 weeks, they rated a significant improvement in the quality of their relationship with the person with dementia [45].

While more data is needed on the quality of online patient communities, there is evidence that high-quality communities exist. In a study on the accuracy and self-correction of an online breast cancer community, researchers found that 10 of 4600 posts (0.22%) were false or misleading; and 7 of these 10 were identified as false or misleading by other community members and corrected within an average of 4 hours 33 minutes [46].

Experts in building and managing online communities recommend the following to build a sustainable and high-quality community [47–49]:

- Model appropriate behavior
- Keep discussions on-topic
- Enforce group norms
- Give members a sense of purpose
- Understand the life cycle of communities
- Allow disagreement and self-correction
- Employ complementary interaction models, eg, in-person support groups

In a public discussion about how to ensure that misinformation is not spread in an online patient community, one community member advised: "Don't build in too many controls, or you will crush the adaptations that squash falsehoods" [50]. Of course, not too many controls does not mean zero controls. In our experience managing online communities, including cancer communities, behind-the-scenes management is critical. Perhaps most importantly, this begins with building an evidence-gathering and evidence-respecting culture so that when questionable information appears, members of the community know which knowledge tools they can use to respectfully challenge the information.

If patients are increasingly using online patient communities for peer support and information gathering, can we be smarter about how we tap into the community to involve them in clinical trials?

17.8 PARTICIPATORY RESEARCH

The idea of more explicitly involving the community in research is not new. In their 2011 book, *Community-Based Participatory Research for Health: From Process to Outcomes*, Minkler and Wallerstein introduce community-based participatory research (CBPR) as follows: "In contrast to more traditional investigator-driven research, CBPR begins with an issue selected by, or of real importance to, the community, and involves community members and other stakeholders throughout the research process, including its culmination in education and action for social change...CBPR is not a method but an orientation to research" [51].

There is a parallel here with the better-known concept of translational research, which aims to translate or apply scientifically meaningful information and make it clinically relevant, that is, relevant to human health. An implicit assumption in much translational research is that clinicians can judge whether the results of a study are relevant to human health, on behalf of both clinicians and patients.

The core assumption of participatory research is that in order to ensure the research matters to the patients and families it is intended to impact, those patients and families must be involved in the research from its outset. While there are many possible ways to involve the "end-user" in the process, the key question, as pointed out by O'Toole et al. [52], is: "How do we distinguish between community-placed and community-based research?" Is a focus group or a patient advisory board sufficient?

Many would argue they are not, and that much of what has been termed participatory research in the past has been traditional research, superficially blessed by a small group of patients. This disconnect between much current research and the possibility of a more collaborative and involved patient population is the motivation behind the recently established Patient-Centered Outcomes Research Institute (PCORI).

PCORI's mission includes "producing and promoting high-integrity, evidence-based information that comes from research guided by patients, caregivers, and the broader health care community." To that end, they state they "incorporate patients and other stakeholders throughout the process more consistently and intensively than others have before" [53].

PCORI has raised awareness in the research community and is providing funds to increase the quantity and quality of participatory clinical research. Smart Patients is involved in a PCORI-funded project, along with Kaiser Permanente, Group Health Cooperative, HealthPartners, and Denver Health, to involve patients in multiple disease areas more closely in research [54]. The approach we are taking is to first build peer-to-peer communities for these patients and families, where one of the explicit goals of the community is to be available for discussions with researchers about research priorities and evolving research plans.

Because our team's core competency is building consumer software, our approach to involving patients in the clinical trial process is informed by the principles of user-centered design. While these principles are not traditionally used in the context of clinical trials, their relevance cannot be overstated.

17.9 BORROWING FROM SILICON VALLEY AND USER-CENTERED DESIGN

Because of his previous role at Google, one of the authors of this chapter (Roni Zeiger) is frequently asked to assess startup ideas. He often gives the following advice: figure out the simplest way to put a prototype of this idea in front of the user you think will benefit from it, find out what they think, then iterate on your prototype with feedback from your users at every step.

One of the early texts that popularized the concept of user-centered design was Don Norman's book, *The Design of Everyday Things* [55]. Here, Norman suggests design of any product or experience should focus on users' needs and simplifying wherever possible. He also explains that failure to design for the user in this way leads to users who make errors, abandon your product, or both. These concepts have been brought to the mainstream by consultancies like IDEO and to web design in particular by Jakob Nielsen and others. The ubiquity of this way of thinking made it straightforward to our team at Smart Patients, when presented with the opportunity to help improve the design of clinical trials, to do so with a user-centered design mindset.

Some have described applying user-centered design to topics like trial design as "crowdsourcing." We make a distinction between crowdsourcing and user-centered design. We think of crowdsourcing as obtaining feedback or services from an arbitrary and usually large group of people. When a member of one of our communities posts a question, it is typically a nonrandom subset of the community who responds: those who have personal experience on the topic or have researched it. For a different question, a different subset will likely respond. In this context, we describe well-functioning online communities as "networks of micro-experts."

Similarly, asking patients to help researchers with trial design is asking them to allow researchers to tap into their experience and expertise as patients. This can be done in a methodical way that allows experts in trial design to tap into the wisdom of their most important stakeholders.

17.10 PARTICIPATORY CLINICAL TRIAL DESIGN

For context, we should share that our involvement in the clinical trial space is somewhat accidental. As we started building our online cancer patient communities at Smart Patients, we elicited feedback from the cancer patients and caregivers initially testing the system. While we expected feedback about the community software itself, we kept hearing that community members wanted a way to search for cancer trials that was more user-friendly than existing tools. We went on to build a trial search engine and incorporated it into the community platform so that patients could find trials of potential interest and start conversations about them.

As a result, we started seeing many conversations about clinical trials, including critiques of existing trials and how patients wished they were different. We subsequently started partnering with researchers in industry and academia to provide them with patient feedback on the design of their trials.

If we consider the clinical trial as the "product" to be designed and the patient as the "user" of that product, let's look at the product development process (Fig. 17.1).

Patients are typically brought into this process at the time patient recruitment begins. From the product design perspective above, we can argue that at this point it's essentially too late. While the product can still be changed based on patient feedback, these changes are expensive—requiring protocol amendments, for example—and are thus unlikely to happen except when required from a regulatory perspective or for near-term business needs. Ironically, the latter often includes the fact that the trial is recruiting too slowly and thus inclusion or exclusion criteria need to be changed because recruitment targets aren't being met.

What we and others have been doing more in the last few years is to invite patients into the trial design process while the protocol is still in draft form. This can be done confidentially, with transparency about the fact that suggestions from patients may or may not be able to be incorporated into the design. The kinds of questions that can be addressed with patients include:

- If you were eligible, would you want to participate in this trial? Why or why not?

- What endpoints would matter most to you?
- What is the most inconvenient aspect of this protocol for you? The scariest?
- What do you wish were different about this trial?
- Is there another question you wish researchers would be asking instead?
- Is there something in the inclusion or exclusion criteria that you think will make accrual difficult in the real world?

An important aspect of user-centered design in general, and its application to clinical trial design in particular, is that feedback from users can be extraordinarily useful even when it comes in the form of a suggestion or request that is impractical or impossible to fulfill. This is because the motivation behind the feedback reveals aspects of the user's perceived needs, concerns, and/or emotional reaction to the product. We can then refine the product's design, within our constraints, to try to address those needs or concerns.

For example, a patient who expresses concern about the overall toll a trial would take on her might inspire a trial design team to reduce the number of not-strictly-required blood draws and to experiment with conducting some of the less critical visits via telemedicine.

An area especially ripe for increased involvement from patients is the area of patient-reported outcomes or PROs. In contrast to traditional outcomes like progression-free survival or tumor diameter, which are measured by clinicians or objective testing, PROs are reported directly by patients such as a patient's assessment of symptoms or satisfaction with treatment. While many assume that simply considering PROs is "patient-centered," the reality is that most PROs are defined by experts without significant input from patients. There can be a vicious cycle here as well because researchers are reluctant to use PROs that have not been previously validated, making it harder to introduce new ones. The FDA is working to encourage more consistent measurement of PROs in the drug development process [56].

A/B testing is a method we have found particularly useful in eliciting from patients their perspective on a variety of issues. A/B testing was popularized in the field of web design [57]. In that context, a set of users is typically shown one of two version of a web site design (version A or version B). The version that results

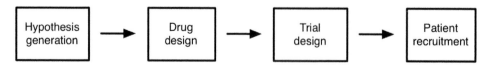

FIGURE 17.1　A generalized workflow for drug development. Based on a scientific hypothesis, a drug is manufactured. One or more trials are designed to test the drug. Generally, patients are directly involved only when a trial starts recruiting subjects.

in a higher percentage of users completing the desired action, such as clicking on the "Join Now" button, is the better version.

In our work obtaining feedback from patients about how to design clinical trials in a more patient-friendly manner, we regularly use A/B testing. For example, we post a summary of a proposed trial, and explain that two potential versions of the trial are identical except for the following (Fig. 17.2).

Trial option A	Trial option B
1 hour driving distance	4 hour driving distance
Visits to site once per week	Visits to site once per month
Optional palliative care offered	Visits to local MD once per week

FIGURE 17.2 A/B testing can be used to elicit patient perspectives on clinical trial design.

We then ask community members (1) to select which they would prefer and (2) to explain why in a conversation with other community members. We refer to this as patient-driven feasibility analysis and have found that it can easily be incorporated the trial design process, if started early enough.

While we know of no data to support this, we hypothesize that involving patients in the trial design process may serve to increase recruitment. Not only might patients who directly participate in the design of a given trial feel a sense of co-ownership of the trial, but also those who learn that patients were involved may view a given trial more favorably.

17.11 WHAT IF TRIAL PARTICIPANTS DISCUSS THE TRIAL IN ONLINE COMMUNITIES?

It should not surprise us that patients in trials may wish to discuss their participation with fellow online community members. A 2014 article in the *Wall Street Journal* summarized understandable concerns from researchers that such public discussion by patients while they are in trials may threaten the integrity of the trial by unblinding patients [58]. However, researchers are also beginning to acknowledge that the proverbial genie is out of the bottle. Craig Lipset, an executive at Pfizer, encourages the research community to study this phenomenon, both for its risks and potential new learning opportunities [59].

Indeed, little data exists about the potential positive and negative impacts of such discussion [60]. Anecdotally, we know that patients teach other about trials they may not have otherwise learned about, and many enroll in trials as a result of such learning. This may be even more widespread in communities for rare cancers because their clinical trials are few or nonexistent, and the trials that do exist are harder to find. It is also reasonable to hypothesize that peer support during a trial might increase trial retention, that is, prevent some participants from dropping out of a trial. Clearly, additional work is needed to determine how such potential benefits might be achieved while avoiding risks such as unblinding.

17.12 CHALLENGES AND NEXT STEPS

We now face important challenges and opportunities in engaging patients in cancer clinical trials. A critical step is that we evolve from thinking about patients as passive participants or *subjects* and consider them active collaborators. By inviting patients to be meaningful contributors to the trial design process, they can become co-owners of the process who want it to succeed. By building feedback loops that enable us to learn more from patients before, during, and after trials, we can improve clinical trials in ways that matter most to the end-users who will then be more likely to participate.

The online tools that patients are increasingly using, including online patient communities and trial search tools, can be leveraged for this kind of patient engagement. What if patients reading information about a trial online could easily initiate a discussion about the trial with experienced peers? (We are experimenting with this now.) What if they could get prompt and thoughtful answers from trial sponsors as well?

Perhaps the biggest near-term challenge lies in increasing participation specifically from underrepresented groups such as the elderly, women, and minorities. In the Black community for example, issues of trust and stigma trump even the issue of awareness. How might we tap into the power of community that exists in many cultures to increase trial participation? The answer may lie in more creatively including them in the process from the start.

LIST OF ACRONYMS AND ABBREVIATIONS

ACOR Association of Cancer Online Resources
BBS Bulletin board system
CBPR Community-based participatory research
COG Children's Oncology Group
CT Computed tomography
FDA Food and Drug Administration
PCORI Patient-Centered Outcomes Research Institute
PRO Patient-reported outcome

References

[1] Bhatt A. Evolution of clinical research: a history before and beyond James Lind. Perspect Clin Res 2010;1(1):6–10.

[2] Institute of Medicine (US) Forum on Drug Discovery, Development, and Translation Transforming clinical research in the United States: challenges and opportunities: workshop summary. Washington, DC: National Academies Press (US); 2010.

[3] The National Cancer Clinical Trials Collaborative Learning Network (CCTCLN). The National Cancer Clinical Trials Collaborative Learning Network (CCTCLN). Retrieved from: <http://www.enacct.org/our-programs/national-cancer-clinical-trials-collaborative-learning-network-ncctcln>; 2014 [accessed 29.04.15].

[4] Wei D. The how-to of clinical trial forecasting, budgeting, and project management, [Chapter 6] Bairu M, Chin R, editors. Global clinical trials playbook: capacity and capability building (1st ed.). San Diego, CA: Academic Press; 2012. p. 58.

[5] McDonald AM, Knight RC, Campbell MK, Entwiste VA, Grant AM, Cook JA, et al. What influences recruitment to randomised controlled trials? A review of trials funded by two UK funding agencies. Trials 2006;7:9.

[6] Bond MC, Pritchard S. Understanding clinical trials in childhood cancer. Paediatr Child Health 2006;11(3):148–50.

[7] CURE-Cure Childhood Cancer. Childhood cancer facts. Retrieved from: <http://www.curechildhoodcancer.org/about-cure/childhood-cancer-facts/>; 2015 [accessed 29.04.15].

[8] Children's Oncology Group. History. Retrieved from: <https://childrensoncologygroup.org/index.php/history>; 2015 [accessed 29.04.15].

[9] Vickers S, Fouad M, Chen MS. Enhancing minority participation in clinical trials (EMPaCT): laying the groundwork for improving minority clinical trial accrual. Cancer 2014;120:i–ii.

[10] Grigsby TJ, Kent EE, Montoya MJ, Sender LS, Morris RA, Ziogas A, et al. Attitudes toward cancer clinical trial participation in young adults with a history of cancer and a healthy college student sample: a preliminary investigation. J Adolesc Young Adult Oncol 2014;3(1):20–7.

[11] Intercultural Cancer Council. Cancer facts: cancer clinical trials: participation by underrepresented populations. Retrieved from: <http://iccnetwork.org/cancerfacts/ICC-CFS11.pdf>; 2008 [accessed 29.04.15].

[12] Unger JM, Hershman DL, Albain KS, Moinpour CM, Petersen JA, Burg K, et al. Health services and outcomes: patient income level and cancer clinical trial participation. J Clin Oncol 2013;31(5):536–42.

[13] Gertz B. Impact of the crisis in clinical research on new drug development. In: Clinical research and new drug development: symposium and meeting reports. American Federation for Medical Research. Retrieved from: <http://www.afmr.org/multimedia/2009/Clinical-Research-Conference/jim200301.pdf>; 2009 [accessed 29.04.15].

[14] Martin SS, Ou F-S, Newby LK, Sutton V, Adams P, Felker GM, et al. Patient- and trial-specific barriers to participation in cardiovascular randomized clinical trials. J Am Coll Cardiol 2013;61(7):762–9.

[15] Meropol NJ, Buzaglo JS, Millard J, Damjanov N, Miller SM, Ridgway C, et al. Barriers to clinical trial participation as perceived by oncologists and patients. J Natl Compr Cancer Netw 2007;5(8):655–64.

[16] Daugherty CK, Ratain MJ, Emanuel EJ, Farrell AT, Schilsky RL. Ethical, scientific, and regulatory perspectives regarding the use of placebos in cancer clinical trials. J Clin Oncol 2008;26(8):1371–8.

[17] Lilly Clinical Open Innovation. Placebos in cancer clinical research: an infographic. Retrieved from: <http://portal.lillycoi.com/2013/12/18/placebos-in-cancer-clinical-research-an-infographic/>; 2013 [accessed 29.04.15].

[18] Katz RV, Kegeles SS, Kressin NR, Green BL, Wang MQ, James SA, et al. The tuskegee legacy project: willingness of minorities to participate in biomedical research. J Health C Poor Underserved 2006;17(4):698–715.

[19] Scharff DP, Mathews KJ, Jackson P, Hoffsuemmer J, Martin E, Edwards D. More than Tuskegee: understanding mistrust about research participation. J Health C Poor Underserved 2010;21(3):879–97.

[20] CSR Inc. Evaluation of patient recruitment strategies—Phase I feasibility study-final report. Retrieved from: <http://aspe.hhs.gov/evaluation/fullreports/06/8384.pdf>; 2006 [accessed 29.04.15].

[21] The Center for Information and Study on Clinical Research Participation (CISCRP). Patient attitudes and perceptions. Retrieved from: <https://www.ciscrp.org/wp-content/uploads/2014/03/ciscrp_data_archive_patient_attitudes_perspectives.pdf>; 2014 [accessed 29.04.15].

[22] Atkinson NL, Saperstein SL, Massett H, Leonard CR, Grama L, Manrow R. Using the internet to search for cancer clinical trials: a comparative audit of clinical trial search tools. Contemp Clin Trials 2008;29(4):555–64.

[23] ClinicalTrials.gov. ClinicalTrials.gov background. Retrieved from: <https://clinicaltrials.gov/ct2/about-site/background>; 2014 [accessed 29.04.15].

[24] Pfiffner PB, Oh J, Miller TA, Mandl KD. Clinicaltrials.gov as a data source for semi-automated point-of-care trial eligibility screening. PLoS One 2014;9(10):e111055.

[25] Pew Research Center. Peer-to-peer health care. Retrieved from: <http://www.pewinternet.org/2011/02/28/peer-to-peer-health-care-2/>; 2011 [accessed 29.04.15].

[26] Pew Research Center. Health online 2013. Retrieved from: <http://www.pewinternet.org/2013/01/15/health-online-2013/>; 2013 [accessed 29.04.15].

[27] ACOR. ACOR.org—Association of Cancer Online Resources. Retrieved from: <http://www.acor.org/>; 2015 [accessed 29.04.15].

[28] American Cancer Society Cancer Survivors Network. Cancer Survivors Network. Retrieved from: <http://csn.cancer.org/>; 2015 [accessed 29.04.15].

[29] Inspire. Inspire. Retrieved from: <http://www.inspire.com/>; 2015 [accessed 29.04.15].

[30] Inspire. About Inspire. Retrieved from: <https://corp.inspire.com/press/inspire-overview.pdf>; 2015 [accessed 29.04.15].

[31] PatientsLikeMe. PatientsLikeMe. Retrieved from: <https://www.patientslikeme.com/>; 2015 [accessed 29.04.15].

[32] Smart Patients. Smart Patients. Retrieved from: <ttps://www.smartpatients.com/>; 2015 [accessed 29.04.15].

[33] Symplur. Healthcare Tweet Chats. Retrieved from: <http://www.symplur.com/healthcare-hashtags/tweet-chats/>; 2015 [accessed 29.04.15].

[34] Internet Society. Brief history of the Internet. Retrieved from: <http://www.internetsociety.org/internet/what-internet/history-internet/brief-history-internet>; 2012 [accessed 29.04.15].

[35] David Carlson's Virtual World. Bulletin board systems. Retrieved from: <http://iml.jou.ufl.edu/carlson/history/bbs.htm>; 2009 [accessed 29.04.15].

[36] Wikipedia. The WELL. Retrieved from: <http://en.wikipedia.org/wiki/The_WELL>; 2015 [accessed 29.04.15].

[37] L-Soft. History of LISTSERV. Retrieved from: <http://www.lsoft.com/corporate/history-listserv.asp>; 2011 [accessed 29.04.15].

[38] David Carlson's Virtual World. The online timeline 1990–1994, first entry for 1994. Retrieved from: <http://iml.jou.ufl.edu/carlson/1990s.shtml>; 2009 [accessed 29.04.15].

[39] L-Soft. LISTSERV mailing list software. Retrieved from: <http://www.lsoft.com/>; 2015 [accessed 29.04.15].

[40] Internet Archive Wayback Machine. ACOR Home Page archive September 18, 2009. Retrieved from: <http://web.archive.org/web/20090918191147/> <http://www.acor.org/>; 2009 [accessed 29.04.15].

[41] Greene J. Online social networking by patients with diabetes: a qualitative evaluation of communication with Facebook. J Gen Intern Med 2011;26(3):287–92.

[42] Shaya FT. Effect of social networks intervention in type 2 diabetes: a partial randomised study. J Epidemiol Commun Health 2014;68:326–32.

[43] Lorig K, Ritter PL, Laurent DD, Plant K, Green M, Jernigan VBB, et al. Online diabetes self-management program: a randomized study. Diabetes Care 2010;33(6):1275–81.

[44] Moskowitz D, Thom DH, Hessler D, Ghorob A, Bodenheimer T. Peer coaching to improve diabetes self-management: which patients benefit most? J Gen Intern Med 2013;28(7):938–42.

[45] McKechnie V, Barker C, Stott J. The effectiveness of an internet support forum for carers of people with dementia: a pre-post cohort study. J Med Internet Res 2014;16(2):e68.

[46] Esquivel A, Meric-Bernstam F, Bernstam EV. Accuracy and self correction of information received from an internet breast cancer list: content analysis. BMJ 2006;332:939.

[47] Meier A, Lyons E, Frydman G, Forlenza M, Rimer B. How cancer survivors provide support on cancer-related internet mailing lists. J Med Internet Res 2007;9(2):e12.

[48] Weiss JB, Berner ES, Johnson KB, Giuse DA, Murphy BA, Lorenzi NM. Recommendations for the design, implementation and evaluation of social support in online communities, networks, and groups. J Biomed Inform 2013;46(6):970–6.

[49] Young C. Community management that works: how to build and sustain a thriving online health community. J Med Internet Res 2013;15(6):e119.

[50] Fox S. Building a research agenda for participatory medicine. Retrieved from: <http://e-patients.net/archives/2010/10/building-a-research-agenda-for-participatory-medicine.html>; 2010 [accessed 29.04.15].

[51] Minkler M, Wallerstein N. Community-based participatory research for health: from process to outcomes. Hoboken, NJ: John Wiley & Sons; 2011.

[52] O'Toole TP, Aaron KF, Chin MH, Horowitz C, Tyson F. Community-based participatory research: opportunities, challenges, and the need for a common language. J Gen Intern Med 2003;18(7):592–4.

[53] Patient Centered Outcomes Research Institute (PCORI). About Us. Retrieved from: <http://www.pcori.org/about-us>; 2014 [accessed 29.04.15].

[54] Patient Centered Outcomes Research Institute (PCORI). Kaiser Permanente & Strategic Partners Patient Outcomes Research To Advance Learning (PORTAL) Network. Retrieved from: <http://www.pcori.org/research-results/2013/kaiser-permanente-strategic-partners-patient-outcomes-research-advance>; 2013 [accessed 29.04.15].

[55] Norman D. The design of everyday things. Retrieved from: <https://archive.org/details/DesignOfEverydayThings>; 1988 [accessed 29.04.15].

[56] Basch E, Geoghegan C, Coons SJ, Gnanasakthy A, Slagle AF, Papadopoulos EJ, et al. Patient-reported outcomes in cancer drug development and us regulatory review: perspectives from industry, the food and drug administration, and the patient. JAMA Oncol 2015;1(3):375–9.

[57] Hanington B, Martin B. Universal methods of design: 100 ways to research complex problems, develop innovative ideas, and design effective solutions. Beverly, MA: Rockport Publishers; 2012, p. 8.

[58] Marcus AD. Researchers fret as social media lift veil on drug trials. Wall Street J 2014. Retrieved from: http://www.wsj.com/articles/researchers-fret-as-social-media-lift-veil-on-drug-trials-1406687404, [accessed 29.04.15].

[59] Lipset CH. Engage with research participants about social media. Nat Med 2014;20:231.

[60] Glickman SW, Galhenage S, McNair L, Barber Z, Patel K, Schulman KA, et al. The potential influence of Internet-based social networking on the conduct of clinical research studies. J Empir Res Hum Res Ethics 2012;7(1):71–80.

18

A New Era of Clinical Research Methods in a Data-Rich Environment

William T. Riley PhD

Office of Behavioral and Social Sciences Research, National Institutes of Health,
Bethesda, MD, United States

O U T L I N E

18.1 Transition From a Data-Poor to
Data-Rich Science   343

18.2 Traditional Trial Designs: What's Wrong
With Continuing to Do What We Do?   344

18.3 Data-Rich Biomedical and Behavioral
Research Environment   345
    18.3.1 Meteorology   346
    18.3.2 Plate Tectonics   346
    18.3.3 Radio Astronomy and Cosmology   346
    18.3.4 Common Attributes of Data-Rich
    Research Science   346

18.4 The Vision of a Data-Rich Biomedical and
Behavioral Research Enterprise   348
    18.4.1 Standard Interoperable Electronic
    Health Record   348
    18.4.2 EHR Integrated With Personal Health
    Information   348
    18.4.3 Integration With Existing Data Sets   348

18.5 Recent Advances That Poise Clinical
Research to Become a Data-Rich
Research Enterprise   348
    18.5.1 Electronic Health Records   348
    18.5.2 Mobile Health Technologies   349
    18.5.3 Patient-Generated Data   349
    18.5.4 Big Data Analytics   349

18.6 New Approaches to Treatment Testing in
Preparation for a Comprehensive Health
Data Research Infrastructure   350
    18.6.1 Single Case Studies   350
    18.6.2 Optimized and Adaptive Interventions   351
    18.6.3 Just-in-Time Adaptive Interventions   351
    18.6.4 Adaptive Designs   352
    18.6.5 Rapid Learning Systems   352

18.7 Conclusion   352

List of Acronyms and Abbreviations   353

References   353

18.1 TRANSITION FROM A DATA-POOR TO DATA-RICH SCIENCE

Clinical treatment research in the biomedical and behavioral sciences has evolved from a data-poor environment. Research plans may be shaped by previously reported research and pilot data, but each new study begins with a blank slate of no data. The clinical trial must be prospectively designed to collect the requisite data to answer the specific, circumscribed study questions. Participant recruitment and data collection are resource and time-intensive. The burden of recurring data collection on

B. Hesse, D. Ahern & E. Beckjord: Oncology Informatics.
DOI: http://dx.doi.org/10.1016/B978-0-12-802115-6.00018-5

the same participants over time results in cross-sectional designs or limited longitudinal designs with as few data collections points as possible (ie, pre, post, follow-up). The burden of data collection also dictates the preference to randomize potential confounds and relegate their variance to error than to specifically measure and control for them. Once initiated, the protocol and the treatment it tests cannot be changed until the study is completed, regardless of advances that might occur during the trial. And after this data collection is completed and the results of the trial published (which is not a certainty), the data from these labor- and time-intensive efforts lay fallow and are seldom if ever used again unless data sharing has been mandated and planned.

Imagine instead what research methods might look like in a data-rich environment in which biomedical and behavioral data are readily available from everyone. Research would not begin from a blank slate but would instead be based on a continuous flow of data on the variables of interest. This would allow naturalistic studies of the covariation of these variables over time and the ability to model how a given outcome might be produced from changes in the mechanisms targeted by a potential treatment. Participants would be identified and invited, not recruited. The treatment would be delivered or "inserted" into this relentless flow of data from the individual or system and the impact of the treatment observed via deviations from the outcomes predicted by the wealth of predictor data available. By leveraging temporally dense data and within subject designs, rapid determinations of the effects of the treatment can be made and the intervention improved and retested iteratively. Any additional data collection and treatment manipulations from a trial would be incorporated into the data stream for others to utilize.

Such a data-rich biomedical and behavioral research environment may seem implausible to those immersed in traditional clinical research methodologies. Recent advances, however, in medical informatics, big data analytics, and mobile and wearable technologies have laid the groundwork for a rich biomedical and behavioral research environment. This chapter will describe:

- the weaknesses of our traditional clinical research methods born from data-poor environments;
- the new methods, designs, and approaches that are conceivable in a data-rich environment, drawing from sciences that have already transitioned to a data-rich environment methodology;
- the recent and future advances that will transform biomedical and behavioral sciences into a data-rich research enterprise;
- alternative designs that facilitate the transition from data-poor methods to a new data-rich methodology for clinical research.

18.2 TRADITIONAL TRIAL DESIGNS: WHAT'S WRONG WITH CONTINUING TO DO WHAT WE DO?

Our traditional clinical trial designs have a long and productive history in the biomedical and behavioral sciences. The randomized controlled trial (RCT) is considered the gold standard of biomedical and behavioral clinical trials. The Consolidated Standards of Reporting Trials (CONSORT) guidelines provide clear and concise direction on designing and conducting RCTs [1]. RCTs have become the standard for inclusion of research findings in meta-analyses such as Cochrane reviews [2], Institute of Medicine (IOM) consensus workshops [3], and various organizational practice guidelines [4]. RCTs represent one of the most common, and some would say only, method for making causal inference about the effects of a treatment.

RCTs, however, are not without limitations. RCTs control for confounds by randomly distributing them between conditions, relegating the variance from these confounds to error. This has important implications, especially for biomedical and behavioral research in which uncontrolled factors often contribute more to health changes than the treatment itself. Patients seek alternative care; take medications not prescribed by the study; and can be affected by serious life events (eg, loss of a job, death of spouse) that can significantly alter their health outcomes [5]. Including the variance from these confounding factors in the error term makes it more difficult to detect the effects of the treatment and necessitates larger sample sizes. More importantly, these confounds may be more important, or at least as important, as the treatment under study. For example, a genetic variant that may influence the effects of a given treatment on a given outcome is a confound that would typically be relegated to error unless the investigator had an a priori precision medicine hypothesis, stratified the conditions on this genetic variant, and incorporated it as a moderator variable in the analyses. Many of these moderators or predictors of treatment outcome are lost in a simple RCT because they are either unmeasured or because the sample size is seldom adequate to detect these moderator effects [6].

RCTs using null hypothesis statistical testing (NHST) or frequentist approaches produce a dichotomous answer—that the null hypothesis (no difference between treatment and control) is either rejected or not rejected. There is considerable debate currently about the pros and cons of NHST versus Bayesian approaches that offer a more probabilistic outcome [7]. There are a number of valid arguments for a transition from NHST to Bayesian analyses of RCTs, but there is little doubt that the ability to use priors to reflect the information available to date on the treatment of interest is consistent with the desire to produce a more cumulative science.

Furthermore, the inferential statistics of RCTs are based on the assumption that the patients in the study are representative of the population of interest [8]. In essence, if we were to do the same trial 20 times, enrolling similar patients from the population, we should find a difference between the treatment and the comparison condition 19 of those 20 times. However, although we are quite fastidious in random assignment to conditions (eg, random number generation for assignment, blinding of assignment), nearly all of the clinical RCTs in the literature are convenience samples drawn from the patients who came to clinic over a specified period or responded to recruitment efforts. These samples clearly cannot be considered representative of the population, so from which population are we inferring with our inferential statistics? One source of the heterogeneity of effects found in meta-analyses of RCTs for various treatments is the differences of the samples that are highly unlikely to be representative of the same population [9].

As a methodology born from a data-poor environment, RCTs are costly and time-consuming to conduct. Recruitment delays are a common occurrence in clinical trials grants supported by the National Institutes of Health (NIH) and have led to increased monitoring of recruitment and enrollment [10]. Recruitment efforts and outcome assessments, especially over long-term follow-ups, are labor intensive and costly to perform well.

RCTs are also slow. Balas and Boren have estimated that it takes 17 years for 14% of the evidence from clinical trials to be implemented in practice [11]. Ioannidis estimated that the clinical trial itself takes approximately 5½ years to conduct and publish [12]. These time frames can be longer if there are recruitment delays or if primary outcomes are long-term occurrences like morbidity or mortality. During this study period, the principal investigator is blind to the treatment conditions and outcomes, and the treatment remains unchanged throughout the study period.

Working from the Ioannidis estimate and adding the time for grant submission and funding, we have estimated that it would take 7 years from grant submission to publication and that during this time a number of major technological achievements would have occurred in the mHealth space that would not be reflected in the study when it is finally published [13]. For example, since smartphones were not introduced until 2007, we should not expect RCT publications of interventions using smartphones until 2014 or later. Indeed, much of what was published prior to 2014 that was a mobile treatment used personal digital assistants (PDAs) with much less capability and functionality than the current smartphone. The recent explosion of passive sensor technologies in the past few years are not likely to be incorporated into treatments and published for a few more years. Similar to the astronomical concept of light-years, when an RCT is published, we are looking back in time and considering the evaluation of technologies and approaches that existed nearly a decade ago. This time lag is not unique to mobile technologies. For example, a recently published trial comparing stents versus medications for stroke was criticized by the surgical community for using dated stent technologies and surgical procedures [14,15].

These criticisms of the RCT are not to say that they should be abandoned altogether. Until a fully functional data-rich environment for biomedical and behavioral research is developed, we will need to continue to rely on the RCT as a primary methodology for assessing the effects of treatments on a variety of clinical outcomes. As a research community, however, we should less easily accept the RCT as the default design for all clinical research questions, consider its weaknesses, and be more open to alternative designs that in some cases are better suited to the question of interest. This will be described further in the section on bridging methodologies that will take us from a data-poor to data-rich environment, but it is first important to consider how other sciences made the transition from a data-poor to data-rich science.

18.3 DATA-RICH BIOMEDICAL AND BEHAVIORAL RESEARCH ENVIRONMENT

In a data-rich environment, a data infrastructure has been put into place to routinely and frequently collect data on the phenomena of interest. The data flowing in can be used to answer a range of research questions instead of having to collect data to answer a given research question. Consider Google or any other search engine and online advertising service as a simple example of research in a data-rich environment. When Google has a question about a graphical user interface (GUI), new search functionality, or different advertising approach, it does not generate the question, then generate the data to answer the question. Instead, it collects all of the data that it can prudently collect from its users on a frequent, longitudinal basis. When it is ready to test a new functionality, it simply drops that functionality into the data stream and analyzes the results. This can be in the form of A–B testing, a rapid form of an RCT [16], or a within subject interrupted time series or ABA design. In a matter of hours or days, the question that Google poses is answered. Granted, their "treatments" are shorter than ours, and their outcomes are more proximate to the treatment than ours, but the availability of a data-rich infrastructure eliminates the need to build a data collection effort from scratch each time they have a question. Google and computer sciences are not alone in taking this data-rich research approach.

18.3.1 Meteorology

As data-rich as meteorology is today, it is important to remember that it was once a data-poor science. Instruments measuring temperature, humidity, and barometric pressure were developed centuries ago, but it took the development of the telegraph to begin sending data from these local instruments to develop weather maps describing wind patterns and storm systems over a wide geographic area. With this new ability to transmit and compile weather data, weather observation stations began to be created across the globe, providing the basis for synoptic weather prediction in the latter half of the 19th century and early half of the 20th century [17].

Synoptic weather prediction, however, was highly inaccurate because it was based only on instruments near the earth's surface. Weather balloons were developed to provide data on weather at higher altitudes. Today, these weather balloons are released twice a day from hundreds of locations across the earth. Around the same time that weather balloons were being employed, early computers were being developed that could handle the computational demands of weather prediction. Basic mathematical calculations for weather forecasting had been developed in the first half of the 20th century, but the calculations were so intensive and time-consuming that the time being forecast would have passed by the time the calculations could be performed [18]. With the computational efficiency of computers, it was now possible to rapidly perform these calculations and predict future weather with reasonable reliability. Today, weather satellites provide not only visual images of weather but also have atmospheric sounders that more completely and continuously measure weather variables than weather balloons. More temporally dense and complete data in combination with greater computer processing speeds able to computationally model all of these data quickly produce the data-rich science of meteorology that we rely on today.

18.3.2 Plate Tectonics

The prediction of earthquakes follows a similar history as the prediction of weather. Seismographs that measure the movement of the earth were developed in the late 19th century. The basic mathematical computations of elastic wave propagation in solids were developed at about the same time. Technological advances in seismographs improved their sensitivity and reliability, Richter created a common metric for the magnitude of earthquakes in the 1930s. Although the readings from

multiple seismographs were transmitted and compiled for some time, it was not until 1961 that the Worldwide Standardized Seismograph Network was established. This network produced a high-quality data set that was instrumental to many of the subsequent advances in the science of seismology and the detection of earthquakes [19].

One of the advances from a data-rich system of networked seismographs was the discovery of plate tectonics. The concept that the crust of the earth consists of plates that gradually crash into one another was posited in the 1960s. Seismic data were consistent with large earthquakes being produced by the movement of these tectonic plates, supporting this theory. As data volume and velocity grew from this worldwide seismic network, computer advances provided the capabilities to store, compile, process, and analyze these data, leading eventually to a central repository for these data [20]. Although accurate earthquake prediction has not been realized, the extensive data produced by this seismic network has greatly advanced our understanding of earthquakes, plate tectonics, and the underlying structure of our planet.

18.3.3 Radio Astronomy and Cosmology

Radio astronomy began in the 1930s with the discovery that the Milky Way was a source of radio emission. Radio astronomy dishes of increasing size were built to detect nonvisual electromagnetic waves. Because of their low resolution, radio telescopes were the first to link data from two or more widely separated antennas to take advantage of interferometry [21].

Radio astronomy would be of little interest to the general public were it not for the cosmological science struggle between a steady state versus expanding model of the universe. The expanding universe or Big Bang model was supported by the discovery of Penzias and Wilson of cosmic microwave background radiation. These findings and subsequent advances in observational techniques (eg, satellite observations of microwave background) have led to ever increasingly precise models of the birth of the universe (eg, cosmic inflation, Lambda Cold Dark Matter (Lambda-CDM)) [22].

18.3.4 Common Attributes of Data-Rich Research Science

The examples from meteorology, seismology, and cosmology provide seven shared processes that resulted in these sciences being data-rich.

1. Measurement Advances. Early measurement instrumentation in these sciences was crude, but the field continuously worked to improve

their precision and efficiency. These sciences were relentless in separating noise from signal, and utilized technological advances, both of the instrumentation itself and of the computational systems needed to filter and compile signals.

2. Data Standards and Integration. Although seismographs changed and improved over time, the metrics for expressing the outputs from these instruments (eg, the Richter scale) remained constant. The same is true for meteorological instruments such as barometric pressure. These standards were critical to the communication and interpretation of findings across a diverse network of measurement instruments as data density increased.

3. Communications and Connectivity. These sciences all benefited from communication advances. While they did not build the telegraph, telephone, or radio, they quickly leveraged these communications technologies to create a shared and connected network of measurement devices that could answer many more questions than isolated measurements at specific locations or times. The development of a shared network resulted in highly impactful findings such as plate tectonics and cosmic inflation that would not have been possible without this connectivity.

4. Temporally Dense Data Collection. These data-rich sciences not only integrated data across space/location, but also across time. Frequent and intensive sampling over time is evident in all of these sciences. Data flow continuously from meteorology, seismology, and radio telescope instruments, not simply because they can but because temporally dense data provide critically important information about variability, patterns, and changes in the systems that they monitor.

5. Data-Intensive Computation. Meteorology is perhaps the best example of the importance of intensive and rapid computations. Until computers became big enough and fast enough, weather predictions could be performed, but too slowly to be any practical use. By the time the computational models had been run, the time for which the weather was being predicted had passed. As with communications technologies, these sciences did not build these computers, but they leveraged them for more rapid and more intensive computational modeling of the phenomena of interest.

6. Computational Modeling. Although statistical modeling is used by these sciences, they rely primarily on computational modeling which makes more specific predictions and better addresses the dynamic complexities of the systems they model.

7. Causal Inference From Explanation and Prediction. These sciences make causal inferences but do so via precise model prediction, not by isolating and controlling the causal agent. We know that large earthquakes are caused by movements of tectonic plates, that jet streams cause the flow of high altitude weather phenomena, and that the current characteristics of our expanding universe are the result of its early inflationary expansion. None of these causal inferences were based on a controlled trial. Furthermore, controlled trials assume a linear causality that is inconsistent with many of the nonlinear phenomena in the biomedical and behavioral sciences. Nonlinearity is particularly clear in meteorology in which numerous weather phenomena (eg, jet streams, low pressure cells, cold fronts) interact with each other mutually and iteratively. These data-rich sciences focus on explanation and prediction, not causation. Instead of attempting to isolate a causal agent, which would be nearly impossible in these sciences anyway, they attempt to understand how the system's components interact to make predictions about new or future observations.

Most importantly, these sciences invested in a data collection and integration informatics infrastructure that could be used to collect and process data and answer a wide and emerging range of research questions. They quickly realized that it was inefficient for the science to pose questions and collect data from scratch only to answer the specific research question of interest. In the biomedical and behavioral sciences, we have some rudimentary data-rich infrastructures, but much of the clinical research enterprise consists of posing questions, prospectively collecting the data to answer those questions, then discarding the data once the questions of that specific study are answered (Box 18.1).

BOX 18.1

COMMON ATTRIBUTES OF A DATA-RICH SCIENCE

- Measurement Advances
- Data Standards and Integration
- Communications and Connectivity
- Temporally Dense Data
- Data-Intensive Computation
- Computational Modeling
- Causal Inference From Explanation and Prediction

18.4 THE VISION OF A DATA-RICH BIOMEDICAL AND BEHAVIORAL RESEARCH ENTERPRISE

Health costs represent a fifth of our gross national product [23] yet health research consists of a patchwork of rudimentary data infrastructures, surveillance systems, and prospective clinical research studies that are fragmented and disconnected. Based on the examples provided above from other areas of science, what might a comprehensive health research data infrastructure look like?

18.4.1 Standard Interoperable Electronic Health Record

Every encounter with the health care system would be captured in a standard and networked format. Similar to the early days of meteorology, the data from electronic health records (EHRs) are isolated within specific EHR vendors and specific health systems [24]. A fully integrated network of health system encounters and data standards for the relevant variables from each encounter would greatly facilitate clinical research. This seamless and integrated EHR system would provide information about every time someone's health was sufficiently compromised for him/her or others to seek medical care, provide a standard snapshot of their health status at each encounter, and note any procedures that were performed to alleviate their compromised health status. As new health care metrics become standard (eg, genetics, metabolomics), these data could be integrated in the system.

18.4.2 EHR Integrated With Personal Health Information

This EHR network needs to be integrated with a patient (or person) generated data system to fill health information gaps, especially from infrequent health care users. Because the EHR provides inadequate data coverage of health status and outcomes, especially in a temporally dense form, data from the health care system would be linked to a range of user generated data including automated and routine administration of self-report health status questions and passive sensor technologies that track various health-related behavioral indices [25]. Some of these passive sensors might track general population risk factors for disease (wireless weight scales) while others might track changes in health status for those with diseases under treatment (eg, wireless glucometers for patients with diabetes). As new technologies are developed and validated, they can be incorporated in the health research infrastructure.

Clearly, respondent burden and participant engagement would need to be addressed, but the value of integrating these data with health records and providing health information feedback to participants would provide benefit to participants. Critically, all of these data would be integrated and compiled, both across these various patient-generated data and with the EHR.

18.4.3 Integration With Existing Data Sets

These EHR and patient generated data inputs would be integrated with other relevant data sets such as death records and with various exposure data sets (eg, air pollution, violence, and poverty) that could be linked to patient location [26]. Connecting location, either home and work address, or more precisely using location capabilities of mobile phones, the exposure to health-related phenomena in the environment could be calculated and compiled for all individuals. Although major contributors to health status, these social determinants of health are frequently ignored in our traditional health informatics systems even though they can often be estimated from location alone if integrated with social exposure data sets [27].

A distributed but integrated network of these health data from all except those who opt-out would produce a complete and comprehensive data-rich health research environment similar to what our natural science colleagues have built for their sciences. Granted, jet streams do not have privacy concerns and tectonic plates do not require Institutional Review Board approval to be studied, but data privacy and security processes continue to improve [28]. More importantly, much of these data already exist, just in a disjointed and disorganized system of surveillance surveys, cohorts, patient registries, numerous EHR systems, and millions of clinical trials that have been conducted over decades. Integration of these data into a comprehensive health research network would provide the basis for an array of big data computational analytics that could answer many of the research questions that we currently answer by the costly and labor-intensive process of gathering yet another data set de novo from a sample of individuals.

18.5 RECENT ADVANCES THAT POISE CLINICAL RESEARCH TO BECOME A DATA-RICH RESEARCH ENTERPRISE

18.5.1 Electronic Health Records

A decade ago when the Office of the National Coordinator for Health Information Technology was created, less than 13% of nonfederal acute care hospitals had EHRs. Today, well over 90% of hospitals and most outpatient clinics have EHRs [29]. While other chapters of this book address EHRs in more detail (see Chapter 4: Engaging Patients in Primary and Specialty Care in this book), there are four points worth noting here. First, there is no question that the EHR is designed for documentation and reimbursement, not for research. Yet, even minimally, the EHR provides reliable data on each clinical encounter; the procedure(s) performed; and vital signs and other quantitative indicators of health status (eg, labs, images). Second, innovative work in predictive algorithms provides for improvements in detecting diagnostic phenotypes from EHRs [30]. Third, efforts to recommend minimal data standards for EHRs, even for less "traditional" medical data, such as behavioral and environmental determinants of health, have been proposed [31]. Fourth, as genomic, metabolomic, and other "-omic" data are integrated with EHR data, a data-rich health research infrastructure begins to emerge and provides the basis for the EHR to become a core aspect of this health research infrastructure.

18.5.2 Mobile Health Technologies

A decade ago, there was no iPhone or Android phone. Today, nearly every adult in the United States owns a cell phone and two-thirds own a smartphone [32]. Like our natural science colleagues, we can leverage new communication and personal computation devices to build an integrated research network infrastructure, filling many of the informational gaps that EHRs are unable to do. Tracking location from cell phones provides a more precise indication of health-related exposures [33]. Using these phones for ecological momentary assessment (EMA) of various health outcomes over time provides a more temporally dense and prospective assessment of health status than currently possible from our traditional health surveys [34]. Additional sensors on the smartphone platform allow for an array of prompted samplings of health indices such as heart rate, motor speed, and cognitive function [35].

A reasonably comprehensive and longitudinal health monitoring system can be produced with smartphones alone (integrated with EHR), but recent advances in wireless health sensor technologies offer even greater monitoring capabilities with less respondent burden. Accelerometers provide data on energy expenditure, sedentary behavior, sleep, and activities [36]. Heart rate, electrodermal activity, and other physiological parameters can be continuously monitored via wearable technologies [37]. Wireless medical devices including weight scales, glucometers, and spirometers provide intensive longitudinal data that fills the time gaps between medical office visits when these data may be obtained or collected [38]. In addition to these sensors, a range of data about activities, social behavior, attitudes, and beliefs can be can be estimated from the digital traces that individuals leave as they interact with computer systems in their daily lives [39]. Leveraging and integrating these data would greatly expand the potential data available to a health research infrastructure.

18.5.3 Patient-Generated Data

Patients have grown impatient waiting for the health research system to generate a patient portal for donating research data, and have taken it upon themselves to do so. Online peer communities such as PatientsLikeMe (see Chapter 16: "Crowdsourcing Advancements in Health Care Research: Applications for Cancer Treatment Discoveries" in this book for an in-depth description) provide a technology-mediated home for patients looking for others dealing with the same disease and has become a repository of patient-generated data and source of potential study participants [40]. Another community called 23andMe has developed an engaging process for genotype–phenotype studies in which individuals not only donate their genetic profile for research but also routinely answer questions about their health [41]. Quantified Self is a movement of individuals who fastidiously track various health indices using mobile and wireless technologies [42]. In addition to using these data to guide their own health decisions, these individuals contribute these data for research purposes. Clearly, there is a pent-up need of individuals to generate, control, use, and donate their data for research purposes.

18.5.4 Big Data Analytics

A health research network infrastructure will require advanced, big data analytics and computational power. Computational advances continue at a rapid pace [43]. Big data approaches offer opportunities to analyze health data similar to the natural science examples from meteorology, seismology, and cosmology. The promise of big data for health research led to the development of the NIH Big Data to Knowledge Initiative, and the creation of the NIH Associate Director for Data Science [44]. As our data sets grow and, as envisioned in this chapter, eventually become an integrated network of all health data, the ability to make sense of these data, and to use them to explain and predict health and illness will be critical. Two examples of big data analytic approaches provide a glimpse into what is possible from these analytic approaches.

One example of big data analytics is pattern recognition analysis. Pattern recognition or machine learning approaches recognize and classify patterns in data. Speech and writing detection software make heavy use of machine learning analytics. These approaches have also been used in medicine to better classify patterns in medical data (please see Chapter 11: Data Visualization Tools for Investigating Health Services Utilization Among Cancer Patients in this book for further discussion on clinical use of pattern recognition). One example is from Beck et al. [45] who used all possible cellular aspects of breast biopsies to predict 5-year mortality. Previous efforts to computerize the diagnostic algorithms of pathologists led to less than optimal predictions. Allowing pattern recognition approaches to generate their own algorithms from the data, however, resulted in superior prediction of 5-year mortality relative to pathologist predictions. More importantly, the pattern recognition analysis revealed characteristics of the cell, particularly the stroma, which had not been part of the pathologists' predictive algorithms but which contributed to the prediction. These findings suggested new directions for basic cellular cancer research.

A second example of big data analytics is computational dynamic modeling. As noted previously, computational modeling is the core analytic approach in the natural sciences. Computational modeling is also a core approach in systems biology, including cancer systems biology which has created in-silico models of various tumors using this approach [46]. These computational modeling approaches have extended beyond systems biology into epidemiology and behavior. Neurophysiological processes have been characterized as computational systems [47]. Agent-based modeling of population dynamics has been instrumental in understanding the spread of infectious diseases [48]. Influences on health behavior have also been approached from a computational modeling perspective [49]. These and other big data analytic approaches provide the ability to model complex health and illness processes to explain, predict, and potentially preempt disease.

18.6 NEW APPROACHES TO TREATMENT TESTING IN PREPARATION FOR A COMPREHENSIVE HEALTH DATA RESEARCH INFRASTRUCTURE

A new approach to health research will require new approaches to treatment development and evaluation. Computational models will allow us not only to better identify the multiple complex mechanisms that contribute to disease, but also to simulate the effects of changes in these mechanisms to change or reverse the disease process. The science can then prioritize the search for agents/treatments that can affect the modeled change in the mechanisms of the disease. This same process hold true for behavioral and environmental determinants of health. By modeling how changes in cigarette taxes, bans on indoor smoking, and availability of smoking

cessation aids affect smoking rates, we can determine how to optimize these environmental factors to reduce smoking [50].

These computational simulations will likely eliminate the need for most pilot trials. Preliminary evidence that the treatment can produce the desired outcome can be based on modeling simulations of the effects of treatments on mechanisms and the effects of mechanisms on outcomes. With rigorous simulations, running 10–30 participants in an open trial of the treatment seems redundant. In addition, Leon and colleagues have argued that pilot trials are not a useful approach for estimating the effect size of the treatment because the confidence intervals around the estimated effect size are so large [51]. Using a pilot trial for feasibility testing also becomes less necessary since an integrated health research network already incorporates most of the data collection infrastructure needed to evaluate the effects of the treatment. Given the growing sense that pilot trials are already overemphasized in the literature [52], alternative methods to the traditional pilot trial appear warranted.

18.6.1 Single Case Studies

Instead of pilot trials, N-of-1 or single case studies can be utilized to test and adapt new treatments. It was difficult to perform these single case studies in a data-poor environment because they require intensive longitudinal data and the establishment of a stable baseline. With the remote measurement and sensor technologies available, these intensive longitudinal data analyses become possible. For treatments in which the effects diminish when withdrawn, reversal designs (eg, ABAB) can be used to test treatment effects [53]. For treatments that will produce sustained effects even after withdrawal, an interrupted time series design can be used [54]. This analysis predicts subsequent data points from a series of baseline data points, and the treatment is considered effective if these subsequent data points are outside of the confidence interval range predicted by the baseline series. These single case designs are not limited to individuals, but can be used to test the effects of health care system and policy "treatments" as well. These designs provide considerable flexibility to test a treatment in a few participants, improve upon the treatment based on these observed effects, and repeat the process in a second series of participants.

One concern regarding single case designs is that they are not generalizable to the population. As noted earlier, one could make the case that even large-scale clinical trials are not generalizable, and it is certainly the case that pilot trials are not generalizable. As the series of single case studies builds and the effects appear reasonably consistent across participants, there is greater ability to generalize the effects to others. Bayesian approaches have been used to predict the probability that a subsequent patient/participant will have effects comparable to those already studied [55]. In addition, single case studies are consistent with a precision medicine approach and can be used to optimize treatments for specific subgroups of patients [56].

18.6.2 Optimized and Adaptive Interventions

Multicomponent treatments are common in the behavioral sciences. Although these multicomponent treatments have been found efficacious for a number of cancer risk behaviors, it is difficult to determine how these treatments can be improved upon when it is unclear after the trial which treatment components worked best. To address this issue, Collins and colleagues outlined a Multiphase Optimization Strategy (MOST) [57]. Core to this framework is an optimization phase in which the various treatment components are tested in isolation and in combination using factorial and fractional factorial designs. For example, this approach has been used to optimize the combination of treatment components for smoking cessation interventions [58]. Although this approach has been used predominantly with behavioral treatments, it is applicable to research questions regarding combination treatments in oncology and other clinical areas as well.

Questions regarding optimal treatment components involve not only what combination of components but also in what sequence. Sequential Multiple Assignment Randomized Trials, or SMART, are designs to answer questions regarding treatment sequence [59]. Based on our traditional RCT approach, clinical practice should offer the treatment that works best on average and if that treatment fails to work for that particular patient, cease attempts to treat the patient. SMART designs are more compatible with actual clinical practice in which secondary treatments are considered after the primary treatment fails. Practice guidelines often provide secondary treatment recommendations, but these secondary treatments are seldom evaluated in those who failed the primary treatment. Instead, the methodology of most practice guidelines defines secondary treatments as those treatments which are effective but less effective than the primary treatment [60]. Therefore, it is possible that the individuals who were nonresponsive to the primary treatment could also be nonresponsive to the secondary treatment. More concerning, a secondary treatment that in the general clinical sample may be deemed ineffective may actually be highly effective for the subset of patients who fail to respond to the primary treatment.

SMART designs involve sequential randomization of participants based on a priori specified decision rules regarding response to the prior intervention. For example, depending on response to the initial treatment, would it be better to continue the current treatment, augment the treatment, switch to a different treatment, or step-down the intensity of the current treatment? After each decision point (eg, responder or nonresponder), participants are rerandomized within these decision categories to receive one of two or more treatments. Based on results from SMART, the field is able to make better decisions about how to optimize the sequencing of treatments.

18.6.3 Just-in-Time Adaptive Interventions

With the advent of mobile technologies, intervention adaptations can be performed much more frequently (multiple times per day) and vary both content and timing in response to a range of variables including physiological states, environmental contexts, and responses to prior intervention prompts [61]. These intensively adaptive interventions have been described as Ecological Momentary Interventions (EMI) or Just-in-Time Adaptive Interventions (JITAI), and although these terms are not synonymous, both describe interventions delivered frequently (daily or greater frequency) and adapted to time, location, context, intrapersonal factors, or other inputs [62]. Heron and Smyth reviewed 27 studies of interventions considered EMIs [63], and there are recent examples of JITAIs for health behaviors such as physical activity [64].

Dynamic and intensively adapting interventions delivered frequently throughout the day in the context of where the behavior occurs and in response to a wide array of inputs on current context, intrapersonal states, and prior intervention responses should prove more effective than static, nonadapting interventions; however, this remains an empirical question, and current research on JITAIs or EMIs are in their infancy. Intensively adaptive interventions generate the need for new research methods. The intensive longitudinal data generated by JITAIs require approaches that are capable of modeling patterns and variability over time such as Time-Varying Effect Models [65] and Mixed-Effect Location Scale Models [66]. Recent extensions of optimization trials such as micro-randomized trials [67], an intensive version of the SMART methods described previously, may be particularly well-suited for evaluating the components of JITAIs delivered via mobile/wireless platforms. Computational modeling simulations also have the potential to provide guidance on when and in which contexts interventions should be delivered. For example, Savage and colleagues used a control systems engineering approach to simulate an adaptive intervention to obtain optimal prenatal weight gain [68].

18.6.4 Adaptive Designs

Adaptive designs and adaptive treatments, evaluated via SMART, are easily confused, but, as their names connote, the distinction is in what is being adapted, the treatment or the design. Technically, SMART can be considered an adaptive design, but it lies at the far end of the range of adaptations that constitute adaptive designs.

When I describe our traditional clinical trial methodology to my engineering colleagues, they are shocked that once a trial is launched, the treatment and design remain unchanged and the investigator remains blind to the data being collected. Adaptive designs are more consistent with engineering designs in that they utilize the accumulating data from the trial to modify certain study characteristics. An adaptive design may allow for dose increases or decreases, dropping or adding a new treatment arm, adjusting the randomization scheme, allocating treatment based on participant characteristics, reestimation of sample size, and/or early stopping of the trial for toxicity, efficacy, or futility. Adaptive trials give investigators the flexibility to use the data at it comes in to improve the trial without undermining the integrity of the intended trial. Adaptive trials typically use Bayesian methods because of their flexibility and adaptability to changes in estimates as data are analyzed. Zang and Lee provide an excellent recent overview of adaptive designs in oncology, including recent examples of adaptive designs in clinical oncology trials [69].

18.6.5 Rapid Learning Systems

Since the concept of a rapid learning health system was advanced in 2007 [70], there has been major investments in databases and learning networks to take advantage of the power of considering every patient as a potential research participant and leveraging the power of EHRs to rapidly answer practical research questions. The US Food and Drug Administration (FDA) mini-Sentinel system accesses hundreds of millions of patient records and generates multiple studies each week on drug safety questions [71]. Recent efforts such as the UK Biobank [64] offer cohort databases that can be used answer a range of clinical questions. Using these and other patient databases, researchers have been able to assess the unintended effects of treatments and produce outcome findings comparable to RCTs [72].

The most recent example of a rapid learning system is the NIH Precision Medicine Initiative (PMI), which seeks to develop a national cohort of more than 1 million participants and combine genetic, EHR, and behavioral and environmental influences on health using the latest technologies to study which individuals respond to which treatments [73]. Existing cohorts are being considered as a partial source of the PMI cohort. This represents an early effort to link all of the various patient cohorts that could serve as a first step toward a truly national and comprehensive health research network infrastructure.

To make maximal use of these large and evolving cohorts, we need to think differently about treatment evaluation within these cohorts. Clearly, we can use these cohorts to identify appropriate study participants and to randomize these participants to treatments. With a sufficiently comprehensive health tracking system, these RCTs can be rapidly implemented. We will seriously underutilize these resources, however, if we use them only as platforms for conducting traditional RCTs more rapidly. Many of the questions traditionally evaluated by RCTs in a data-poor environment can be answered differently in a data-rich environment. Some of these alternative approaches have been discussed in this section. As cohort data become more temporally dense, rigorous within subject designs can be performed, either on single participants or large groups. Computational modeling of health changes within these large cohorts allows researchers to assess the effect of a treatment by inserting it into the system and observing how it impacts the computational model.

As we transition from a data-poor to a data-rich health research environment, our methods need to change as well. The approaches discussed here are not all conceptually new, but advances in informatics in the service of supporting more intensive longitudinal data collection, reliable and efficient measurement; and computational capabilities have made these approaches more accessible than ever before.

18.7 CONCLUSION

Clinical research is rapidly entering a transition from a data-poor environment in which data must be prospectively obtained to a data-rich environment in which data are made readily available within a health research network infrastructure. The absence of a health research infrastructure is starkly contrasted with natural sciences such as meteorology, seismology, and cosmology that have developed integrated, temporally dense data systems that provide for a comprehensive platform for rapidly answering research questions and better understanding and predicting phenomena. Health expenditures represent a fifth of the gross domestic product in the United States [23], yet we do not have an integrated health research system that would allow us to better understand the complex determinants of health and improve the health of the nation.

A number of recent advances in informatics have laid the groundwork for such a health research infrastructure. EHRs are now used by most health care systems and, if augmented to be a better research platform and integrated across health care systems, EHRs could serve as the base for a comprehensive health research infrastructure. Large research cohorts have been developed that combine genetic, EHR, and other data sources to provide a data-rich approach to a variety of health questions. Mobile and wireless communications and computing provide the opportunity to monitor health indices and determinants between clinic visits and provide intensive longitudinal perspectives on the patterns and variability of health and health influences. Pockets of patient groups have already begun to collect these data on themselves and donate these data for research. If we can then integrate location data from individuals with the range of databases about exposures in those locations, the components of a comprehensive health research infrastructure are in place.

As clinical research transitions from a data-poor to data-rich science, it is imperative that we recognize the weaknesses of our current methods, born from a data-poor environment, and seriously consider and experiment with alternative methods more well-suited for a data-rich environment. As this transition continues, our methods will need to become more adaptive, intensively longitudinal, and dynamically computational. Fortunately, other sciences have made this transition, and with a thoughtful understanding of the differences between these sciences and ours, we can follow their example for developing a new data-rich clinical research science.

Disclaimer: The content of this chapter represent the views of the author and do not represent the views of the National Institutes of Health.

LIST OF ACRONYMS AND ABBREVIATIONS

CONSORT Consolidated Standards of Reporting Trials
EHR Electronic health record
EMA Ecological momentary assessment
EMI Ecological Momentary Interventions
FDA Food and Drug Administration
GUI Graphical user interface
IOM Institute of Medicine
JITAI Just-in-Time Adaptive Interventions
Lambda-CDM Lambda Cold Dark Matter
MOST Multiphase Optimization Strategy
NHST Null hypothesis statistical testing
NIH National Institutes of Health
PDA Personal digital assistant
PMI Precision Medicine Initiative
RCT Randomized controlled trial
SMART Sequential Multiple Assignment Randomized Trial

References

[1] Altman DG, Schulz KF, Moher D, Egger M, Davidoff F, Elbourne D, et al. The revised CONSORT statement for reporting randomized trials: explanation and elaboration. Ann Intern Med 2001;134(8):663–94.

[2] Higgins JPT, Green S. Cochrane handbook for systematic reviews of interventions. West Sussex: John Wiley and Sons; 2008.

[3] Graham R, Mancher M, Wolman DM, Greenfield S, Steinberg E. Clinical practice guidelines we can trust. Committee on standards for developing trustworthy clinical practice guidelines. Washington, DC: National Academies Press; 2011.

[4] National Comprehensive Cancer Network. NCCN guidelines. <http://www.nccn.org/professionals/physician_gls/f_guidelines.asp> [accessed 01.05.15].

[5] Clark DB, Taylor CB, Roth WT, Hayward C, Ehlers A, Margraf J, et al. Surreptitious drug use by patients in a panic disorder study. Am J Psychiatry 1990;147(4):507–9.

[6] Aguinis H, Beaty JC, Boik RJ, Pierce CA. Effect size and power in assessing moderating effects of categorical variables using multiple regression: a 30-year review. J Appl Psychol 2005;90:94–107.

[7] Skrepnek GH. The contrast and convergence of Bayesian and frequentist statistical approaches in pharmacoeconomic analysis. Pharmacoeconomics 2007;25(8):649–64.

[8] Wolff N. Using randomized controlled trials to evaluate socially complex services: problems, challenges and recommendations. J Ment Health Policy Econ 2000;3:97–109.

[9] Thompson SG. Why sources of heterogeneity in meta-analysis should be investigated. BMJ 1994;309:1351–5.

[10] NIMH policy for the recruitment of participants in clinical research. <http://www.nimh.nih.gov/funding/grant-writing-and-application-process/nimh-policy-for-the-recruitment-of-participants-in-clinical-research.shtml> [accessed 01.05.15].

[11] Balas EA, Boren SA. Managing clinical knowledge for health care improvement: yearbook of medical informatics. Stuttgart: Schattauer; 2000.

[12] Ioannidis JP. Effect of statistical significance of results on time to completion and publication of randomized efficacy trials. JAMA 1998;279:281–6.

[13] Riley WT, Glasgow RE, Etheredge L, Abernethy AP. Rapid, responsive, relevant (R3) research: a call for a rapid learning health research enterprise. Clin Transl Med 2013;2:10.

[14] Chimowitz MI, Lynn MJ, Derderyn CP, Turan TN, Fiorella D, for the SAMMPRIS Trial Investigators Stenting versus aggressive medical therapy for intracranial arterial stenosis. NEJM 2011;265:993–1003.

[15] Qureshi AI. Interpretations and implications of the prematurely terminated stenting and aggressive medical management for preventing recurrent stroke in the intracranial stenosis (SAMMPRIS) trial. Neurosurgery 2012;70:E264–8.

[16] Kohavi R, Longbotham R, Sommerfield D, Henne RM. Controlled experiments on the web: survey and practical guide. Data Min Knowl Disc 2009;18:140–81.

[17] Lutgens FK, Edward JT. Weather analysis and forecasting The atmosphere: an introduction to meteorology, 7th ed. Upper Saddle River, NJ: Prentice Hall; 1998, pp. 278–302.

[18] Shuman FG. History of numerical weather prediction at the National Meteorological Center. Wea Forecasting 1989;4:286–96.

[19] Ben-Menahem A. A concise history of mainstream seismology: origins, legacy, and perspectives. Bull Seismol Soc Am 1995;85(4):1202–25.

[20] Gubbins D. Seismology and plate tectonics. Cambridge: Cambridge University Press; 1990.

[21] Hey JS. The radio universe, 2nd ed. Oxford, NY: Pergamon Press; 1975.

[22] Woolfson M. Time, space, stars and man: the story of big bang, 2nd ed. London: World Scientific Publishing; 2013.

[23] World Bank. Health expenditure as a percent of GDP. <http://data.worldbank.org/indicator/SH.XPD.TOTL.ZS> [accessed 01.05.15].

[24] Köpcke F, Trinczek B, Majeed RW, Schreiweis B, Wenk J, Leusch T, et al. Evaluation of data completeness in the electronic health record for the purpose of patient recruitment into clinical trials: a retrospective analysis of element presence. BMC Med Inform Decis Mak 2013;13:37.

[25] Sarasohn-Kahn J. Making sense of sensors: how new technologies can change patient care. California Healthcare Foundation; 2013. <http://www.chcf.org/~/media/MEDIA%20LIBRARY%20Files/PDF/M/PDF%20MakingSenseSensors.pdf> [accessed 01.05.15].

[26] Nuckols JR, Ward MH, Jarup L. Using geographic information systems for exposure assessment in environmental epidemiology studies. Environ Health Perspect 2004;112(9):1007–15.

[27] Braveman P, Egerter S, Williams DR. The social determinants of health: coming of age. Annu Rev Public Health 2011;32:381–98.

[28] Abbas A, Khan SU. A review on the state-of-the-art privacy-preserving approaches in the e-health clouds. IEEE J Biomed Health Inform 2014;18(4):1431–41.

[29] Charles D, Gabriel M, Furukawa MF. Adoption of electronic health record systems among U.S. Non-federal acute care hospitals: 2008–2013, ONC Data Brief, no. 16. Washington, DC: Office of the National Coordinator for Health Information Technology; 2014.

[30] Ng K, Ghoting A, Steinhubl SR, Stewart WF, Malin B, Sun J. PARAMO: a PARAllel predictive MOdeling platform for healthcare analytic research using electronic health records. J Biomed Inform 2014;48:160–70.

[31] IOM (Institute of Medicine) Capturing social and behavioral domains and measures in electronic health records: Phase 2. Washington, DC: The National Academies Press; 2014.

[32] Pew Research Center. US smartphone use in 2015. <http://www.pewinternet.org/2015/04/01/us-smartphone-use-in-2015/> [accessed 01.05.15].

[33] Su JG, Jerrett M, Meng YY, Pickett M, Ritz B. Integrating smartphone based momentary location tracking with fixed site air quality monitoring for personal exposure assessment. Sci Total Environ 2015;506–507:518–26.

[34] Shiffman S, Stone AA, Hufford MR. Ecological momentary assessment. Annu Rev Clin Psychol 2008;4:1–32.

[35] Topol EJ, Steinhubl SR, Torkamani A. Digital medical tools and sensors. JAMA 2015;313(4):353–4.

[36] Dobkin BH. Wearable motion sensors to continuously measure real-world physical activities. Curr Opin Neurol 2013;26(6):602–8.

[37] Chan M, Estève D, Fourniols JY, Escriba C, Campo E. Smart wearable systems: current status and future challenges. Artif Intell Med 2012;56(3):137–56.

[38] Russell-Minda E, Jutai J, Speechley M, Bradley K, Chudyk A, Petrella R. Health technologies for monitoring and managing diabetes: a systematic review. J Diabetes Sci Technol 2009;3(6):1460–71.

[39] Alshaikh F, Ramzan F, Rawaf S, Majeed A. Social network sites as a mode to collect health data: a systematic review. J Med Internet Res 2014;16(7):e171.

[40] PatientsLikeMe. <https://www.patientslikeme.com> [accessed 01.05.15].

[41] 23andMe. <https://www.23andme.com/research/> [accessed 01.05.15].

[42] Quantified self. <http://quantifiedself.com> [accessed 01.05.15].

[43] Jin Y, Hammer B. Computational intelligence in big data. Comput Intell Mag IEEE 2014;9:12–13.

[44] Margolis R, Derr L, Dunn M, Huerta M, Larkin J, Sheehan J, et al. The National Institutes of Health's Big Data to Knowledge (BD2K) initiative: capitalizing on biomedical big data. J Am Med Inform Assoc 2014;21(6):957–8.

[45] Beck AH, Sangoi AR, Leung S, Marinelli RJ, Nielsen TO, van de Vijver MJ, et al. Systematic analysis of breast cancer morphology uncovers stromal features associated with survival. Sci Transl Med 2011;3(108):108–13.

[46] Byrne HM. Dissecting cancer through mathematics: from the cell to the animal model. Nat Rev Cancer 2010;10:221–30.

[47] Freestone DR, Karoly PJ, Nešić D, Aram P, Cook MJ, Grayden DB. Estimation of effective connectivity via data-driven neural modeling. Front Neurosci 2014;8:383.

[48] Siettos CI, Russo L. Mathematical modeling of infectious disease dynamics. Virulence 2013;4(4):295–306.

[49] Timms KP, Rivera DE, Piper ME, Collins LM. A hybrid model predictive control strategy for optimizing a smoking cessation intervention. Proc Am Control Conf 2014;2014:2389–94.

[50] Vugrin ED, Rostron BL, Verzi SJ, Brodsky NS, Brown TJ, Choiniere CJ, et al. Modeling the potential effects of new tobacco products and policies: a dynamic population model for multiple product use and harm. PLoS One 2015;10(3):e0121008.

[51] Leon AC, Davis LL, Kraemer HC. The role and interpretation of pilot studies in clinical research. J Psychiatr Res 2011;45(5):626–9.

[52] Tomlinson M, Rotheram-Borus MJ, Swartz L, Tsai AC. Scaling up mHealth: where is the evidence? PLoS Med 2013;10(2):e1001382.

[53] Barlow DH, Nock MK, Hersen M. Single case experimental designs. Strategies for studying behavior change, 3rd ed. Boston, MA: Allyn & Bacon; 2009.

[54] Jandoc R, Burden AM, Mamdani M, Lévesque LE, Cadarette SM. Interrupted time series analysis in drug utilization research is increasing: systematic review and recommendations. J Clin Epidemiol 2015;S0895–4356(15):00123–7.

[55] Zucker DR, Ruthhazer R, Schmid CH. Individual (N-of-1) trials can be combined to give population comparative treatment effect estimates: methodologic considerations. J Clin Epidemiol 2010;63(12):1312–23.

[56] Dallery J, Raiff BR. Optimizing behavioral health interventions with single-case designs: from development to dissemination. Transl Behav Med 2014;4(3):290–303.

[57] Collins LM, Murphy SA, Nair VN, Strecher VJ. A strategy for optimizing and evaluating behavioral interventions. Ann Behav Med 2005;30(1):65–73.

[58] Collins LM, Baker TB, Mermelstein RJ, Piper ME, Jorenby DE, Smith SS, et al. The multiphase optimization strategy for engineering effective tobacco use interventions. Ann Behav Med 2011;41(2):208–26.

[59] Almirall D, Nahum-Shani I, Sherwood NE, Murphy SA. Introduction to SMART designs for the development of adaptive interventions: with application to weight loss research. Transl Behav Med 2014;4(3):260–74.

[60] von Dinklage JJ, Ball D, Siilvestri GA. A review of clinical practice guidelines for lung cancer. J Thorac Dis 2013;5(Suppl. 5):S607–22.

[61] Collins LM, Murphy SA, Bierman KL. A conceptual framework for adaptive preventive interventions. Prev Sci 2004;5(3):185–96.

[62] Riley WT, Serrano KJ, Nilsen W, Atienza AA. Mobile and wireless technologies in health behavior and the potential for intensively adaptive interventions. Curr Opin Psychol 2015;5:67–71.

[63] Heron KE, Smyth JM. Ecological momentary interventions: incorporating mobile technology into psychosocial and health behaviour treatments. Br J Health Psychol 2010;15(Pt 1):1–39.

[64] Adams MA, Sallis JF, Norman GJ, Hovell MF, Hekler EB, Perata E. An adaptive physical activity intervention for overweight adults: a randomized controlled trial. PLoS One 2013;8(12):e82901.

[65] Lanza ST, Vasilenko SA, Liu X, Li R, Piper ME. Advancing the understanding of craving during smoking cessation attempts: a demonstration of the time-varying effect model. Nicotine Tob Res 2014(16 Suppl. 2):S127–34.

[66] Hedeker D, Mermelstein RJ, Demirtas H. Modeling between-subject and within-subject variances in ecological momentary assessment data using mixed-effects location scale models. Stat Med 2012;31(27):3328–36.

[67] Liao P, Klasnja P, Tewari A, Murphy SA. Micro-randomized trials in mHealth; 2015. <http://arxiv.org/pdf/1504.00238.pdf>.

[68] Savage JS, Downs DS, Dong Y, Rivera DE. Control systems engineering for optimizing a prenatal weight gain intervention to regulate infant birth weight. Am J Public Health 2014;104(7):1247–54.

[69] Zang Y, Lee JJ. Adaptive clinical trial designs in oncology. Chin Clin Oncol 2014;3(4):49.

[70] Etheredge LM. A rapid-learning health system. Health Aff 2007;26:W107–18.

[71] Psaty BM, Breckenridge AM. Mini-Sentinel and regulatory science—big data rendered fit and functional. N Engl J Med 2014;370(23):2165–7.

[72] Sudlow C, Gallacher J, Allen N, Beral V, Burton P, Danesh J, et al. UK biobank: an open access resource for identifying the causes of a wide range of complex diseases of middle and old age. PLoS Med 2015;12(3):e1001779.

[73] Tannen RL, Weiner MG, Xie D. Use of primary care electronic medical record database in drug efficacy research on cardiovascular outcomes: comparison of database and randomized controlled trial findings. Br Med J 2009;338:b81.

[74] Collins FS, Varmus H. A new initiative on precision medicine. N Engl J Med 2015;372(9):793–5.

CHAPTER

19

Creating a Health Information Technology Infrastructure to Support Comparative Effectiveness Research in Cancer

Susan K. Peterson PhD, MPH[1] and Kevin Patrick MD, MS[2]

[1]Department of Behavioral Science, University of Texas MD Anderson Cancer Center, Houston, TX, United States [2]Department of Family Medicine and Public Health, The Qualcomm Institute/Calit2, University of California-San Diego, San Diego, CA, United States

OUTLINE

19.1 Introduction	358		19.7.2 Use Case 2: Intervention to Manage Radiation Treatment-Related Side Effects in Head and Neck Cancers	366
19.2 Cancer CER: Gaps and Opportunities	358		19.7.3 Use Case 3: Survivorship Management, Specifically, Improving QOL in Colorectal Cancer Survivors	366
19.3 Health Information Technology Infrastructure for Improving CER	359		19.7.4 Use Case Results	367
19.4 Enhancing the Collection of Evidence to Inform Patient Care and CER Through Distance Medicine Technology	360		19.8 Strengthening the Capacity of the CER Infrastructure Through EHRs	367
19.5 Distance Medicine Technology in Cancer Care and Research	361		19.8.1 Use of Patient Portals in Oncology for Data Exchange and Retrieval	368
19.6 CYCORE: CYberinfrastructure for Cancer COmparative Effectiveness REsearch	361		19.8.2 Integrating Data From Multiple Sources to Support CER	368
19.6.1 CYCORE Architecture	364		19.9 Conclusion	369
19.7 Application of CYCORE Across the Cancer Prevention and Control Continuum to Accelerate CER	364		List of Acronyms and Abbreviations	369
			Acknowledgments	369
19.7.1 Use Case 1: Prevention of Cancer Risk and Sequelae Through Remote Monitoring of Long-Term Outcomes of Smoking Cessation Treatment	364		References	370

B. Hesse, D. Ahern & E. Beckjord: Oncology Informatics.
DOI: http://dx.doi.org/10.1016/B978-0-12-802115-6.00019-7

19.1 INTRODUCTION

Informatics infrastructures that integrate data from multiple traditional (ie, clinical trials) and nontraditional (eg, mobile, wearable, and home-based technologies) sources can inform comparative effectiveness research (CER) across the cancer prevention and care continuum. This includes information on care practices, patient engagement, and elucidation of patient-reported outcomes (PROs). Development of these platforms is in the early stages. Recent policy developments to expand coverage for health care and promote new methods of patient-centered CER have set the stage for accelerated efforts in this arena. This chapter outlines the background for these developments, provides examples of prototype systems that support new forms of CER, and discusses future directions and policy in supporting the creation and utilization of integrated informatics infrastructures.

19.2 CANCER CER: GAPS AND OPPORTUNITIES

In 2014, approximately 1.66 million Americans were diagnosed with cancer and 585,000 deaths were attributed to cancer-related pathologies [1]. Cancer-related health care expenditures approximate $228 billion annually [2]. There were an estimated 13.7 million cancer survivors in the United States in 2012 and the number is expected to increase to 18 million by 2022, including a growing number who will be on long-term therapy for the management of their disease [3,4]. While some breakthroughs in cancer prevention and treatment have occurred, advances in this complex disease lag far behind the progress seen in other diseases, such as cardiovascular disease [2]. Part of the problem may be that adherence to schedules of treatment or oral medication may interfere with the ability to ascertain the most effective treatments. For example, medication nonadherence is estimated to occur in approximately 50–75% of patients [5,6]. Genetic variability also may play a large role in response to treatment and remains largely unaccounted for, although the pace of discovery in this area is accelerating rapidly. Increasing evidence that lifestyle factors, such as diet, exercise, body weight status, supplement use, alcohol use, and continuing tobacco use (or exposure to secondhand smoke), significantly impacts the course of disease yet these are typically unaccounted for between and across trials [7–12]. Thus, greater progress in the prevention and treatment of cancer may be achieved if we can better assess and intervene on these factors, many of which are grounded in behavior.

The Institute of Medicine (IOM) has defined CER as "the generation and synthesis of evidence that compares the benefits and harms of alternative methods to prevent, diagnose, treat, and monitor a clinical condition or to improve the delivery of care. The purpose of CER is to assist consumers, clinicians, purchasers, and policy makers to make informed decisions that will improve health care at both the individual and population levels" [13]. CER is based on evaluating outcomes of an intervention in real-world settings and with populations that are broader than those typically included in randomized controlled trials that are the gold standard for evaluating efficacy. CER typically compares at least two interventions or approaches and results are intended to facilitate decision making by multiple groups, including but not limited to patients and the public, health care providers, and policy makers.

Rigorous methodological standards for CER were proposed in the Patient Protection and Affordable Care Act and the new Patient-Centered Outcomes Research Institute (PCORI) [14]. The emphasis on patient-centeredness in CER focuses research on the engagement of patients along with other key stakeholders throughout the entire research process. Importantly, it recognizes the need to account for diverse patient characteristics and health outcomes across diverse settings [15]. These efforts are consistent with the mission of PCORI and with other national policy efforts such as the Investing in Innovations Initiative by the Office of the National Coordinator for Health Information Technology (ONC) [16].

In the American Recovery and Reinvestment Act (ARRA) of 2009 (P.L. 111-5), the US Congress appropriated $1.1 billion to provide strong federal support of CER. IOM's 2009 report from the Committee on Initial National Priorities for CER [13] identified 100 priority health questions to be addressed by CER, including cancer-specific questions focused on behaviors and prevention, as follows:

- Compare the effectiveness of incorporating information about new biomarkers (including genetic information) with standard care in achieving health behavior change and improving clinical outcomes.
- Compare the effectiveness of interventions (eg, community-based multilevel interventions, simple health education, usual care) to reduce health disparities in multiple diseases and conditions, including cancer.
- Compare the effectiveness of different benefit design, utilization management, and cost-sharing strategies in improving health care access and quality in patients with cancer and other chronic diseases.
- Compare the effectiveness of film-screen or digital mammography alone and mammography plus

magnetic resonance imaging in community practice-based breast cancer screening in high-risk women at varying ages and race or ethnicity, and with different risk factors.

A more widespread application of CER approaches provides an opportunity to improve health outcomes and quality of care. However, gaps and limitations in CER research have been noted [17–19]. Many patient-centered research questions that could benefit from CER remain unanswered. Dissemination and translation of CER findings to patients and clinicians is suboptimal, resulting in missed opportunities for applying CER findings to improve patient outcomes. Traditionally, the data infrastructure for CER has been highly fragmented with sources of data limited in terms of clinical robustness, their ability to capture data longitudinally, and their ability to capture data at—and enable feedback or decision making at—the point of care. The ability to interconnect and integrate data sources with each other in a way that can inform health care decision-making also has been limited. There has been a limited focus in CER research on priority populations, and minimal attention has been paid to behavior change important for both the prevention and treatment of cancer. The need to focus on these latter issues in CER has been called out as a priority recommendation [17]. These have the potential to impact risk factors that are important in cancer prevention and survivorship, including decreasing obesity and increasing physical activity, decreasing tobacco use, and increasing adherence to medical therapies [17].

These gaps and limitations are apparent in cancer CER. Although the causes of over half of all cancers have been attributed to behaviors such as tobacco use, lifestyle behaviors, and low adherence to preventive recommendations, the routine collection of data related to behavioral factors is often not included in oncology clinical trials and clinical care [7]. It may be the case that our inability to make full progress against the prevention and treatment of cancer is due to our limitations in accounting for these factors. A broader and more robust effort to collect data related to behavioral risk factors and outcomes is needed to more fully realize the full benefits and impact of CER.

19.3 HEALTH INFORMATION TECHNOLOGY INFRASTRUCTURE FOR IMPROVING CER

As the emphasis on CER increases, and as expectations rise for the contributions of this research in the context of diminishing health care resources, gaps in both knowledge and the research infrastructure are emerging [13]. These gaps include limitations in methods for data capture, storage, integration, and analysis. To fully realize the promise of CER in achieving more informed decisions and better outcomes, the need to address these gaps will become more urgent [16,17].

In 2010, a presidential commission report noted the need for an integrated approach for health information technology (HIT) that links physicians, patients, consumers, researchers, and institutions within an information technology (IT)-enabled system [20,21]. Advantages to IT-enabled health care include reducing fragmented information, ensuring safer and better quality care, and aggregating data at the point of care as well as at the population level to assure meaningful use [20]. Fig. 19.1 provides an overview of IT applications in cancer care, highlighting their roles in supporting and empowering patients, and in supporting linkages and exchanges between patients and providers, between providers themselves, and between providers and health care systems. A technologically innovative cancer care environment that incorporates data from web-enabled mobile devices, integrated patient phenotype, and genotype databases for personalized treatment, and applications for real-time clinical decision support was envisioned over a decade ago [20,22]; yet technical, structural, ethical/legal, and cultural barriers to adopting this structure persist [20].

Goals of a HIT infrastructure to enhance CER include the following:

- Broadening the scope and quality of data that can be collected on factors that may contribute to prevention, treatment, and control outcomes, both for persons with a cancer diagnosis, as well as those at increased risk for the disease;
- Exploiting and improving upon software and database systems utilized in other scientific domains to efficiently increase capacity for larger and more complex data sets;
- Enabling the pursuit of new research questions not addressable using current systems by improving the integration of patient data captured through objective monitoring (ie, sensor capture) and/or self-reporting, and the subsequent analysis of those data;
- Providing decision support and patient adherence-monitoring for care providers; and
- Enabling patients to participate actively in their prevention and treatment regimens.

Achieving these goals can facilitate the conduct of CER, and in turn provide an opportunity to improve the quality and outcomes of health care by generating more and better information to support decisions by the public, patients, caregivers, clinicians, payers, and policy makers.

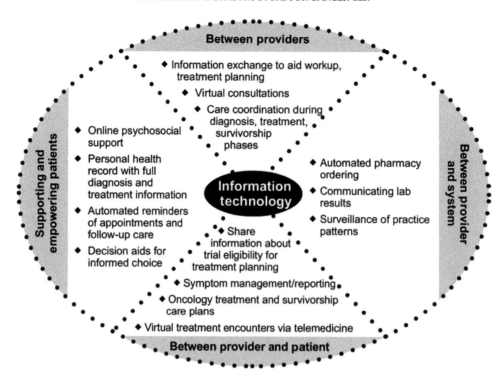

Between providers
- ◆ Information exchange to aid workup, treatment planning
- ◆ Virtual consultations
- ◆ Care coordination during diagnosis, treatment, survivorship phases

Supporting and empowering patients
- ◆ Online psychosocial support
- ◆ Personal health record with full diagnosis and treatment information
- ◆ Automated reminders of appointments and follow-up care
- ◆ Decision aids for informed choice

Information technology

Between provider and system
- ◆ Automated pharmacy ordering
- ◆ Communicating lab results
- ◆ Surveillance of practice patterns

- ◆ Share information about trial eligibility for treatment planning
- ◆ Symptom management/reporting
- ◆ Oncology treatment and survivorship care plans
- ◆ Virtual treatment encounters via telemedicine

Between provider and patient

FIGURE 19.1   An overview of IT applications in cancer care.

19.4 ENHANCING THE COLLECTION OF EVIDENCE TO INFORM PATIENT CARE AND CER THROUGH DISTANCE MEDICINE TECHNOLOGY

The ability to remotely monitor and intervene outside of the traditional clinic visit can be an added value to cancer care. Remote monitoring, or even consultations using telemedicine approaches, can allow health care providers to care for those patients who may have difficulty traveling or to provide enhanced follow-up care. The telemedicine sector is expected to grow at a rate of 18% through 2018, suggesting that such platforms could become standard of care in the future [23]. These systems can enable clinicians to identify potential problems early on, prior to a crisis point, and may facilitate prevention of problems through early intervention. These systems may be particularly useful in times of acute care when patients may benefit from additional support, such as following a hospital discharge after surgery. For example, patients who are discharged postsurgery can be sent home with a tablet so that clinicians can follow up via remote visits [24], enabling remote examination of surgical wounds and early detection of any potential problems. Coupled with physical activity monitors, clinicians can also monitor patients postsurgery to identify whether patients are making appropriate progress with their recovery. These technologies can increase patient engagement with their care, can

improve treatment outcomes, and can potentially reduce costs. This issue has become more important as a result of the Affordable Care Act. Recently discharged patients can incur on average $30,000 in nonreimbursable costs when they are readmitted within 30 days of an initial hospital discharge [25].

Systems that enable remote, real-time monitoring of patients' symptoms and other health-related outcomes may offer cost-effective strategies to optimize cancer care outside of the clinic setting [26,27]. Devices and systems that remotely collect and transmit health-related data that enable clinical decision making have been used successfully in the management of chronic diseases, including diabetes, asthma, heart failure, chronic obstructive pulmonary disease, and chronic wound management [28–33]. In conditions other than cancer, there is support for the use of remote monitoring to achieve improved patient quality of life (QOL), better symptom control and wound healing, reduced lower limb amputations, decreased emergency room visits and unplanned hospitalizations, fewer bed days of care, decreased nursing home admissions in the elderly, and decreased overall costs to the health system [32–35]. In contrast, recent evidence also suggested that home tele-monitoring in older adults with multiple chronic health conditions was not superior to usual care in reducing emergency room visits or inpatient hospitalizations [36], and surprisingly resulted in higher mortality among those who were tele-monitored. This suggests that there are many details to be worked out to ensure that these systems operate in a consistently productive way to improve health outcomes. The complex settings in which remote monitoring systems are deployed involve physician, patient, and health system factors, and how a monitoring program is organized, choice of technology, and staff and patient training also may influence their effectiveness [37]. Thus, there is a need for additional empiric research [37,38] to help define for which group of patients and under which circumstances remote monitoring is most appropriate and effective. This need may be particularly pronounced in oncology because of the multiple medical, behavioral, social, and contextual factors involved in cancer care.

19.5 DISTANCE MEDICINE TECHNOLOGY IN CANCER CARE AND RESEARCH

Much of cancer care occurs in the ambulatory care setting. Common treatments such as radiation therapy and chemotherapy are delivered on an outpatient basis. The increasing shift to oral chemotherapy and hormonal therapy for several cancers is leading to more cancer care being provided with reduced clinical contact with health care providers, and a greater reliance on patient adherence and management of day to day care. At the same time, many common treatments for cancer are associated with related toxicities that can often result in psychologically distressing and even potentially life-threatening side effects (eg, nausea, vomiting, mucositis, diarrhea, and febrile neutropenia) [39–45]. While some common side effects of cancer treatment, such as fatigue, are not necessarily life threatening, they have been associated with poorer treatment adherence and reduced QOL, and compromised psychological functioning [46–48]. Side effects such as fatigue also can persist well into survivorship and can have longer term effects on QOL well past the end of treatment. Given that most cancer care is delivered on an outpatient basis, patients are responsible for monitoring and managing a range of potentially diverse and complicated side effects without readily available clinical support. Patients are responsible for making potentially complex decisions about when to contact the treatment team in the event of new, escalating, or unexpected side effects.

Remote monitoring of cancer-related symptoms and similar outcomes may be a cost-effective strategy to optimize care for cancer survivors, particularly during times of acute care. As noted above, remote monitoring of health-related outcomes has been used on an increasing basis in other chronic diseases such as heart disease and hypertension. Thus, the technological capability to remotely and objectively capture data on patient symptoms as well as PROs, and to transmit those data for monitoring and interpretation by a member of the clinical care team, may become a powerful disease management tool in cancer. Enabling this data capture in real time or near real time may become a particularly valuable feature in cancer care and survivorship, as many patients may live at significant distances from specialized centers where they receive cancer care.

Prototype systems for the remote real-time monitoring of cancer patients have been described and positive outcomes reported [26]. However, these findings exist primarily for systems that collect PROs via telecommunications technologies [38,49]. These systems have commonly used a smartphone or automated interactive telephone calls for the reporting of adverse effects by patients to their primary cancer treatment centers. When the adverse effects reach a predefined threshold of severity, the systems often generate alerts for response.

While prototype remote monitoring systems that combine biometric and self-reported data for cancer patients have been conceptualized [50,51], few studies report the efficacy of such systems. The ability to effectively engage patients outside of the traditional clinic setting using distance medicine technologies has multiple advantages, including:

- Increased efficiency in clinical trials through new methods of continuous data collection (and thus potentially the need for fewer participants);
- Collection of new types of data to yield a greater understanding of treatment effects;
- Improved ability to monitor treatment adherence, symptoms, side effects, and toxicities, both objectively as well as through PROs; and
- The ability to generate, synthesize, and fuse different types of data to identify trends relevant to prevention and survivorship, which in turn can inform CER and rapid learning systems in oncology.

19.6 CYCORE: CYBERINFRASTRUCTURE FOR CANCER COMPARATIVE EFFECTIVENESS RESEARCH

Recognition is growing about the need to incorporate behavioral, environmental, and psychological data into cancer prevention and care whenever possible; for example, data on adherence to treatment protocols or lifestyle behaviors [9]. The CYberinfrastructure for COmparative effectiveness REsearch (CYCORE) project has been working toward this goal to develop a prototype cyberinfrastructure (CI) that enables more comprehensive and valid collection and analyses of data from a multitude of domains [5]. Supported by the National Cancer Institute (NCI), CYCORE directly addresses several primary gaps in cancer CER as noted in the Report to the President and Congress on CER [17], namely: (1) the limited focus on behavior change interventions reflected in CER; and (2) limitations in data infrastructure, including fragmented data, lack of clinical robustness, and lack of a data capture and feedback loop at the point of care. As a result, the work accomplished in the initial CYCORE project has begun to advance the science of incorporating behavioral and other health-related outcome assessment methods in the context of cancer prevention and control research. CYCORE's design utilizes a novel approach of objective, home-based assessment of cancer patients, their caregivers, and their health care providers, which has resulted in a more robust and complete picture of health-related outcomes at a time when patients are on active treatment yet away from the clinic setting. The approach to developing CYCORE is user-centered in that it promotes the active engagement of patients, caregivers, and clinicians by establishing user-friendly, patient-accessible platforms for direct entry of their personal health information as well as interfaces that enable clinicians, researchers, and patients to track these data and view trends, which facilitates assessment of research endpoints and supports clinical decision making [5]. CYCORE accomplishes these goals through the following features: (1) patient accessible platforms for direct entry of data; (2) remote patient monitoring and management; (3) sensors, ecological momentary assessment (EMA), video interfaces that allow clinicians and researchers to track data in real time and view trends; (4) interoperable data systems that support integration with electronic health records (EHRs) and research data sources; (5) reduced reliance on manual aggregation of data which in turn increases efficiency of analysis; and (6) infrastructure that enables the collection and analysis of data from new sources so that study questions can evolve over time.

The overarching goal of the CYCORE project has been to develop a comprehensive, state-of-the-art cyber-platform that will enable large-scale and robust CER across the cancer continuum, that is, from cancer prevention, to cancer treatment, and ultimately to cancer control and survivorship care. The need for such an infrastructure is great given that cancer is a complex disease and we are still a long way from cure. Overcoming the cancer challenge likely lies in our ability to conduct CER in a way that enables synthesis of data from multiple sources: not only data from clinical trials, but those data that exist in other domains and have not yet been collected in the most rigorous fashion. Some domains may exist outside of health care settings where data may be less standardized but nonetheless potentially valuable. For example, lifestyle behaviors captured via consumer-focused technologies may be of unproven validity and reliability, but may be better than current methods of self-report. Also, data on

supplement use and potential exposure to environmental carcinogens may add to an understanding of the totality of influences on cancer treatment and outcomes.

In the long run, this effort will require integrating information obtained from many heterogeneous sources, including electronic medical records (EMRs), sensing and imaging devices, data sets from multiple studies, web-based user interfaces, and more. For the information to be analyzed in meaningful ways, and the results disseminated in a user-friendly fashion to medical providers and their patients, the data structures for the information must then be made compatible. As a start to this process, CYCORE combines a home-based technology (eg, the Home Health Hub (HHH)) with mobile phone or tablet-based assessments to permit passive data capture and two-way exchange between doctor and patient in support of monitoring physiological, behavioral, and experiential parameters outside of the clinic setting. CYCORE also incorporates algorithms and statistically rigorous analytical tools that drive data collection rules and provide decision support, in near real time, to researchers and medical providers, in support of optimizing cancer treatment and prevention of negative sequelae.

CYCORE has been developed to be fully compatible with other large-scale IT support systems that currently exist in oncology, and has begun to fill important gaps present in today's systems; for example, how data are collected from cancer patients outside of the clinical setting, such as in their homes and communities. CYCORE also has taken an innovative approach to aggregating, analyzing, and using those data.

The combination of human and environmental interfaces for CYCORE; infrastructure processes (eg, secure, scalable transportation, storage, and processing of data); various data analysis tools; and stakeholders' policy requirements continues to yield significant scientific insight not only on the clinical side, but also into the construction and maintenance of systems at this scale. In developing CYCORE, we have directly addressed the following research questions:

- How to respond to changes in requirements over time?
- What architectural patterns would work to provide an extensible framework to deal with new data sources?
- How to distribute information, while addressing cross-cutting concerns such as privacy and security?
- How to manage the lifecycle of all resources, such as sensors, data, studies, policies, and algorithms, in a scalable and adaptable manner throughout the life span of the system?
- How to collect and integrate data from various kinds of sensors, which might experience failures,

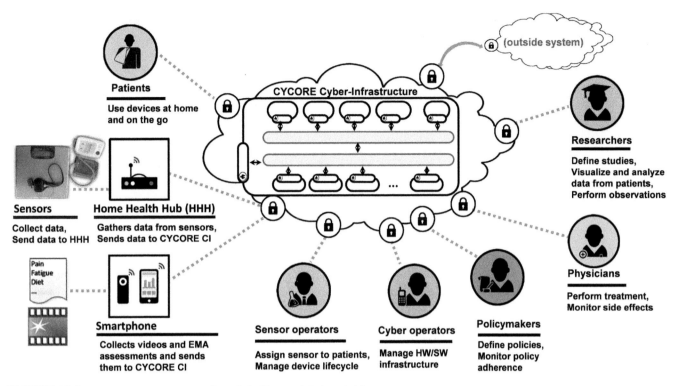

FIGURE 19.2 CYCORE's use case-specific stakeholders and their activities.

intermittent connectivity with the system, and unreliable data transfer?

- How to abstract from the complexity of the hardware and networking infrastructure and expose their services in a transparent way?

Fig. 19.2 depicts CYCORE's use case-specific stakeholders and their activities. As an example, consider the scenario of a head and neck cancer patient who has just completed the first of 35 daily radiation therapy sessions she will have over the next 7 weeks. As her therapy proceeds, her symptoms will rapidly worsen: at weeks 2–3, she can expect a sore throat, irritated skin, and decreased taste; by weeks 4–5, she will face pain at rest and when swallowing, resulting in decreased eating; by week 6 through 2–3 weeks posttreatment, she will experience intense pain, mouth sores, and peeling of the skin. Although this patient will see her radiation oncology physician on a weekly basis, her greatly diminished swallowing capability places her at high risk for dehydration while she is at home, which can—and frequently does—lead to an emergency room visit or hospitalization. With CYCORE, the patient takes daily measurements related to dehydration risk (blood pressure, pulse, and weight); and uses a smartphone to self-report dehydration-related symptoms, urine color, and dietary and fluid intake. These self-report

questions, called EMAs, are triggered by the smartphone according to a schedule determined by the researcher. Plugged in at her home is a miniature computer (the HHH) that collects the data wirelessly from the various devices and sends it to CYCORE's backend services. Clinicians and researchers monitor these data daily to determine if intervention is warranted. After securing an Institutional Review Board (IRB)-approved protocol, researchers use CYCORE to collect, store, and visualize their participant data. As sensor operators, research staff members register new sensors and assign sensors to participants, while CYCORE's cyberinfrastructure correctly maps the data to participants, and elucidates sensor malfunctions. A researcher following a head and neck cancer patient may wish to monitor adherence to swallowing exercises or smoking cessation protocols. CYCORE's smartphone programming allows the participant to self-record videos from home, which are then uploaded for monitoring. This scenario shows how each stakeholder has a unique way of interacting with the system to achieve their goals. The CI supports user roles and provides access to CYCORE capabilities according to the access rights of each role. Fig. 19.3 shows that people, devices, or outside systems connect to CYCORE securely and that each has a tailored entry point to the system, such that only the relevant subset of capabilities is accessed.

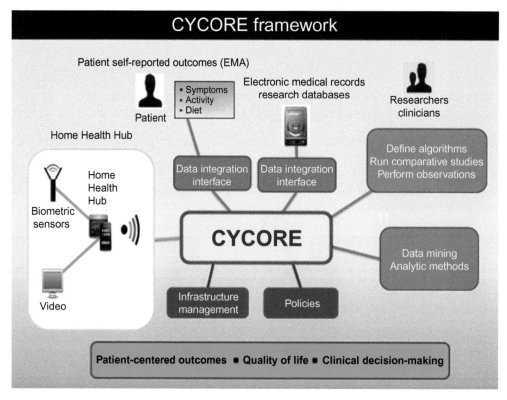

FIGURE 19.3   People, devices, or outside systems connect to CYCORE securely and each has a tailored entry point to the system.

19.6.1 CYCORE Architecture

To facilitate the integration of system capabilities into a scalable infrastructure, CYCORE has been built as a service-oriented architecture, a paradigm of software development that provides loose coupling between its various system services. Services are the mechanism by which specific needs (eg, a researcher's need to visualize data in a web browser) and capabilities (eg, obtaining data from sensors) are brought together within a single software system [18]. Service-oriented architectures promote independent development and reuse of software components that, in turn, reduce development cost. In addition, they provide the means to offer, discover, and interact with CYCORE's capabilities (eg, acquiring sensor data, storing and linking data from various sensors, processing data and displaying graphs, or exporting data to software packages normally used for CER outcomes assessment). All functional capabilities and resources are represented as services in CYCORE, with precisely defined service–access protocols based on message exchange. Moreover, the CYCORE system has requirements for privacy, security, fault tolerance, dependability, scalability, and flexibility. The system also ensures scalability, so CYCORE can grow as new needs are identified, and new users engage with the system without changes to the underlying CI.

19.7 APPLICATION OF CYCORE ACROSS THE CANCER PREVENTION AND CONTROL CONTINUUM TO ACCELERATE CER

We initially demonstrated the capabilities of CYCORE in use cases that represented real-world, challenging problems across the cancer prevention and control continuum (Fig. 19.4) [50]. The overall system design was informed by an intensive requirements gathering process that involved more than 120 stakeholders, including research investigators and staff; clinicians (eg, physicians, physician assistants, nurses, speech pathologists, dietitians); administrators; policy makers; and informatics/IT experts [5]. Based on these findings, we formulated use cases in three patient and survivor populations that represented different phases across the cancer continuum (Fig. 19.4), as described in the following sections.

19.7.1 Use Case 1: Prevention of Cancer Risk and Sequelae Through Remote Monitoring of Long-Term Outcomes of Smoking Cessation Treatment

Tobacco is the most preventable cause of death in the United States [1], and is associated with increased risk

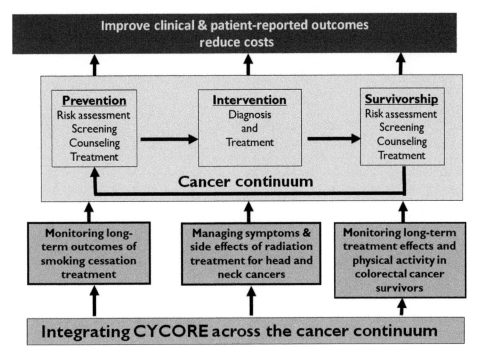

FIGURE 19.4 Different phases across the cancer continuum.

of at least 15 types of cancer. Tobacco use is responsible for more than 440,000 deaths annually, including those caused by secondhand smoke, and is responsible for at least 30% of all cancer deaths [1]. Cancer patients who continue to smoke after their diagnosis are at risk for increased complications during treatment, increased risk for developing other cancers, and decreased survival compared to nonsmokers [52].

The University of Texas MD Anderson Cancer Center's Tobacco Treatment Program (TTP) is an evidence-based program that provides comprehensive, state-of-the-art tobacco cessation services to MD Anderson Cancer Center patients and their family members [53,52]. Services include in-person, phone-based, and/or webcam behavioral counseling; nicotine replacement therapies; and tobacco-treatment prescription medication [54]. Typically, patients receive six to eight counseling sessions with long-term follow-up at 3-month intervals for up to a year following completion of tobacco treatment [55].

The goal of this use case was to evaluate the feasibility of using CYCORE to engage patients who had completed the TTP in daily monitoring of expired carbon monoxide (CO). During smoking, CO is readily absorbed from the lungs into the bloodstream. A unique feature of CO exposure is that the carboxyhemoglobin (COHb) in the blood represents a useful biological marker of the dose that the individual has received, making it a useful measure of the degree of smoke intake. The level of COHb in the blood is commonly determined indirectly by measuring CO levels in expired air. The measurement of expired air has the advantages of ease, speed, and relatively good subject acceptance.

CO monitors are widely used for validating self-reported smoking status in clinical and community trials. However, given the elimination half-life time of COHb, regular smokers who abstain for several hours at a time may present expired CO readings that do not accurately reflect their true smoking behavior. The ability to measure CO several times a day as part of CYCORE reduces the error, increases the precision of measurement of smoking, and strengthens validation of the self-reported smoking status.

CYCORE supported the use of a small, lightweight and portable CO monitor for home use by patients in this study. Patients who had completed their 1-year follow-up time point for the TTP, and who self-reported as current or former smokers were recruited to the study. The monitor used a single switch operation with an LED display that displayed carbon monoxide levels parts per million and percent COHb to users. Patients were instructed to use these monitors three times daily by blowing into a disposable mouthpiece over two nonconsecutive 1-week time periods. Patients also completed daily EMAs regarding smoking behavior via a smartphone application. Data from the CO monitor and smartphone EMA application were uploaded daily via the HHH to CYCORE, where the data were available for viewing and analysis.

19.7.2 Use Case 2: Intervention to Manage Radiation Treatment-Related Side Effects in Head and Neck Cancers

Radiation-based treatment for head and neck cancers has been associated with 20–30% rates of ≥ grade 3 mucositis and 40–90% rates in patients receiving concomitant chemotherapy [56,57]. Radiation-initiated mucositis occurs within 3 weeks of treatment inducement, peaks during weeks 5–7, and can result in painful swallowing and chronic dysphagia for an extended period [57]. It rarely occurs in isolation. Rather, mucositis typically appears concomitant with pain, difficulty swallowing and speaking, fatigue, and taste alterations, triggering altered eating and drinking capabilities, which in turn, create a climate for nutritional deficiencies and dehydration [57–60] and prompt increased expenditures on supportive care, hospitalizations, and emergency room visits [57,61]. Patients experiencing mucositis may risk having cancer-related treatment dose reductions and delays required for tissue recovery [57]. Risk factors for malnutrition and dehydration during radiation treatment include severe pretreatment weight loss, tumor site of nasopharynx or base of tongue, and concurrent chemotherapy.

Typically, standard of care for head and neck cancer patients undergoing radiation treatment includes a once weekly clinical evaluation by the radiation oncologist (vital signs, pain, nutritional/hydration status). The nutritionist is seen as needed, with the first time typically occurring during the initial 2 weeks of treatment. In addition, a speech therapist consults with patients as needed. Clinical considerations during each visit include supportive care and alterations in pain medications and need for feeding tube or intravenous fluids based on nutrition/hydration status. Unfortunately, the onset of dehydration can rapidly develop between weekly visits, resulting in increased emergency room visits and inpatient admissions. Earlier identification of physiological decline via home assessments of blood pressure, heart rate, weight, and eating or drinking difficulties can enable preemptive clinic-based treatments, while reducing hospitalization-associated costs and interruptions in cancer-related radiation treatments [61].

The goal of this use case was to evaluate the feasibility of using CYCORE to enable head and neck cancer patients in sensor-based home monitoring for risk of dehydration during their radiation treatment period. With CYCORE, patients took daily measurements related to dehydration risk (blood pressure, pulse, and weight); and used a smartphone to self-report dehydration-related symptoms, urine color, and dietary and fluid intake. The HHH transmits the data from the various devices and sends it to CYCORE's backend services. The patient's physician then monitored these diverse data that same day via his computer or mobile device, and was able to determine if clinical intervention might be warranted. Data were collected during weeks 1 or 2, and weeks 4 or 5, during the typical 6-week radiation treatment period.

19.7.3 Use Case 3: Survivorship Management, Specifically, Improving QOL in Colorectal Cancer Survivors

Colorectal cancer is the third most common cancer for both men and women in the United States, with more than 136,000 new cases diagnosed in 2014 [1]. Although long-term survival for patients diagnosed with metastasis is typically low [62], many patients live for several years after diagnosis. Median survival for patients with unresectable metastatic disease who receive multiagent chemotherapy regimens ranges from 23 to 32 months [63,64]. There are an increasing number of chemotherapeutic agents available [62]; as treatment options increase and survival time lengthens, it becomes even more critical to focus on enhancing the functioning and QOL of patients with metastatic disease. This group represents a growing population of cancer survivors whose disease will be managed long term by successive chemotherapy regimens and/or maintenance chemotherapy. The cancer survivorship issues of this population are understudied, and interventions are needed to help them address needs such as maintenance of physical functioning and symptom and toxicity management.

While health-related QOL after colorectal cancer diagnosis appears to be similar or only slightly lower than in the general population [65,66], certain symptoms such as depression, diarrhea, fatigue, and insomnia remain problems for survivors [66], and younger patients seem to suffer the greatest QOL deficits. In studies of health-related QOL among long-term survivors, however, patients with advanced disease are underrepresented. Assessment of QOL among stage IV colorectal patients receiving chemotherapy indicates increased fatigue, sleep disturbance, and side effects, and decreases in physical functioning and global QOL during the treatment process [67]. Physical well-being is lower in survivors with stage IV colorectal cancer compared with those who have earlier stage disease [68]. Longitudinal studies show that the overall health-related QOL of survivors of stage I, II, and III colorectal cancer either improves after diagnosis or declines and then subsequently improves, but QOL of survivors with stage IV disease declines after diagnosis and remains low [68]. Issues associated with toxicity, such as diarrhea, nausea, vomiting, and fatigue, may vary according to treatment regimen; the impact of treatment-related toxicity may affect a patient's treatment decisions, QOL, and activities of daily living [69]. While considerable progress is being made in treating advanced colorectal cancer, increased research attention is needed on interventions to improve the quality, as well as quantity of life for this survivor group.

Physical activity has been found to improve QOL in cancer survivors and also can positively impact recurrence risk and survival [11,70–72]. This use case demonstrated the feasibility of having colorectal cancer survivors engage in self-monitoring of parameters relevant to physical activity, including time periods during treatment and while off active treatment. Survivors used multiple sensors over 2 nonconsecutive weeks, including an accelerometer, heart rate monitor, and global positioning system monitor. In addition, survivors completed assessments on physical activity and cancer-related symptoms on a varying daily schedule using an EMA application delivered via a smartphone. These data were transmitted to CYCORE via HHH's in survivors' homes.

19.7.4 Use Case Results

Across all three use cases, an average of 96% of patients completed the studies, demonstrating that it is highly feasible to expect that patients across a diverse range of diseases and treatment conditions will successfully engage in remote monitoring [73]. We administered questionnaires assessing patients' perspectives regarding usability and feasibility of remote monitoring, and responses indicated a very high degree of satisfaction with using the sensors and devices for collection and transmission of the data. Mean scores on ratings of ease of use, self-efficacy regarding remote monitoring, provision of data to health care providers, and perceived utility of the data typically exceeded 9 on scales that rated satisfaction from 0 (lowest) to 10 (highest) scale.

In addition, the head and neck cancer use case yielded important preliminary findings [74]. Sensor data revealed that dehydration-related events occurred in at least 60% of patients who engaged in remote monitoring, with 35% of patients experiencing two or more such events. Dehydration events also were significantly associated with several symptoms including nausea ($p = 0.004$), vomiting ($p = 0.004$), and swallowing difficulty ($p = 0.004$), with pain approaching statistical significance ($p = 0.74$). These findings indicated that, in addition to being a feasible and acceptable assessment method, CYCORE also identified important signs and symptoms in near real time that may warrant clinical intervention. Systems such as CYCORE that collect data to address current gaps in CER also may offer more immediate clinical benefit to patients and providers and may enable more rapid clinical decision making and responsiveness. We are presently conducting an NCI-funded randomized controlled trial to identify whether the use of CYCORE during radiation therapy for head and neck cancer reduces hospitalizations and emergency care visits related to dehydration, compared to usual care.

19.8 STRENGTHENING THE CAPACITY OF THE CER INFRASTRUCTURE THROUGH EHRs

In recent years, transition to EMRs has emerged as a key priority for the US health care system [75,76]. The advantages of EMRs are widely embraced in oncology care, and include improved documentation and data availability, streamlined order entry to decrease medical errors, and facilitation of clinical reminders to increase rates of recommended screening [77]. Further, the ability to electronically mine vast amounts of clinical data available through these records is a tremendous advantage for researchers, policy makers, payers, and others including CER investigators. To accelerate progress in the transition from paper charts to electronic records, the US Department of Health and Human Services initiated financial incentives beginning in 2011 for health care providers who demonstrated meaningful use of HIT.

Systems that engage patients and enable the collection of their data, along with the ability to integrate those data with EMRs, also can serve as robust data sources for CER. Patient portals are web-based or mobile applications that enable patients to access selected data from their EHRs, and in some cases, communicate with their health care providers [78]. Often, the portal is a component of the HER and may include lab reports, imaging studies, pathology reports, medication lists, and in some cases, doctors' and hospital notes. Early prototypes enabled viewing of clinical data from the medical record, and later enhancements included opportunities for patients to schedule appointments, refill prescriptions, and engage in secure messaging with health care providers. Some portals enable online "virtual visits" between health care providers and patients to evaluate health conditions. Such visits are likely to be limited to simple, straightforward conditions like respiratory infections and back pain; however, this type of use is not widespread in oncology care.

The utility of patient portals may be strengthened when the two-way exchange of information is amplified to enable patients to provide information relevant to their ongoing care and management of their disease, such as information regarding medication adherence and adverse effects. In regard to adverse effects from medications, patients experiencing such effects may not attribute those symptoms to the drugs that they are taking. This may be particularly true for cancer patients who often use multiple medications for both managing their primary disease as well as comorbid conditions that are related or unrelated to their cancers. It is not uncommon for patients to underreport adverse drug effects to their physicians, even if they suspect that their symptoms are related to their medications, and physicians also may not routinely and actively solicit such information [79,80]. Nevertheless, information on adverse drug effects and adherence can be important in CER as it can better inform findings related to medication effectiveness. Systems that engage patients and enable the collection of data related to problems and barriers to medication adherence, along with the ability to integrate those data with EHRs, also can serve as robust data sources for CER.

One example of such a system implemented in primary care is Patient Gateway, a patient portal linked to an EHR, developed by Partners HealthCare, an integrated delivery network formed by Massachusetts General Hospital and Brigham and Women's Hospital [81]. Patient Gateway includes a medications module that allows patients to view and modify their medication and allergy information in the EHR, and report medication side effects, nonadherence and other medication-related problems. These PROs can be communicated to the health care team and updated within the EHR as needed. Integrating behavioral data such as medication adherence along with other PRO data such as drug-related symptoms enhances the quality of data that can be obtained from EMRs for CER.

19.8.1 Use of Patient Portals in Oncology for Data Exchange and Retrieval

Patient-facing data capture applications, such as patient portals within EHR systems, have the potential to enhance CER and ultimately the quality of care; [82] however, their full potential and impact have not yet been realized. In oncology, patient portals are increasingly available and are a consistent feature in commercially available EMR systems that are used by cancer centers and other cancer health care providers. Providers and patients are still becoming accustomed to how portals fit into the traditional cancer care model, although patients indicate a high degree of interest in having direct access to information such as test results provided through these portals, and in using them to engage with their clinicians [75]. The use of patient portals have not been well-studied in oncology [83–87]. One of the initial studies to examine the use of portals in a cancer center setting found that patients' adoption and use doubled on an annual basis [88]. However, this study, like similar studies conducted in care settings other than oncology, suggests disparities in portal use based on age, education, and race or ethnicity. For example, older, less educated, and non-White patients may be less likely to use portals and/or to use them less frequently [89]. These disparities in portal use are similar to those observed in adoption or use of other technological applications

and offer evidence of a continuing "digital divide" in fuller adoption of such technologies in cancer care. When considering the role of portals as patient-facing data collection methods, the limitations introduced by such disparities in use must be considered, as well as the resulting impact on data quality and representativeness.

Nonetheless, data exchange through patient portals interconnected with EMRs in oncology care may introduce particular advantages for CER. Because longitudinal outpatient care in oncology may be more intensive compared with other medical specialties, there is an opportunity for increased and more continuous flow of data between portal-based patient health records and the EMR. As noted earlier, the expansion of CI within the health care IT environment can expand the capacity for the amount and type of data collected, capabilities for storage and analytics, interoperability within and between systems, and opportunities for patient engagement [90]. In addition to expanding the capacity for conducting CER, a CI-enabled system also could serve as an intervention platform for patients and providers. Such a system could integrate patient facing portals for the intake of multiple forms of data, such as objectively collected sensor-based data on behavioral, physiological and environmental outcomes as well as PROs. In turn, these data could generate opportunities for behavioral support and change interventions for patients as well as decision support for clinicians.

The actual impact that portals integrated with EMRs have on clinical care has not been well established. Use of patient portals has resulted in modest improvements in treatment adherence in diseases or conditions other than cancer and patient perception of control, and little if any change in other health-related outcomes [91,92]. As in other medical specialties, implementing this technology in cancer care practice raises questions of cost, security, assignment of rights and responsibilities, and liability. From a clinical perspective, disease complexity and severity in cancer populations raise additional considerations for patients and providers [88].

19.8.2 Integrating Data From Multiple Sources to Support CER

For EHRs to transform care and improve CER, they will need to include measures on a much wider range of health-relevant parameters than they do presently [93]. A promising approach to improving measurement capabilities in CER is the integration of health behavior and PROs, and environmental data from population surveys into research data warehouses to support patient-centered CER. The Washington Heights/Inwood Informatics Infrastructure for Comparative Effectiveness Research (WICER) is an example of a patient-centered research data warehouse that links electronic clinical data from

New York Presbyterian Hospital's clinical data warehouse with the same data from ambulatory care, long-term care, and home health settings, and with data from a population-based health survey that is focused on social determinants of health and health behaviors [94]. A goal of WICER is to facilitate CER for improving community health in Washington Heights and Inwood, a primarily Latino community of New York City. WICER's approach facilitates the ability to conduct CER utilizing the unique contributions of a variety of data sources. The application of geocoding to link data in the WICER research data warehouse could further enhance patient-centered CER by integrating potentially important socioeconomic and physical environment influences on health outcomes.

19.9 CONCLUSION

The American Society of Clinical Oncology (ASCO) has emphasized the need to more fully integrate communication and IT into cancer care so that patients' experiences can more readily inform clinical research and improve patient care [76]. This will require a systems approach that enables greater and more rapid access of patients' health data to better understand therapeutic responses, side effects, QOL, comorbidities and general health status. Such an approach will undoubtedly benefit, and may potentially transform, the conduct of CER and its ability to more effectively translate findings into improving the care that we provide to persons throughout the cancer continuum, from primary prevention through management of challenging treatments and into survivorship care. In turn, this approach also may accelerate discovery of useful and practical information concerning the most effective interventions and health care services for particular situations, and thus better inform decision making by both health care providers and patients.

This chapter has highlighted several recent technological advances that have begun to illuminate new ways of assessing outcomes that are important to both patients and providers. The advent of sensor technology brings tremendous opportunities for expanding our ability to collect more robust data related to health behaviors, treatment impact, survivorship, and QOL. The evidence base for these technologies in cancer care and prevention is still limited. However, the highly encouraging findings from projects like CYCORE demonstrate that implementing sensor and related technology for remote monitoring and assessment is highly feasible and acceptable to patients and providers, adds value to patient care and to the patient experience, and that it may be cost-effective as well. In turn, data captured via these systems permit an unprecedented opportunity to examine, from a more granular perspective, important outcomes that can directly impact CER. Meeting the HIT goals proposed by

organizations such as ASCO is not without challenges, however. IT infrastructure must be responsive to data capture needs across the cancer continuum, including support for longitudinal and continuous data collection while managing legal and policy concerns, including but not limited to the Health Insurance Portability and Accountability Act of 1996 (HIPAA) and patient privacy. This suggests a need for adaptive technologies and agile development methods that continuously incorporate patient and provider feedback. As with any technology or practice shift, there are bound to be barriers to acceptability, which may be best overcome through user-centered research and development. To that end, resources will be needed to identify the opportunities and constraints in accelerating the use and implementation of new health IT approaches to expand the evidence base for implementation. Finally, sustainability is a long-term goal that requires attention throughout the technology adoption and evaluation process. Many questions exist about how these technologies fit into—and indeed perhaps transform—work flows for the cancer prevention and treatment community and cancer-related outcomes at a population level. The work described in this chapter sets the stage to answer some of these questions.

LIST OF ACRONYMS AND ABBREVIATIONS

ASCO American Society of Clinical Oncology
CER Comparative effectiveness research
CI Cyberinfrastructure
CYCORE Cyberinfrastructure for comparative effectiveness research
HER Electronic health record
EMA Ecological momentary assessment
EMRs Electronic medical records
HIPAA Health Insurance Portability and Accountability Act of 1996
HIT Health information technology
HHH Home health hub
IOM Institute of Medicine
IRB Institutional Review Board
IT Information technology
NCI National Cancer Institute
ONC Office of the National Coordinator for Health Information Technology
PCORI Patient-Centered Outcomes Research Institute
PROs Patient-reported outcomes
QOL Quality of life
TTP Tobacco Treatment Program at The University of Texas MD Anderson Cancer Center
WICER Washington Heights/Inwood Informatics Infrastructure for Comparative Effectiveness Research

Acknowledgments

The authors wish to acknowledge the following sources of support for work that is described in this chapter: the National Cancer Institute, National Institutes of Health (RC2A 148263-01, R01CA177914-01,

R01CA177996-01); and, the Patient-Reported Outcomes, Survey, and Population Research Shared Resource (CA 16672) as well as e-Health Technology (Duncan Family Institute for Cancer Prevention and Risk Assessment), at the University of Texas MD Anderson Cancer Center.

References

[1] American Cancer Society. Cancer Facts and Figures 2014. Atlanta: American Cancer Society; 2014.

[2] Allan J, Barwick TA, Cashman S, Cawley JF, Day C, Douglass CW, et al. Clinical prevention and population health: curriculum framework for health professions. Am J Prev Med 2004;27(5):471–6.

[3] Rowland JH, Kent EE, Forsythe LP, Loge JH, Hjorth L, Glaser A, et al. Cancer survivorship research in Europe and the United States: where have we been, where are we going, and what can we learn from each other? Cancer 2013;119(Suppl. 11):2094–108.

[4] de Moor JS, Mariotto AB, Parry C, Alfano CM, Padgett L, Kent EE, et al. Cancer survivors in the United States: prevalence across the survivorship trajectory and implications for care. Cancer Epidemiol Biomarkers Prev 2013;22(4):561–70.

[5] DiMatteo MR. Variations in patients' adherence to medical recommendations: a quantitative review of 50 years of research. Med Care 2004;42(3):200–9.

[6] Vermeire E, Hearnshaw H, Van Royen P, Denekens J. Patient adherence to treatment: three decades of research. A comprehensive review. J Clin Pharm Ther 2001;26(5):331–42.

[7] Gritz ER, Dresler C, Sarna L. Smoking, the missing drug interaction in clinical trials: ignoring the obvious. Cancer Epidemiol Biomarkers Prev 2005;14(10):2287–93.

[8] Bairati I, Meyer F, Jobin E, Gelinas M, Fortin A, Nabid A, et al. Antioxidant vitamins supplementation and mortality: a randomized trial in head and neck cancer patients. Int J Cancer 2006;119(9):2221–4.

[9] Chlebowski RT, Aiello E, McTiernan A. Weight loss in breast cancer patient management. J Clin Oncol 2002;20(4):1128–43.

[10] Holmes MD, Chen WY, Feskanich D, Kroenke CH, Colditz GA. Physical activity and survival after breast cancer diagnosis. JAMA 2005;293(20):2479–86.

[11] Meyerhardt JA, Heseltine D, Niedzwiecki D, Hollis D, Saltz LB, Mayer RJ, et al. Impact of physical activity on cancer recurrence and survival in patients with stage III colon cancer: findings from CALGB 89803. J Clin Oncol 2006;24(22):3535–41.

[12] Velicer CM, Ulrich CM. Vitamin and mineral supplement use among US adults after cancer diagnosis: a systematic review. J Clin Oncol 2008;26(4):665–73.

[13] Institute of Medicine Initial national priorities for comparative effectiveness research. Washington, DC: The National Academies Press; 2009.

[14] Selby JV, Beal AC, Frank L. The Patient-Centered Outcomes Research Institute (PCORI) national priorities for research and initial research agenda. J Amer Med Assoc 2012;307(15):1583–4.

[15] Washington AE, Lipstein SH. The Patient-Centered Outcomes Research Institute—promoting better information, decisions, and health. N Engl J Med 2011;365(15):e31.

[16] Department of Health and Human Services, Office of the National Coordinator for Health Information Technology. Health 2.0: investigating in innovations initiative. <http://www.health-2con.com/devchallenge/2015>.

[17] U.S. Department of Health and Human Services. Federal Coordinating Council for Comparative Effectiveness Research, Report to the President and Congress; 2009.

[18] Alemayehu D, Sanchez RJ, Cappelleri JC. Considerations on the use of patient-reported outcomes in comparative effectiveness research. J Manag Care Pharm 2011;17(9 Suppl. A):S27–33.

[19] Lohr KN. Comparative effectiveness research methods: symposium overview and summary. Med Care 2010;48(Suppl. 6): S3–S6.

[20] Clauser SB, Wagner EH, Aiello Bowles EJ, Tuzzio L, Greene SM. Improving modern cancer care through information technology. Am J Prev Med 2011;40(5):S198–207.

[21] Executive Office of the President of the United States, President's Council of Advisors on Science and Technology. Realizing the Full Potential of Health Information Technology to Improve Healthcare for Americans: The Path Forward. December 2010.

[22] Sittig DF. Potential impact of advanced clinical information technology on cancer care in 2015. Cancer Causes Control 2006;17(6):813–20.

[23] Kakria P, Tripathi NK, Kitipawang P. A real-time health monitoring system for remote cardiac patients using smartphone and wearable sensors. Int J Telemed Appl; 2015.

[24] Ventola CL. Mobile devices and apps for health care professionals: uses and benefits. P T 2014;39(5):356–64.

[25] Medicare Payment Advisory Commission. Health Care Spending and the Medicare Program. Washington, D.C., 2014.

[26] Kofoed S, Breen S, Gough K, Aranda S. Benefits of remote real-time side-effect monitoring systems for patients receiving cancer treatment. Oncol Rev 2012;6(1):e7.

[27] Hicks LL, Fleming DA, Desaulnier A. The application of remote monitoring to improve health outcomes to a rural area. Telemed J E Health 2009;15(7):664–71.

[28] Barnett TE, Chumbler NR, Vogel WB, Beyth RJ, Qin H, Kobb R. The effectiveness of a care coordination home telehealth program for veterans with diabetes mellitus: a 2-year follow-up. Am J Manag Care 2006;12(8):467–74.

[29] Chumbler NR, Neugaard B, Kobb R, Ryan P, Qin H, Joo Y. Evaluation of a care coordination/home-telehealth program for veterans with diabetes: health services utilization and health-related quality of life. Eval Health Prof 2005;28(4):464–78.

[30] Rasmussen LM, Phanareth K, Nolte H, Backer V. Internet-based monitoring of asthma: a long-term, randomized clinical study of 300 asthmatic subjects. J Allergy Clin Immunol 2005;115(6):1137–42.

[31] Louis AA, Turner T, Gretton M, Baksh A, Cleland JG. A systematic review of telemonitoring for the management of heart failure. Eur J Heart Fail 2003;5(5):583–90.

[32] Bartoli L, Zanaboni P, Masella C, Ursini N. Systematic review of telemedicine services for patients affected by chronic obstructive pulmonary disease (COPD). Telemed J E Health 2009;15(9):877–83.

[33] Santamaria N, Carville K, Ellis I, Prentice J. The effectiveness of digital imaging and remote expert wound consultation on healing rates in chronic lower leg ulcers in the Kimberley region of Western Australia. Primary Intention 2004;12:62–72.

[34] Bartoli G, Cipolletti R, Di Antonio G, Giovannini R, Lanari S, Marcolini M, et al. A convergent approach to (R)-Tiagabine by a regio-and stereocontrolled hydroiodination of alkynes. Org Biomol Chem 2010;8(15):3509–17.

[35] Noel HC, Vogel DC, Erdos JJ, Cornwall D, Levin F. Home telehealth reduces healthcare costs. Telemed J E Health 2004;10(2): 170–83.

[36] Takahashi PY, Pecina JL, Upatising B, Chadhry R, Shah ND, Van Houten H, et al. A randomized controlled trial of telemonitoring in older adults with multiple health issues to prevent hospitalizations and emergency department visits. Arch Intern Med 2012;172(10):773–9. archinternmed. 2012.256 v1.

[37] Wilson SR, Cram P. Another sobering result for home telehealth—and where we might go next: comment on "a randomized controlled trial of telemonitoring in older adults with multiple health issues to prevent hospitalizations and emergency department visits." Arch Intern Med 2012;172(10):779–80. archinternmed. 2012.685 v1.

[38] Martin S, Kelly G, Kernohan WG, McCreight B, Nugent C. Smart home technologies for health and social care support. Cochrane Database Syst Rev 2008(4):CD006412.

[39] Hesketh PJ, Sanz-Altamira P, Bushey J, Hesketh AM. Prospective evaluation of the incidence of delayed nausea and vomiting in patients with colorectal cancer receiving oxaliplatin-based chemotherapy. Support Care Cancer 2012;20(5):1043–7.

[40] Jones JM, Qin R, Bardia A, Linquist B, Wolf S, Loprinzi CL. Antiemetics for chemotherapy-induced nausea and vomiting occurring despite prophylactic antiemetic therapy. J Palliat Med 2011;14(7):810–4.

[41] Blanke CD, Bot BM, Thomas DM, Bleyer A, Kohne CH, Seymour MT, et al. Impact of young age on treatment efficacy and safety in advanced colorectal cancer: a pooled analysis of patients from nine first-line phase III chemotherapy trials. J Clin Oncol 2011;29(20):2781–6.

[42] Ridolfi L, Bertetto O, Santo A, Naglieri E, Lopez M, Recchia F, et al. Chemotherapy with or without low-dose interleukin-2 in advanced non-small cell lung cancer: results from a phase III randomized multicentric trial. Int J Oncol 2011;39(4):1011–7.

[43] Kuderer NM, Dale DC, Crawford J, Cosler LE, Lyman GH. Mortality, morbidity, and cost associated with febrile neutropenia in adult cancer patients. Cancer 2006;106(10):2258–66.

[44] Du XL, Osborne C, Goodwin JS. Population-based assessment of hospitalizations for toxicity from chemotherapy in older women with breast cancer. J Clin Oncol 2002;20(24):4636–42.

[45] Richardson A, Ream E. The experience of fatigue and other symptoms in patients receiving chemotherapy. Eur J Cancer Care (Engl) 1996;5(Suppl. 2):24–30.

[46] Scully C, Sonis S, Diz PD. Oral mucositis. Oral Dis 2006;12(3):229–41.

[47] Sonis ST, Oster G, Fuchs H, Bellm L, Bradford WZ, Edelsberg J, et al. Oral mucositis and the clinical and economic outcomes of hematopoietic stem-cell transplantation. J Clin Oncol 2001;19(8):2201–5.

[48] Glaus A. Assessment of fatigue in cancer and non-cancer patients and in healthy individuals. Support Care Cancer 1993;1(6):305–15.

[49] McCann L, Maguire R, Miller M, Kearney N. Patients' perceptions and experiences of using a mobile phone-based advanced symptom management system (ASyMS) to monitor and manage chemotherapy related toxicity. Eur J Cancer Care (Engl) 2009;18(2):156–64.

[50] Patrick K, Wolszon L, Basen-Engquist KM, Demark-Wahnefried W, Prokhorov AV, Barrera S, et al. CYberinfrastructure for COmparative effectiveness REsearch (CYCORE): improving data from cancer clinical trials. Transl Behav Med 2011;1(1):83–8.

[51] Cheng C, Stokes TH, Wang MD. caREMOTE: the design of a cancer reporting and monitoring telemedicine system for domestic care. Conf Proc IEEE Eng Med Biol Soc 2011;2011:3168–71.

[52] Blalock J, Lam C, Minnix JA, Karam-Hage M, Gritz ER, Robinson JD, et al. The effect of mood, anxiety, and alcohol use disorders on smoking cessation in cancer patients. J Cogn Psychother 2011;25:82–96.

[53] Mallen MJ, Blalock JA, Cinciripini PM. Using technology to serve patients and practitioners: a comprehensive tobacco-cessation program for cancer patients. Counse Psychother Res 2006;6(3):196–201.

[54] Karam-Hage M, Cinciripini P, Gritz ER. Tobacco use and cessation for cancer survivors: an overview for clinicians. Cancer J Clin 2014;64(4):272–90.

[55] Wippold R, Karam-Hage M, Blalock J, Cinciripini P. Selection of optimal tobacco cessation medication treatment in patients with cancer. Clin J Oncol Nurs 2015;19(2):170–5.

[56] Trotti A, Bellm LA, Epstein JB, Frame D, Fuchs HJ, Gwede CK, et al. Mucositis incidence, severity and associated outcomes in patients with head and neck cancer receiving radiotherapy with or without chemotherapy: a systematic literature review. Radiother Oncol 2003;66(3):253–62.

[57] Murphy BA. Clinical and economic consequences of mucositis induced by chemotherapy and/or radiation therapy. J Support Oncol 2007;5(9 Suppl. 4):13–21.

[58] Cady J. Nutritional support during radiotherapy for head and neck cancer: the role of prophylactic feeding tube placement. Clin J Oncol Nurs 2007;11(6):875–80.

[59] Gaziano JE. Evaluation and management of oropharyngeal Dysphagia in head and neck cancer. Cancer Control 2002;9(5):400–9.

[60] Givens DJ, Karnell LH, Gupta AK, Clamon GH, Pagedar NA, Chang KE, et al. Adverse events associated with concurrent chemoradiation therapy in patients with head and neck cancer. Arch Otolaryngol Head Neck Surg 2009;135(12):1209–17.

[61] Elting LS, Cooksley C, Chambers M, Cantor SB, Manzullo E, Rubenstein EB. The burdens of cancer therapy. Clinical and economic outcomes of chemotherapy-induced mucositis. Cancer 2003;98(7):1531–9.

[62] National Cancer Institute. Surveillance Research Program CSBS, Epidemiology, and End Results (SEER) program stat database: incidence-SEER; 2007.

[63] Grothey A, Sugrue MM, Purdie DM, Dong W, Sargent D, Hendrick E, et al. Bevacizumab beyond first progression is associated with prolonged overall survival in metastatic colorectal cancer: results from a large observational cohort study (BRiTE). J Clin Oncol 2008;26(33):5326–34.

[64] Lang I, Kohne CH, Folprecht G, Rougier P, Curran D, Hitre E, et al. Quality of life analysis in patients with KRAS wild-type metastatic colorectal cancer treated first-line with cetuximab plus irinotecan, fluorouracil and leucovorin. Eur J Cancer 2013;49(2):439–48.

[65] Arndt V, Merx H, Stegmaier C, Ziegler H, Brenner H. Quality of life in patients with colorectal cancer 1 year after diagnosis compared with the general population: a population-based study. J Clin Oncol 2004;22(23):4829–36.

[66] Ramsey SD, Berry K, Moinpour C, Giedzinska A, Anderson MR. Quality of life in long term survivors of colorectal cancer. Am J Gastroenterol 2002;97:1228–34.

[67] Arraras Urdaniz JI, Vera Garcia R, Martinez Aguillo M, Manterola Burgaleta A, Arias de la Vega F, Salgado Pascual E. Quality of life assessment through the EORTC questionnaires of colorectal cancer patients in advanced disease stages. Clin Trans Oncol Off Publ Federation Span Oncol Soc Natl Cancer Inst Mexico 2006;8(9):664–71.

[68] Ramsey SD, Andersen MR, Etzioni R, Moinpour C, Peacock S, Potosky A, et al. Quality of life in survivors of colorectal carcinoma. Cancer 2000;88(6):1294–303.

[69] Goldberg RM, Rothenberg ML, Van Cutsem E, Benson III AB, Blanke CD, Diasio RB, et al. The continuum of care: a paradigm for the management of metastatic colorectal cancer. Oncologist 2007;12(1):38–50.

[70] McNeely ML, Campbell KL, Rowe BH, Klassen TP, Mackey JR, Courneya KS. Effects of exercise on breast cancer patients and survivors: a systematic review and meta-analysis. CMAJ 2006;175(1):34–41.

[71] Cox M, Carmack C, Hughes D, Baum G, Brown J, Jingran A, et al. Antecedents and mediators of physical activity in endometrial cancer survivors: increasing physical activity through steps to health. Health Psychol 2015;34(10):1022–32.

[72] Bluethmann SM, Basen-Engquist K, Vernon SW, Cox M, Pettee Gabriel K, Stansberry SA, et al. Grasping the "teachable moment": time since diagnosis, symptom burden and health behaviors in breast, colorectal and prostate cancer survivors. Psychooncology 2015;24(10):1250–7.

[73] Peterson SK, Basen-Engquist K, Demark-Wahnefried W, Prokhorov AV, Shinn EH, Martch SL, et al. Feasibility of using home-based mobile sensors for remote patient monitoring in cancer care and prevention. J Clin Oncol 2014;32(15):p. 5.

[74] Peterson SK, Shinn EH, Basen-Engquist K, Demark-Wahnefried W, Prokhorov AV, Baru C, et al. Identifying early dehydration risk with home-based sensors during radiation treatment: a feasibility study on patients with head and neck cancer. J Natl Cancer Inst Monographs 2013;2013(47):162–8.

[75] Feeley TW, Shine KI. Access to the medical record for patients and involved providers: transparency through electronic tools. Ann Intern Med 2011;155(12):853–4.

[76] Kris MG, Meropol NJ, Winer EP, (Eds.). American Society of Clinical Oncology. Accelerating progress against cancer: ASCO's blueprint for transforming clinical and translational cancer research. Alexandria, Virginia; 2011.

[77] Levit L, Balogh E, Nass S, Ganz PA, editors. Delivering high-quality cancer care: charting a new course for a system in crisis. Washington DC: 2013 by the National Academy of Sciences; 2013.

[78] Ammenwerth E, Schnell-Inderst P, Hoerbst A. Patient empowerment by electronic health records: first results of a systematic review on the benefit of patient portals. Stud Health Technol Inform 2011;165:63–7.

[79] Gandhi TK, Weingart SN, Borus J, Seger AC, Peterson J, Burdick E, et al. Adverse drug events in ambulatory care. N Engl J Med 2003;348(16):1556–64.

[80] Nightingale G, Hajjar E, Swartz K, Andrel-Sendecki J, Chapman A. Evaluation of a pharmacist-led medication assessment used to identify prevalence of and associations with polypharmacy and potentially inappropriate medication use among ambulatory senior adults with cancer. J Clin Oncol 2015;33(13):1453–9.

[81] Schnipper JL, Gandhi TK, Wald JS, Grant RW, Poon EG, Volk LA, et al. Design and implementation of a web-based patient portal linked to an electronic health record designed to improve medication safety: the patient gateway medications module. Inform Prim Care 2008;16(2):147–55.

[82] Zhou YY, Kanter MH, Wang JJ, Garrido T. Improved quality at Kaiser Permanente through e-mail between physicians and patients. Health Aff (Millwood) 2010;29(7):1370–5.

[83] Goel MS, Brown TL, Williams A, Cooper AJ, Hasnain-Wynia R, Baker DW. Patient reported barriers to enrolling in a patient portal. J Am Med Inform Assoc 2011;18(Suppl. 1):i8–12.

[84] Palen TE, Ross C, Powers JD, Xu S. Association of online patient access to clinicians and medical records with use of clinical services. J Amer Med Assoc 2012;308(19):2012–9.

[85] Honeyman A, Cox B, Fisher B. Potential impacts of patient access to their electronic care records. Inform Prim Care 2005;13(1):55–60.

[86] Byczkowski TL, Munafo JK, Britto MT. Variation in use of internet-based patient portals by parents of children with chronic disease. Arch Pediatr Adolesc Med 2011;165(5):405–11.

[87] Fisher B, Bhavnani V, Winfield M. How patients use access to their full health records: a qualitative study of patients in general practice. J R Soc Med 2009;102(12):539–44.

[88] Gerber DE, Laccetti AL, Chen B, Yan J, Cai J, Gates S, et al. Predictors and intensity of online access to electronic medical records among patients with cancer. J Oncol Pract Am Soc Clin Oncol 2014;10(5):e307–12.

[89] Sarkar U, Karter AJ, Liu JY, Adler NE, Nguyen R, Lopez A, et al. Social disparities in internet patient portal use in diabetes: evidence that the digital divide extends beyond access. J Am Med Inform Assoc 2011;18(3):318–21.

[90] Hesse BW, Croyle RT, Buetow KH. Cyberinfrastructure and the biomedical sciences. Am J Prev Med 2011;40(5 Suppl. 2):S97–S102.

[91] Davis Giardina T, Menon S, Parrish DE, Sittig DF, Singh H. Patient access to medical records and healthcare outcomes: a systematic review. J Am Med Inform Assoc 2014;21(4):737–41.

[92] Ammenwerth E, Schnell-Inderst P, Hoerbst A. The impact of electronic patient portals on patient care: a systematic review of controlled trials. J Med Internet Res 2012;14(6):e162.

[93] Bates DW, Bitton A. The future of health information technology in the patient-centered medical home. Health Aff (Millwood) 2010;29(4):614–21.

[94] Yoon S, Wilcox AB, Bakken S. Comparisons among health behavior surveys: implications for the design of informatics infrastructures that support comparative effectiveness research. EGEMS (Wash DC) 2013;1(1):1021.

20

Editors' Conclusion: Building for Change

Bradford W. Hesse PhD[1], David K. Ahern PhD[2,3,4] and Ellen Beckjord PhD MPH[5]

[1]Health Communication and Informatics Research Branch, Division of Cancer Control and Population Sciences, National Cancer Institute, Rockville, MD, United States
[2]Health Communication and Informatics Research Branch, Healthcare Delivery Research Program, National Cancer Institute, Rockville, MD, United States [3]Program in Behavioral Informatics and eHealth, Department of Psychiatry, Brigham & Women's Hospital, Boston, MA, United States [4]Harvard Medical School, Boston, MA, United States [5]Population Health Program Design and Engagement Optimization, UPMC Health Plan, Pittsburgh, PA, United States

O U T L I N E

20.1 Introduction   373

20.2 The Bright Spots in Oncology Informatics   375
  20.2.1 Learning Oncology Systems   375
  20.2.2 Population Health Informatics   376
  20.2.3 Technology to Improve Care Coordination
         and Delivery   377
  20.2.4 The Rise of Consumer Engagement and
         Participation   378
  20.2.5 Turning Data Into Actionable Knowledge
         Through Interdisciplinary Science   379

20.3 Living in a Post HITECH World   380
  20.3.1 Evolution of New Care and Payment
         Models Enabled by Informatics Technology   381

  20.3.2 Coevolution of Payment Reform
         and HIT   382

20.4 Building the Future Together   382
  20.4.1 Providers   382
  20.4.2 Researchers   383
  20.4.3 Developers   383
  20.4.4 Consumers   384

20.5 Conclusion   384

List of Acronyms and Abbreviations   385

References   385

Few will have the greatness to bend history itself, but each of us can work to change a small portion of events. It is from numberless diverse acts of courage and belief that human history is shaped. **Robert F. Kennedy.**

20.1 INTRODUCTION

We began our journey together in the first chapter of this book by confronting the uncomfortable diagnosis of an "oncology care system in crisis" as described within a

B. Hesse, D. Ahern & E. Beckjord: Oncology Informatics.
DOI: http://dx.doi.org/10.1016/B978-0-12-802115-6.00020-3

report published by the US-based Institute of Medicine (IOM) (now referred to as the National Academy of Medicine) [1]. Within that context, we encountered a disquieting prognosis that with an aging population domestically and internationally [2], and with the recognition that cancer is a disease associated with aging [3], pressures on the oncology system from an unprecedented demand for services will increase [4]. We also noted, paradoxically, that as treatments improve in effectiveness, the number of people who can count themselves as cancer survivors will also be growing, exerting yet another strain on systems to offer better support for disease surveillance, coping with distress, and ameliorating late stage sequelae from antineoplastic treatments. Furthermore, as the oncology care system pivots toward precision medicine—a movement set into higher gear through its inclusion in the 2015 Presidential "State of the Union" speech on January 20, 2015—the demands of a heavily data-driven treatment protocol are predicted to outstrip individual clinicians' and patients' cognitive capacities unless efforts are made to preprocess the raw data in ways that will produce actionable information suitable for clinical decision making [5].

A concerted effort is needed, we concluded, to alleviate the projected strains on the oncology system through an aggressive, but strategic, use of health information technology (HIT). We are not alone in that conclusion. In his book *The Quality Cure*, David Cutler observed that *"health care is among the most information-intensive processes in the economy. And yet, the information basis on which health care makes these decisions is among the least sophisticated of any industry in the economy"* [6]. Economic data have been clear in demonstrating a return on investment for strategically deploying information technologies (IT) in other sectors of the economy, with measurable increases in productivity noted in the technology, finance, manufacturing, and other sectors [7,8]. Those data have also been clear in showing that health care has been slow in adopting IT for quality improvement purposes, and as a consequence productivity has stagnated while administrative costs have been escalating. Literally billions of dollars in wasted expenses can be conserved, Cutler argued, just by using networking and HIT to automate redundant tasks and improve connections between crucial components in the health production supply chain. This was one of the reasons why the 111th Congress in the United States passed the Health Information Technology for Economic and Clinical Health (HITECH) Act in 2009. Adoption of HIT was considered to be a necessary, albeit not sufficient, prelude to health care improvement and cost containment [9].

Going into this book, we suspected that the strategic use of informatics technologies would pay extra dividends in supporting the multifaceted goals of clinical and preventive oncology. According to a number of

early data reports and task force meetings, we knew that an interoperable informatics infrastructure would be needed to support the information demands of molecular medicine in cancer prevention and treatment [10], to ensure continuity of care between primary and specialty care [11,12], to enable a bed-to-bench feedback loop for research [13], to enable better cancer control and prevention [14,15], and to serve as a lifeline for cancer survivors [16]. What we did not know, until we solicited recognized experts in their respective fields to author significant portions of this book, was just how much thinking and progress had been made already within in each of these areas.

To be sure, the relatively rapid diffusion of HIT in the wake of the HITECH Act has come with a prolonged period of growing pains and needs for system reengineering. As Robert Wachter quipped in his 2015 book *The Digital Doctor: Hope, Hype, and Harm at the Dawn of Medicine's Computer Age*, "the wiring of healthcare has proven to be the Mother of all Adaptive Problems" [17]. Competing business interests have led to reported instances of "data blocking" between components of the health production supply chain; early technologies deployed for clinical use can often appear "kludgy" or cumbersome if they are not optimized to integrate well in supporting teams of practice; the novelty of incorporating computer technologies within patient encounters can lead to a sense of distraction or depersonalization within the patient–provider encounter; while a relentless need for data entry can suck up staff time and consume hospital resources [18]. These are just a few of the problems brought to a series of Senate subcommittee hearings on the problems encountered during the fallout from a national conversion to health digital record keeping.

Still, in the midst of this massive experimentation there are bright spots of success that can help guide the way forward. In this concluding chapter, we begin with those bright spots as we look to the early successes and experiments of our authors as they report from the frontlines of the digital revolution in cancer. We will not be Pollyannaish in our review of these highlights. We recognize that these victories have been hard won, and that obstacles remain before these techniques scale up. That is why we dedicated one section of the book to the sciences—old and new—that are stepping up to the plate to assist these experiments in reaching their tipping point. We will then be candid in our appraisals of where the future of oncology informatics may lie in a post-HITECH world, taking into account the evidence-based conclusions of academic consortia and government-funded scientific reviews of the current state of informatics deployment in the United States. We conclude with our observations of next steps for the multiple constituencies who must work together in forging a new system of oncology care that delivers on the "triple aim" of better patient experience, improved population health, and reduced costs. There is work to be done, we argue, for all stakeholders in oncology informatics from researchers to developers, and from practicing clinicians to the patients they serve.

20.2 THE BRIGHT SPOTS IN ONCOLOGY INFORMATICS

As we looked across the chapters included in this text, we were gratified to see certain themes emerge time and time again. These are emblematic areas of development that resonate well with the national discussions occurring as health care systems reorient themselves toward practices that inculcate the principles of predictive, preemptive, personalized, and participative care. They stand as an integrative background against which the many individual informatics implementation experiments are playing out in the areas of clinical and preventive oncology. We recount five of those thematic areas below.

20.2.1 Learning Oncology Systems

In 2007, the National Academies Press published the results of an IOM Roundtable on Evidence-Based Medicine titled "The Learning Healthcare System" [19]. Released before the flurry of adoption that would be a hallmark of the HITECH Act days, the report was forward-thinking in the way that it described how an interoperable lattice of electronic health record (EHR) systems could change the culture of biomedical research and practice. First, the authors of the report explained, data harvested from EHRs could provide feedback to health care administrators and clinical practitioners on how to improve the quality and efficiency of their operational systems. The concept is directly analogous to the ways in which savvy operations managers use statistical process control to improve the quality and efficiency of their operations in manufacturing or business. Second, the physiologic sensors and electronic laboratory data needed to monitor the efficacy of treatment protocols in an electronically wired health care system could be tapped to serve as conduits of scientific data back into the biomedical research enterprise. The translational continuum from bench to bedside to population health could be dramatically shortened with a greater contiguity between intervention, monitoring, reassessment, and discovery [20].

These two facets of a learning health care system—using data to improve the quality of care and using biologic monitoring to accelerate discovery—are echoed through several chapters of this text. In the opening chapter to this text, Schilsky and Miller describe a significant investment from the American Society of Clinical Oncology (ASCO) into the Cancer Learning Intelligence Network for Quality, or CancerLinQ. This physician-led quality improvement initiative embraces the IOM vision for creating a learning health care system by capturing data from the complete longitudinal record of cancer patients' experience, and then mining those data for best-practice links between process and outcomes, and then providing the distilled intelligence scraped from thousands of records back to individual oncologists through a practical set of practice-management tools. The initiative is cutting-edge in its vision, and sector-wide in its scope. With such a high profile, the initiative is sure to run afoul of all the obstacles inherent in the nation's struggle to bring together disparate data streams for the purpose of improving medical practice through evidence-based intelligence. When successful, though, the project should bring the power of "big data" directly into cancer care.

Likewise, Kibbe in his chapter describes work being done at the National Institutes of Health (NIH) to enable a national learning health care system for research in cancer. Enabling a stronger partnership between computer scientists and informaticists on the one hand, and biomedical researchers and practitioners on the other hand was a core tenet of NIH director Francis Collins' research agenda when he took the helm of the nation's premiere biomedical research agency in 2009 [21]. Kibbe provides detail to that vision by explaining how the National Cancer Institute (NCI) is working directly with other data scientists at the NIH to ensure that the appropriate incentives are in place to encourage professional sharing of genomic, clinical, and eventually behavioral/environmental data through "micro-attribution" of credit by contributing software and data sets; by standardizing ontologies and streamlining workflows; by connecting data streams from both traditional laboratory sources and new mobile technologies; by taking advantage of plummeting costs for molecular testing; and for building more sophisticated computational models of cancer biology. In an even more timely way, Kibbe is at the center of the NCI's efforts to operationalize the nation's shift to precision medicine and he offers insight into how a distributed data system built on a foundation of coordinated standards, data liquidity, and an emerging sense of "data altruism" will help power the next wave of clinical research studies in cancer.

Within the *Cancer Care Continuum* section, oncologists Hirsh and Abernethy provide a glimpse of how data liquidity and the realization of a learning health care system in cancer are beginning to benefit real clinical teams and patients in the life-critical environments of evidence-based care. These authors confronted the information-intensive nature of oncology head-on, describing how practitioners struggle to keep up with a cacophony of incoming signals from structured and unstructured data, from an exploding and at times contradictory evidence base, professional guidelines, patient-generated data, and genomics. Their careful articulation of the use case across the clinical spectrum of care, combined with their own frontline experience retooling the decisional architectures of oncology through a meticulous engineering of informatics systems, offers a glimpse of what the learning oncology system of the future might look like in practice.

Similarly, in the last section of the book—which is intended to be a glimpse forward in time—Peterson and Patrick illustrate how a partnership between the MD Anderson Comprehensive Cancer Center and the UC San Diego's Center for Wireless and Population Health Systems was able to produce a functioning cyberinfrastructure upon which to conduct comparative effectiveness research (CER) in cancer. The health care system is fraught, according to the IOM's report *Knowing What Works in Healthcare: A Blueprint for the Nation*, with variable medical practices around the country that can lead to a misuse and abuse of resources [22]. It can also create unreliability in the delivery of care from one region of the country to the next, or even from one practice to the next. As payment models shift toward value-based reimbursements and consumer-directed practices, an ability to compare the cost-effectiveness of comparable treatments will be an essential component of the learning oncology system. Peterson and Patrick utilize advanced computing technologies, seeded by investments from the National Science Foundation, to create a working prototype of a platform that would support comparative effectiveness studies.

A limiting factor for progress within the learning health care system, as expressed repeatedly by participants in the IOM roundtable series, is the ability of our research methods to keep up with the opportunities for accelerated discovery in a data-rich clinical system. In his chapter, Riley highlights a bright spot in the thinking of methodologists and statisticians on how to transcend the multiple limitations of traditional null hypothesis testing, and the randomized clinical trial (RCT), both of which had been crafted during a time of data paucity. Riley highlights compelling examples from the worlds of astronomy, geophysics, and meteorology to abstract common aspects of how data-rich environments can be exploited to catalyze scientific discovery and accelerate the path from big data to knowledge.

20.2.2 Population Health Informatics

Another bright spot is the movement that many of our authors have shown in linking together the previously disparate worlds of public health and clinical health care services. In a *Health Affairs* Blog posted on September 16, 2015, pediatrician and health disparities researcher Ivor Horn declared that a perfect confluence of policy and technology may finally make it possible to make significant progress in the communities in which health care plans and hospitals are located. On the policy side, she noted that reimbursement strategies from the Federal government favor the production of health and wellness as a cost savings, preventive measure against the coffer-draining expenses of chronic disease or late-stage care. The Centers for Medicare & Medicaid Services (CMS), the largest payer for medical services, has begun codifying these changes through its emphasis on "value" and "accountable care" rather than traditional fee-for-service. Likewise, meaningful use incentives from the HITECH Act have enabled the ability of medical practices and hospitals to monitor the welfare of all their patients through dashboards, and then identify actions that can be taken to improve population health outcomes. Finally, a movement in the marketplace for affordable consumer technologies is beginning to facilitate a more equitable penetration of behavioral support tools for those who have been the most vulnerable.

Throughout the text our authors have reflected on how oncology informatics can be deployed to boost population health and ensure health equity "by design" [23]. In her chapter on reducing cancer disparities through community engagement, Oh and her colleagues described two case studies in which the power of an informatics-infused care system was combined with the problem-solving strategies of a community-based participatory research program to protect against inequitable care. In one example, EHR and cancer registry data were combined to establish a baseline in treatment completion for both African Americans and their Caucasian counterparts. A feedback system was then constructed to warn care teams when appointments or milestones in care were missed for whatever reason. A team of nurse navigators would then act on the early warning system to facilitate care completion. In their other example, a group of population health engineers were able to create electronic linkages to community resources and then embed that intelligence into the clinical encounter through the EHR. The subthemes echoed throughout their chapter emphasized the ability of the informatics technology to make progress toward population health goals transparent, to make data relevant and actionable, to build capacity among community partners, and to enable a bottom-up approach for community health.

Two of our chapters in the continuum of care section highlighted some of these same population health themes. The chapter on primary prevention, by Morgan and Fiore, acknowledged that the explosion in consumer-facing health applications has the profound potential of equipping individuals with personalized support for smoking cessation, diet and exercise, sun safety, and adherence to human papillomavirus (HPV) vaccination recommendations. Although that market is expanding by unanticipated leaps and bounds, the role of health practitioners and scientists will be to guide consumers toward those applications that have an evidence base for initiating and maintaining behavior change. Morgan and Fiore also presented data on how EHR systems can be used to monitor consistent access to prevention services, as needed to qualify for reimbursement under value-based care models, and illustrated how transparent data from disease registries to local health departments helped community planners emphasize obtainable population health prevention goals. In a reassuring display of interoperability, the authors even described a closed loop feedback system in which the data from patients who had been referred to state-run quit lines were reincorporated into an EHR as a status check on quitters' progress.

In a similar vein, the chapter on early detection described how HIT could be engineered into primary care workflows to support age and risk informed recommendations for routine screening. These authors were careful in describing the meticulous process that standards boards, such as the US Preventive Services Taskforce, must go through to determine who in a given population would receive a mortality benefit after going through the monetary and psychological costs of screening. The HIT solutions can be engineered to ensure that the right populations receive the appropriate attention to assure that they are adherent to those recommendations. Screening is a process, they argued, that must begin with an appropriate judgment of suitability for initial recommendation, followed by a coordination of testing and laboratory services, and then followed by prompt discussion with patients regarding next steps. Perturbations of that process can lead to a loss of follow-up, with potentially fatal downstream consequences. HIT can serve as a bulwark against such failures, and can strengthen communities with data on adherence throughout a given population. Because computer-hosted guidance can be updated in real time, the recommendations generating prompts for screening tests can be kept current based on the state of epidemiologic science and can be personalized to represent individual needs.

In the contributing sciences section of the book, authors Penberthy, Winn, and Scott illustrate how the public health practice of cancer surveillance can be expanded through strategic informatics approaches to provide a more comprehensive, data-driven view of incidence, prevalence, etiology, and context. As progress is made on national goals for interoperability of care systems, data will begin to flow between hospitals, laboratories, oncology practices, and many other ancillary links in the oncology services supply chain. These can be assembled to complete the epidemiologic profile on genomically classified variants of the disease as patients go from diagnosis, to treatment, to ongoing monitoring, and eventually to death or survivorship. The progression is a movement away from the cumbersome and highly restrictive techniques prevalent within most cancer registry systems today, to the more expansive and nimble electronic systems being assembled to associate electronic pathology reports with other components of the EHR and pharmacologic record systems. It should enable a more comprehensive approach to cancer surveillance, while creating a springboard for a learning public health system.

20.2.3 Technology to Improve Care Coordination and Delivery

In their chapter on *Coordination at the Point of Need*, Kim and her colleagues illustrated what the distributed landscape of care looks like for a cancer patient. Within this landscape, a single patient and his or her family may be expected to interact with a primary care provider; with several specialists at various points of diagnosis and treatment; with community services for financial and socially supportive help if needed; with in-patient and out-patient hospital services; with individually managed clinics; with home care; and at some point perhaps with hospice care. If the patient is older, with multiple chronic conditions, the number of providers in the patient's contact list will grow even larger. Until now, the patient may have been expected to be the sole coordinator of these myriad services, following a long and lonely road saddled with reams of paper-based printouts, care plans, pharmaceutical information, insurance forms, and laboratory reports.

A bright spot we are beginning to see throughout this book is the role that health information technologies can play in supporting coordination of services from multiple perspectives. Kim and her colleagues highlighted the successes of informaticists working with cancer specialists to create a functional EHR in oncology that would allow multiple care providers to obtain a coordinated view of a patient's status and care delivery as an aid in the "total management of cancer patients" [24]. Similarly, Krist and his coauthors describe how the "patient-centered medical home (PCMH)" model has been evolving in the primary care setting. The model makes extensive use of HIT to coordinate information about a given patient so that the information can be made accessible to primary care office staff serving essentially as the case manager for a patient's goals and progress for care. Krist et al. acknowledge that when a patient is diagnosed with cancer, the coordinating function for care is often passed over to the oncology team, but continues to emphasize the importance of interoperability between oncology records and primary care records as the patient transitions into the survivor phase. In that vein, Beckjord and her colleagues highlight the ways in which HIT has been used to support long-term health needs after cancer treatment by extending monitoring capabilities along with cumulative planning. Dubenske and her colleagues describe work being prototyped through the Comprehensive Health Enhancement Support System (CHESS) in Wisconsin that succeeded in prolonging life through clinician reports, and helped guide ancillary services in coordinating end-of-life planning and care.

Although much of the initial engineering work for coordinating care has been done on the provider side, new bright spots are emerging in informaticists' efforts to empower patients as a crucial linking pin in their own care. In their chapter on communication science, Hesse and his colleagues recount the success of communication management systems to keep track of clinical milestones based on personalized care plans and then generate communications to patients and their care teams. In work reported from the Kaiser Permanente system in Southern California, such a system was able to achieve a four-fold increase in pap and mammography screening, along with a 10-fold increase in colorectal cancer screening. Secure messaging systems to patients have been utilized to achieve greater efficiencies in coordinating appointments, in ordering and reconciling medications, and in improving the quality of patient data in the medical record. In the final section of the book, Zeiger and Frydman relate the ongoing story of how the Internet has helped cancer patients find each other to obtain both instrumental and emotional support from online communities, and how willing those online patients are in helping to coordinate the research and care enterprise. Their illuminating development came from their own efforts in using the power of online communities to tackle the perennial challenge of recruitment to clinical trials.

20.2.4 The Rise of Consumer Engagement and Participation

The Zeiger and Frydman chapter brings to the fore another significant theme running through the book: with the participative nature of connected systems, patients are embracing the opportunity to become more involved in their own health care and to be involved as equal partners in accelerating the research enterprise. Data from the NCI's Health Information National Trends Survey (HINTS) revealed that in 2003, the first time the survey was fielded in the general population, an estimated 66,735,918 Americans reported going online to look for health-related topics. By 2013, that number had risen to an estimated 144,523,246 Americans going online to look for health information either for themselves or loved ones. In 2014, for those who searched for health information from any source, 69% or an estimated 117,172,798 Americans reported going online first before going anywhere else. Contrast that number to the mere 14.8% who went to their doctors first. At the same time, HINTS data suggest that trust in providers has not gone down with a rise in Internet searching, but in some respects has increased [25–27].

What is evolving is a new relationship between health care consumers and health care providers, in which consumers are becoming more actively involved as motivated patients and are relying on their care teams to be trusted partners in guiding their care. Krist and his colleagues in their chapter on "Engaging Patients in Primary and Specialty Care" emphasize this theme. Citing data on how important patient engagement is to reduce costs and improve outcomes in both primary and cancer care, the chapter aptly describes how HIT can be engineered to empower patients and caregivers in taking a proactive stance toward managing their own health conditions. The chapter reiterates a popular blueprint Krist published in the Journal of the American Medical Association for how informaticists may build systems that successively increase levels of patient empowerment [28]. At the highest level of functionality, informed patients would be given the electronic tools to review vetted health information, interact with decision aids, utilize risk calculators, personalize messages, and provide logistical support for appointments and follow-up. In going beyond talk, and walking the walk, Krist and his colleagues are currently building and testing systems that achieve this high level support through funding from the NCI.

Ahern, Braun, Cooley, and Bickmore take on the challenge of building systems that are directly supportive of patients' health-oriented behaviors by doing a deep dive into the science of behavioral medicine. What was especially illuminating from their chapter was to learn how principles of behavioral support have been piloted with evidentiary success in efforts to engage patients in preventive behaviors, to maintain adherence to complex therapeutic regimens, to screen for psychosocial distress, to promote vigilance for survivors, and to cross literacy boundaries in personalizing support equitably across populations. Encouraging greater participation by patients in their own health care is part-and-parcel of the meaningful use criteria for incentives under HITECH, they reminded us; while paying attention to psychological sequelae from cancer treatment will rise in priority as reimbursements shift from fee-for-service to value-based care and population health management. The authors describe efforts underway to standardize measurements and ontologies to fully capture the experience of the whole cancer patient, including efforts supported by the IOM.

Not only are patients becoming more engaged in their own health care, but there has also been a rise in motivation by patients to accelerate progress in cancer by contributing as citizen scientists to the research enterprise. Kibbe referred to this observation in his chapter by describing ways in which cancer researchers can encourage "data altruism," built on channels designed to support data liquidity. Indeed, efforts to build a cohort of patient volunteers will be a central strategy to enable the research needed to advance precision medicine, and Kibbe is instrumental in creating the infrastructure to support that effort on the national stage. Chiauzzi, Eichler, and Wicks build further on the concept by describing the building blocks needed to accelerate science through patient-fueled, "crowdsourcing" concepts. Crowdsourcing—or the creation of new data, information, knowledge, or innovations resulting from engaging a large group (ie, crowd) of individuals outside of a traditional organization to problem-solve—is not necessarily a new concept. The English Oxford Dictionary was built from the voluntary contributions of literati dispersed throughout the English-speaking world. What makes the current era so opportune is the way that electronic platforms can accelerate knowledge building exponentially through massively distributed electronic networks. Wikipedia, they noted, generated upwards of 34 million articles in 287 languages over the course of a mere decade. PatientsLikeMe, the authors' home organization, is setting its own exemplary pace by offering a safe haven for patients to contribute the data that will help conquer their disease. What the authors have given to the readers of this book is a well-researched formula for capturing the accelerative advantages of crowdsourcing in the area of cancer.

20.2.5 Turning Data Into Actionable Knowledge Through Interdisciplinary Science

A final theme that echoes throughout the book is that as cancer care gets more complex, and as HIT in the service of oncology gets more robust, there will be a rising need to cross scientific boundaries in moving evidence into practice within informatics-enabled environments. We worked carefully to acknowledge this need in our creation of the list of authors of chapters in this book. The Schilsky and Miller chapter at the beginning of the book set the tone for this theme by illustrating how the nation's largest professional society for practicing oncologists has committed to an inclusion of advanced data science principles within the Society's armamentarium to accelerate diffusion of best practice in clinical care. Warren Kibbe, in his chapter, demonstrated how an advanced understanding of molecular genetics coupled with a leadership role in biomedical informatics and an intuitive feel for organizational dynamics can be woven

together to promote a new era of data liquidity and data sharing. Others in the *Extraordinary Opportunity* section follow suit by combing expertise in informatics with training in public health, primary care, specialty care, nursing, and health communication to improve the flow and utilization of data to accelerate successes against cancer across multiple fronts.

In the *Informatics Support Across the Care Continuum* section, authors with complementary areas of expertise come together to detail ways of improving the utilization of data at the various points of influence along the trajectory from prevention to survivorship and end-of-life. For example, in the prevention chapter, authors with expertise in health psychology and clinical practice outline a blueprint for utilizing data to modify individual patient behavior, to inform medical practice, and even to create a bridge between care systems and state or community public health resources. Similarly, the early detection chapter combines epidemiologic and medical expertise to illustrate how a system that is sensitive to the tradeoffs between false positives and false negatives can use informatics solutions to improve the screening performance of primary care practices, hospitals, regional networks, and even international research and standards setting organizations. In the remaining chapters, experts in health services delivery, systems engineering, psychosocial counseling, patient advocacy, and medical oncology combine their perspectives to illustrate how data will be used to support cancer patients across their journeys from diagnosis on.

The *Science of Informatics* section was our attempt to go even further in bringing new expertise to the table as we consider the research agenda ahead for the field. In their chapters, Ahern et al. and Hesse worked with experts in clinical oncology, behavioral medicine, communication science, human computer interaction, and ontology development in order to create a framework for how data could be utilized to improve on meaningful use goals of improved safety, enhanced patient engagement, reliable continuity of care, and accountability over population health. In another pair of complementary chapters, Horowitz and Onukwugha brought scientific knowledge from neuropsychology, epidemiology, and human system integration together to lay a foundation for a new era of information utilization based on data visualization techniques. These data visualization techniques will likely be needed to enable the future of cancer surveillance as described by experts in medical informatics, epidemiology, public health, and statistical methodology for the final chapter of the section.

Silicon Valley publisher Tim O'Reilly famously quipped that "data will be the new Intel Inside" when communicating a vision for the future of health care—that is, Health 2.0—in an era of interconnected computing platforms [29]. This observation is illustrated aptly within the final section of the book on *Accelerating Discovery Through Oncology Informatics*. Zeiger and Frydman in their chapter, along with Chiauzzi, Eichler, and Wicks in their chapter, described how innovative developments in crowdsourcing platforms could be marshaled to create a platform for participation between patients and researchers. Within these platforms, data will indeed be the coin of the realm, with security and policy measures in place to protect patients' investments in science reinforcing the patient cry of "no data about me without me." Upping the ante on transdisciplinary work even further, Peterson and Patrick illustrate what happens when leading technology experts from the UC San Diego Supercomputer Center marry their expertise with the research priorities articulated by scientists at an NCI-awarded comprehensive cancer center to improve oncology care. As an aside, these investigators were some of the first to envision the role of cloud computing in medicine, a concept that has become commonplace in the wake of the HITECH Act. As data flows improve, Riley completes the section by offering a roadmap for moving big data into knowledge through the use of new analytic methodologies, new technologies, and new approaches to connected science.

20.3 LIVING IN A POST HITECH WORLD

As described above, much has been accomplished in the last six years since the passage of the HITECH Act and as a direct result of the substantial financial investments in electronic medical records (EMRs). There has been a 60% increase in the use of EMRs from 2013 [30] and the upward trend is likely to be maintained with the continuation of financial incentives through the Meaningful Use (MU) Program. Overall, most hospitals and physicians have responded favorably to the MU incentive program and adopted at least a basic EMR. HITECH enabled the construction of a foundational information infrastructure, especially within hospitals and for small, priority primary care practices, which serve as the building blocks for a more coordinated and efficient health care system. Finally, the "bright spots" highlighted above show the enormous potential for HIT to do public good when carefully designed with ongoing end user input and when implemented effectively.

These notable accomplishments notwithstanding, several recent credible and influential reports raise serious concerns about the unintended consequences of HITECH. The authors of these reports conclude that the original goals of HITECH were too ambitious and the enormity of the challenges to adoption of HIT was greatly underestimated. Indeed, the general consensus from these experts is that HITECH as originally conceived failed to achieve its goal of creating a robust information infrastructure necessary to support a 21st century, learning health care system.

Perhaps the most vexing problem encountered was the unwillingness among health systems and EMR vendors to agree on and adopt established standards for data sharing such that health information would flow unimpeded beyond the walls of individual practices, hospitals, and health systems. Ironically it was not that the necessary standards were not available, including ASCO's multiyear effort to develop cancer-specific standards to improve oncology care [31]; rather, the business case for the various stakeholders was not aligned such that interoperability would become the de facto model for practice. Hence, in 2016 we now face the situation where critical health information remains trapped within silos of provider practices, hospitals, and health systems and unavailable to patients in easily digested formats without overcoming considerable obstacles. Moreover, the policy of "information blocking" has been revealed as a deceptive and defensive response by some vendors of HIT programs and services where data fluidity is not consistent with their business models. Recently, ASCO published a policy brief on its website identifying a number of barriers to information blocking reported by its members and makes a series of recommendations for Congress to enact legislation to ensure that widespread interoperability is achieved [32]. In response, Congress has taken note of this disturbing trend and is considering offering potential legislation to prohibit such actions going forward as not in the public interest.

The lack of interoperability of health information is particularly troublesome for oncology. The inability to seamlessly share information from one oncology practice to another, or from one cancer center to another, creates serious delays in care coordination and decision making where the stakes are often very high: life or death. The IOM report, *Delivering High Quality Cancer Care: Charting a New Course for a System in Crisis* [1], contends that current HIT tools and resources are inadequate to address the delivery system challenges, with the lack of interoperability as a major barrier. ASCO acknowledges that this problem has reached a crisis level and has invested significant resources in CancerLinQ (see Schilsky and Miller's chapter) to enable data fluidity and create a continuous feedback loop to enable a learning system to emerge. As a countervailing force to this intransigence among HIT vendors and health systems a number of public–private collaboratives have emerged to stimulate and support data sharing [33]. These multistakeholder collaboratives seek to foster open and transparent systems, which incent and support data fluidity to improve quality of care. These organizations and their members also are committed to addressing the issue of sustainability so that information sharing remains a priority and can be consistent with business success and growth.

Fortunately, the Office of the National Coordinator has released the Interoperability Roadmap report [34], which lays out a detailed plan for achieving a fully interoperable health system by 2025. The major goals of this plan are:

1. Send, receive, find, and use priority data domains to improve health care quality and outcomes (2015–17);
2. Expand data sources and users in the interoperable HIT ecosystem to improve health and lower costs (2018–20); and
3. Achieve nationwide interoperability to enable a learning health system, with the person at the center of a system that can continuously improve care, public health, and science through real-time data access (2021–24).

This report generally has been well received by the various stakeholder groups and endorsed by many organizations as a viable approach to achieving full interoperability. It includes specific milestones and metrics, calls to action, and documented commitments to take appropriate action from key stakeholders. Despite overall enthusiasm for this Plan, however, several medical societies and provider organizations have expressed serious concern that the Plan is not aggressive enough in its timeline and milestones [35]. They note that what is needed at this critical juncture is not a roadmap but rather "action now." These provider groups are responding to the thunderous complaints of many of their members who rail against the disruptive influence of EMRs and other HIT products which often fail to accommodate preferred workflows and clinical processes [36]. Indeed, 111 major medical societies including the American Medical Association and the Medical Group Management Association also have raised serious concerns about the MU Stage 3 proposed rule and have asked Congress to refocus MU Stage 3 on promoting interoperability and enabling innovation [37]. They argue that the provisional MU Stage 3 rule should not be implemented without adequately addressing overarching concerns about impact on patient safety, privacy and security, interoperability, and, relevant to this discussion, physician access to high performing EMRs.

There is also the sentiment expressed that because technology has become pervasive in the clinical setting it has undermined the provider–patient relationship by interfering with human-to-human interaction necessary to establishing a trusting relationship, so essential to healing and improved health. The current generation of EMRs and HIT products are largely retrofitted electronic documentation systems, which suffer from poor end-user design and limited functionality. Although these systems collect voluminous and potentially critical information for informed decision making there are serious limitations in their capabilities to extract relevant information at the point of care and in a usable fashion. Usability of most current EMRs is rated as poor by providers and typically doesn't augment the clinical encounter but rather disrupts and interferes with optimal workflow. In an effort to adapt to the demands of EMRs, providers have shifted their EMR-related work to outside of the clinical encounter and use templates to streamline documentation [38]. The expectation for HITECH was that EMRs would evolve with greater adoption and use, moving from a basic version to a more comprehensive platform that would provide just-in-time clinical decision support and also enable population health and clinical research. Few EMRs today achieve those objectives but could be vastly improved by drawing knowledge and expertise from the informatics community around user-centered design (UCD), agile development, and human-computer interaction (see the chapters by Shneiderman and Horowitz et al.).

A recent paper described a study where a research team visited 11 different EMR vendors in order to analyze their UCD processes. Not surprisingly, results indicated that there was a diverse range of practices ranging from basic to well-developed in the approach to UCD. The authors concluded that vendors could benefit from studies that provide greater contextual analysis of clinical workflows, encourage enrollment of providers in usability studies, and engage leadership in support of such work [39].

Fully integrated health systems with aligned payment structures (eg, Kaiser, Geisinger, Intermountain Health) recognize the potential for combining comprehensive EMRs as clinical data repositories that when coupled with agile, IT-based decision support tools, can enable greater uptake and end user satisfaction as well as more timely and effective clinical decision support [40].

20.3.1 Evolution of New Care and Payment Models Enabled by Informatics Technology

Concurrent with the massive scope of HIT deployment a fundamental shift in health care delivery models has emerged, transforming from individual and multispecialty group practices to PCMHs and Accountable Care Organizations (ACOs). The former structure focuses on team-based and coordinated care with an emphasis on promoting both individual and population health. The latter structure attempts to achieve improvements in health care quality while simultaneously controlling costs and also taking on risk sharing as a model for sustainability. Both structures leverage HIT as critical components for business operations and clinical management.

20.3.2 Coevolution of Payment Reform and HIT

The ACO model is viewed currently as the preferred approach to achieving the triple aim, namely, improve individual and population health, reduce incremental costs, and improve health care quality. Recently, CMS launched this approach to specialty care under the authority of the Affordable Care Act with the Oncology Care Model as one key area [41]. Given that historically oncology practices have been responsible for dispensing chemotherapeutic agents, CMS is seeking to engage oncology practices in innovative experiments testing new payment models for achieving higher performance for enhanced chemotherapy administration. The major aims for this model are to enhance the quality and coordination of oncology care while simultaneously reducing the costs to Medicare. Private payers are encouraged to participate with Medicare to broaden incentives for care transformation to occur at the practice level.

Central to the ultimate success of this approach is the ability of practitioners to use the most current evidence at the point of care and to engage in shared decision making with patients. Both of these processes require the effective use of HIT that is well designed with provider and patient input, easily accessible, and fits seamlessly into the clinical encounter. Many of the chapters in the book highlight the ways in which HIT can optimize evidence-based oncology care delivered by providers, and enable meaningful shared decision making between patients and providers. Despite the many challenges that remain, the future for cancer care is hopeful. The final section below illustrates the many ways in which HIT and informatics can help the various stakeholders achieve a higher quality health care system.

20.4 BUILDING THE FUTURE TOGETHER

Our journey with this book started on the heels of the identification of a "crisis" in cancer care by the IOM [1], and we end feeling hopeful that multiple efforts are underway to equip the system to step up to the crisis, and ultimately, avert it. With so many bright spots surfaced by the authors of the chapters in this book, and with accompanying changes in policies and strategy at multiple levels of the cancer care system, significant change is at hand.

What will these changes mean for key stakeholders working with and within the cancer care system and HIT? How will these changes empower them to leverage informatics in pursuit of the "triple aim"—optimized health outcomes at lower costs while providing high-quality patient experiences [42]—for people affected by cancer? Here, we consider four stakeholder groups—providers, researchers, developers, and consumers—with respect to what the future of HIT has to offer them, and what challenges they will have to overcome to realize the full potential of HIT.

20.4.1 Providers

Perhaps more than any other stakeholders, providers have endured the most unintended negative consequences of the introduction of HIT into their daily workflow. As noted above by many professional societies, abysmal failures in the usability of EHRs implemented into practice have given rise to examples of clinical practice being weakened—not optimized—by the introduction of informatics. Beyond usability issues, simply the introduction of a computer as a key feature of the clinical encounter has had negative results. In his blog post titled "My Recent Hospital Stay and the Care of the Computer," Dr Alan Spiro powerfully captures this phenomenon, saying "For those of you worried about depersonalization of medical and nursing care I want to reassure you. The commitment to caring for the computer is front and center. The nurse and the doctor are diligent in paying attention to the computer, frequently touching the computer to show concern, and feeding it frequently" [43].

When the provider is forced to attend to the EHR's needs more than to the patient's needs, something has gone terribly wrong. At the same time, it is providers who stand to be enormously empowered to deliver the best care possible to patients because of the integration of HIT into clinical care. Ensuring that HIT supports providers to "work at the top of their license" requires careful attention to three issues, each of which is addressed in this book. The issues are (1) ensuring that HIT is being leveraged to bring clinically useful data to the point-of-care; (2) ensuring that the clinically useful data introduced at the point-of-care is adequately visualized and contextualized so as to be actionable; and (3) ensuring that the system containing the data and presenting it in an actionable format is highly usable and implemented in a way that supports, and does not disrupt, the provider's workflow—including their interactions with their patients.

Providers are keenly aware of the disparity between the potential of HIT to benefit their practice and current suboptimal experiences, and they are advocating for themselves in impressive ways. In response to the Interoperability Roadmap document described above, Dr Robert Wergin, Chair of the Board of the American Academy of Family Physicians penned a letter to the Director of the Office of the National Coordinator for Health Information Technology [35]. In it, he made an impassioned plea for more resources to be devoted to achieving interoperability, and to prioritize interoperability as a superordinate goal over and above any standards within the meaningful use criteria. Dr Wergin made reference to the "inadequate products" from developers that have found their way into the workflow of health care providers, and suggested that developers, not providers, be held financially accountable for achieving the clinical goals their HIT solutions are designed to address. Dr Wergin shines a light on a critical issue in this letter—that the incentives for developers and the providers who use their systems are significantly misaligned. When vendors propose transactional costs associated with information exchange via EHRs (ie, "information blocking") [32], their potential for profit increases but provider incentives—whether volume- or value-based—are negatively affected by the disastrous workflow and efficiency implications. Another negative consequence is animosity that brews between these two stakeholder groups who ultimately have to work together to realize the full potential of HIT. As providers continue to advocate for themselves and their patients, partnerships with developers that "begin with the end in mind" and align incentives wherever possible will be critical to making progress.

20.4.2 Researchers

For the researcher working to accelerate scientific discovery in cancer; translation of that science into interventions delivered in clinical care; and the human experience of the disease and its treatment, HIT creates tremendous opportunities related to the collection and availability of data. With the integration of data systems from clinical, community, and consumer-generated sources, the informatics-enabled data ecosystem that is available for use as a foundation for research is broader and deeper than ever before.

These new opportunities are not without their challenges. More sources of data mean more responsibility to be diligent about privacy and security and a greater need to carefully scrutinize the reliability and validity of data from various sources. Additionally, the pace at which HIT applications are developed and become new sources of data for researchers generally outpaces the speed at which research has traditionally occurred [44]. To fully capitalize upon the new opportunities afforded to them by the changes in the data ecosystem of cancer fueled by HIT, researchers will have to embrace the new and innovative methods described in this book for making reliable, yet efficient, inferences about ways to enhance outcomes at all levels of cancer care.

Doing so will necessitate more multi- and transdisciplinary collaborations between researchers from disciplines such as behavioral medicine, clinical science, data science, engineering, computer science, and behavioral

economics. Federal funding for researchers will continue to be a core component of supporting HIT research and its translation into practice, but researchers will also likely find themselves having to pursue less traditional forms of funding to support more agile and smaller scale projects. To be competitive in the "challenges" and high-risk, potentially high-yield short-term investment funding opportunities that are increasingly common at local, state, national, and international levels, researchers will need to diversify their fundraising skill sets to include more entrepreneurial skills that will serve them well in supporting a robust and high-impact program of HIT research.

20.4.3 Developers

Developers seeking to create innovations that will positively impact cancer care are now frequently being met with demands from clinical stakeholders for scalable, usable informatics solutions. In June of 2014, Apple announced its release of HealthKit, which not only allows iPhone users to grant HealthKit access to health-relevant data they generate just by using their device (eg, number of steps taken during the day), but the open source platform also creates a point of entry for mobile application developers to integrate their health-related solutions into a consumer's mobile device.

Another point of integration, perhaps even more significant, was the partnership between Apple's HealthKit with Epic Systems and Mayo Clinic. This signified a new opportunity for developers to have visibility into the data collected and generated by clinical systems of care. Not only does this visibility have huge potential to increase the relevance and impact of consumer-facing HIT solutions by tying them directly to the medical system, but it also created more room for developers to think about health care providers as consumers of their solutions. By integrating into the fabric of clinical care, developers have new opportunities to craft solutions that are contextually relevant, workflow-friendly, and user-centered—three features that are critical to the success of both provider- and consumer-facing informatics tools.

Perhaps the biggest challenge facing developers is finding ways of being commercially successful in the health care ecosystem. As discussed earlier, arriving at commercially viable business models that align with the needs of providers, researchers, and consumers is not always intuitive. Developers are instrumental in advancing cancer care—and all health care—to new levels via increased use of HIT, and they should be incentivized to produce innovative solutions and rewarded for their contributions. Reconciling these reasonable expectations with increased calls for open source platforms and business models that do not monetize clinical transactions in ways that negatively impact provider workflows will not be easy. Developers will be most successful and efficient if they conceive their solutions from the beginning in collaboration with end-users, supported by the best evidence available from research.

20.4.4 Consumers

Health care consumers—and, in particular, consumers personally affected by cancer—were top of mind for us throughout all stages of completing this book. We are indebted to the cancer survivors who took time to share with us their perspectives during focus groups and interviews we conducted at the formative stage of the book, as well as to the individuals who have contributed over the years to the NCI's HINTS [45], the nationally representative data source that has been incredibly useful to guiding our understanding of Americans' uses and expectations of HIT. The guidance we have received from consumers, which should be carefully considered as providers, researchers, and developers continue their push to realize the full potential of HIT, points to three areas in which consumers are looking for HIT to offer benefit. They are: using HIT to reduce the "work" associated with health; using HIT to benefit others; and using HIT as a source of support.

The stressors associated with cancer are not only a function of being diagnosed with a life threatening illness that is accompanied by significant physical, emotional, and practical concerns [46], but also of having to manage the information and navigate the medical system that are inevitably part of one's cancer journey. This has been appropriately characterized as "work" associated with illness [47], and for most people, adding more work to an already busy and fast-paced life is not a welcome addition. Maintaining health even when one is not sick requires a significant amount of work, as many facets of modern American life are not well-aligned with meeting nutrition, physical activity, or preventive health care guidelines.

Consumers want HIT to reduce the "work" of health and illness. They expect that HIT will make it easier for them to acquire, process, and make use of needed health information. They want HIT to shift the burden of responsibility for communicating their health history and data within their medical records from them to the health care system. They are tired of hand-carrying piles of paper records from one provider to another, and now expect that all providers in their personal health care ecosystem should be able to know what the others are recommending. Making this work more efficient and convenient will not only require consumer-facing solutions that address these issues, but also system-side solutions that support information sharing and care coordination, and continued shifts in policies that make

the clinical information consumers desire more available to them (eg, [48]).

Second, consumers want HIT to empower them to benefit others. This is largely in the form of sharing their data for the purposes of both research and to lend support and insight to other consumers in a comparable clinical situation. Initially, consumers looked to HIT to enable sharing their deidentified medical record data to benefit the clinical enterprise. Now that consumers are using HIT outside of the clinical context to generate clinically meaningful data via the use of health-relevant mobile applications, the "data altruism" movement encompasses an even broader opportunity for consumers to use their data in the service of helping others. While not unique to the cancer survivor community, we note that cancer survivor advocates have been some of the most historically active in finding creative ways to support one another, and expect that survivors will play a significant role in shaping how HIT can become optimally useful in the service of helping others affected by cancer.

Finally, consumers look to HIT as a source of support. Cancer, like any life-threatening illness, has the hallmark characteristic of shining a spotlight on the uncertainty that is inherent in everyday life, though easier to ignore when in good health. HIT stands to ease the anxiety associated with this uncertainty in many ways, including through facilitating the connection of consumers to needed information, to their health care team, to others experiencing similar clinical circumstances, and to the family members and friends working to support them. In this way, HIT can truly serve as a lifeline for consumers. As such, we can come to a new appreciation for the urgency of realizing the full potential of HIT. Failures at any level—whether technical, operational, or in implementation—ultimately impact consumers. When facing an illness like cancer, consumers must endure a significant level of vulnerability. One of the most tragic consequences of missteps in HIT is when HIT exacerbates this vulnerability. One of its most important roles and potentials is to ameliorate it.

20.5 CONCLUSION

Although we are at the end of the book, we view this time as just the nascent stage of what will become a mature field of oncology informatics. Much has been accomplished over the last decade but we have much more to achieve to realize the benefits of HIT and informatics. We are eternally grateful to all our authors whose contributions provide the core learnings and insights of the book. We remain optimistic that oncology care will improve through the strategic use of HIT, and believe HIT will be foundational to a much improved health care system to the benefit of all citizens.

LIST OF ACRONYMS AND ABBREVIATIONS

ACO Accountable Care Organization
ASCO American Society of Clinical Oncology
CancerLinQ Cancer Learning Intelligence Network for Quality
CER Comparative effectiveness research
CHESS Comprehensive Health Enhancement Support System
CMS Centers for Medicare & Medicaid Services
EHR Electronic health record
EMR Electronic medical record
HINTS Health Information National Trends Survey
HIT Health information technology
HITECH Health Information Technology for Economic and Clinical Health
HPV Human papillomavirus
IOM Institute of Medicine
IT Information technology
MU Meaningful Use
NCI National Cancer Institute
NIH National Institutes of Health
PCMH Patient-centered medical home
RCT Randomized clinical trial
UCD User centered design

References

[1] Levit LA, Balogh E, Nass SJ, Ganz P. Institute of Medicine (U.S.). Committee on improving the quality of cancer care: addressing the challenges of an aging population. Delivering high-quality cancer care: charting a new course for a system in crisis. Washington (DC): The National Academies Press; 2013. xxviii, p. 384.

[2] Fishman TC. Shock of gray: the aging of the world's population and how it pits young against old, child against parent, worker against boss, company against rival, and nation against nation, 1st Scribner hardcover ed. New York, NY: Scribner; 2010. 401 pp.

[3] American Cancer Society Cancer facts & figures 2015. Atlanta, GA: American Cancer Society; 2015.

[4] Shulman LN, Jacobs LA, Greenfield S, Jones B, McCabe MS, Syrjala K, et al. Cancer care and cancer survivorship care in the United States: will we be able to care for these patients in the future? J Oncol Pract 2009;5(3):119–23.

[5] Institute of Medicine (U.S.). Meeting (37th: 2007: Washington, DC). McClellan MB. Evidence-based medicine and the changing nature of health care: 2007 IOM annual meeting summary. Washington (DC): The National Academies Press; 2008.

[6] Cutler DM. The quality cure: how focusing on health care quality can save your life and lower spending too. Berkeley, CA: University of California Press; 2014. xviii, 214 pp.

[7] Cutler DM, Davis K, Stremikis K. Why health reform will bend the cost curve. Issue Brief (Commonw Fund) 2009;72:1–16.

[8] Cutler DM, Davis K, Stremikis K. The impact of health reform on health system spending. Issue Brief (Commonw Fund) 2010;88:1–14.

[9] Buntin MB, Jain SH, Blumenthal D. Health information technology: laying the infrastructure for national health reform. Health Aff (Millwood) 2010;29(6):1214–9.

[10] Institute of Medicine A foundation for evidence-driven practice: a rapid learning system for cancer care. Workshop summary. Washington, DC: The National Academies Press; 2010.

[11] Patlak M, Balogh E, Nass SJ, National Cancer Policy Forum (U.S.) National Coalition for Cancer Survivorship (U.S.) Institute of Medicine (U.S.) Patient-centered cancer treatment planning: improving the quality of oncology care: workshop summary. Washington, DC: National Academies Press; 2011. xii.

[12] Taplin SH, Clauser S, Rodgers AB, Breslau E, Rayson D. Interfaces across the cancer continuum offer opportunities to improve the process of care. J Natl Cancer Inst Monogr 2010;2010(40):104–10.

[13] Nass SJ, Wizemann TM, National Cancer Policy Forum (U.S.) Informatics needs and challenges in cancer research: workshop summary. Washington, DC: National Academies Press; 2012. xvi, 129 pp.

[14] Institute of Medicine Capturing social and behavioral domains and measures in electronic health records: phase 2. Washington, DC: National Academies Press; 2015.

[15] Hesse BW. Public health informatics Gibbons MC, editor. eHealth solutions for healthcare disparities. New York, NY: Springer; 2007, p. 109–29.

[16] Hewitt ME, Ganz PA, Institute of Medicine (U.S.). American Society of Clinical Oncology (U.S.) From cancer patient to cancer survivor: lost in transition: an American Society of Clinical Oncology and Institute of Medicine symposium. Washington, DC: National Academies Press; 2006. vi.

[17] Wachter RM. The digital doctor: hope, hype, and harm at the dawn of medicine's computer age. New York, NY: McGraw-Hill Education; 2015.

[18] DesRoches CM, Painter MW, Jha AK. Health information technology in the United States: progress and challenges ahead. Princeton, NJ Princeton, NJ: Robert Wood Johnson Foundation; 2014 2014. Health information technology in the United States: progress and challenges ahead. Princeton, NJ Princeton, NJ: Robert Wood Johnson Foundation; 2014, 2014.

[19] Olsen L, Aisner D, McGinnis JM, Institute of Medicine (U.S.) Roundtable on evidence-based medicine. The learning healthcare system: workshop summary. Washington, DC: National Academies Press; 2007. xx.

[20] Shaikh AR, Butte AJ, Schully SD, Dalton WS, Khoury MJ, Hesse BW. Collaborative biomedicine in the age of big data: the case of cancer. J Med Internet Res 2014;16(4):e101.

[21] Collins F. Newsmaker interview. Francis Collins: looking beyond the funding deluge. Interview by Jocelyn Kaiser. Science 2009;326(5950):214.

[22] Eden J, Institute of Medicine (U.S.) Committee on reviewing evidence to identify highly effective clinical services. Knowing what works in health care: a roadmap for the nation. Washington, DC: National Academies Press; 2008. xxii.

[23] Wong WF, LaVeist TA, Sharfstein JM. Achieving health equity by design. JAMA 2015;313(14):1417–8.

[24] Galligioni E, Berloffa F, Caffo O, Tonazzolli G, Ambrosini G, Valduga F, et al. Development and daily use of an electronic oncological patient record for the total management of cancer patients: 7 years' experience. Ann Oncol 2009;20(2):349–52.

[25] Hesse BW, Nelson DE, Kreps GL, Croyle RT, Arora NK, Rimer BK, et al. Trust and sources of health information: the impact of the Internet and its implications for health care providers: findings from the first Health Information National Trends Survey. Arch Intern Med 2005;165(22):2618–24.

[26] Hesse BW, Moser RP, Rutten LJ. Surveys of physicians and electronic health information. N Engl J Med 2010;362(9):859–60.

[27] Eysenbach G. From intermediation to disintermediation and apomediation: new models for consumers to access and assess the credibility of health information in the age of Web2.0. Stud Health Technol Inform 2007;129(Pt 1):162–6.

[28] Krist AH, Woolf SH. A vision for patient-centered health information systems. JAMA 2011;305(3):300–1.

[29] Hesse BW, Hansen D, Finholt T, Munson S, Kellogg W, Thomas JC. Social participation in health 2.0. IEEE Comput 2010;43(11):45–52.

[30] DesRoches CM, Painter MW, Jha AK, (editors). Health information technology in the United States, 2015: transition to a post-HITECH world. Princeton (NJ): Robert Wood Johnson Foundation; 2015.

[31] Cancer-specific data sharing standards for communication, collaboration, and coordination of care. American Society of Clinical Oncology; 2015. Available from: <http://www.asco.org/practice-research/cancer-specific-data-sharing:standards-communication-collaboration>.

[32] American Society of Clinical Oncology, Position paper. Available from: <http://www.asco.org/sites/www.asco.org/files/position_paper_for_clq_briefing_09142015.pdf>; 2015.

[33] Jacob JA. On the road to interoperability, public and private organizations work to connect health care data. JAMA 2015;134(12):3.

[34] Technology TOotNCfHI. Connecting health and care for the nation: a shared nationwide interoperability roadmap. 2015; Final Version 1.0: 77.

[35] Wergin R. <http://www.aafp.org/dam/AAFP/documents/advocacy/health_it/interoperability/LT-ONC-INterOp-100515.pdf>; 2015.

[36] Rosenbaum L. Transitional chaos or enduring harm? The EHR and the disruption of medicine. N Engl J Med 2015;373(17):4.

[37] Letter to Senate from 111 medical associations: AMA; 2015. Available from: <http://assets.fiercemarkets.net/public/004-Healthcare/internal/senatemuletter11-3.pdf>.

[38] Zhang J, Chen Y, Ashfaq S, Bell K, Calvitti A, Farber NJ, et al. Strategizing EHR use to achieve patient-centered care in exam rooms: a qualitative study on primary care providers. J Am Med Inform Assoc 2016;23:137–43.

[39] Ratwandi RM, Fairbanks RJ, Hettinger AZ, Benda NC. Electronic health record usabilty: analysis of the user-centered design processes of eleven electronic health record vendors. J Am Med Inform Assoc 2015;22:4.

[40] Mandl K, Mandel J, Kohane I. Driving innovation in health systems through an apps-based information economy. Cell Syst 2015;1(1):11.

[41] Medicare CfMa. Oncology Care Model 2015. Available from: <https://innovation.cms.gov/initiatives/Oncology-Care/>.

[42] Berwick DM, Nolan TW, Whittington J. The triple aim: care, health, and cost. Health Aff (Millwood) 2008;27(3):759–69.

[43] Spiro A. <http://healthwealthandlife.blogspot.com/2015/06/my-recent-hospital-stay-and-care-of.html>; 2015.

[44] Mohr DC, Cheung K, Schueller SM, Hendricks Brown C, Duan N. Continuous evaluation of evolving behavioral intervention technologies. Am J Prev Med 2013;45(4):517–23.

[45] Nelson DE, Kreps GL, Hesse BW, Croyle RT, Willis G, Arora NK, et al. The Health Information National Trends Survey (HINTS): development, design, and dissemination. J Health Commun 2004;9(5):443–60.

[46] Beckjord EB, Reynolds KA, van Londen GJ, Burns R, Singh R, Arvey SR, et al. Population-level trends in posttreatment cancer survivors' concerns and associated receipt of care: results from the 2006 and 2010 LIVESTRONG surveys. J Psychosoc Oncol 2014;32(2):125–51.

[47] Valdez RS, Holden RJ, Novak LL, Veinot TC. Transforming consumer health informatics through a patient work framework: connecting patients to context. J Am Med Inform Assoc 2015;22(1):2–10.

[48] Delbanco T, Walker J, Darer JD, Elmore JG, Feldman HJ, Leveille SG, et al. Open notes: doctors and patients signing on. Ann Intern Med 2010;153(2):121–5.

Glossary

Accountable Care Organization Groups of clinicians, hospitals, and other health care providers who come together voluntarily to give coordinated high quality care to their patients. An official recognition and payment model from the Centers for Medicare and Medicaid Services.

Adaptive Clinical Trial A type of clinical trial in which the diagnosis, lab values, and genetic features identified as clinical actionable mutations are used to assign a patient to a specific treatment arm.

Adjuvant Therapy Also called adjunct therapy or adjunctive therapy or care, is therapy that is given in addition to the primary, main, or initial therapy to maximize its effectiveness. As an adjuvant agent modifies the effect of another agent, so adjuvant therapy modifies other therapy. In cancer therapy, the surgeries and complex treatment regimens used have led the term to be used mainly to describe adjuvant cancer treatments.

Advance Care Planning Making decisions about the care you would want to receive if you happen to become unable to speak for yourself, including consideration of what types of life-sustaining treatments align with your preferences, preparation of an advance directive, and preparation of a durable power of attorney.

Advance Directive A formal legal document specifically authorized by state laws that allows patients to continue their personal autonomy and that provides instructions for care in case they become incapacitated and cannot make decisions.

Advanced Cancer Cancer that has spread to other places in the body and usually cannot be cured or controlled with treatment.

Adverse Event Management An approach to controlling the side effects of a given treatment approach.

Adverse Event Reporting Any undesirable experience associated with the use of a medical product in a patient. The event is serious and should be reported to the Food and Drug Administration (FDA) when it results in death, hospitalization, disability, birth defect, intervention to prevent permanent impairment, threat to life, or other medical events.

Agile Technology Technology, such as software, developed to meet the time pressures of a real world operating environment.

Aging in Place Defined as "the ability to live in one's own home and community safely, independently, and comfortably, regardless of age, income, or ability level" by the Centers for Disease Control and Prevention. The "Aging in Place" movement has been invigorated by informaticists who are building remote supports for seniors to thrive at home with the assistance of technology.

Algorithm A step-by-step procedure for solving a problem or accomplishing some end especially by a computer.

Annual Wellness Visit A yearly office visit paid for by the Centers for Medicare and Medicaid Services for beneficiaries focused on developing and updating a personalized prevention plan based on a patient's current health and risk factors.

Apomediation Is a new scholarly sociotechnological term that describes the ways in which information surrounds both traditional intermediaries, such as physicians in medicine, and consumers. Apomediation was used to describe the effects of an electronic environment in health care which does not serve to displace intermediaries (ie, disintermediation) but to describe the phenomenon in which patients frequently bring information culled from the Internet to their care teams for interpretation.

Asset-Based Community Development Asset-Based Community Development (ABCD) is a strategy for sustainable community-driven development. Beyond the mobilization of a particular community, ABCD is concerned with how to link microassets to the macroenvironment. The appeal of ABCD lies in its premise that communities can drive the development process themselves by identifying and mobilizing existing, but often unrecognized assets, and thereby responding to and creating local economic opportunity.

Asset-Based Community Engaged Research Asset-based community engaged research is a research strategy whereby community and university members work as equal partners to: (1) identify community priorities; (2) track community assets; (3) leverage community assets; (4) conduct research; and (5) generate new knowledge that is then used to reset priorities.

Attentional Blink Deficit in reporting the second of two targets presented in a rapid succession.

Bad Death A dying and death experience that is inconsistent with one's preferences and values and extends unnecessary physical or psychological suffering for the dying individual and/or his or her loved ones.

Bayesian Approach A statistical inference approach in which the true state is expressed in terms of degrees of belief called Bayesian probabilities based on the specification of prior distributions.

Bereavement A period of mourning after a loss, especially after the death of a loved one.

Big Data A branch of health care informatics that pools large and disparate data sets and applies a suite of mathematical approaches that derives associations, facilitates comparisons, and generates insights that are otherwise not possible using standard mono-source analytics.

Big Data Analytics The process of examining large data sets containing a variety of data types to uncover hidden patterns and unknown correlations.

Biobank A collection or bank of biological samples, such as blood, urine, tissue, and DNA that are linked to health information, and are used for scientific research.

Biorepository A facility that collects, catalogs, and stores samples of biological materials, such as urine, blood, tissue, cells, DNA, RNA, and protein, from humans, animals, or plants for laboratory research. If the samples are from people, medical information may also be stored along with a written consent to use the samples in laboratory studies.

Blue Button A tool, frequently found within patient portals and other secure websites, which provides patients with the ability to access and share their health record.

Bundled Payments A single payment to providers or facilities for all services related to treatment of a given condition.

Cancer Abstract Format The arrangement of information fields or elements in a cancer abstract. A cancer abstract is a summary, abridgement, or abbreviated record that identifies pertinent cancer information about the patient, the disease, the cancer-directed treatment, and the disease process from the time of diagnosis until the patient's death. The abstract is the basis for all of the registry's functions.

Cancer Control Continuum The cancer control continuum describes the various points of cancer control: prevention, early detection, diagnosis, treatment, survivorship, and end-of-life. The cancer control continuum is a useful framework on which to view plans, progress, and priorities. It helps identify research gaps, areas for collaboration and assessing impact, and where more resources may be needed.

Cancer Learning Intelligence Network for Quality (CancerLinQ) A technology platform developed by the American Society of Clinical Oncology to aggregate and analyze cancer patient data with the goal of providing feedback and insights to clinicians and to improve care.

CancerLinQ see Cancer Learning Intelligence Network for Quality.

Cancer Surveillance The collection of data on cancer cases to provide population-based trends and outcomes for cancer, typically representing a complete census of all cases within a defined geographic region such as a state. Traditional functions of cancer surveillance include reporting incidence, prevalence, survival, and mortality trends for populations covered.

Cancer Survivor Has been defined in two different ways. One refers to a cancer patient who has no evidence of disease after completion of treatment. Another refers to persons from the time of diagnosis throughout any treatment, remission, and/or recurrence. The latter definition emphasizes the process of living with, through, and beyond cancer.

Care Coordination The deliberate organization of patient care activities between two or more participants (including the patient) involved in a patient's care to facilitate the appropriate delivery of health care services. Organizing care involves the marshaling of personnel and other resources needed to carry out all required patient care activities, and is often managed by the exchange of information among participants responsible for different aspects of care.

Change Blindness A lack of awareness of the existence of change blindness and change simultanagnosia in everyday life.

Change Simultanagnosia The inability of an observer to see more than one distinct change among the attended items.

Chemotherapy The treatment of disease by means of chemicals that have a specific toxic effect on the disease-producing microorganisms (antibiotics) or that selectively destroy cancerous tissue (anticancer therapy).

Choropleth Map A thematic map that uses graded differences in shading or color or the placing of symbols inside pre-defined, aggregated units (or areas) on a map in order to indicate differences in the average values of some measure in those areas.

Citizen Science In general terms, the concept of citizen science refers to the participative inclusion of data and input from lay persons into the scientific enterprise. It has gained new currency in the age of the Internet, as scientists investigate methods for "crowd sourcing" solutions to scientific problems.

Clinical Data Research Networks (CDRNs) A project supported by the Patient-Centered Outcomes Research Institute aimed at forming partnerships between various health systems in order to use the collective data infrastructure to streamline clinical research.

Clinical Decision Support (CDS) A health information technology that assists clinicians at the point of care in optimizing care delivery by providing guidance and evidence to support the decisions being made in real time.

Clinical Summaries An after-visit summary that provides a patient with relevant and actionable information and instructions. Electronic health records (EHRs) are mandated to support a clinician creating these as part of Meaningful Use.

Clinical Trial A formal study carried out according to a prospectively defined protocol that is intended to discover or verify the safety and effectiveness of procedures or interventions in humans.

Common Rule A short name for The Federal Policy for the Protection of Human Subjects which sets forth requirements for human subjects research, such as the use of informed consent

Communication Management System An informatics-enabled data system that allows care providers to monitor communications between staff and outreach efforts to patients in order to ensure that no one is left "out of the loop" on essential communications.

Communication Science The interdisciplinary mix of theory and empirical evidence that contributes to a more informed understanding of how humans convey information to each other across multiple channels, in multiple contexts, and in differing time frames to achieve desired goals.

Community-Based Participatory Research (CBPR) In contrast to more traditional investigator-driven research, CBPR begins with an issue selected by, or of real importance to, the community, and involves community members and other stakeholders throughout the research process, including its culmination in education and action for social change.

Community Health Improvement Plan A community health improvement plan (or CHIP) is a long-term, systematic effort to address public health problems based on the results of community health assessment activities and the community health improvement process.

Community Health Needs Assessment A community health needs assessment (CHNA), also known as a community health assessment (sometimes called a CHA), refers to a state, tribal, local, or territorial health assessment that identifies key health needs and issues through systematic, comprehensive data collection and analysis.

Comorbidities A disease or condition that coexists with a primary disease but also stands on its own as a specific disease. For example, someone can have cancer and heart disease.

Comparative Effectiveness Research (CER) Has been defined by the Institute of Medicine as "the generation and synthesis of evidence that compares the benefits and harms of alternative methods to prevent, diagnose, treat, and monitor a clinical condition or to improve the delivery of care. The purpose of CER is to assist consumers, clinicians, purchasers, and policy makers to make informed decisions that will improve health care at both the individual and population levels."

Computational Modeling A mathematical modeling approach that requires extensive computational resources to study the behavior of a complex system, often a complex nonlinear system.

Computer-Assisted Detection The use of computer software to analyze tissue patterns in an image in order to identify those with some probability of being abnormal. The technology can be manipulated to vary the sensitivity and specificity, and to mark areas of abnormality. Also known as computer aided detection.

Connected Health As used by the President's Cancer Panel in 2014, the concept of "connected health" refers to the use of wireless sensors, Internet applications, wearable technologies, telephones, and mobile computing devices to support patients as they take charge of their general health, their cancer treatments, and their chronic conditions as cancer survivors.

Continuous Quality Improvement Continuous quality improvement is the process-based, data-driven approach to improving the quality of a product or service. It operates under the belief that there is always room for improving operations, processes, and activities to increase quality.

Conversational Agent A medium for automated communication with patients and consumers that uses simulated face-to-face counseling with an animated health counselor.

Cost-Effectiveness A formal method for comparing the benefits of a medical intervention (measured in terms of clinical outcome or utility) with the costs of the medical intervention to determine which alternative provides the maximum aggregate health benefits for a given level of resources, or equivalently, which alternative provides a given level of health benefits at the lowest cost.

Crowdsourcing The creation of new data, information, knowledge or innovations that result from the engagement of a crowd of individuals through a call for achieving a specific objective for potential rewards of personal development, recognition, personal satisfaction, and/or monetary awards.

Cyberinfrastructure This "is the coordinated aggregate of software, hardware, and other technologies, as well as human expertise, required to support current and future discoveries in science and engineering. The challenge of [CI] is to integrate relevant and often disparate resources to provide a useful, usable, and enabling framework for research and discovery characterized by broad access and 'end-to-end' coordination."

Data Altruism A form of participation in clinical research in which the patient contributes or "donates" his or her clinical data broadly or to specific projects.

Data Lake Clinical data (comprised of PHI and PII), practice management data, and potentially data from other sources, that flows through an ingestion gateway into a storage database.

Data Liquidity Referring to the fluid nature of data, such that it flows through the health care system to the appropriate stakeholders in a useful manner.

Datamart Often a subset of a data warehouse that contains data specific to a particular subject or for a particular function.

Data Science Scientific domain involving the conversion of data into information and knowledge.

Data Standards A documented agreement on representations, formats, and definitions of common data.

Decision Aid A tool that provides patients with evidence-based, objective information on all treatment options for a given condition. Decision aids present the risks and benefits of all options and help patients understand how likely it is that those benefits or harms will affect them. Decision aids can include written materials, Web-based tools, videos, and multimedia programs. Some decision aids are targeted at patients, and others are targeted for clinician use with patients.

Deidentified Referring to aggregate statistical data or data stripped of individual identifiers.

Depression A mental condition marked by ongoing feelings of sadness, despair, loss of energy, and difficulty dealing with normal daily life. Other symptoms of depression include feelings of worthlessness and hopelessness, loss of pleasure in activities, changes in eating or sleeping habits, and thoughts of death or suicide. Depression can affect anyone, and can be successfully treated.

Digital Health Literacy Digital health literacy is the ability to seek, find, understand, and appraise health information from electronic sources and apply the knowledge gained to addressing or solving a health problem.

Digital Mammography The use of radiation to create an image that is then captured and translated into an image on a computer (digital) monitor.

Disease Progression The cancer disease becomes worse or spreads in the body.

Disintermediation A reduction in the use of intermediaries between producers and consumers. Electronic platforms, such as the Internet, often shaped new business models wherein traditional intermediaries were replaced by direct access to producers.

Distant Disease The tumor has spread beyond the original site, traveled to other parts of the body, and begun to grow in the new location(s).

Double-Blind Controlled Trial A study in which some participants are given an experimental treatment and some are given a placebo and/or a known treatment, but neither the participants nor the researchers know which participants receive which treatment until the study is over.

Ecological Momentary Assessment (EMA) Repeated sampling of a person's current behaviors and experiences in real time and in the natural environment.

Ecological Momentary Interventions (EMI) The extension of intervention delivery by mobile technologies to deliver interventions during an individual's daily life and in his/her natural environment.

eHealth Gunther Eysenbach, the founding editor of the *Journal of Medical Internet Research*, defines ehealth as "an emerging field at the intersection of medical informatics, public health, and business." It refers to the delivery of medical services or knowledge through the Internet and related technologies.

Electronic Health Record An electronic health record, or EHR, refers to a systematic collection of health information pertinent to an individual patient or population collected in real-time. The American Hospital Association distinguishes between a "basic EHR," which should encompass an implementation of at least 10 pre-specified functions and be deployed in at least one clinical unit of the hospital, and a "comprehensive EHR," which includes 14 additional functions and is implemented in at least seven clinical units in the hospital. They often contain information about a patient's medical history, diagnoses, medications, immunization dates, allergies, radiology images, and lab and test results.

Electronic Pathology Report (e-path) Copy of the pathology report is transmitted electronically to the central cancer registry. The process begins when the pathologist completes the pathology report, marking it as "final"; the process ends when the electronic pathology report data are loaded into the central registry's information system and are ready for use in the central registry (ie, casefinding, updating existing records with additional information, special studies, etc.)

Electronic Patient-Reported Outcomes Any electronically captured, patient-reported health status for physical, mental, and social-wellbeing that can be used to measure research, clinical, or quality outcomes.

Electronic Prescribing The use of computing devices to enter, modify, review, and output or communicate drug prescriptions; the physician or other health care provider sends an accurate, error-free, and understandable prescription directly to a pharmacy from the point of care; replaces paper and faxed prescriptions.

End-of-Life Care A term used to describe the support and medical care given during the time surrounding death.

Endogenous Control Allocation of attention according to high-level factors such as the viewer's interest in a particular object, and his/her expectations about it.

Exogeneous Control Allocation of attention on the basis of the physical properties in the image.

Factorial and Fractional Factorial Designs An experimental design that consists of two or more discrete factors and tests all possible combinations of all levels of all factors. Fractional factorial designs test only a carefully chosen subset of all combinations of all levels of all factors possible from a full factorial design.

False Negative When a test (or an observer) incorrectly indicates that a disease (or a target) is absent; also known as a "Miss."

False Positive When a test (or an observer) incorrectly indicates that a disease (or a target) is present; also known as a "False Alarm."

Family Caregivers Relatives, friends, or neighbors who provide assistance related to an underlying physical or mental disability but are unpaid for those services.

Fatigue A condition marked by extreme tiredness and inability to function due to lack of energy. Fatigue may be acute or chronic.

Fee for Service (FFS) A payment model in which health care providers are paid for each service performed.

Healthcare Common Procedure Coding (HCPC) Produced by the Centers for Medicare and Medicaid Services (CMS), HCPC is a collection of standardized codes that represent medical procedures, supplies, products and services. The codes are used to facilitate the processing of health insurance claims by Medicare and other insurers.

Health Care Safety Net System The health care safety net includes health care providers that deliver care in a variety of settings including public hospitals, community health centers, local health departments, free clinics, special service providers, and in some cases, physician networks and school-based clinics that deliver care to low-income and/or vulnerable patients. Although many receive state and federal funding, safety nets are locally organized and managed, and they serve unique local needs and are attuned to the needs of the population they serve.

Health Certificate Effect When patients receiving negative screening results (eg, no cancer) are given a false sense of security and may feel there is no need to modify their lifestyle.

Health Disparities A type of difference in health that is closely linked with social or economic disadvantage. Health disparities negatively affect groups of people who have systematically experienced greater social or economic obstacles to health. These obstacles stem from characteristics historically linked to discrimination or exclusion, such as race or ethnicity, religion, socioeconomic status, gender, mental health, sexual orientation, or geographic location. Other characteristics include cognitive, sensory, or physical disability.

Health Information Technology In its broadest usage, the term refers to the systematic application of information technology to health care. It can encompass ehealth, mhealth, EHRs, and other facets of information technology to improve the delivery of care.

Health Insurance Portability and Accountability Act (HIPAA) Privacy Rule Establishes national standards to protect individuals' medical records and other personal health information and applies to health plans, health care clearing houses, and those health care providers that conduct certain health care transactions electronically. The Rule requires appropriate safeguards to protect the privacy of personal health information, and sets limits and conditions on the uses and disclosures that may be made of such information without patient authorization. The Rule also gives patients rights over their health information, including rights to examine and obtain a copy of their health records, and to request corrections.

Health-Related Quality of Life A multidimensional concept including physical, mental, emotional, and social functioning and the associated impact of health status on quality of life.

Health Risk Assessment Plus Process Also known as a patient-centered health risk assessment, it is a tool to systematically assess patients' health behaviors and mental health and provide follow-up activities and monitoring of progress toward achieving health improvement goals.

Hospice Care The most intensive form of palliative care; a service delivery system that provides palliative care for patients who have a limited life expectancy and require comprehensive biomedical, psychosocial, and spiritual support as they enter the terminal stage of an illness or condition. It also supports family members coping with the complex consequences of illness, disability, and aging as death nears. Hospice care further addresses the bereavement needs of the family following the death of the patient.

Illusory Conjunction When an observer perceives an object to have two or more features which actually belong to different objects in the image.

Inattentional Blindness The failure to detect, or properly perceive, objects or events that occur unexpectedly while one is processing other stimuli.

Informed Decision Making A process that can occur in the health care setting or community with the intention of informing an individual's decision.

Inreach Reminders Reminders that are provided during the course of patient encounters that inform clinicians a patient is due for a screening test.

Internet of Things The network of physical objects or "things" embedded with electronics, software, sensors, and connectivity to enable objects to exchange data with the manufacturer, operator and/or other connected devices.

Interoperability In the context of health care, interoperability refers to the informatics infrastructure of one system to connect with the informatics infrastructure of another for the purposes of communication, data sharing, and other essential activities.

Interrupted Time Series A type of time series analyses in which the series of data are "interrupted" by the introduction of the treatment, and causal impact is inferred by differences in the posttreatment series data from that predicted by the pre-treatment series.

Just-in-Time Adaptive Interventions (JITAI) Interventions designed to address the dynamically changing needs of individuals by adapting the content and timing of intervention delivery to optimize its effects.

Late Effects Side effects of cancer treatment that do not manifest until after treatment has ended.

Lead Time Bias The perception that people live longer because of screening when in fact it is simply because there is additional time between when a cancer is found by screening and when it would appear symptomatically.

Learning Community Health System A learning community health system is a system that incorporates multiple data sources to generate ongoing cycles of analysis for new knowledge to allow communities to have updated and tailored community health system feedback. The system is dynamic and will grow and change as it gains and responds to new knowledge.

Learning Health Care Information Technology (IT) System A health care system that uses advances in information technology to continuously and automatically collect and compile the evidence needed to deliver the best, most up-to-date personalized care for each patient from clinical practice, disease registries, clinical trials, and other information sources. That evidence is made available as rapidly as possible to users of a learning health care IT system, which include patients, physicians, academic institutions, hospitals, insurers, and public health agencies. A learning health care IT system ensures that this data-rich system learns routinely and iteratively by analyzing captured data, generating evidence, and implementing new insights into subsequent care.

Learning System A system in which the data that are collected inform the performance of the system or the decision rules that define its performance in a continuous fashion.

Localized Disease The tumor has extended beyond the original site but has not spread to other organs and begun to grow in the new location(s).

Machine Learning (ML) A computer science discipline in which algorithms are developed and can learn from data, ultimately being used to make predictions.

Meaningful Use According to the American Recovery and Reinvestment Act of 2009, Meaningful Use has three main components: (1) use of a certified electronic health record (EHR) in a meaningful manner; (2) electronic exchange of health information to improve quality of health care; (3) use of certified EHR technology to submit clinical quality and other measures.

Providers need to show they're using certified EHR technology in ways that can be measured significantly in quality and in quantity.

Metadata Data, commonly found in sensor data, which describes or provides context for other data. For instance, geolocation data, accelerometer data, battery data, and GPS information can act as metadata, contributing further meaning to the data.

Metastases The spread of cancer from one part of the body to another. A tumor formed by cells that have spread is called a "metastatic tumor" or a "metastasis." The metastatic tumor contains cells that are like those in the original (primary) tumor. The plural form of metastasis is metastases.

Mhealth The term mhealth is usually used as an abbreviation of "mobile health," and usually refers to the use of mobile telecommunications and information technology devices to support health-related goals.

Micro-Attribution Applying credit or recognition for contribution and use of information resources including software, data sets, and annotations of data sets into derived works.

Micro-Experts People who have deep knowledge and/or experience in a specific area, typically without formal scientific or medical training.

Mixed Effect Location Model An extension of the standard mixed model statistical approach in which specific types of general mixed model statistical approaches add a subject-level random effect to the within-subject variance specification, permitting subjects to have influence not only on the mean but also on variability over time.

Mobile Application (App) A software program that can be downloaded and accessed directly using a telephone or another mobile device, like a tablet or music player.

Multicomponent Treatments Treatments consisting of more than one active ingredient.

Multilevel Ecological Framework (Biopsychosocial Model) A heuristic popularized by George Engel MD that conceives of individuals as living in a dynamic system that seeks equilibrium and includes nested levels of human aggregation. Depending upon the situation being explained different levels can be identified. Commonly in health care we identify the individual within a health care team, within a health care organization, within a community, state, and nation. The family can also be considered as a level.

MultiUser Notes An electronic document that can be viewed and edited by multiple parties, usually with protocols set for read and write access. A public-facing example in health care is the "Open Notes" initiative, which began as a pilot project between Beth Israel Deaconess Medical Center, Geisinger Health System, and Harborview Medical Center in Seattle, and was designed to give patients access to the clinical notes written by their doctors and nurses.

Natural Language Processing (NLP) Process by which digital text from online documents stored in the organization's information system is read directly by software and automatically coded.

NCI Metathesaurus The unified medical language system for CancerLinQ. It is based on the Unified Medical Language System (UMLS) of the National Cancer Institute, part of the National Library of Medicine, a large multipurpose vocabulary database that contains information about biomedical and health-related concepts, such as the Systematized Nomenclature of Medicine-Clinical Terms (SNOMED-CT).

Needs A patient's physical or emotional requirements.

Net Neutrality A principle referring to the openness of the Internet which maintains that accessibility to content is not subject to discrimination by Internet providers.

Null Hypothesis Statistical Testing (NHST) A statistical inference approach in which the null hypothesis (eg, no difference between treatments) is assumed true and rejected only if the observed data have a low likelihood, typically 5% or less, that the alternative hypothesis (eg, a true difference between treatments) of being the result of sampling error.

Oncology Medical Home Models A coordinated, efficient model for the delivery of quality cancer care. While not specific, the focus is on quality and cost.

Ontology An ontology is a content theory about the sorts of objects, properties of objects, and relations between objects that arise within a domain of knowledge; a structured vocabulary of terms and their interrelationships.

Outreach Reminders Reminders sent to patients' homes to remind them they are due for a screening test.

Overdiagnosis The diagnosis of a condition or disease that will never cause symptoms or death if left undetected.

Palliative Care Patient- and family-centered care that optimizes quality of life by anticipating, preventing, and treating suffering. Palliative care throughout the continuum of illness involves addressing physical, intellectual, emotional, social, and spiritual needs and facilitating patient autonomy, access to information, and choice.

Participatory Design An approach to the assessment, design, and development of technological and organizational systems that places a premium on the active involvement of potential or current users.

Passive Sensors Devices that detect and respond to input from physiology, behavior, and/or environment without any active effort on the part of the participant or system to detect the data being collected.

Patient-Centered Cancer Care Patient-centered cancer care considers the patient as a whole person, beyond their disease, from the time of diagnosis through the balance of their life; is respectful of the patient's preferences, needs, and values related to the involvement of their family and friends in their care; empowers the patient to participate in their care in a way that is consistent with their preferences, needs, and values; and requires that multiple levels of the cancer care delivery are designed to accommodate the needs of patients and caregivers, acknowledging that the care delivery system must support providers to function effectively.

Patient-Centered Care Providing care that is respectful of and responsive to individual patients, needs, values, and preferences and ensuring that patient values guide all clinical decisions.

Patient-Centered Medical Home (PCMH) A model of the organization of primary care that delivers the core functions of primary health care encompassing five essential functions and attributes: comprehensive care, patient-centered, coordinated care, accessible services, and quality and safety.

Patient-Generated Data A description of health data that are gathered from a patient or caregiver to help manage a given condition. Sources may include approaches such as sensors or surveys.

Patient-Led Research Research projects that are initiated or guided by patients.

Patient Navigator Patient navigators educate and assist patients in receiving and comprehending health care services and resources to improve their health. Although their roles might overlap, patient navigators are not specifically community health workers or health advocates; rather, their activities are focused on improving patient access to care, self-management skills and abilities.

Patient Portal A patient portal is a secure online website that gives patients convenient 24-hour access to personal health information from anywhere with an Internet connection. Using a secure username and password, patients can view health information, such as recent doctor visits, discharge summaries, medications, immunizations, allergies, and lab results. Some patient portals also allow patients to exchange secure email with their health care teams, request prescription refills, schedule nonurgent appointments, check benefits and coverage, and update contact information.

Patient-Powered Research Networks (PPRNs) A project supported by the Patient-Centered Outcomes Research Institute aimed at forming partnerships across patients and/or caregivers to drive patient-centered comparative effectiveness research via the resulting networks.

Patient-Reported Outcomes (PROs) Any patient-reported health status for physical, mental, and social-wellbeing that can be used to measure research, clinical, or quality outcomes.

Patient-Reported Outcome Measures Questionnaires completed by patients in order to assess single or multiple constructs related to symptoms, functional status, quality of life, and other aspects of health.

Patient Safety Freedom from accidental injury; ensuring patient safety involves the establishment of operational systems and processes that minimize the likelihood of errors and maximizes the likelihood of intercepting them when they occur.

Pattern Recognition A branch of machine learning that classifies data (patterns) based on either a priori knowledge or on statistical information extracted from the patterns.

Phase IV Surveillance The process monitoring of the safety of a medication after it has been released on the market.

PHR A longitudinal patient health record (PHR) owned by the individual, incorporating elements of the EMR including clinician notes, care plans, tests, and results, and populated by data from interoperable monitoring devices.

Placebo A treatment that is nonactive and not intended to have any clinical effect.

Polyps An abnormal collection of cells that forms on the lining of any organ that has blood vessels; they are generally found in the colon. The cells can be of various types on a spectrum from being completely inconsequential (benign) to being cancerous.

Preattentive Processes Perceptual processes that operate automatically, without any need for attention or limited resources. These processes are spatially parallel (operating locally on each point of the input) and rapid (ie, completed within 100–200 ms).

Precision Medicine Form of medicine that uses information about a person's genes, proteins, and environment to prevent, diagnose, and treat disease. In cancer, precision medicine uses specific information about a person's cancer to help diagnose, plan treatment, find out how well treatment is working, or make a prognosis. Examples of precision medicine include using targeted therapies to treat specific types of cancer cells, such as HER2-positive breast cancer cells, or using tumor marker testing to help diagnose cancer. Also called personalized medicine.

Preferences A patient's concerns, expectations, and choices regarding health care, based on a full and accurate understanding of care options.

Privacy In the context of health information technology, privacy refers to an individual's confidence in having a say in who is allowed to collect, use, or share their medical information.

Prognosis The likely outcome or course of a disease; the chance of recovery or recurrence.

Prostate-Specific Antigen A protease that is secreted by the epithelial cells of the prostate gland.

Protected Health Information (PHI) Information that is protected under the HIPAA Privacy Rule; the Privacy Rule protects all "individually identifiable health information" held or transmitted by a covered entity or its business associate, in any form or media, whether electronic, paper, or oral. "Individually

identifiable health information" is information, including demographic data, that relates to: the individual's past, present, or future physical or mental health or condition; the provision of health care to the individual, or the past, present, or future payment for the provision of health care to the individual, and that identifies the individual or for which there is a reasonable basis to believe it can be used to identify the individual. Individually identifiable health information includes many common identifiers (eg, name, address, birth date, Social Security Number). The Privacy Rule excludes from protected health information employment records that a covered entity maintains in its capacity as an employer and education and certain other records subject to, or defined in, the Family Educational Rights and Privacy Act, 20 U.S.C. §1232g.

Protocol Specifications that describe the details of an experiment or study and how they are to be carried out in a standardized fashion.

Proto-Objects Localized precursors of objects with at least some degree of structure.

Prototype An early, usually not fully-functional, version of a technology that is used for testing in the process of developing a final technology suitable for use at scale.

Public Health Informatics (PHI) The systematic application of information and computer science and technology to public health practice, research, and learning.

Quality of Life The overall enjoyment of life. Many clinical trials assess the effects of cancer and its treatment on the quality of life. These studies measure aspects of an individual's sense of well-being and ability to carry out various activities.

Quantified Self The process of incorporating measurement of oneself into daily functioning to track health or performance.

Quitline A tobacco cessation service available through a toll-free telephone number. Quitlines are staffed by counselors trained specifically to help smokers quit. Quitlines deliver information, advice, support, and referrals to tobacco users.

Randomization The process of making something random; in the context of clinical research, study participants are often randomly allocated to different conditions of a study.

Randomized Clinical Trial A study in which the participants are assigned by chance to separate groups that compare different treatments; neither the researchers nor the participants can choose the group to which they are assigned. Using chance to assign people to groups means that the groups will be similar and the treatments they receive will be compared objectively. At the time of the trial, it is not known which treatment is best. It is the patient's choice to participate in a randomized trial.

Randomized Controlled Trials (RCTs) A scientific experiment in which people are randomly assigned to different treatments to assess their efficacy, independent of any biases. Considered to be the gold standard.

Rapid Learning System An approach borrowed from engineering and applied to health in which electronic health records can be merged into research databases and rapid-learning networks that contain clinical information on millions of patients, allowing the health system to learn from real-world experience and rapidly develop new evidence and apply it to health care.

Recurrence Cancer that has returned after a period of time during which the cancer could not be detected. The cancer may come back to the same place as the original (primary) tumor or to another place in the body. Also called recurrent cancer.

Registry A repository of uniform data for a specified population.

Relational Coordination Communicating and relating for the purpose of task integration. This concept was developed by Jody Gittell PhD and includes a theory that makes visible the social processes and human interactions that underlie the coordination of complex work.

Reminder System A system to remind or encourage health professionals to support health behaviors. The systems can provide trainings, organizational protocols or referral processes, financial remuneration for providers, and materials such as self-help.

Remission A decrease in or disappearance of signs and symptoms of cancer. In partial remission, some, but not all, signs and symptoms of cancer have disappeared. In complete remission, all signs and symptoms of cancer have disappeared, although cancer still may be in the body.

Reversal Designs A type of single-case design to examine the effect of a treatment on a single participant by delivering and then subsequently withdrawing the treatment.

Screen-Film Mammography The use of radiation to create and capture a breast image on photographic film.

Screening The use of a test on individuals who do not exhibit signs or symptoms of disease to identify those who are at increased risk for that disease. These individuals must then be evaluated to determine if disease is present. Since screening consists of screening and evaluation, it is more appropriate to think of screening as a process not just a test.

Shared Care Planning Shared care planning is a process that involves collaboration among patients, family and caregivers, health care teams, and others to develop a shared understanding of both the goals and interventions that make up the trajectory of care. During planning, tools for assessing risk are helpful in identifying those patients who may require more intensive coordination.

Secure Messaging A server-based approach to protect sensitive data, especially when allowing patients to communicate with their care teams through a patient portal. Secure messaging approaches are designed to comply with industry standards such as HIPAA, GLBA, and SOX.

Security In the context of health information technology, security refers to an individual's confidence that safeguards are in place to protect his or her medical information from being seen by people who do not have permission.

Self-Efficacy An individual's belief in his/her ability to perform behaviors necessary to achieve a goal or produce an outcome.

Sensitivity The likelihood a test will be positive for disease when a disease is present. Also known as the true positive rate.

Sequential Multiple Assignment Randomized Trial (SMART) An experimental design to test and optimize adaptive interventions. The approach randomly assigns participants to each treatment option at each critical decision stage of an adaptive intervention (eg, if no response to treatment A after 6 weeks, continue treatment A or switch to treatment B).

Shared Decision Making (SDM) A process in which patients are engaged as active partners with their clinician in clarifying medical options and choosing a preferred course of care.

Short Message Service (SMS) A text messaging service component of phone, web, or mobile communication systems. It uses standardized communications protocols to allow fixed line or mobile phone devices to exchange short text messages.

Side Effects Physical or emotional effects (usually undesirable) secondary to exposure to treatment for a clinical issue.

Social Networks Social networks are online communities that provide instrumental, emotional, and social support. These networks may be focused on a specific health condition and may include the individuals with that condition as well as their family, caregivers, or other interested individuals. With respect to cancer, social networks that allow for both within-family team

and community team collaboration can have a significant impact on health care throughout the cancer continuum.

Specificity The likelihood a test will be negative for disease when a disease is not present. Also known as the true negative rate.

Stages of Change (or Transtheoretical Model) A model that describes the series of stages that patients progress through when making a health behavior change.

Statistical (or Ensemble) Summaries Perceptual information about the statistical properties of a set of objects (eg, mean orientation, standard deviation of size) distinct from information about individual object properties.

Subitizing Rapid and accurate apprehension of small quantities.

Surrogate Decision-Maker If a patient is unable to make decisions or speak for themselves about personal health care, someone else must provide direction in decision making, as the surrogate, or proxy, decision maker.

Targeted Therapies In oncology, a treatment that is more specific for cancer cells than normal cells. Compared with traditional chemotherapy, this ideally results in more effective treatment of the cancer with fewer side effects.

Technology-Mediated Social Participation The use of technology to actively or passively capture input from a number of sources to more comprehensively reflect the perspectives of multiple stakeholders, usually in the service of driving consensus or surfacing insights.

Telemedicine The use of telecommunications technologies—including telephones, video conferencing, smartphones, and mobile computers—to support the delivery of medical services, messages, and knowledge to patients remotely.

Time Varying Effect Model A statistical model that uses intensive longitudinal data (ILD) to observe change over time not only in the outcome but also in the factors that influence the outcome (ie, does not assume that the factors or their effects are time-invariant).

Translational Research Aims to translate or apply scientifically meaningful information and make it clinically relevant, that is, relevant to human health.

Treatment Summaries and Survivorship Care Plans (TS/SCPs) An individualized care plan for cancer survivors that includes guidelines for monitoring and maintaining health.

Treemap Treemap, coined by Dr Ben Shneiderman, is the name for a space-constrained visualization of hierarchical structures that splits the screen into rectangles in alternating horizontal and vertical directions as you traverse the screen from top to bottom.

True Negative When a test (or an observer) correctly indicates that a disease (or a target) is absent; also known as a "Correct Rejection."

True Positive When a test (or an observer) correctly indicates that a disease (or a target) is present; also known as a "Hit."

Unstructured Data Information that cannot be easily stored, queried, recalled, analyzed, and manipulated by machine; examples include office medical records, handwritten physician and nurse notes, hospital admission and discharge records, paper prescriptions, radiograph films, magnetic resonance imaging (MRI) images, computed tomography (CT) images, and other images.

User-Centered Design An approach to design that puts the needs and preferences of end-users at the center of the design and development process throughout the lifecycle of product development.

U.S. Preventive Services Task Force (USPSTF) An independent panel of national experts in prevention that makes evidence-based recommendations about screenings, counseling services, and preventive medications.

Virtual Registry A linkage of multiple population-based cancer registries, permitting a centralized, automated, and efficient way to access patient data, pooled from those registries, for research purposes; uses advanced IT security protocols, with the data remaining behind separate security firewalls at each participating registry; increases accuracy and completeness of information, relative to traditional cancer registries.

Weber Fraction In psychophysics, the ratio of the smallest detectable difference between quantities to the magnitude of the smaller quantity; equivalently, the ratio of the standard deviation of an estimate to its mean.

Within-Subject Design A type of experimental design in which all participants are exposed to every treatment or condition and repeatedly evaluated.

Workflow The processes required to complete a task by an industry, company, department, or employee.

Index

Note: Page numbers followed by "*b*," "*f*," and "*t*" refer to boxes, figures, and tables, respectively.

A

A/B testing, 338–339, 339*f*
ABCD approach. *See* Asset-Based Community Development approach (ABCD approach)
"Abnormal gist", 291
ACA. *See* Affordable Care Act (ACA)
Accessibility, 154
"Accountability for Cancer Care through Undoing Racism and Equity" study (ACCURE study), 29–32
Accountable Care Organization model (ACO model), 60–61, 257, 381–382
ACO model. *See* Accountable Care Organization model (ACO model)
ACOR. *See* Association of Cancer Online Resources (ACOR)
ACoS. *See* American College of Surgeons (ACoS)
ACS. *See* American Cancer Society (ACS)
ACTIVE. *See* Assessing Caregivers for Team Intervention through Videophone Encounters (ACTIVE)
Adaptive designs, 352
Adaptive instruments, 47
ADE. *See* Adverse drug event (ADE)
Advanced cancer, 182
  bereavement, 184
  caregiving, 184
  CHESS, 190–197
  decision making, 183–184
  future directions for development and implementation, 200
  future directions for research, 197
    decision making research, 198–199
    economic outcomes, 199
    family involvement, 199–200
    patient outcomes, 197–198
    research design, 197
  opportunities for eHealth, 184–190
  symptom management, 182–183
Adverse drug event (ADE), 261
Adverse event (AE), 325
  detection and drug safety, 325
Adverse health behaviors and emotional distress, screening and intervention for
  screening for emotional distress and unmet needs, 243–244
  screens for emotional distress in oncology, 244*t*
Affordable Care Act (ACA), 26, 114–115, 360

Agency for Healthcare Research and Quality (AHRQ), 132–133, 169, 260–261
Agent-based modeling of population dynamics, 350
Agile technology, 280
AHIMA. *See* American Health Information Management Association (AHIMA)
AHRQ. *See* Agency for Healthcare Research and Quality (AHRQ)
AJCC. *See* American Joint Committee on Cancer (AJCC)
Alcohol consumption, 107, 117
ALS. *See* Amyotrophic Lateral Sclerosis (ALS)
ALS Functional Rating Scale (Extension Items) (ALSFRS-EX), 320
ALS Functional Rating Scale (Revised) (ALSFRS-R), 319
Althea Health, 316
American Cancer Society (ACS), 24, 163, 214–216
American College of Surgeons (ACoS), 243
American Health Information Management Association (AHIMA), 149
American Joint Committee on Cancer (AJCC), 224
American Medical Informatics Association (AMIA), 239
American Recovery and Reinvestment Act (ARRA), 358–359
American Society of Clinical Oncology (ASCO), 4, 50, 62, 82–83, 146–147, 232, 307–308, 369, 375
AMIA. *See* American Medical Informatics Association (AMIA)
Amyotrophic Lateral Sclerosis (ALS), 312, 319
Analytic approaches, 153–154
API. *See* Asian and Pacific Islander (API)
Approximate number system, 291
ARPANET, 334
Asian and Pacific Islander (API), 24
Assessing Caregivers for Team Intervention through Videophone Encounters (ACTIVE), 186
Asset-Based Community Development approach (ABCD approach), 32
Asset-based community-engaged research approach, 32
Association of Cancer Online Resources (ACOR), 268–269, 334–335
Attentional control, 293–294

Attentional system, 289. *See also* Preattentive system; Nonattentional systems
  control, 290
  in perceptual experience, 289–290
  precise estimation of number, 290

B

Balancing survival, 147–148
Bayesian approaches, 350–351
BCSC. *See* Breast Cancer Surveillance Consortium (BCSC)
BCT. *See* Boot Camp Translation (BCT)
BD2K. *See* Big Data to Knowledge (BD2K)
Behavior change
  Behavior Change Wheel, 233
  taxonomy, 239
    excerpt from, 240*f*
    excerpt from ontology, 240*f*
Behavioral informatics, 232, 239. *See also* Informatics; Oncology informatics
  applications of resources and tools in cancer care
    implementing psychosocial screening, 244–248
    low literacy support, 248
    physical activity promotion, 242–243
    screening and intervention, 243–244
    tobacco use and informatics-based interventions, 241–242
    virtual exercise coach, 243*f*
  behavioral ontologies, 239
  Reusable Knowledge in Health Counseling Dialog System, 241*f*
  taxonomies, 239–241
Behavioral Intervention Technologies (BITs), 233
Behavioral science, 232
Behavioral/psychological sciences in advancing informatics, 232
  behavior-health linkages, 235*t*–236*t*
  behavioral measures in EHRs, 237–238
  cognitive processes and CDS, 236–237
  contribution to mHealth, 238–239
  HIT infrastructure, 238
  theories and models of behavior change, 232–236
  types of evidence for fuzzy-Trace theory, 237*t*
  YAP#DFCI, 238*b*
Bereavement, 184
  CHESS and, 192–193
  opportunities for, 189–190

Big Data, 151
  analytics, 349–350
  Initiative, 208–209
Big Data to Knowledge (BD2K), 46
Biomarker discovery, 324
Biomedical Research Integrated Domain
    Group model (BRIDG model), 47
Biorepositories, 282–283
BITs. *See* Behavioral Intervention
    Technologies (BITs)
Body mass index (BMI), 163
Bone metastasis (BM), 223
Boot Camp Translation (BCT), 60
Bottom-up approach, 35
Breast cancer, 124–125
  screening, 126–127
Breast Cancer Surveillance Consortium
    (BCSC), 134
BRIDG model. *See* Biomedical Research
    Integrated Domain Group model
    (BRIDG model)
Bright spots in oncology informatics, 375
  actionable knowledge through
    interdisciplinary science, 379–380
  learning oncology systems, 375–376
  population health informatics, 376–377
  rise of consumer engagement and
    participation, 378–379
  technology to improving care coordination
    and delivery, 377–378
"Build and evaluate loops", 76
Building future, 382
  consumers, 384
  developers, 383–384
  providers, 382–383
  researchers, 383

C

C-CDA. *See* Consolidated-Clinical Document
    Architecture (C-CDA)
CAD. *See* Computer-assisted detection
    (CAD)
Canadian Virtual Hospice, 186
"Cancer atlas" system, 212
Cancer Care and Racial Equity Study
    (CCARES), 30–31
Cancer Care Continuum section, 375–376
Cancer Genome Characterization Initiative
    (CGCI), 50
Cancer Health Enhancement Support System
    (CHESS), 168–169
Cancer Learning Intelligence Network for
    Quality (CancerLinQ), 10, 50, 149, 232
  ASCO'S vision for rapid learning system
    in oncology, 10
  data architecture, 10–12
  data ingestion, 11*f*
  history and current status
    background and prototype
      development, 12
    development, 12–13
    SAP, 13
  portal, 14
  regulatory underpinnings of, 17
    data governance guiding principles and
      policies, 18

solution operating characteristics
    CDS, 14–15
    data ingestion, 13–14
    observational CDS use case, 17*b*
    personalized medicine CDS use case,
      15*b*–16*b*
    quality benchmarking, 14
    secondary uses of deidentified and/or
      limited data sets, 16–17
    user types, 14
Cancer surveillance, 277
  current status and opportunities for
    informatics in
    automation through NLP, 280
    data linkages for surveillance, 280–282
  data domains, 279*f*
  new areas for
    biorepositories, 282–283
    clinical trials case identification in real
      time, 283
    expanded ability to assessing quality of
      care, 283
    expanded ability to making sense of
      cancer patterns and trends,
      283–284
    national virtual registry, 283
  sources of data, 278*f*
  tumor characterization, 279
Cancer Target Discovery and Development
    project (CTD² project), 50
Cancer Text Information Extraction System
    (caTIES), 219
Cancer treatment, 145–146
  balancing survival and quality of life,
    147–148
  data aggregation, 148–149
  data optimization, 149–151
  evidentiary uncertainty, 146–147
  genomics in care continuum, 153
  limitations of guidelines, 147
  market evolution, 148
  novel organizational approaches, 155
  patient insights to optimizing care, 151–153
    PROs, 151–152
    sensors, 152
    use case, 152
  RCTs, 146
  tooling, 153–155
Cancer(s), 269. *See also* Advanced cancer;
    CYberinfrastructure for COmparative
    effectiveness REsearch (CYCORE)
  applications of data visualization in
    cancer science, 214
    clinical applications, 216–219
    population statistics, 214–216
  cancer-related health care expenditures, 358
  CER, 358–359
  clinical research
    adaptive instruments, 47
    building national learning health care
      system for cancer, 46
    capturing patient experience across
      continuum of care, 46
    connected health and mobile
      technologies, 48
    data access, 43–44

    data liquidity, 42
    data packet, 42*f*
    data science, 42–43
    drivers, 41–42
    empowering patient as full participant
      in research, 46
    incentives for data sharing, 46–47
    lowering barriers to data access for
      cancer research, 48–49
    ontologies and workflow systems, 47
    precision medicine drivers, 49–50
    translational research, 44–46
  cluster, 209–210
  communication, 261–262
  continuum, 160
  data system, 4
  disparities reducing through community
    engagement, 29–32
    ACCURE study, 29–32
    CBPR, 27–29
    challenges for field, 35–36
    PHIs, 24–27, 32–34
    strengths of PHI applications in health
      disparities, 36–37
  distance medicine technology in care and
    research, 361
  epidemiology, 104
  foraging for, 299–300
  health disparities, 24–25
  informatics, 200
  IT applications in cancer care, 360*f*
  mortality, 124–125
  patterns and trends, 283–284
  prevention, 104
  science, 214
  screening registry, 136
  survivors, 159–161
  survivorship, 159–162
CancerLinQ. *See* Cancer Learning
    Intelligence Network for Quality
    (CancerLinQ)
CAP. *See* College of American Pathologists
    (CAP)
Capacity-building component, 35
Carbon monoxide (CO), 365
Carboxyhemoglobin (COHb), 365
Care coordination, 83, 164–165
  challenge of, 82*f*
  and delivery, 377–378
  frameworks for, 83, 85*t*–86*t*
    CCM, 84
    CWCC, 86–88
    elements, 83–84
    IPC, 84–86
  HIT functions for, 88
    within and across health care
      teams, 89
    across multiple teams, 90
    person-centered coordination, 89
    shared care planning, 89
Care planning, 84
Caregiver, 183–184, 210–211
Caregiving, 184
  CHESS and, 192–193
caTIES. *See* Cancer Text Information
    Extraction System (caTIES)

CBPR. *See* Community-based participatory research (CBPR)
CCARES. *See* Cancer Care and Racial Equity Study (CCARES)
CCD. *See* Continuity of Care Document (CCD)
CCI. *See* Charlson Comorbidity Index (CCI)
CCM. *See* Chronic care model (CCM)
CDISC. *See* Clinical Data Interchange Standards Consortium (CDISC)
CDS. *See* Clinical decision support (CDS)
CEEI. *See* Continuous evaluation of evolving interventions (CEEI)
Center for Primary Care Informatics (CPCI), 136
Centers for Disease Control and Prevention (CDC), 24, 107, 136, 148–149, 210, 277–278
Centers for Medicare & Medicaid Services (CMS), 9, 34, 68, 82, 148, 280, 376
CER. *See* Comparative effectiveness research (CER)
Cervical cancer, 125
  screening, 127
CGCI. *See* Cancer Genome Characterization Initiative (CGCI)
CHAARTED. *See* Chemohormonal Therapy *vs.* Androgen Ablation Randomized Trial for Extensive Disease in Prostate Cancer (CHAARTED)
Change
  blindness, 290
  simultanagnosia, 290
Charlson Comorbidity Index (CCI), 224
CHC. *See* Community health center (CHC)
CHCANYS. *See* Community Health Care Association of New York State (CHCANYS)
Chemohormonal Therapy *vs.* Androgen Ablation Randomized Trial for Extensive Disease in Prostate Cancer (CHAARTED), 146–147
Chemotherapy, 151, 199
CHESS. *See* Cancer Health Enhancement Support System (CHESS); Comprehensive Health Enhancement Support System (CHESS)
CHH. *See* Community Health Hub (CHH)
CHI. *See* Consumer health informatics (CHI)
Chicago health, 32–34
Children's Oncology Group (COG), 332
CHIP. *See* Community Health Implementation Plan (CHIP)
CHNA. *See* Community Health Needs Assessment (CHNA)
CHOP. *See* Cyclophosphamide, adriamycin, vincristine, and prednisone (CHOP)
Choropleth mapping, 209–210
Chronic care model (CCM), 71–72, 84
CI. *See* Confidence interval (CI); Cyberinfrastructure (CI)
Cigar smokers, 105
Cinematch, 44–45
Circos software, 214
Citizen
  contributions, 48–49

science, 48–49
Claims data, 281–282
Clear Health Costs, 315
"Clear Value Plus" program (CVP program), 154
ClinGen. *See* Clinical Genome Resource (ClinGen)
Clinic-based environmental scan, 138
Clinic-community resource scan, 138
Clinical and Translational Science Awards (CTSA), 48
Clinical applications, 216–219
Clinical Data Interchange Standards Consortium (CDISC), 47, 150
Clinical decision support (CDS), 5, 14–15, 136, 154, 232, 236–237, 270–271
Clinical Genome Resource (ClinGen), 50
Clinical Measure Analysis (CMA), 14
Clinical Measurement Library (CML), 14
Clinical Oncology Treatment Plan and Summary (eCOTPS), 13–14
Clinical quality measure (CQM), 14
Clinical trials, 7
  case identification in real time, 283
  as foundation of evidence-based medicine in cancer, 7–8
  limitations of conventional, 8–9
Clinician Report (CR), 93–94, 192
ClinVar, 50
Closed-loop functionality, 112
Clustering Based on Density Distribution Function (DENCLUE), 210
CMA.. *See* Clinical Measure Analysis (CMA)
CML. *See* Clinical Measurement Library (CML)
CMS. *See* Centers for Medicare & Medicaid Services (CMS)
CO. *See* Carbon monoxide (CO)
CoC. *See* Commission on Cancer (CoC)
Cochrane review, 110
Coevolution of payment reform, 382
COG. *See* Children's Oncology Group (COG)
Cognitive
  computing, 154
  processes, 236–237
  schemata, 257
COHb. *See* Carboxyhemoglobin (COHb)
Cohort Comparison (CoCo), 219–223
College of American Pathologists (CAP), 280
Colonoscopy Reporting System (CoRS), 137
Colorectal cancer (CRC), 24, 125
  QOL in, 366–367
  screening, 294–296
Colorectal screening, 127–128
Commission on Cancer (CoC), 243
Common Rule, 17, 321–322
Communication, 164–165
  management systems, 256–257
  revolution, 253–254
    communication science, 254–255
    "dot. com implosion", 254
    informatics enabled communication tools, 256*t*
    interdefining facets of informatics-supported communication, 255*f*
    inventory of informatics tools, 255–260
  technology, 185–186

Communication error(s), 254
  in oncology, 260–261
Communication science
  communication revolution, 253–260
  functional approach to patient-centered communication, 263–271
  to improving quality of cancer care, 260
    cancer communication, 261–262
    communication error in oncology, 260–261
    core functions of patient-centered communication, 263*f*
    rules for realigning health care, 262–263, 262*t*
Community
  engagement, 29–32
  navigation, 93
  setting, 60
Community Health Care Association of New York State (CHCANYS), 136
Community health center (CHC), 110
Community Health Hub (CHH), 138
Community Health Implementation Plan (CHIP), 26
Community Health Needs Assessment (CHNA), 26
Community-based participatory research (CBPR), 24, 27, 73, 337
  community organizations and movement towards population health, 29
  design and delivery, 28
  ethical considerations, 28
  implementation and continuous improvement, 28
  orientation to research, 27–28
  public involvement in health, research, and science, 29
Community-wide care coordination (CWCC), 84, 86–88, 88*f*
CommunityRx partners, 32, 33*f*
  asset-based community-engaged research approach, 32
  community
    engagement, 32
    and university collaborators, 32–33
  Health Care Innovation Award, 34
  HealtheRx, 34
  MapApp, 33
Comparative effectiveness research (CER), 4, 146, 323, 358, 376. *See also* CYberinfrastructure for COmparative effectiveness REsearch (CYCORE)
  cancer, 358–359
  distance medicine technology
    in cancer care and research, 361
    through CER, 360–361
  evidence collection to inform patient care, 360–361
  health information technology infrastructure for improving, 359
  IT applications in cancer care, 360*f*
  strengthening capacity through EHRs, 367
  integrating data from multiple sources, 368–369
  patient portals in oncology, 368

Comprehensive assessment, 83–84
Comprehensive health data research
    infrastructure, treatment testing in
    preparation for, 350
  adaptive designs, 352
  just-in-time adaptive interventions, 351
  optimized and adaptive interventions, 351
  rapid learning systems, 352
  single case studies, 350–351
Comprehensive Health Enhancement
    Support System (CHESS), 93–94,
    186–187, 190, 232–233, 258, 377–378
  for caregiving and bereavement, 192–193
  elderly woman, 194*b*
  lessons
    from development and implementation,
      193–195
    from evaluation, 196
  services, 191*t*
  and symptom management, 191–192
Computational modeling, 347, 350
Computed tomography (CT), 128, 335
Computer-aided detection systems (CAD
    systems). *See* Computer-assisted
    detection (CAD)
Computer-assisted detection (CAD), 131, 298
Computer-assisted interventions, 187–188
Confidence interval (CI), 116, 264
Connected health, 48
Consent, 42, 46
  consent-derived access, 48
Consolidated Standards of Reporting Trials
    (CONSORT), 344
Consolidated-Clinical Document
    Architecture (C-CDA), 13–14, 49,
    149–150
Consumer health informatics (CHI), 234
Consumer(s), 384
  consumer-facing applications, 169
  culture, 308
  engagement and participation, rise of,
    378–379
  genetic testing services, 313
Context-aware, 171–172
Continuity of Care Document (CCD), 13–14,
    149–150
Continuous evaluation of evolving
    interventions (CEEI), 118
"Continuous patient engagement", 316
Continuous quality improvement (CQI), 34
Conventional clinical trials, limitations of,
    8–9
Conversational agents, 248
Coordination of systems, 291
  coordination of interacting systems, 292*f*
  implications, 292
  virtual representation, 291–292
Cordata Oncology, 93
CoRS. *See* Colonoscopy Reporting System
    (CoRS)
CPCI. *See* Center for Primary Care
    Informatics (CPCI)
CPT. *See* Current Procedural Terminology
    (CPT)
CQI. *See* Continuous quality improvement
    (CQI)

CQM. *See* Clinical quality measure (CQM)
CR. *See* Clinician Report (CR)
CRC. *See* Colorectal cancer (CRC)
Crowd, 310
CrowdMed, 314
Crowdsourcing, 308, 337
  clinical trial challenges, 308
  conflicts of interest and IP, 323
  data privacy, 322–323
  distributed problem-solving projects, 308
  ethical issues, 321–322
  with examples, 308
  future
    adverse event detection and drug safety,
      325
    biomarker discovery, 324
    patient partnership in clinical research,
      323–324
    phase IV surveillance, 325
    phenomics, 324–325
    real world CER, 325
  in health care, 312
    for diagnostics and drug discovery,
      312–314
    for health care delivery improvements,
      314–315
    for optimizing treatment, 314
    patient as researcher, 315–320
    PLM renal cell cancer patient, 318*f*
    steps in continuous engagement, 317*t*
  history, 308–309
  methodological issues, 320–321
  parameters, 309–312
  types, 309*t*
CT. *See* Computed tomography (CT)
CTD² project. *See* Cancer Target Discovery
    and Development project (CTD²
    project)
CTSA. *See* Clinical and Translational Science
    Awards (CTSA)
Current Procedural Terminology (CPT), 311
CVP program. *See* "Clear Value Plus"
    program (CVP program)
CWCC. *See* Community-wide care
    coordination (CWCC)
Cyberinfrastructure (CI), 361–362
CYberinfrastructure for COmparative
    effectiveness REsearch (CYCORE),
    361–362
  architecture, 364
  across cancer prevention and control
    continuum, 364
    cancer risk and sequelae prevention,
      364–365
    phases across cancer continuum, 365*f*
    QOL in colorectal cancer, 366–367
    radiation-based treatment for head and
      neck cancers, 366
    survivorship management, 366–367
    use case results, 367
  case-specific stakeholders and activities,
    362–363, 363*f*
  infrastructure processes, 362–363
  people, devices, or outside systems, 364*f*
Cyclophosphamide, adriamycin, vincristine,
    and prednisone (CHOP), 150–151

D
DARPA. *See* United States Defense
    Advanced Research Programs
    Administration (DARPA)
Data
  access, 43–44
  aggregation, 148
    providers and networks, 148
    secondary data sources, 149
    translating data into action, 149
    tumor registries, 148–149
  altruism, 48–49, 375, 379, 384
  characteristics, 311
  data sets, integration with existing, 348
  data sharing, incentives for, 46–47
    meaningful use of common data
      elements, 47
    standardization of common data
      elements, 47
  donors, 49
  exploration, 292–293
    attentional control, 293–294
    visual variables, 293
    visualization as extended vision, 293
  ingestion, 13–14
  lake, 11
  linkages for surveillance, 280–281
    claims data, 281–282
    data from industry partners, 282
    infusion chemotherapy, 281
    new challenges to surveillance data
      quality, 282
  liquidity, 42, 171
  optimization, 149
    addressing gap in codified, standardized
      data, 149–150
    NLP and ML, 150–151
    use case, 151
  science, 42
    impact of mHealth, 42–43
  standards and integration, 347
  warehousing, 43
Data visualization, 154
  applications of data visualization in cancer
    cancer science, 214
    clinical applications, 216–219
    population statistics, 214–216
  case studies, 219
    algorithm development using claims
      data, 223–224
    CoCo, 219–223
    EventFlow, 219–223
    patient comorbidity and health services
      utilization, 224–227
  software systems, 210–212
  strengths of available tools, 212
  techniques, 209–210
  tools, 208–209
  weaknesses of available tools, 214
Data-intensive computation, 347
Data-rich
  advances in data-rich research enterprise,
    348–350
  data-rich biomedical and behavioral research
    enterprise, 348
  environment, 345–348

enterprise, 348
 EHR integration with personal health information, 348
 integration with existing data sets, 348
 standard interoperable electronic health record, 348
 environment, 345–346
  attributes of data-rich research science, 346–347, 347b
  meteorology, 346
  plate tectonics, 346
  radio astronomy and cosmology, 346
 research enterprise, advances in
  Big Data analytics, 349–350
  EHRs, 348–349
  mobile health technologies, 349
  patient-generated data, 349
  research science attributes, 346–347, 347b
 science, transition from data-poor to, 343–344
 traditional trial designs, 344–345
 transition from data-poor to data-rich science, 343–344
 treatment testing in preparation for comprehensive health data research infrastructure, 350–352
Database of Genotypes and Phenotypes (dbGAP), 48
DBSCAN. See Density Based Spatial Clustering of Applications with Noise (DBSCAN)
Decision
 aids, 70
 making, 183–184
  models, 69–70
   opportunities for, 187–189
   research, 198–199
 rules, 245–246
 support, 267f
Dehydration events, 367
Deidentified data sets, 12
DENCLUE. See Clustering Based on Density Distribution Function (DENCLUE)
Density Based Spatial Clustering of Applications with Noise (DBSCAN), 210
Depressed mood, 182–183
Developers, 383–384
Diagnostic and Statistical Manual of Mental Disorders (DSM-5), 239
Diagnostic Imaging Report (DIR), 149–150
Digital divide, 63, 174
Digital Imaging and Communications in Medicine (DICOM), 149–150
Distance medicine technology
 in cancer care and research, 361
 CER through, 360–361
Distributed problem-solving projects, 308
DIYGenomics, 316
Do Not Resuscitate (DNR), 188
"dot. com implosion", 254
Double Divide, 36
Draft Standard for Trial Use (DSTU), 13–14
Drilling, 300
Drivers, 41–42

Drug discovery, crowdsourcing for, 312–314
DSTU. See Draft Standard for Trial Use (DSTU)

E
E consent, 48
e-path. See Electronic pathology (e-path)
Early detection, 124–126
 breast cancer screening, 126–127
 cervical cancer screening, 127
 challenge, 129–131
  failure during follow-up, 131–132
  failure to detect, 131
  failure to screen, 131
 colorectal screening, 127–128
 communication challenges, 132–133
  HIT, 133
  information systems, 133
  screening, 133
  use of IT in early detection, 134
 epidemiology
  breast cancer, 124–125
  cervical cancer, 125
  colorectal cancer, 125
  lung cancer, 125
 evidence-based solutions, 134–139
 high-risk individuals, 128
 lung cancer screening, 128
 process of care, 128
  organized vs. opportunistic screening programs, 129
  screening, 128–129
 screening, 126
Easy-to-use data repositories, 48
EBI. See European Bioinformatics Institute (EBI)
Ecological momentary assessment (EMA), 171–172, 349, 361–363
Ecological momentary interventions (EMI), 171–172, 351
Ecology of medical care, 73
Economic outcomes, 199
eCOTPS. See Clinical Oncology Treatment Plan and Summary (eCOTPS)
Edmonton Symptom Assessment Scale (ESAS), 192
eHealth, 259. See also mHealth
 application, 233
 opportunities for, 184–185
  bereavement, 189–190
  channels of communication, 185f
  decision making, 187–189
  informatics, 185–186
  for symptom management, 186–187
Electronic CQM (eCQM), 14
Electronic health record (EHR), 6, 26, 44, 61, 82, 105–106, 134, 146, 186, 208, 234, 256, 280, 348–349, 361–362, 375
 behavioral measures in, 237–238
 CER strengthening capacity through, 367–369
 challenges, 113–114
 changing regulatory and policy environment, 114
  ACA, 114–115
  federal incentive program, 114

  guidance on treating tobacco dependence, 114–115
 EHR-enabled SCP, 169–170
 engaging physicians to improving patients' health, 112–113
 integration with personal health information, 348
 linking patients to state tobacco quitlines and closed-loop functionality, 112
 using lung cancer screening, 111–112
 patient registries, 113
 system, 216–219, 289–290
 and tobacco cessation, 108–111
  additional studies, 110–111
  advising all smokers to quit and assess interest in quitting, 110
  asking smoker identification, 109–110
  assist with cessation, 110
Electronic medical record (EMR), 24–25, 43, 131, 237, 316, 362, 380
Electronic pathology (e-path), 280
Electronic patient-reported outcome system (ePRO), 91, 171, 268
Electronic personal health record (ePHR), 114
Electronic Self-Report Assessment-Cancer (ESRA-C), 92, 186
Electronically collected Patient Reported Outcomes (e-PRO). See Electronic patient-reported outcome system (ePRO)
Elixir Sulfanilamide, 321
EMA. See Ecological momentary assessment (EMA)
EMI. See Ecological momentary interventions (EMI)
Emotions
 coping with, 269–270
 emotional
  contagion study, 322
  effects, 162–163
  screening for, 243–244
EMPI. See Enterprise master patient index (EMPI)
EMR. See Electronic medical record (EMR)
End-of-life care, 182–184
Endogenous control, 290
Ensemble summaries. See Statistical summaries
Enterprise master patient index (EMPI), 12
Environmental scan, 138
EORTC. See European Organization for Research and Treatment of Cancer (EORTC)
ePHR. See Electronic personal health record (ePHR)
Epidemiological studies, 242–243
ePRO. See Electronic patient-reported outcome system (ePRO)
ER positive. See Estrogen positive (ER positive)
ESAS. See Edmonton Symptom Assessment Scale (ESAS)
ESMO. See European Society of Medical Oncology (ESMO)
ESRA-C. See Electronic Self-Report Assessment-Cancer (ESRA-C)

Estrogen positive (ER positive), 124–125
European Bioinformatics Institute (EBI), 48
European Organization for Research and
    Treatment of Cancer (EORTC), 92
European Prospective Investigation into
    Cancer and Nutrition cohort study
    (EPIC cohort study), 106
European Society of Medical Oncology
    (ESMO), 4
Evaluation, 84
EventFlow, 219–223
Evidence-based
    medicine, 43
        in cancer, clinical trials as foundation
            of, 7–8
        solutions
            challenges with using IT, 139
            Nebraska Department of health and
                human services, 138–139
            NYSDOH, 136–137
            OCHIN, 134–136
            overcoming disparities, 139
            Parkland health and hospital system,
                137–138
            strategies, 138
Evidentiary uncertainty, 146–147
Exchanging information, 264–265
Existential issues, 163
Exogenous control, 290
Expert
    crowds, 310
    designers, 76
    "determination" method, 12
Extensible Markup Language (XML), 13–14,
    245–246

F

FAIR. See Findable, Accessible, Interoperable,
    Reusable (FAIR)
Family
    Health History tool, 49
    involvement, 199–200
    teams, 91
FCC. See Federal Communications
    Commission (FCC)
FDA. See Food and Drug Administration
    (FDA); US Food and Drug
    Administration (FDA)
Fear of recurrence, 163
Fecal immunochemical test (FIT), 126
Fecal occult blood testing (FOBT), 127–128
Federal Communications Commission
    (FCC), 35–36
Federal incentive program, 114
Federally Qualified Health Center (FQHC),
    134
Fee for service (FFS), 146
Financial rewards, 310–311
Findable, Accessible, Interoperable, Reusable
    (FAIR), 42
FIT. See Fecal immunochemical test (FIT)
Fitbit, 117
"5 A's" approach, 108, 109f
Florida Cancer Data System, 281
FOBT. See Fecal occult blood testing (FOBT)

Foldit, 313
FOLFIRINOX, 147, 152
Food and Drug Administration (FDA), 8–9,
    47, 321, 335
    Patient-Focused Drug Development
        Initiative, 324
Foraging for cancer, 299–300
Fostering healing relationships, 263–264
FQHC. See Federally Qualified Health Center
    (FQHC)
Frictionless data, 42–43
Fruit and Vegetable Scan (FVS), 241
Functional approach to patient-centered
    communication, 263–271
Functional needs, 263, 271–272
Fuzzy-Trace theory, types of evidence for,
    237, 237t

G

GA4GH. See Global Alliance for Genomics
    and Health (GA4GH)
Gamification, 312–313
GDB Compare system, 212
GEM platform. See Grid-Enabled Measures
    platform (GEM platform)
Generalized Anxiety Disorder Symptom
    7-item (GAD-7), 244
Genetic variability, 358
Genomic Data Commons (GDC), 48
Genomics Data Sharing (GDS), 46–47
    policy, 42
Geographic Information Systems (GIS),
    209–210
Global Alliance for Genomics and Health
    (GA4GH), 49–50
Global positioning system (GPS), 43
Graphical user interface (GUI), 345–346
Greensboro Health Disparities Collaborative
    (GHDC), 29, 32f
    Cone Health's commitment to, 30
    fledgling GHDC's first task, 30
Grid-Enabled Measures platform (GEM
    platform), 173–174
Growing Hierarchical Self-Organizing Map
    (GHSOM), 214

H

HADS. See Hospital Anxiety and Depression
    Scale (HADS)
HCE. See Hierarchical Clustering Explorer
    (HCE)
HCIL. See Human Computer Interaction
    Laboratory (HCIL)
HCPC. See Healthcare Common Procedure
    Coding (HCPC)
Health
    affairs, 376
    certificate effect, 111
    disparities, strengths of PHI applications
        in, 36–37
    eQuits program, 110–111
    equity in survivorship, 174
Health and Human Services (HHS), 106
Health care
    consumers, 384

crowdsourcing in, 312
    for diagnostics and drug discovery,
        312–314
    for health care delivery improvements,
        314–315
    for optimizing treatment, 314
    patient as researcher, 315–320
    PLM renal cell cancer patient, 318f
    steps in continuous engagement, 317t
health care delivery improvements,
    crowdsourcing for, 314–315
operations, 17
rules for realigning, 262–263, 262t
teams, 91–92
    within and across, 89–90
Health Information Exchange (HIE), 238
Health Information National Trends Survey
    (HINTS), 161, 216, 257, 378
Health information technology (HIT), 4, 26,
    56, 82, 114, 124, 209, 234, 256–257, 359,
    374. See also Information technology
    (IT)
for decision making, 70–71
functions for care coordination, 88
    within and across health care teams, 89
    multiple teams, 90
    person-centered coordination, 89
    shared care planning, 89
implementation to promoting patient
    engagement, 73–76
for improving CER, 359
infrastructure, 238
three ways, 66–67
tools to patient engagement, 61
    EHRs, 61
    general limitations of current systems,
        63
    model for making HIT more patient-
        centered, 63–66, 64f
    national strategy to promoting, 62–63
    patient e-health tools, 62
    patient portals, 61–62
    PHR, 61–62
Health Information Technology for Economic
    and Clinical Health Act (HITECH
    Act), 11, 31, 114, 134, 146, 234, 256,
    374, 376
HITECH world, living in post, 380
    coevolution of payment reform, 382
    health IT, 382
    information blocking, 380
    new care and payment models
        evolution, 381
    Office of National Coordinator, 381
Health Insurance Portability and
    Accountability Act (HIPAA), 11,
    43–44, 108, 278, 315
Health IT, 382
Health Level Seven (HL7), 13–14, 47,
    149–150, 315
Health maintenance organization (HMO),
    257
Health Quality Measures Format (HQMF), 14
Health risk assessment (HRA), 65
    Plus, 68

Health-related quality-of-life (HRQOL), 25, 152, 161
Healthcare Common Procedure Coding (HCPC), 281–282
HealtheRx, 34
HealthKit, 383
HER2. *See* Human epidermal growth factor receptor 2 (HER2)
HHS. *See* Health and Human Services (HHS); U. S. Department of Health and Human Services (HHS)
HIE. *See* Health Information Exchange (HIE)
Hierarchical Clustering Explorer (HCE), 210–211
High-risk individuals, 128
HINTS. *See* Health Information National Trends Survey (HINTS)
HIPAA. *See* Health Insurance Portability and Accountability Act (HIPAA)
HIT. *See* Health information technology (HIT); Human Intelligence Task (HIT)
HITECH Act. *See* Health Information Technology for Economic and Clinical Health Act (HITECH Act)
HL7. *See* Health Level Seven (HL7)
HMO. *See* Health maintenance organization (HMO)
Home Health Hub (HHH), 362
Hospice, 183–184, 188–189
Hospital Anxiety and Depression Scale (HADS), 244
Hospital setting, 58–60
HQMF. *See* Health Quality Measures Format (HQMF)
HRA. *See* Health risk assessment (HRA)
HRQOL. *See* Health-related quality-of-life (HRQOL)
HTML. *See* HyperText Markup Language (HTML)
Human Computer Interaction Laboratory (HCIL), 209
Human epidermal growth factor receptor 2 (HER2), 124–125
Human Intelligence Task (HIT), 313
Human number perception, 294
  and quantitative data, 294
Human papillomavirus (HPV), 28, 107, 127, 376–377
Human phenotype (HP), 45
Human-systems integration, 209
HyperText Markup Language (HTML), 216

I

IARC. *See* International Agency for Research on Cancer (IARC)
IBM. *See* International Business Machines (IBM)
ICD. *See* International Classification of Diseases (ICD)
ICD-10 (ICD-10). *See* International Statistical Classification of Diseases and Related Health Problem, 10th Revision
ICD-9-CM. *See* International Classification of Diseases, Ninth Revision, Clinical Modification (ICD-9-CM)

ICD-O. *See* International Classification of Diseases for Oncology (ICD-O)
ICSG. *See* Internet cancer support group (ICSG)
Illusory conjunction, 290
Impact of Pain Scale, 320
Implementation activities, 84
Inattentional blindness, 257, 289–290
Industry partners, data from, 282
Informatics, 164, 166–167, 185–186
  current efforts in, 90–96
  informatics tools, inventory of, 255–256
    cancer therapies, 259
    communication management systems, 256–257
    informatics enabled communication tools, 256*t*
    interactive conferencing, 259–260
    medical ethicists, 260
    patient portals, 257–258
    self-management and coaching tools, 259
    videoconferencing, 256
  infrastructures, 358
  new areas for cancer surveillance through biorepositories, 282–283
    clinical trials case identification in real time, 283
    expanded ability to assessing quality of care, 283
    expanded ability to making sense of cancer patterns and trends, 283–284
    national virtual registry, 283
  systems, 187
  technology
    new care and payment models evolution, 381
Informatics-based approach, 244–248
Informatics-based interventions, 241–242
Informatics-based solutions, opportunities for, 167
  data liquidity and interoperability, 171
  informatics-enabled survivorship care plans and care planning, 169
    EHR-enabled SCPs, 169–170
    internet-enabled SCPs, 170
  internet and informatics using among cancer survivors, 167–169
    consumer-facing applications, 169
    ICSGs, 168–169
    mHealth and context-aware, real-time intervention, 171–172
    rapid learning systems in survivorship care, 172–173
  standardization measurement, 173–174
Informatics-infused health care system, 208
Information blocking, 380
Information seeking and processing, 163–164
Information technology (IT), 107, 124, 374. *See also* Health information technology (HIT)
  for cancer prevention, 107–108
  IT-enabled system, 359
  skin cancer prevention, 108
Informed consent, 48, 321–322

Informed decision making, 69
InfoZoom, 210–211
Infusion chemotherapy, 281
InnoCentive platform, 312
Innovative analytical techniques, 324
Institute of Medicine (IOM), 4, 29, 43, 57, 83, 161, 182–183, 237, 254, 323, 344, 358, 373–374
Institutional Review Board (IRB), 18, 44, 282, 316, 363
Integrated patient care framework (IPC framework), 84–86
Integrated PHR, 61–62
Intensive longitudinal data, 349–351
Interactive conferencing, 259–260
Interactive Parallel Bar Charts (IPBC), 211–212
Interactive preventive health record (IPHR), 65
Interactive voice response service (IVRS), 116
Interdisciplinary science, actionable knowledge through, 379–380
International Agency for Research on Cancer (IARC), 124
International Business Machines (IBM), 258
International Classification of Diseases (ICD), 239
International Classification of Diseases, Ninth Revision, Clinical Modification (ICD-9-CM), 223
International Classification of Diseases for Oncology (ICD-O), 280
International Organization for Standardization (ISO), 47
International Physical Activity Questionnaire (IPAQ), 241
International Statistical Classification of Diseases and Related Health Problem, 10th Revision (ICD-10), 311
Internet
  internet-enabled SCP, 170
  and online cancer communities, 334
  shaped online cancer communities, 334–335
Internet cancer support group (ICSG), 168–169
"Internet of Things", 258
Internet-related technologies, 255–256
Interoperability, 171
IOM. *See* Institute of Medicine (IOM)
IPAQ. *See* International Physical Activity Questionnaire (IPAQ)
IPBC. *See* Interactive Parallel Bar Charts (IPBC)
IPC framework. *See* Integrated patient care framework (IPC framework)
IPHR. *See* Interactive preventive health record (IPHR)
IRB. *See* Institutional Review Board (IRB)
ISO. *See* International Organization for Standardization (ISO)
IT. *See* Information technology (IT)
IVRS. *See* Interactive voice response service (IVRS)

J

Janet Freeman-daily's care coordination story, 87*b*
Just-in-Time Adaptive Interventions (JITAI), 351
"Just-in-time" fashion, 291–292

K

Kaggle, 315
KarmaLegoSification framework (KLS framework), 211–212
"Killer app", 171–172

L

Late effects, 162–163
Layout, 291
LDCT. *See* Low-dose computed tomography (LDCT)
Learning community health system, 37
Learning health care system creation in oncology
    CancerLinQ, 10, 12–17
    challenges of delivering quality cancer care, 4
        cancer data system, 4
        complexity and cost of cancer care delivery, 6–7
        components of cancer, 4
        consensus statement, 4
        diversity of cancer and cancer patient population, 5
        IOM committee, 4–5
        key recommendations, 4
        NCPB, 4
        need for multidisciplinary cancer care, 5–6
    quality, value, and learning interface, 9–10
    traditional learning in cancer medicine, 7
        clinical trials as foundation of evidence-based medicine in cancer, 7–8
        conventional clinical trials, limitations of, 8–9
Learning Health System Training Program (LHSTP), 154–155
Learning Healthcare System, 43, 375
Learning interface, 9–10
LED. *See* Light emitting diode (LED)
LHRH. *See* Luteinizing hormone-releasing hormone (LHRH)
LHSTP. *See* Learning Health System Training Program (LHSTP)
"Library card" access model, 48
Lifelines, 211–212
Light emitting diode (LED), 259
Limited data sets, 12
LIVESTRONG Centers, 165–166
Logical decomposition, 45
Long-term health status, 163
Lotsa Helping Hands, 91
Low-dose computed tomography (LDCT), 111
Lowering barriers to data access for cancer research, 48
    data altruism and citizen contributions, 48–49

easy-to-use data repositories, 48
informed consent and consent-derived access, 48
Lung cancer, 125
    screening, 111–112, 128
Luteinizing hormone-releasing hormone (LHRH), 219

M

M & M. *See* Morbidity and Mortality (M & M)
Machine learning (ML), 149–151
    approaches, 349–350
Magnetic resonance imaging (MRI), 127
Making decisions, 265–267
Mammalian phenotype (MP), 45
Mammography, 126
MapApp, 33
Marginal Value Theorem (MVT), 299
Market evolution, 148
Massachusetts Institute of Technology (MIT), 309
Meaningful, Active, Productive Science in Service to Community program (MAPSCorps program), 32–33
Meaningful Use (MU), 107–108, 113–114, 134, 136
    Program, 380
Measurement advances, 346–347
Medical decision making, engaging patients in, 68–69
    decision-making models, 69–70
    examples of decisions, 69
    using HIT for decision making, 70–71
Medical image perception, 294–299
Medical Information Visualization Assistant (MIVA), 211–212
Medicare's Hospital Value-Based Purchasing Program, 9
Medication reconciliation, 90
Melanoma skin cancer, 107
Meteorology, 346
mHealth, 42–43, 171–172. *See also* eHealth application, 233
    and cancer prevention, 115–116
    contribution to, 238–239
    research gaps and opportunities, 117–118
Milliseconds (ms), 288
Minnesota study, 112
Miscommunication, 261–262
MIT. *See* Massachusetts Institute of Technology (MIT)
MIVA. *See* Medical Information Visualization Assistant (MIVA)
ML. *See* Machine learning (ML)
MMS. *See* Multimedia message service (MMS)
Mobile
    health technologies, 349
    technologies, 48
Moderate to vigorous physical activity (MVPA), 152
MOHR study. *See* My Own Health Report study (MOHR study)
Monarch Initiative, 45
Morbidity and Mortality (M & M), 260–261

Moses Cone Community Foundation, 30
MOST. *See* Multiphase optimization strategy (MOST)
MP. *See* Mammalian phenotype (MP)
MRI. *See* Magnetic resonance imaging (MRI)
ms. *See* Milliseconds (ms)
MS. *See* Multiple sclerosis (MS)
MU. *See* Meaningful Use (MU)
Multicomponent treatments, 351
Multidisciplinary cancer care, need for, 5–6
Multimedia message service (MMS), 115
Multimodality therapies, 7–8
Multiphase optimization strategy (MOST), 118, 351
Multiple sclerosis (MS), 320
Multiple teams, 90, 92–94
Multiuser notes, 258
MVPA. *See* Moderate to vigorous physical activity (MVPA)
MVT. *See* Marginal Value Theorem (MVT)
My Own Health Report study (MOHR study), 68
MyHealtheVet, 43–44
MyPreventiveCare, 65–66

N

"*n*-of-1" studies, 319
National Academy of Medicine, 373–374
National Cancer Institute (NCI), 7, 25, 44, 104, 148–149, 160, 210, 232, 257, 277–278, 308, 361–362, 375
    NCI Metathesaurus, 11–12
National Cancer Policy Board (NCPB), 4
National Center for Advancing Translational Sciences (NCATS), 48
National Center for Biomedical Ontology (NCBO), 47
National Center for Biotechnology Information (NCBI), 50
National Coalition of Cancer Survivorship (NCCS), 160
National Comprehensive Cancer Network (NCCN), 30, 145–146, 244, 281
National Council for Prescription Drug Programs (NCPDP), 149–150
National Health Interview Survey (NHIS), 127
National Institutes of Health (NIH), 30, 42, 155, 232, 345, 375
National learning health care system, 46
National Library of Medicine, 11–12
National Oceanic and Atmospheric Administration (NOAA), 270
National Program of Cancer Registries (NPCR), 148–149, 277–278
National Research Council (NRC), 209
National virtual registry, 283
Natural language processing (NLP), 11, 149–151, 279
NCATS. *See* National Center for Advancing Translational Sciences (NCATS)
NCBI. *See* National Center for Biotechnology Information (NCBI)
NCBO. *See* National Center for Biomedical Ontology (NCBO)

NCCN. *See* National Comprehensive Cancer Network (NCCN)

NCCS. *See* National Coalition of Cancer Survivorship (NCCS)

NCI. *See* National Cancer Institute (NCI)

NCI-Molecular Analysis for Therapy Choice (NCI-MATCH), 45, 45*f*

NCPB. *See* National Cancer Policy Board (NCPB)

NCPDP. *See* National Council for Prescription Drug Programs (NCPDP)

Nebraska Department of health and human services, 138–139

Net neutrality, 41–42

Netflix, 44–45

Networks, 148

Neuro-QoL. *See* Quality of Life in Neurological Disorders (Neuro-QoL)

Neurophysiological process, 350

New care and payment models evolution, 381

New York State (NYS), 136

New York State Department of Health (NYSDOH), 136–137

NewChoiceHealth, 315

NGO. *See* Nongovernmental organization (NGO)

NHIS. *See* National Health Interview Survey (NHIS)

NHST. *See* Null hypothesis statistical testing (NHST)

Nicotine metabolism, 104

Nicotine replacement therapy (NRT), 106

NIH. *See* National Institutes of Health (NIH)

NIH BD2K-funded Data Discovery Index, 46–47

NLP. *See* Natural language processing (NLP)

NMC. *See* Novel Molecule Challenge (NMC)

NOAA. *See* National Oceanic and Atmospheric Administration (NOAA)

Nonattentional systems, 290. *See also* Attentional system; Preattentive system
  approximate number system, 291
  layout, 291
  scene gist, 291
  sensing, 291
  statistical summaries, 290–291

Nonexpert crowds, 310

Nongovernmental organization (NGO), 311

Nonmonetary factors, 311

Nontraditional data streams, 311–312

Novel Molecule Challenge (NMC), 312

Novel organizational approaches, 155

NPCR. *See* National Program of Cancer Registries (NPCR)

NRC. *See* National Research Council (NRC)

NRT. *See* Nicotine replacement therapy (NRT)

Null hypothesis statistical testing (NHST), 344–345

NurseNav, 93

Nurture patient autonomy, 268

Nutrition, 116–117

NYS. *See* New York State (NYS)

NYSDOH. *See* New York State Department of Health (NYSDOH)

O

Obamacare. *See* Affordable Care Act (ACA)

Obesity, 106

OCHIN. *See* Oregon Community Health Information Network (OCHIN)

Odds ratio (OR), 116, 241–242, 264

Office of National Coordinator (ONC), 62, 381

Office of National Coordinator for Health Information Technology (ONC), 114, 236, 314–315, 358

-omics data streams, 311

ONC. *See* Office of National Coordinator (ONC); Office of National Coordinator for Health Information Technology (ONC)

OncoKompass, 172

OncoLife, 170

Oncology, 145–146, 287–288
  care system in crisis, 373–374
    HITECH Act, 374
  clinical trial protocols, 248
  communication error in, 260–261
  frontiers of perceptual science and oncology informatics, 299
    foraging for cancer, 299–300
    strategies for volumetric search, 300
  human number perception and quantitative data, 294
  patient portals in, 368
  vision works, 288
    attentional system, 289–290
    coordination of systems, 291–292
    nonattentional systems, 290–291
    preattentive system, 288–289
    visual attention and medical images, 294–299
    visualization and data exploration, 292–294

Oncology Care Model, 82–83, 148

Oncology informatics
  behavioral informatics, 232, 239–241
    applications of resources and tools in cancer care, 241–248
    behavioral/psychological sciences in advancing informatics, 232–239
  bright spots in, 375
    actionable knowledge through interdisciplinary science, 379–380
    learning oncology systems, 375–376
    population health informatics, 376–377
    rise of consumer engagement and participation, 378–379
    technology to improving care coordination and delivery, 377–378
  frontiers of perceptual science and, 299
    foraging for cancer, 299–300
    strategies for volumetric search, 300

Oncology Research Information Exchange Network (ORIEN), 311

OncoNav, 93

"One size fits all" approach, 28

One-on-one training, 186

Online cancer communities
  impact, 336
  internet shaped, 334–335
  patients talk about, 336
  trial participants, 339

Ontology, 47. *See also* Oncology informatics

Open data, 42–43

Open Notes, 258

Open Research Exchange (ORE), 319–320

Open science, 46–47

Opportunistic screening programs, 129

Optimal foraging theory, 299–300

Optimized and adaptive interventions, 351

OR. *See* Odds ratio (OR)

Ordering Points to Identify Clustering Structure (OPTICS), 210

ORE. *See* Open Research Exchange (ORE)

Oregon Community Health Information Network (OCHIN), 134–136, 135*f*

Organizational interactions, 128–129

Organized screening programs, 129

ORIEN. *See* Oncology Research Information Exchange Network (ORIEN)

Overweight, 106

P

Pain management, 182

Palliation, 182

Palliative care, 182, 186, 190, 197, 200

Parkland health and hospital system, 137–138

Participant characteristics, 310

Participant-Centered Consent (PCC), 46, 322
  toolkit, 48

Participant-led research (PLR), 316

Participatory
  clinical trial design, 338–339
  design, 76, 337, 381
    principles, 28
  research, 337

Partnership for Health (PFH), 242

Patient
  cohorts, 352
  comorbidity and health services utilization, 224–227
  crowd, 324
  mastery enhancement, 268
  navigation, 71, 92–93
  outcomes, 197–198
  partnership in clinical research, 323–324
  patient e-health tools, 62
  patient/provider record matching, 12
  portals, 61–62, 257–258
    in oncology, 368
  registries, 113
  as researcher, 315–316
    ALS study, 319
    ALSFRS-EX, 320
    ORE, 319
    PLM, 316
    PLM renal cell cancer patient, 318*f*
    PLR, 316
    quantified self studies, 320
    steps in continuous engagement, 317*t*
  users, 76

"Patient Care Monitor" (PCM), 91
Patient engagement, 57
  community setting, 60
  HIT implementation to promoting, 73–76
  HIT tools, 61
    EHRs, 61
    general limitations of current systems, 63
    model for making HIT more patient-
      centered, 63–66, 64f
    national strategy to promoting, 62–63
    patient e-health tools, 62
    patient portals, 61–62
    PHR, 61–62
  key patient engagement activities
    empowering patients with health
      information, 66–67
    gathering patient reported information,
      67–68
    medical decision making, 68–71
    three ways HIT, 66–67
  to managing transitions of care, 71–72
    CMS, 71
  primary care setting, 57–58
  rethinking care delivery system, 60–61
  specialty and hospital setting, 58–60
  survivorship planning, engaging patients
    and caregivers for, 72–73
  value across cancer control continuum,
    56–57
Patient Health Questionnaire-9 (PHQ-9), 92,
  244
Patient health record (PHR), 61–62, 89
Patient Powered Research Network (PPRN),
  311
Patient Protection and Affordable Care Act,
  358
Patient reported outcome (PRO), 43, 62,
  151–152, 265, 269, 358
Patient Reported Outcomes Measurement
  Information System (PROMIS), 46, 68
Patient Reported Outcomes Version of the
  Common Terminology Criteria for
  Adverse Effects (PRO-CTCAE), 46
Patient-centered
  barriers to trial participation, 332
    distrust of research process, 332
    fear of jeopardizing relationship with
      physician, 333
    fear of side effects, 332
    inconvenience and expense of frequent
      travel, 333
    lack of awareness of trials, 333
    perceived complexity of protocol, 333
    randomization and in fear of receiving
      placebo, 332
  functional approach to communication,
    263
    communication context surrounding
      oncology care, 266f
    coping with emotions, 269–270
    decision support, 267f
    enabling self-management, 267–269
    exchanging information, 264–265
    fostering healing relationships, 263–264
    making decisions, 265–267
    managing uncertainty, 270–271

internet and online cancer communities,
  334
Internet shaped online cancer
  communities, 334–335
medical home, 84–86
oncology care, 82–83
online cancer communities
  impact, 336
  patients talk about, 336
  trial participants, 339
participatory clinical trial design, 338–339
participatory research, 337
patients searching for trials online, 333–334
silicon valley, 337
trials, 331–332
user-centered design, 337
workflow for drug development, 338f
Patient-Centered Medical Home (PCMH), 58,
  136, 377–378
Patient-Centered Outcomes Research
  Institute (PCORI), 57, 151, 323, 337,
  358
Patient-generated data, 151, 349
Patient-powered research network, 316
Patient-provider interactions, 128
Patient-reported outcome (PRO), 7, 239, 308,
  338
PatientsLikeMe (PLM), 311, 316
PatientViewpoint, 91
Pattern recognition approaches, 349–350
Payer-driven approaches, 148
Payoff matrix, 298
PCAST. See President's Council of Advisors
  on Science and Technology
  (PCAST)
PCC. See Participant-Centered Consent
  (PCC)
PCM. See "Patient Care Monitor" (PCM)
PCMH. See Patient-Centered Medical Home
  (PCMH)
PCORI. See Patient-Centered Outcomes
  Research Institute (PCORI)
PCORNet, 155
PCPs. See Primary care physicians (PCPs);
  Primary care providers (PCPs)
PDQ database. See Physician Data Query
  database (PDQ database)
PDUFA V. See Prescription Drug User Fee
  Act fifth authorization (PDUFA V)
Perceptual science and oncology informatics,
  299
  foraging for cancer, 299–300
  strategies for volumetric search, 300
"Perceptual set" effect, 299
Person teams, 91–92
Person-centered coordination, 89
Personal digital assistants (PDAs), 115, 345
Personal health information
  EHR integration with, 348
Personal Health Network (PHN), 94, 95f
Personally identifiable information (PII), 11
PFH. See Partnership for Health (PFH)
Phase IV surveillance, 325
Phenomics, 324–325
PHI. See Protected health information (PHI)
PHIs. See Public health informatics (PHIs)

PHN. See Personal Health Network (PHN)
PHQ-9. See Patient Health Questionnaire-9
  (PHQ-9)
PHRs. See Patient health record (PHR)
Phylo, 313
Physical activity, 106, 116–117
  promotion, 242–243
Physical effects, 162–163
Physical inactivity, 106
Physician Data Query database (PDQ
  database), 257–258
Physician Quality Reporting System (PQRS),
  9
PII. See Personally identifiable information
  (PII)
Plate tectonics, 346
PLC. See Portable Legal Consent (PLC)
PLM. See PatientsLikeMe (PLM)
PLR. See Participant-led research (PLR)
PMI. See Precision Medicine Initiative (PMI)
PMSs. See Practice management systems
  (PMSs)
PNAS. See Proceedings of National Academy
  of Sciences (PNAS)
POA. See Power of attorney (POA)
Point of need, 83, 86
  coordination at, 90–96
  opportunities for oncology informatics at,
    96–97
Poor nutrition, 106
Population statistics, 214–216
Population-based cancer registry systems, 282
Population-based Research Optimizing
  Screening through Personalized
  Regimens (PROSPR), 134
Population-based screening programs, 126
Portable Legal Consent (PLC), 322
Positive health behaviors, adopting and
  maintaining, 163
Positive predictive value (PPV), 223, 296
Post-traumatic stress disorder (PTSD), 162
Posttreatment, 163, 165
Power of attorney (POA), 188
PPRN. See Patient Powered Research
  Network (PPRN)
PPS. See Prospective Payment System (PPS)
PPV. See Positive predictive value (PPV)
PQRS. See Physician Quality Reporting
  System (PQRS)
PR positive. See Progesterone positive (PR
  positive)
Practical sequelae effects, 162–163
Practice management systems (PMSs), 10
Preattentive processes, 288
Preattentive system, 288. See also Attentional
  system; Nonattentional systems
  complex properties, 289
  simple properties, 289
  visual features, 288
Precision medicine drivers, 49–50
Precision Medicine Initiative (PMI), 352
Predictive, preventive, personalized, and
  participatory medicine (P4 medicine),
  312, 320
Prescription Drug User Fee Act fifth
  authorization (PDUFA V), 324

President's Council of Advisors on Science and Technology (PCAST), 258
Prevention of cancer, 104
    current use of information technology for, 107–108
    EHRs, 108–115
    key behaviors of interest for, 104
        alcohol consumption, 107
        behavioral risk factors, 104
        cancer sites, 105t
        challenges of maintaining behavioral change, 104–105
        overweight and obesity, 106
        physical inactivity, 106
        poor nutrition, 106
        smoking and tobacco use, 105–106
        sun damage, 107
        viral infection, 107
    mobile, web, and wearable applications, 115
        alcohol consumption, 117
        mHealth and cancer prevention, 115–116
        mHealth research gaps and opportunities, 117–118
        nutrition and physical activity, 116–117
        sun protection, 117
        tobacco and smoking behaviors, 116
Price Check, 315
Primary care physicians (PCPs), 108, 258
Primary care providers (PCPs), 164
Primary care setting, 57–58, 58f
Primary prevention, 104
Privacy, 171
"Privacy policy", 322
Privacy Rule, 11
PRO. See Patient-reported outcome (PRO)
PRO-AEs, 325
Proceedings of National Academy of Sciences (PNAS), 319
Progesterone positive (PR positive), 124–125
PROMIS. See Patient Reported Outcomes Measurement Information System (PROMIS)
PROs. See Patient reported outcome (PRO)
Prospective Payment System (PPS), 9
PROSPR. See Population-based Research Optimizing Screening through Personalized Regimens (PROSPR)
Prostate-specific antigen (PSA), 216–219
    PSA testing, 113
Protected health information (PHI), 11, 278
Prototype remote monitoring systems, 361
Providers, 148, 382–383
    interactions, 128
Psychological science in advancing informatics, 232
Psychometric process, 319–320
Psychosocial Screen for Cancer (PSSCAN), 244
PTSD. See Post-traumatic stress disorder (PTSD)
Public health informatics (PHIs), 24, 32–34
    cancer health disparities, 24–27
    CBPR, 24
    examples, 29–34
    strengths of PHI applications in health disparities, 36–37

Q
QOL. See Quality of life (QOL)
QOPI. See Quality Oncology Practice Initiative (QOPI)
Quality Adjusted Life Year (QALY), 234–236
Quality benchmarking, 14
Quality cancer care, challenges of delivering, 4
    cancer data system, 4
    complexity and cost of cancer care delivery, 6–7
    components of cancer, 4
    consensus statement, 4
    diversity of cancer and cancer patient population, 5
    IOM committee, 4–5
    key recommendations, 4
    NCPB, 4
    need for multidisciplinary cancer care, 5–6
Quality improvement, 10, 12–13
Quality interface, 9–10
Quality of life (QOL), 147–148, 161, 360–361
Quality of Life in Neurological Disorders (Neuro-QoL), 46
Quality Oncology Practice Initiative (QOPI), 10
Quantified Self, 349
    quantified self-data streams, 311
    studies, 320
Quantitative data, 294

R
Radiation to bone (RtB), 219
Radiation-initiated mucositis, 366
Radio astronomy and cosmology, 346
Randomized clinical trial (RCT), 7, 84, 325, 376
Randomized controlled trial (RCT), 146, 238, 344
Rapid cycle iteration (RCI), 34
Rapid learning health care system, 9–10
Rapid learning systems, 352
    in survivorship care, 172–173
        value propositions of learning system, 173
RCI. See Rapid cycle iteration (RCI)
RCT. See Randomized clinical trial (RCT); Randomized controlled trial (RCT)
Reach Effectiveness Adoption Implementation Maintenance (RE-AIM), 196
Reaction time, 290
    functions, 299
Real world CER, 325
Real-time intervention, 171–172
Redacted data sets, 12
Relative risk (RR), 116
Research design, 197
Researchers, 383
Response time (RT). See Reaction time
Robust patient engagement, 71
RtB. See Radiation to bone (RtB)

S
"Safe harbor" method, 12
SAMI. See Symptom assessment and management Intervention (SAMI)
SAP software, 13
Scene gist, 291
Science, technology, engineering, and mathematics training program (STEM training program), 33
Science of Informatics, 379
SCP. See Survivorship care plan (SCP)
"Screen and intervene" approach, 245
Screening, 126, 128–129, 377
    and intervention for adverse health behaviors and emotional distress
        screening for emotional distress and unmet needs, 243–244
        screens for emotional distress in oncology, 244t
SDM. See Shared decision making (SDM)
SDOs. See Standard development organizations (SDOs)
SDT. See Self-Determination Theory (SDT); Signal detection theory (SDT)
SEBASTIAN. See System for Evidence-Based Advice through Simultaneous Transaction with Intelligent Agent Across Network (SEBASTIAN)
Secondary data sources, 149
Secure messaging, 62, 257
Security, 171
Security Rule, 11
Sedentary time (SED), 152
SEER Program. See Surveillance, Epidemiology, and End Results Program (SEER Program)
Self-Determination Theory (SDT), 232–233
Self-management, 71–72
    and coaching tools, 259
    enabling, 267–269
Self-Organizing Map (SOM), 210
Sensing, 291
Sensors, 152
Sequential Multiple Assignment Randomized Trials (SMART), 351
"Share My Journey" app, 258–259
Shared care plan(s), 89, 94–96
    process, 86, 89
Shared decision making (SDM), 69, 265–266
    tools, 56
SHARP. See Strategic Health IT Advanced Research Projects (SHARP)
Short message service (SMS), 115
Signal detection theory (SDT), 296–298
Silicon valley, 337
Single case studies, 350–351
Single nucleotide polymorphism (SNP), 313
Skilled nursing facility (SNF), 224
Skin cancer(s), 107
    prevention, 108
SMART. See Sequential Multiple Assignment Randomized Trials (SMART)
SMART goals. See Specific, measurable, achievable, realistic, and timely goals (SMART goals)

smokefree.gov website, 116
Smoking, 105–106
    behaviors, 116
    cessation interventions, 111–112
    cessation treatment
        cancer risk and sequelae prevention,
            364–365
SMS. *See* Short message service (SMS)
SNF. *See* Skilled nursing facility (SNF)
SNOMED. *See* Systemized Nomenclature of
    Medicine (SNOMED)
SNOMED-CT. *See* Systemized Nomenclature
    of Medicine–Clinical Terms
    (SNOMED-CT)
SNP. *See* Single nucleotide polymorphism
    (SNP)
Social Cognitive Theory, 233, 242–243
SOM. *See* Self-Organizing Map (SOM)
SPARCCS study. *See* Survey of Physician
    Attitudes Regarding the Care of Cancer
    Survivors study (SPARCCS study)
SPARQL Protocol and RDF Query Language
    (SPARQL), 47
Specialty setting, 58–60
Specific, measurable, achievable, realistic,
    and timely goals (SMART goals), 68
SSM. *See* Subsequent search misses (SSM)
STAMPEDE. *See* "Systemic Therapy in
    Advancing or Metastatic Prostate
    Cancer: Evaluation of Drug Efficacy"
    (STAMPEDE)
Stand-alone PHRs, 61–62
Standard development organizations (SDOs),
    149–150
Standardization, 150
    measurement, 173–174
State tobacco quitlines, 112
State-run quit lines, 376–377
State/federal policies, 129
Statistical opinion method, 12
Statistical summaries, 290–291
STEM training program. *See* Science,
    technology, engineering, and
    mathematics training program (STEM
    training program)
Stop Smoking with Mobile Phones (STOMP),
    116
Strategic Health IT Advanced Research
    Projects (SHARP), 236
Strategies and Opportunities to Stop
    Colorectal Cancer study (STOP CRC
    study), 134–135
Subsequent search misses (SSM), 298–299
Sun damage, 107
Sun protection, 117
Surgeon General's Family Health Portrait, 49
Surveillance, Epidemiology, and End Results
    Program (SEER Program), 44, 210,
    270, 277–278
Surveillance data, 277–278
Survey of Physician Attitudes Regarding
    the Care of Cancer Survivors study
    (SPARCCS study), 166
Survivorship, 160
    care, 167
        model, 164–165

challenges in, 162
    adopting and maintaining positive
        health behaviors, 163
    care coordination and survivorship care
        model, 164–165
    information seeking and processing,
        163–164
    physical, emotional, and practical
        sequelae and late effects, 162–163
    SCP, 165–167
    survivorship care planning, 165–167
community, 73
engaging patients and caregivers for
    planning, 72–73
envisioning future state, 174
    informatics-based solutions, 174–176
    leveraging "long data" in survivorship,
        174
management, 366–367
opportunities for informatics-based
    solutions, 167–174
population data on, 160–161
recommendations for, 161
Survivorship care plan (SCP), 59–60, 72,
    165–167
    challenges to delivery of, 165–166
    intersection of, 166–167
Symptom assessment
    component, 245
    lung cancer report, 246*f*, 247*f*
Symptom assessment and management
    Intervention (SAMI), 245*b*
    system, 245
Symptom management, 182–183
    CHESS and, 191–192
    opportunities for, 186–187
System for Evidence-Based Advice through
    Simultaneous Transaction with
    Intelligent Agent Across Network
    (SEBASTIAN), 245
"Systemic Therapy in Advancing or Metastatic
    Prostate Cancer: Evaluation of Drug
    Efficacy" (STAMPEDE), 146–147
Systemized Nomenclature of Medicine
    (SNOMED), 49, 311
Systemized Nomenclature of Medicine–
    Clinical Terms (SNOMED-CT), 150

T
TARGET. *See* Therapeutically Applicable
    Research to Generate Effective
    Treatments (TARGET)
Task
    characteristics, 309
    motivational structure, 310
Telemedicine sector, 360
"Telephone tag", 262
Temporally dense data collection, 347
The Cancer Genome Atlas (TCGA), 50
The Partnership Project (TPP), 29
Theories and models of behavior change,
    232–236
Therapeutically Applicable Research to
    Generate Effective Treatments
    (TARGET), 50
"Three A's" strategy, 62

Three V's. *See* Velocity, variety, volume
    (Three V's)
Time–motion study, 113–114
Tobacco, 364–365
    behaviors, 116
    cessation, 108–111
    dependence, 105
        guidance on treating, 114–115
    use, 105–106, 241–242
Tobacco Treatment Program (TTP), 365
Top influencers, 44
TPP. *See* The Partnership Project (TPP)
Traditional data streams, 311
Traditional learning in cancer medicine, 7
    clinical trials as foundation of evidence-
        based medicine in cancer, 7–8
    conventional clinical trials, limitations of,
        8–9
Traditional trial designs, 344–345
Translational research, 44–46
Transparency, 34–35
Treatment summary (TS), 59–60, 72, 165
Trial recruitment, 332
TTP. *See* Tobacco Treatment Program (TTP)
Tumor registries, 148–149
23andMe's approach, 321

U
Ultraviolet light (UV light), 107
UMLS. *See* Unified medical language system
    (UMLS)
UNC. *See* University of North Carolina
    (UNC)
Uncertainty, managing, 270–271
Undoing racism principles, 29
Unified medical language system (UMLS),
    11–12
United States Defense Advanced Research
    Programs Administration (DARPA),
    309
United States Preventive Services Task Force
    (USPSTF), 65, 111, 124, 266–267
University of North Carolina (UNC), 29
Unmet needs, screening for, 243–244
US Department of Health and Human
    Services (HHS), 9, 25
US Food and Drug Administration (FDA),
    114, 151–152, 311, 352
US health care system, 12
US Public Health Service (USPHS), 105
Usability testing, 76
User-centered design (UCD). *See*
    Participatory design
USPHS. *See* US Public Health Service
    (USPHS)
USPSTF. *See* United States Preventive
    Services Task Force (USPSTF)
UV light. *See* Ultraviolet light (UV light)

V
Value interface, 9–10
Value propositions of learning system, 173
Velocity, variety, volume (Three V's), 151
Veteran's Administration (VA), 268, 320
    health care system, 171

VIA. *See* Visual inspection with acetic acid (VIA)
Viral infection, 107
Virtual exercise coach, 243*f*
Virtual registry, 283
Vision works, 288
  attentional system, 289–290
  coordination of systems, 291–292
  nonattentional systems, 290–291
  preattentive system, 288–289
VisPap, 210–211
Visual attention, 289
  icon arrays and human number perception, 295*f*
  and medical images, 294–296
  prevalence effect, 296–298
  SSM, 298–299
  visual search displays, 297*f*
Visual inspection with acetic acid (VIA), 127

Visual search task, 296
Visual variables, 293
Visualization, 292–293
  attentional control, 293–294
  as extended vision, 293
  visual variables, 293
VISualization of Time-Oriented RecordS system (VISITORS system), 212
Volumetric search, strategies for, 300

W
Washington Heights/Inwood Informatics Infrastructure for Comparative Effectiveness Research (WICER), 368–369
Watson Health team, 154
Weber fraction, 291
Weber's Law, 291
Weight loss

increased physical activity for, 117
  support for, 117
Wellutainment, 152
"Wiki" style approach, 72
Wireless medical devices, 349
Workflow systems, 47
Workforce training, 154–155
World Health Organization (WHO), 126–127, 239

X
XML. *See* Extensible Markup Language (XML)

Y
Young Adult Program at Dana-Farber Cancer Institute (YAP@DFCI), 238*b*